Elite Techniques in Shoulder Arthroscopy

John D. Kelly IV
Editors

Elite Techniques in Shoulder Arthroscopy

New Frontiers in Shoulder Preservation

Springer

Editor
John D. Kelly IV, MD
Director, Shoulder Sports Medicine
Director, Penn Center for Throwing Athletes
University of Pennsylvania
Department of Orthopedics
Philadelphia, PA, USA

ISBN 978-3-319-25101-1 ISBN 978-3-319-25103-5 (eBook)
DOI 10.1007/978-3-319-25103-5

Library of Congress Control Number: 2015958660

Springer Cham Heidelberg New York Dordrecht London

Printed on acid-free paper

Springer International Publishing AG Switzerland is part of Springer Science+Business Media (www.springer.com)

I dedicate this book to my family.

To my daughters, Mary Elizabeth and Ann Marie: I thank God for you daily. I could not have "scripted" better daughters. You both exude kindness, compassion, and dignity. You both will truly effect meaningful change in your lifetimes.
To Marie, the love of my life, the answers to my prayers: You are the greatest exemplar of compassion I have known. You continually provide me with wise counsel, unwavering loyalty, and steadfast support.
You will always be my soul mate.

Foreword

One of the big challenges in teaching shoulder arthroscopy today is that many of the techniques are so sophisticated that the craftsmanship necessary to perform these procedures can be difficult to convey. Yet the burden of craft that is incumbent upon arthroscopic shoulder surgeons is greater than ever.

Dr. John D. Kelly IV has assembled a formidable group of authors to elucidate the fine points of *Elite Techniques in Shoulder Arthroscopy*, incorporating the title of his book into the mission of this important work. However, the subtitle of his book, *New Frontiers in Shoulder Preservation*, is equally a statement of this mission. In my opinion, shoulder arthroscopy is the single greatest tool that the orthopedic surgeon can implement toward the goal of joint preservation for any joint in the body. And joint preservation is particularly important in this day of conflicting expert opinions in which the surgeon may be confused as to whether to treat a large or massive rotator cuff tear with arthroscopic repair (joint preserving) or reverse total shoulder replacement (joint sacrificing).

John Kelly has been my friend for more than 15 years, and I have always admired his determination to do the right thing for his patients. He does the right thing whether or not it is easy. And as my fellows have often heard me say, "There's the easy way and there's the cowboy way." I am glad to confirm that Dr. Kelly is preserving and advancing the "cowboy way" of shoulder arthroscopy with his excellent new book. Strong work!

San Antonio, TX
June 28, 2015

Stephen S. Burkhart, MD

Preface

This book is a mere reflection of the graces and blessings I have received from my teachers, mentors, and those involved in my formation.

I wish to acknowledge the sage teachers who enriched my ability to provide ethical and up-to-date care of my patients.

John Lachman taught me the ethics of patient care like no other. Ray Moyer was the greatest exemplar of integrity and loving patient care I have ever known. Joseph Torg is perhaps the wisest counselor on matters of life and orthopedics on earth.

Steven Burkhart taught me how to view a shoulder in mechanical terms, while Felix "Buddy" Savoie continues to instruct me in the most revolutionary shoulder arthroscopic techniques.

I have had the "gift" of a tried and true friend and colleague, Brian Sennett, who has been a continual supportive force in my career, in addition to a superlative source of shoulder knowledge.

My chairman, L. Scott Levin, has supported my academic endeavors without question and has proven time and time again that leadership is all about "walking the talk."

Finally, I wish to acknowledge my editor, Jenn Schneider, who demonstrated the "patience of Job" in seeing this work to completion.

Philadelphia, PA John D. Kelly IV, MD

Contents

Part III Glenohumeral Arthritis

Part IV Rotator Cuff

Contributors

Jason B. Anari, MD Department of Orthopaedic Surgery, University of Pennsylvania, Philadelphia, PA, USA

Daniel C. Austin, MD Department of Orthopaedic Surgery, Dartmouth Hitchcock Medical Center, Lebanon, NH, USA

Luke Austin, MD Department of Orthopaedic Surgery, Thomas Jefferson University Hospital, Sewell, NJ, USA

Nicole S. Belkin, MD Department of Orthopaedic Surgery, Hospital of the University of Pennsylvania, Philadelphia, PA, USA

James P. Bradley, MD Department of Orthopaedic Surgery, University of Pittsburgh School of Medicine, Pittsburgh, PA, USA

Eric Breitbart, MD Department of Orthopaedic Surgery, University of Pennsylvania Health Systems, Philadelphia, PA, USA

Stephen S. Burkhart, MD The San Antonio Orthopaedic Group, San Antonio, TX, USA

Jon-Michael E. Caldwell, MD Department of Orthopaedic Surgery, New York Presbyterian—Columbia University Medical Center, New York, NY, USA

Nancy A. Chauvin, MD Department of Radiology, The Children's Hospital of Philadelphia, Philadelphia, PA, USA

Perelman School of Medicine at the University of Pennsylvania, Philadelphia, PA, USA

Brian J. Cole, MD, MBA Department of Orthopaedics, Rush University Medical Center, Chicago, IL, USA

Patrick J. Denard, MD Southern Oregon Orthopedics, Medford, OR, USA

Dinesh Dhanaraj, MD, MSPH Department of Orthopaedic Surgery, Princeton HealthCare System, Plainsboro, NJ, USA

Arash A. Dini, MD Department of Orthopaedics, Tulane University School of Medicine, New Orleans, LA, USA

Brian C. Domby, MD Orthopaedic Sports Medicine and Spine Center, Florida Medical Clinic, Tampa, FL, USA

David Glaser, MD Department of Orthopaedic Surgery, University of Pennsylvania, Philadelphia, PA, USA

Joshua Asher Gordon, MD Department of Orthopaedic Surgery, Hospital of the University of Pennsylvania, Philadelphia, PA, USA

Joshua A. Greenspoon, BSc Vail Valley Medical Center, Steadman Philippon Research Institute, Vail, CO, USA

C. Edward Hoffler II, PhD, MD The Miami Hand and Upper Extremity Institute, Miami, FL, USA

John G. Horneff III, MD Rothman Institute Orthopaedics, Thomas Jefferson University, Philadelphia, PA, USA

G. Russell Huffman, MD, MPH Department of Orthopaedic Surgery, University of Pennsylvania, Philadelphia, PA, USA

Ann Marie Kelly, BA Department of Orthopedics, University of Pennsylvania, Philadelphia, PA, USA

John D. Kelly IV, MD Department of Orthopaedics, University of Pennsylvania, Philadelphia, PA, USA

Viviane Khoury, BSc, MD Division of Musculoskeletal Imaging, University of Pennsylvania Health System, Philadelphia, PA, USA

W. Ben Kibler, MD Lexington Clinic, Shoulder Center of Kentucky, Lexington, KY, USA

Stuart D. Kinsella, MD, MTR Department of Orthopaedic Surgery, Massachusetts General Hospital, Boston, MA, USA

Marc Labbé, MD Department of Orthopaedic Surgery, Baylor College of Medicine, Houston, TX, USA

University of Texas Medical Branch, Galveston, TX, USA

Brian Leggin, PT, DPT, OCS Penn Therapy and Fitness at Valley Forge, Berwyn, PA, USA

William N. Levine, MD Department of Orthopaedic Surgery, New York Presbyterian—Columbia University Medical Center, New York, NY, USA

Helen H. Lu, PhD Department of Biomedical Engineering, Columbia University, New York, NY, USA

Eric C. McCarty, MD Department of Orthopaedic Surgery, University of Colorado School of Medicine, Aurora, CO, USA

Michael H. McGraw, MD Department of Orthopaedic Surgery, Hospital of the University of Pennsylvania, Philadelphia, PA, USA

Kevin J. McHale, MD Department of Orthopaedic Surgery, Hospital of the University of Pennsylvania, Philadelphia, PA, USA

Peter J. Millett, MD, MSc Vail Valley Medical Center, The Steadman Clinic, Vail, CO, USA

Michele Monaco, DSc, ATC Department of Human Movement Science, Immaculata University, Immaculata, PA, USA

Jose M. Morey, MD Department of Radiology and Biomedical Imaging, University of Virginia, Hampton, VA, USA

Department of Internal Medicine, Eastern Virginia Medical School, Hampton, VA, USA

Department of Radiology, Hampton VA Medical Center, Hampton, VA, USA

Almaden Research Lab, IBM Watson, Hampton, VA, USA

Craig D. Morgan, MD Morgan Kalman Clinic, Wilmington, DE, USA

Michael J. O'Brien, MD Department of Orthopaedics, Tulane University School of Medicine, New Orleans, LA, USA

Min Jung Park, MD, MMSc Department of Orthopaedic Surgery, Southern California Permanente Medical Group, Lancaster, CA, USA

Stephanie C. Petterson, MPT, PhD Orthopaedic Foundation, Stamford, CT, USA

Christos D. Photopoulos, MD Department of Orthopaedic Surgery, Hospital of the University of Pennsylvania, Philadelphia, PA, USA

Kevin D. Plancher, MD, MS Clinical Professor, Department of Orthopaedic Surgery, Albert Einstein College of Medicine, New York, NY, USA

Marisa Pontillo, PT, DPT, SCS GSPP Penn Therapy and Fitness, Penn Sports Medicine Center, Philadelphia, PA, USA

Sohale Sadeghpour, MD Department of Orthopaedics, Tulane University School of Medicine, New Orleans, LA, USA

Felix H. Savoie III, MD Department of Orthopaedics, Tulane University School of Medicine, New Orleans, LA, USA

Vishal Saxena, MD Department of Orthopaedic Surgery, University of Pennsylvania, Philadelphia, PA, USA

Aaron Sciascia, MS, ATC, PES Lexington Clinic, Should Center of Kentucky, Lexington, KY, USA

Brian J. Sennett, MD Department of Orthopaedic Surgery, University of Pennsylvania, Philadelphia, PA, USA

Penn Sports Medicine Center, Philadelphia, PA, USA

Nathan W. Skelley, MD Department of Orthopaedic Surgery, Barnes-Jewish Hospital/Washington University in St. Louis, Saint Louis, MO, USA

Matthew V. Smith, MD, MSc Department of Orthopaedics, Washington University in St. Louis, Saint Louis, MO, USA

Barbara Steele, MD Orthopaedic Surgery Sports Medicine, University of Pennsylvania Health System, Philadelphia, PA, USA

Joshua Sykes, MD Department of Orthopaedic Surgery, University of Pennsylvania, Philadelphia, PA, USA

Stephen J. Thomas, PhD, ATC Department of Kinesiology, Temple University, Philadelphia, PA, USA

Fotios P. Tjoumakaris, MD Department of Orthopaedic Surgery, The Rothman Institute, Thomas Jefferson University Hospital, Egg Harbor Township, NJ, USA

Pramod B. Voleti, MD Department of Orthopaedic Surgery, Hospital of the University of Pennsylvania, Philadelphia, PA, USA

Ryan J. Warth, MD Department of Orthopaedic Surgery, University of Texas Health Sciences Center, Houston, TX, USA

Lauren Wessel, BS Department of Orthopaedic Surgery, Washington University in St. Louis, Houston, TX, USA

Robert W. Westermann, MD Department of Orthopaedics and Rehabilitation, University of Iowa Hospitals and Clinics, Iowa City, IA, USA

Brian R. Wolf, MD, MS Department of Orthopaedics and Rehabilitation, University of Iowa Hospitals and Clinics, Iowa City, IA, USA

Miltiadis H. Zgonis, MD Department of Orthopaedic Surgery and Sports Medicine, University of Pennsylvania, Philadelphia, PA, USA

Penn Sports Medicine Center, Philadelphia, PA, USA

Xinzhi Zhang, PhD Department of Biomedical Engineering, Columbia University, New York, NY, USA

Part I

Overhead Athlete

Pathophysiology of Throwing Injuries

1

Stephen J. Thomas, W. Ben Kibler, and Aaron Sciascia

Introduction

The throwing motion is one of the most unique motions the human body can produce. It incorporates both extreme velocities and impeccable accuracies into one fluid motion [1, 2]. The ability to generate velocity and maintain accuracy is dependent on the synergistic motion of multiple linked body segments. This synergistic motion can be related to the physics that describes waves. Wave mechanics states that if timed correctly, two waves can sum together or completely cancel each other out [3]. The generation of energy with throwing can be thought as waves of energy, which when timed correctly can continually build throughout each body segment. However, if the motion is not synergistic or coordinated, the waves of energy may cancel each other out (Fig. 1.1). When this occurs, distal segments are required to make up for the energy lost at the proximal segments [4]. The driving force in this system is the muscle. Muscles are the actuators of our body that create both motion and force production at the joint segments. The neural activation of muscle is a key component of the ability to not only throw with high velocities but also have pinpoint accuracy. As stated previously, during throwing, waves of energy are created starting with the lower extremity and moving through the core and upper extremity and finally to the ball [5]. Two main components of neural activation can be modulated to throw harder and more accurate. First, the timing of neural impulses is of paramount importance in throwing. If the sequenced activation of muscles is not conducted properly, then waves of energy will cancel out and the resulting kinematics will suffer [6]. Second, the amplitude of neural impulses will dictate the amount of force that is generated at each segment and, therefore, if timed properly, will sum together and be placed on the ball to create maximal velocity [6, 7]. Since throwing is a repetitive act, with major league pitchers averaging 80–100 pitches per game, muscles do undergo fatigue. Fatigue generally has two components that occur simultaneously: neural and mechanical [8]. Neural fatigue will cause nonoptimal firing patterns and reduced amplitudes of neural impulses. Instead of having very complex firing patterns that lead to optimal activation of muscles, the activation becomes less complex with large groups of motor units within muscles firing simultaneously [9, 10]. This is an attempt to make up for the reduced neural amplitude. This compensation pattern results in uncoordinated kinematics that leads to waves of energy being canceled.

S.J. Thomas, PhD, ATC (✉)
Department of Kinesiology, Temple University, Philadelphia, PA, USA
e-mail: sjthomasatc@gmail.com

W.B. Kibler, MD • A. Sciascia, MS, ATC, PES
Lexington Clinic, Shoulder Center of Kentucky, Lexington, KY, USA

J.D. Kelly IV (ed.), *Elite Techniques in Shoulder Arthroscopy*,
DOI 10.1007/978-3-319-25103-5_1

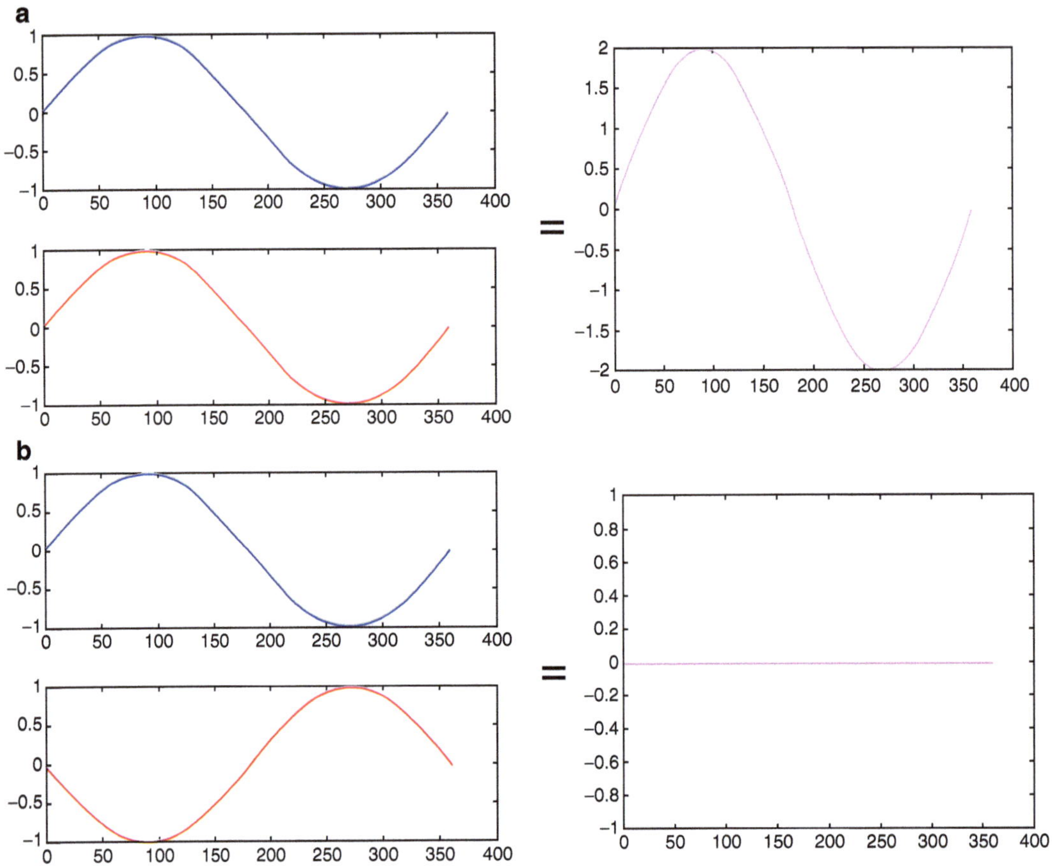

Fig. 1.1 (**a**) An illustration of two individual waves that are in phase. When summed together, the resulting wave is doubled. (**b**) An illustration of two individual waves that are 180° out of phase. When summed together, the resulting wave is completely canceled out

Mechanical fatigue is typically caused by the microdamage of myosin and actin bonds during eccentric muscular contractions [11]. As the amount of damaged myosin and actin increases, the ability to mechanically generate force is reduced. This will also cause a negative feedback loop into the neural component, thereby creating nonoptimal neural firing [10]. It is therefore clear that throwing is a high-velocity act that requires intricate neuromuscular control and timing to achieve optimal performance. In addition, the repetitive nature of throwing can easily lead to fatigue that will disrupt both the kinematics and kinetics. These components are the basis for understanding the pathophysiology of throwing injuries and will be discussed in more detail throughout this chapter.

Due to the complexity of the topic, we will incorporate both basic science and clinical principles to represent the full spectrum of understanding. The role of proper mechanics is very important and often difficult to master; therefore, both normal and abnormal throwing biomechanics will be covered in detail. In addition, the stress of throwing, even with proper kinematics, will cause structural adaptations to both the bone and soft tissues. These adaptations are often the key in both preventing and treating throwing athletes. Therefore, upper extremity structural adaptations will be discussed. Lastly, we will tie all of this information together to gain a more complex understanding of the clinical presentation of several common injuries that occur in throwing athletes.

Mechanics of the Overhead Motion: What Makes the Ball Go?

The overhead throwing motion is developed and regulated through a sequentially coordinated and task-specific kinetic chain of force development and a sequentially activated kinematic chain of body positions and motions [12]. The kinematics of the baseball throw have been well described and may be broken down into phases [13–15]. The most widely accepted descriptions of the phases of throwing include the wind-up, stride, arm cocking, arm acceleration, arm deceleration, and follow-through [15]. These descriptions portray how muscles can move the individual segments, demonstrate the temporal sequence of the motions, and describe the joint angles achieved. The shoulder has been shown to obtain between 160 and 185° of maximal external rotation and 14° of maximal horizontal adduction during the cocking phase, while humeral abduction reaches 90–95° at ball release during arm acceleration [14].

The kinetics have also been described. Moderate anterior shear (380 N) and compressive forces (660 N) occur during arm cocking with internal rotation and horizontal adduction torque reaching up to 90 and 110 Nm, respectively [14]. The forces and torques enable the high internal rotation velocity of approximately 7000° per second to occur during the arm acceleration phase. Consequentially, high posterior shear, inferior shear, and compressive forces occur (310–1090 N) as the body attempts to decelerate the arm [14]. These forces and motions are applied to all of the body segments to allow their summation, regulation, and transfer throughout the segments to result in the performance of the task of throwing. The muscle activation sequencing to produce these kinematics and kinetics demonstrates a proximal-to-distal activation to optimize efficiency [5, 16–19]. In the early phases of throwing (wind-up and stride phases), scapular muscle activity (serratus anterior and upper trapezius) commences prior to larger global shoulder muscle activity (deltoid and pectoralis major) [17, 20]. As the throwing motion progresses from the stride phase to the arm cocking phase, the rotator cuff muscles, specifically the supraspinatus and infraspinatus, have a large amount of activity primarily to align the humeral head with the glenoid [20]. The high activity expands to the remaining rotator cuff muscles during the cocking phase in order to maintain concavity compression and to resist distraction [21, 22]. The cocking phase is also characterized by moderate to high concentric and eccentric activity in larger muscles such as the anterior deltoid, pectoralis major, latissimus dorsi, teres major, biceps brachii, and triceps brachii activity [22]. All of these muscles continue to work both concentrically and eccentrically throughout the remainder of the throwing phases in order to resist unnecessary translations, maintain proper positioning, and direct the ball to its target. The term "kinetic chain" is used collectively to describe the mechanical linkages. Using these definitions and terminology allows a unifying concept to understand the overall mechanics.

An effective athletic kinetic chain is characterized by three components [23]: (1) optimized anatomy in all segments, (2) optimized physiology (muscle flexibility and strength and well-developed, efficient, task-specific, motor patterns for muscle activation), and (3) optimized mechanics (sequential generation of forces appropriately distributed across motions that result in the desired athletic function).

The kinetic chain has several functions: (1) It uses integrated programs of muscle activation to temporarily link multiple body segments into one functional segment (e.g., the back leg in cocking stance and push-off, the arm in long-axis rotation prior to ball release or ball impact) to decrease the degrees of freedom in the entire motion [13, 24, 25], (2) it provides a stable proximal base for distal arm mobility, (3) it maximizes force development in the large muscles of the core and transferring it to the hand [13, 26, 27], (4) it produces interactive moments at distal joints that develop more force and energy than the joint itself could develop and decrease the magnitude of the applied loads at the distal joint [5, 14–17, 28], and (5) it generates torques that decrease deceleration forces [14–16, 29, 30].

Multiple studies have clearly established the basic roles of the kinetic chain, both in baseball and tennis [5, 15, 17, 26, 28, 31–35]. Each body part has specific roles in the entire motion [13]. The feet are contact points with the ground and allow maximum ground reaction force for proximal stability and force generation. The legs and core are the mass for the stable base and the engine for the largest amount of force generation. The scapula must move in specific motions to provide a stable base for muscle activation and congruent ball and socket kinematics. During the initiation of throwing, the scapula is positioned in 40° of internal rotation in the plane of the scapula with slight anterior tilt [36]. As the phases progress, posterior tilt occurs until peaking at maximal humeral external rotation which then transitions to anterior tilt at ball release. Scapular external rotation occurs with maximal horizontal abduction which is likely why the highest serratus anterior activity is seen during the cocking phase [20, 36]. At ball release, the scapula begins in slight upward rotation but reaches a maximum of 40° upward rotation at humeral external rotation [36]. The high amount of lower trapezius activity coincides not as a prime mover of upward rotation but instead as a control for deceleration [22]. The shoulder is the funnel for force regulation and transmission and the fulcrum for stability during the rapid motion of the arm. The arm and hand is the rapidly moving delivery mechanism of the force to the ball or racquet.

To achieve its role in kinetic chain function, the shoulder must develop precise ball and socket kinematics to create maximum concavity compression [21] that optimizes functional stability throughout the entire range of rapid motion. Static restraints include the ligaments (at end ranges of motion) and the limited ball and socket anatomy of the humerus and glenoid. These static constraints must be limited to allow for the wide range of motions. Most of the constraints are dynamic, allowing wide ranges of motion but still conferring functional stability throughout the motions. Requirements for functional stability include optimum alignment of the humerus and glenoid within ±30° angulation [30], co-contraction and compression force couples of the rotator cuff and shoulder muscles [20, 37], a stable scapular base [38], adequate balanced rotational range of motion [39–41], and labral integrity to act as a washer, allowing "best fit" of the humerus into the glenoid [42].

Tasks performed in baseball and tennis occur as a result of the summation of speed principle which states that in order to maximize the speed at the distal end of a linked system, the movement should start with the proximal segments (the hips and core) and progress to the distal segments (shoulder, elbow, wrist) [16]. Each segment in this linked system can influence motions of its adjacent segments. For example, during a baseball pitch, stability of the back and stride legs allow rotation of the trunk which in turn allows for maximal throwing arm external rotation. The stable lower extremity serves as a platform for trunk and upper extremity motion where the amount of trunk rotation is proportionate to the amount of arm motion which can occur. Variations in motor control and physical fitness components such as strength, flexibility, or muscle endurance can affect the efficiency and effectiveness of all segments of the linked system [24, 25, 43].

Efficient mechanics can be improved by decreasing the possible degrees of freedom (DOF) throughout the entire motion [24, 25, 44, 45]. There are 244 possible DOF in the body from the foot to the hand [24]. Most models of maximum efficiency in body motions find that limiting DOF to about 6–8 maximizes the total force output and minimizes effort and load [45]. The DOF can be limited by coordinated muscle activation coupling, called integrative complexes, that constrain and couple positions and motions so that several segments move as one [44]. Examples include the back leg stance position in baseball cocking, where the body is stabilized over the planted leg [13], and the long axis rotation motion in baseball or tennis, where shoulder internal rotation, a minimally moving elbow, and forearm pronation allow the hand to rotate around the long axis from shoulder to wrist [34].

The limited number of independent DOF are called nodes and represent key positions and motions in the overhead tasks [13]. These key positions have been correlated with optimum force development and minimal applied loads and can be considered the most efficient methods of coor-

Table 1.1 Baseball nodes and possible consequences

	Node	Normal mechanics	Pathomechanics	Result	To be evaluated
1	Foot position	Directly toward home plate	Open or closed	Increased load on the trunk or shoulder	Hip and/or trunk flexibility and strength
2	Knee motion	Stand tall	Increased knee flexion	Decreased force to arm	Hip and knee strength
3	Hip motion	Facing home plate	Rotation away from home plate	Increased load on shoulder and elbow	Hip and trunk strength
4	Trunk motion	Controlled lordosis	Hyperlordosis and back extension	Increased load on abdominals and "slow arm"	Hip and trunk strength
5	Scapular position	Retraction	Scapular dyskinesis	Increased internal and external impingement with increased load on rotator cuff muscles	Scapular strength and mobility
6	Shoulder/scapular motion	Scapulohumeral rhythm with arm motion (scapular retraction/humeral horizontal abduction/humeral external rotation)	Hyperangulation of the humerus in relation to the glenoid	Increased load on the anterior shoulder with potential internal impingement	Scapular and shoulder flexibility and strength
7	Elbow position	High elbow (above 90° abduction)	Dropped elbow (below 90° abduction)	Increased valgus load on elbow	Scapular position and strength, trunk and hip flexibility and strength
8	Hand position	On top of the ball	Under or on side of the ball	Increased valgus load on the elbow	Shoulder and elbow position

dinating kinetic chain activation. There may be multiple individual variations in other parts of the kinetic chain, but these are the most basic and the ones required to be present in all motions. The baseball pitching motion can be evaluated by analyzing a set of eight progressive positions and motions (Table 1.1) [32]. These include trunk control over the back leg, hand in pronation "on top of the ball" in cocking, front leg directly toward home plate, control of lumbar lordosis in acceleration, hips facing home plate, arm cocking (scapular retraction/arm horizontal abduction/shoulder external rotation to maintain cocked arm in the scapular plane, "high" elbow above shoulder, and long axis rotation) coupled shoulder internal rotation/forearm pronation, at ball release [5, 13, 15, 17, 28, 31, 46]. The tennis serve motion can be evaluated by analyzing a set of eight "nodes" or positions and motions that are correlated with optimum biomechanics (Table 1.2) [13]. These include optimum foot placement, adequate knee flexion in cocking progressing to knee extension at ball impact, hip/trunk counter rotation away from the court in cocking, back hip tilt downward in cocking, hip/trunk rotation with a separation around 30°, coupled scapular retraction/arm rotation to achieve cocking in the scapular plane, back leg to front leg motion to create a "shoulder over shoulder" motion at ball impact, and long axis rotation into ball impact and follow-through [13, 23, 48]. These nodes can be evaluated by visual observation or by video recording and analysis. Tennis-specific pathomechanics with detailed descriptions of the deleterious motions are listed in Table 1.2.

Adequate performance of the kinetic chain requires optimum anatomy and physiology. Optimum anatomy must be present in all of the joints in the kinetic chain. Joint injury (such as sprained ankles, unresolved knee injury or stiffness, hip tightness, or back injury) can have deleterious effects for core stability, force production, interactive moment production, and arm position [23, 43]. Optimum physiology requires adequate

Table 1.2 Tennis nodes and possible consequences

	Node	Normal mechanics	Pathomechanics	Result	To be evaluated
1	Foot position	In line, foot back	Foot forward	Increased load on trunk or shoulder	Hip and/or trunk flexibility and strength
2	Knee motion	Knee flexion greater than 15°	Decreased knee flexion less than 15°	Increased load on the anterior shoulder and medial elbow	Hip and knee strength
3	Hip motion	Counterrotation with posterior hip tilt	No hip rotation or tilt	Increased load on shoulder and trunk; inability to push through increasing load on abdominals	Hip and trunk flexion flexibility and strength
4	Trunk motion	Controlled lordosis; X-angle ~30°	Hyperlordosis and back extension; X-angle <30° (hypo), X-angle >30° (hyper)	Increased load on abdominals and "slow arm"; Increased load on the anterior shoulder	Hip, trunk, and shoulder flexibility
5	Scapular position	Retraction	Scapular dyskinesis	Increased internal and external impingement with increased load on rotator cuff muscles	Scapular strength and mobility
6	Shoulder/ scapular motion	Scapulohumeral rhythm with arm motion (scapular retraction/ humeral horizontal abduction/humeral external rotation)	Hyperangulation of the humerus in relation to the glenoid	Increase load on the anterior shoulder with potential internal impingement	Scapular and shoulder strength and flexibility
7	Shoulder over shoulder	Back shoulder moving up and through the ball at impact and then down into follow-through	Back shoulder staying level	Increased load on abdominals	Front hip strength and flexibility, back hip weakness
8	Long-axis rotation	Shoulder internal rotation/forearm pronation	Decreased shoulder internal rotation	Increased load on medial elbow	Glenohumeral rotation

X-angle = measurement of hip/trunk separation angle, the angle between a horizontal line between the anterior aspect of both acromions and the horizontal line between both ASIS when viewed from above first described by McLean and Andrisani [151]

Note: Numbers 1–6 occur prior to the acceleration phase of the service motion, while numbers 7–8 occur after ball impact

muscle strength, flexibility, and endurance throughout the kinetic chain. It also requires proper muscle activation patterns for core stability, force development, integrative complexes, joint stabilization, and segment deceleration [23]. The optimized anatomy can then be acted upon by the optimized physiology to create task-specific mechanics to achieve the kinematics and kinetics that produce the desired result of optimal performance in throwing or hitting the ball and create the lowest possible risk of injury.

Abnormal Biomechanics Caused by Structural and Neuromuscular Adaptations

Due to the large repetitive stress of throwing that was described previously, several tissues go through structural and neuromuscular adaptations. These adaptations are different for each tissue type, location, and function. Ultimately, these adaptations cause abnormal pitching biomechanics, which will increase the stress on tissues. This will cause a downward spiral effect, which leads to further tissue adaptations and additional alterations in pitching biomechanics. The combination and continual progression will ultimately lead to shoulder or elbow injuries, which commonly require surgical intervention. In this section, we will cover each of the adaptations that occur due to throwing and the effect they have on pitching biomechanics.

Range of Motion

The most common adaptation that is seen clinically in throwers is a shift in the arc of shoulder motion bilaterally. Throwers often present with a decrease in glenohumeral internal rotation (IR) and a concurrent increase in glenohumeral external rotation (ER) on the throwing arm compared to the nonthrowing arm [49–58] (Fig. 1.2). Wilk et al. [41] has developed the total motion concept which adds IR and ER together to calculate the total arc range on each side. Wilk et al. [41] states that if the *total* motion is equal bilaterally regardless of the shift in motion pattern, then the clinician should not be concerned. When total motion is equal bilaterally, it has been suggested that the shift in the arc of motion is only caused by a bony adaptation called humeral retroversion. However, if there is a loss of total motion on the throwing side, there is usually a soft tissue tightness present which may be reversible with treatment. Recently, this has been supported demonstrating that baseball players with a loss of total motion of 5° or more had a higher rate of shoulder injury [59, 60]. In addition to the total motion concept, there has been much research investigating glenohumeral internal rotation deficits (GIRD). This is a term that has been developed to describe the loss of IR on the throwing arm [52]. There are several hypotheses for the cause of GIRD; however, evidence is still lacking to fully understand the specific tissue adaptations. The three main hypotheses are humeral retroversion, posterior rotator cuff tightness, and posterior capsule tightness/thickness. Each of these tissue adaptations will be discussed in detail in upcoming sections. Regardless of the source of GIRD, it was demonstrated that baseball players with a GIRD of 20° or more were two times more likely to be injured [59].

Bone

The bone is a tissue that is known to have adaptable properties to mechanical load [61]. As such, throwing causes several bony adaptations that are important in understanding the throwing athlete. First, humeral retroversion is described as the bony rotation between the proximal and distal ends of the humerus [62] (Fig. 1.3). Traditionally, it is measured with CT or MRI; however, ultrasound has been demonstrated to be as accurate and have much more accessibility [63, 64]. To understand humeral retroversion in throwers, we first need to discuss the developmental process in normal individuals. At birth, the humerus is in an excessively retroverted position [65]. Clinically this equates to increased glenohumeral ER and decreased glenohumeral IR [66]. Throughout normal development, the humerus undergoes a rotation process that decreases the amount of humeral retroversion. It has been shown that 80 % of the normal developmental rotation process is completed by 8 years old and the remaining 20 % extends to 18 years old [65]. Throwing prior to the completion of this normal developmental rotation process seems to diminish or halt the process, thereby creating side to side differences in humeral retroversion. Most throwers will have more humeral retroversion on the throwing side compared to the nonthrowing side. The association between humeral retroversion and injury is still being heavily researched. Initially, it was suggested to be a positive adaptation. Early researchers reasoned that increase retroversion would afford ER without stretching the anterior capsule and would theoretically inhibit tuberosity/glenoid contact in ER (internal impingement) [47]. However, some recent research suggests that baseball players with greater humeral retroversion have a history of elbow injury [67]. Others have found that baseball players with greater humeral retroversion

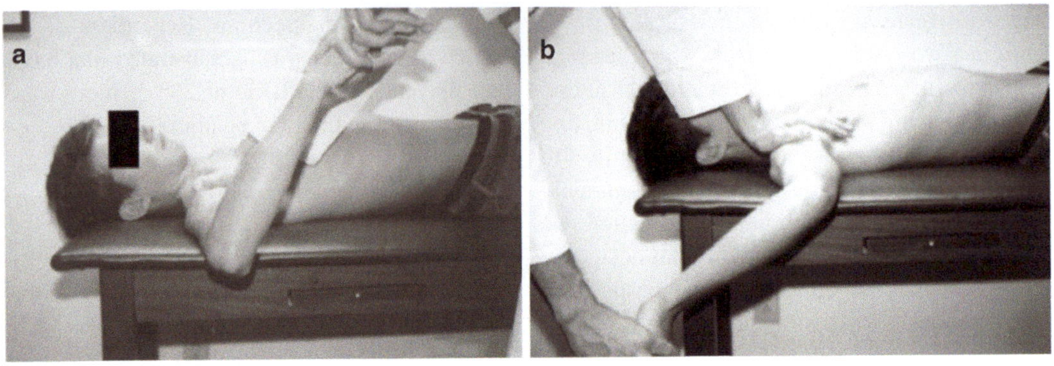

Fig. 1.2 (**a**) Internal rotation is measured with the patient's shoulder in 90° abduction and the elbow in 90° flexion while the examiner stabilizes the scapula. The end point of internal rotation is taken as the point at which the scapula begins to rotate posteriorly. (**b**) External rotation is also measured while stabilizing the scapula. Note that the neutral position (0°) is that in which the forearm is perpendicular to the patient's body (12 o'clock position in the supine patient) (Reprinted from Burkhart SS, Morgan CD, Kibler WB. The disabled throwing shoulder: spectrum of pathology Part I: pathoanatomy and biomechanics. Arthroscopy. 2003 Apr;19(4):404–20, with permission from Elsevier)

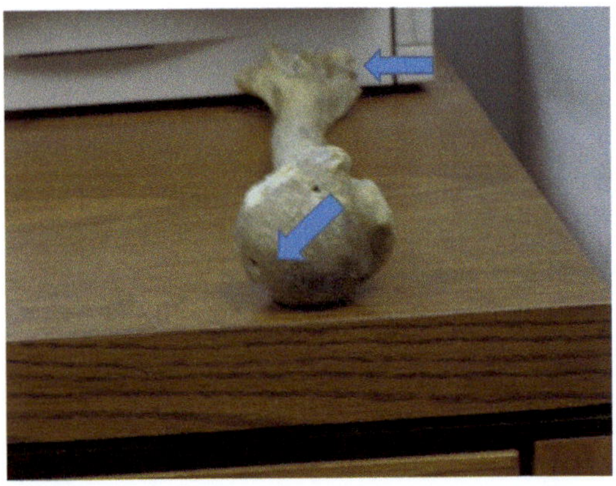

Fig. 1.3 Humeral retroversion (HRT). HRT can be measured as the angle formed by a *line* drawn through the center of the longitudinal axis of the humeral head and neck meeting a *line* drawn along the transverse axis of the condyles, when looking proximal to distal along the humerus (Reprinted from Kinsella SD, Thomas SJ, Huffman GR, Kelly JD 4th. The thrower's shoulder. Orthop Clin North Am. 2014 Jul;45(3):387–401, with permission from Elsevier)

have a thicker posterior capsule of the shoulder [68], which has been implicated in causing shoulder and elbow injuries [52]. Currently, the evidence suggesting that humeral retroversion is either helpful or deleterious to long-term performance is inconclusive.

Next, bone mineral density has been examined bilaterally in baseball players. The results of these studies suggest that the proximal and mid shaft of the humerus on the throwing arm has increased bone mineral density [69, 70]. This finding would be hypothesized based on Wolf's law [61] and the rotational stress of throwing. These results suggest that throughout development, the humerus will adapt in a manner equal to the mechanical loads that are placed on it. This information is important in adolescent throwers due to the open epiphyseal plate at the proximal humerus and the increased propensity for little leaguer's shoulder. Adolescent throwers need to progress in throwing at a much slower pace and also limit the amount of pitches per game and season to allow the bone to adapt at a healthy rate.

The last bony adaptation that can occur in throwers is morphological changes to the bicipital groove. The bicipital groove can develop stenosis from bone ingrowth or spurs [71] (Fig. 1.4). The increased growth of bone within the groove will cause mechanical irritation to the synovial sheath of the biceps tendon and over time cause significant injury. Although bicipital grove stenosis hasn't been documented much in the literature, it likely occurs more frequently in throwing athletes than has previous been suspected.

Soft Tissue

There are many different types of soft tissues in the shoulder that can adapt due to the stress of throwing. Each tissue is different in terms of its

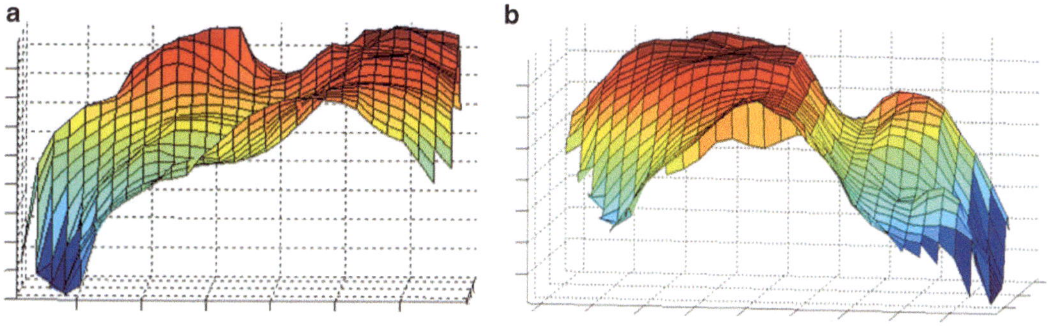

Fig. 1.4 A three-dimensional reconstruction of a bicipital groove viewed from distal to proximal through the bicipital groove. (**a**) This demonstrates the development of bicipital groove stenosis. (**b**) This demonstrates a normal bicipital groove area

composition, structure, and function. In this section, we will discuss all of the different types of soft tissue that are important when treating throwing athletes.

The first category is the joint capsule. The capsule is composed of an inner and outer layer. The inner layer is known as the synovial layer and is responsible for secreting synovial fluid to maintain joint health. The outer layer is composed of dense irregular connective tissue [72]. This layer provides the strength and stabilizing component to the capsule. Throwers can develop adaptations in both the anterior and posterior locations of the joint capsule [68, 73]. During the late cocking and acceleration phase of throwing, large anterior forces occur [14]. Due to these repetitively large forces, it is often thought that the connective tissue of the capsule plastically deforms and is left in a lengthened position. Structurally, the anterior capsule will be unable to center the humeral head on the glenoid at the end ranges of motion. This will allow increased joint translations in the anterior direction, which has been thought to cause secondary impingement or labral injury [74]. During throwing, the athlete will have excessive ER and pain during the late cocking phase of the throw. However, a detailed examination is necessary to discern whether the ER seen during throwing is caused by a combination of glenohumeral, scapular, thoracic, and lumbar motion. It is important to note that anterior capsular laxity does not occur to every throwing athlete. It is often used as a generic diagnosis due to the player having excessive ER and shoulder pain. For example, a recent study by Borsa et al. [75] demonstrated that healthy college throwers did not have side to side differences in anterior translation. This suggests that when this increased anterior humeral translation does occur, it is likely pathologic and may require surgical intervention.

Next, the posterior capsule also undergoes structural adaptations; however, these adaptations are much different than the anterior capsule. When examining pitching kinetics, research has shown that during the deceleration phase, the distraction force is on average 1.5 times body weight [14]. Typically, during the deceleration and follow-through phase, the posterior rotator cuff muscles and scapular stabilizers can absorb the energy [76]. However, throughout a game, these muscles will likely fatigue, thereby reducing the amount of energy that can be absorbed [77]. In this situation, the shoulder will continue to internally rotate to the end range, which will place the remaining force on the posterior capsule. According to Wolf's law [61], the posterior capsule may adapt to the increased stress by hypertrophying. It has been hypothesized that the posterior capsule will ultimately become thick and fibrotic with repetitive throwing, which will create noncompliant tissue and limit glenohumeral IR. Thomas et al. [68] has measured this thickness with ultrasound and found that the throwing shoulder's posterior capsule is thicker compared to the nonthrowing shoulder and the thickness correlates with the loss of glenohumeral IR. In addition, several cadaver studies have shown that a tight posterior capsule will shift the center of the humeral head in a posterior-superior direction during the late cocking phase of the throw [78, 79]. A posterior-superior shift of the humeral head has been demonstrated to cause internal impingement and place increased stress at the insertion of the long head of the biceps tendon at the superior labrum [52] (Fig. 1.5). It is expected that the posterior capsule thickens due to throwing; however, it is currently unknown when this adaptation becomes excessive and problematic.

The next category of soft tissue that is a concern with throwers is muscle/tendon units. There are several muscle/tendon units that develop similar adaptations at the shoulder girdle. The muscles that will be discussed include the posterior rotator cuff (infraspinatus and teres minor), pectoralis minor, triceps brachii, latissimus dorsi, and the teres major.

First, the infraspinatus and teres minor are the two muscles that comprise the posterior rotator cuff. As stated previously, these two small muscles attempt to repetitively absorb a large amount of the 1.5 times body weight force that occurs during the deceleration phase of the throw [14]. To absorb energy, muscles function eccentrically which entails a forceful breaking of the myosin and actin bonds [80]. Several studies have found that repetitive eccentric contractions of the muscle cause significant damage, often called delayed-onset muscle soreness (DOMS) [81–83]. Several studies have also identified that repetitive eccentric contractions cause an increase in passive stiffness and reduced range of motion that peaks at 24 h and typically takes 4–5 days to return to baseline [84, 85]. It is hypothesized that this clinical presentation is caused by damaging of the sarcoplasmic reticulum, which releases excessive calcium [84]. This has been demonstrated in throwers following a simulated game and is characterized by a decrease in glenohumeral IR immediately following the game [86]. Recently, it has been shown that the loss of IR is still present up to 3 days following pitching [87]. This physiologic phenomenon of muscle would

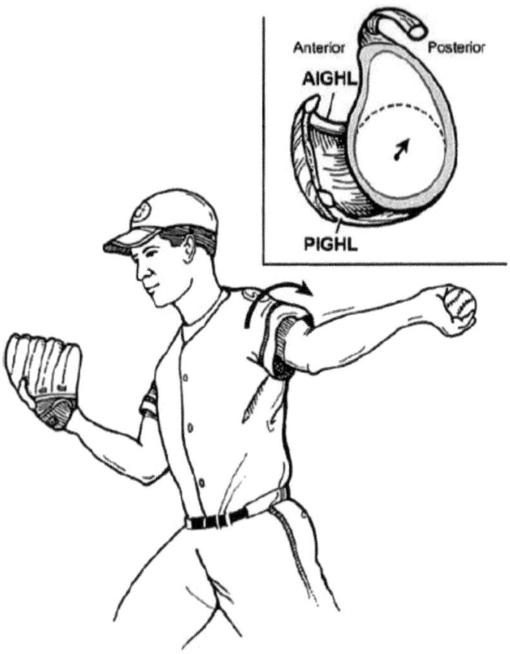

Fig. 1.5 In abduction and external rotation (late cocking), the posterior band of the IGHL is bowstrung beneath the humeral head, causing a posterosuperior shift in the glenohumeral rotation point. Also in late cocking, the biceps vector shifts posteriorly and twists at its base, maximizing peel-back forces. As a result of the tight postero-inferior capsule, this pitcher shows classic derangements of pitching mechanics: hyperexternal rotation, hyperhorizontal abduction (out of the scapular plane), dropped elbow, and premature trunk rotation (Reprinted from Burkhart SS, Morgan CD, Kibler WB. The disabled throwing shoulder: spectrum of pathology Part I: pathoanatomy and biomechanics. Arthroscopy. 2003 Apr;19(4): 404–20, with permission from Elsevier)

not be a concern if throwing did not occur until after the muscle tissue returned to a normal state. However, most throwers initiate throwing before the muscle tissue returns to normal. Over time, the posterior rotator cuff muscles may develop excessive tightness. The hypothesis is that the immediate loss of glenohumeral IR following throwing will still be present before the next bout of throwing, thereby adding to the total loss of motion. This can continue to occur over the season leading to excessive tightness, characterized by a loss of glenohumeral IR. Posterior rotator cuff tightness is thought to be problematic and is hypothesized that it will alter normal throwing biomechanics [52]. During normal throwing, the shoulder is positioned in the scapular plane (30° anterior to the frontal plane) during the late cocking phase [1, 88]. A tight posterior rotator cuff may position the shoulder in the frontal plane or even in excessive horizontal abduction to release the tension in the posterior rotator cuff. This position will place increased valgus stress on the medial elbow and increased anterior stress on the anterior capsule and cause internal impingement [15, 89]. To address this situation, clinicians should focus on treating the excessive posterior rotator cuff tightness [90–92] and not attempt to change the altered throwing biomechanics. As the muscle tightness is resolved, the altered biomechanics will return to normal.

There are additional muscles that are often overlooked in throwing athletes but do develop significant tightness that can affect throwing biomechanics. The next group of muscles includes the pectoralis minor, triceps brachii, latissimus dorsi, and the teres major. One commonality of these muscles is that they have an attachment on the scapula and therefore can have an effect on scapular motion. The latissimus dorsi is one exception to that rule, but the research isn't entirely clear. According to most anatomy textbooks, the latissimus dorsi does not have a common attachment site on the scapula, although one cadaver study did recognize that 40 % of the cadavers had an attachment to the tip of the inferior angle [93]. However, the age of the cadavers was not reported, and the attachment may have developed as an adhesion due to patients being bedridden. Future research should identify the prevalence of this attachment in overhead athletes. The pectoralis minor is a thin broad muscle that originates at the third to fifth ribs and inserts on the coracoid process of the scapula. The muscle functions to depress and protract the scapula, although it does not create large ranges of motion. Throwing athletes commonly develop excessive tightness of this muscle with unknown origin [94]. It is thought that the tightness corresponds with inhibition/weakness of the posterior scapular stabilizing muscles, such as the lower trapezius and rhomboids [95]. Since serratus anterior inhibition/weakness is often observed [96, 97] and is the major scapular protractor, pectoralis minor tightness might develop due to compensation for the serratus anterior during throwing. Regardless of the mechanism, pectoralis minor tightness will cause excessive scapular protraction and anterior tilting at rest and during overhead motions [98]. This position has been shown to decrease the subacromial space, which increases the likelihood of developing subacromial and subcoracoid impingement [99]. It also can cause increased anterior stress on the anterior capsule during the late cocking phase of throwing [100]. Stretching is often difficult due to the anatomy of the pectoralis minor, and preventative stretching is likely more effective than waiting until tightness develops [101, 102]. Next, the triceps brachii has a broad origin due to three heads; however, the long head originates on the inferior glenoid and inserts with the other two heads distally on the olecranon process. Therefore, the long head of the triceps brachii is a two-joint muscle and functions at both the elbow and the shoulder. The triceps is very unique since it must coordinate motion at both the shoulder and elbow simultaneously during throwing. This is especially important during the deceleration and follow-through phase of the throw when the muscle is functioning eccentrically to absorb energy. Since the triceps must stabilize and absorb energy at two joints, the stress will be increased within the muscle, thereby creating more eccentric muscle damage during throwing. Similar to the posterior rotator cuff, the triceps will also experience an increase in passive muscle tension and reduced range of motion that requires 4–5 days to recover [85, 103]. Throwing prior to complete recovery will cause the triceps to continually develop tightness throughout the season. Triceps tightness will directly affect scapular motion since its origin is on the inferior glenoid. When the triceps is tight, it has the potential to pull the scapula into excessive protraction and anterior tilting during the deceleration and follow-through phase of throwing. This will cause excessive eccentric loading on the scapular retractors and serratus anterior, which are muscles that often develop inhibition/fatigue. In addition, triceps tightness also has the potential to decrease glenohumeral IR due to the origin on the inferior glenoid. As previously stated, GIRD can be caused from various sources (bone, capsule, posterior rotator cuff, and triceps) and can increase the likelihood of injury [59]. Examining for triceps tightness involves measuring elbow flexed and elbow extended forward flexion with the scapula stabilized [104]. If there is a large increase in forward flexion with the elbow extended, then the loss of motion is caused by triceps tightness. The final group of muscles to be discussed is the internal rotators. Throwing athletes typically have very strong internal rotators [105], which allow them to throw with high velocities. However, the overdevelopment of these muscles often causes excessive tightness. The two major internal rotators that develop adaptive tightness are the latissimus dorsi [106] and the teres major [107]. Both muscles share a common insertion site on the medial aspect of the bicipital groove of the humerus and therefore will affect glenohumeral motion in a similar way when tight. Tightness of these muscles will limit forward flexion and glenohumeral ER. During the late cocking phase of the throw, ER is essential to impart maximal velocity [2, 108]. Typically the thrower is still able to achieve normal ER by compensating at other locations. First, tightness within the latissimus dorsi may cause an excessive lordotic curve within the lower back to ultimately achieve the same glenohumeral ER [31, 106]. Second, tightness within the teres major can directly affect scapular motion [109] to ultimately achieve the same glenohumeral ER, further contributing to the inhibition/weakness of the scapular stabilizers. The tightness can be assessed clinically by examining forward flexion and glenohumeral ER with the scapula stabilized. Stabilizing the scapula is important to isolate the muscular tightness since the scapula can often compensate. The teres major does have a direct attachment on the scapula, making stabilization very important. The latissimus dorsi may have an attachment on the scapula, but it is still debatable. Tightness of the internal rotators has not been greatly recognized in the literature, and therefore, the association with shoulder and elbow injuries is not known.

Tendinous tissue also adapts to the stress of throwing in time. Throwing athletes often develop tendon-related injuries, which include tendinopathy and tears. The most common tendons affected are the rotator cuff and the long head of the biceps [110, 111]. The act of throwing is typically classified as overuse due to the repetitive nature and the high loads. It is thought that overuse activity causes tendon degeneration and damage. Many basic science studies have been performed examining the biologic consequences of overuse activity on the rotator cuff [112–114]. These studies have collectively found that overuse activity causes the tendon to express more cartilage-related genes (collagen II and aggrecan) and less tendon-related genes (collagen I) [114–117]. Essentially, the tendon becomes more like cartilage and less like tendon. It is thought that the overuse activity causes changes in joint mechanics, which places increased compression and sheer loads on the tendon [115]. Tendons are designed to resist tensile loads and in normal conditions rarely experience compression or sheer loads. The tendons will adapt based on the mechanical loading and therefore will become more cartilage-like [118]. It has also been shown that very high tensile loads within the tendon can also cause the tendon to express more cartilage genes and less tendon genes [119]. This is counterintuitive since tensile loading is thought to produce tendon-related genes and not cartilage-related genes. However, we need to consider what is occurring to the tendon cells during high tension and not just the overall tendon. As the tendon is loaded in tension, a phenomenon called Poisson's ratio occurs [120]. As the tendon is stretched, it increases in length, therefore causing the width and thickness to decrease. When this occurs under high amounts of tension, the cells within the middle of the tendon experience compression instead of the tension [119] (Fig. 1.6). When the loading switches from tension to compression or even sheer, the tendon will weaken, resulting in damage or even tears during throwing. This phenomenon has been demonstrated clinically and is called chondrometaplasia [121]. It is also possible that calcium deposit formation within tendon may be the further progression of this condition [122]. The best current treatment to allow the tendon to recover from overuse

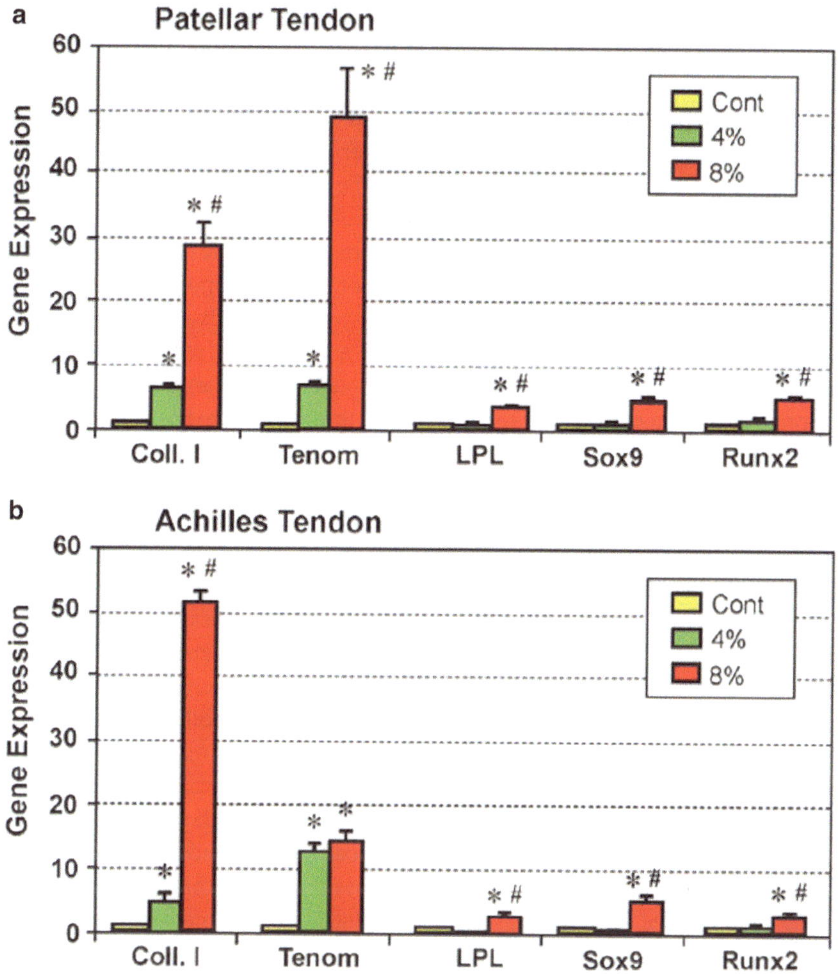

Fig. 1.6 The expression of tenocyte and non-tenocyte-related genes in patellar (**a**) and achilles (**b**) TSCs in response to mechanical loading in vitro. Total RNA were collected from TSCs stretched to 4 % or 8 % for qRT-PCR analysis. In PTSCs under low mechanical loading (*green*, 4 % stretching), only those genes related to tenocytes (Coll. I, or collagen type I; Tenom or tenomodulin) were highly expressed, but under high mechanical loading (*red*, 8 % stretching), both tenocyte and non-tenocyte-related genes increased their expression. Similar results were obtained for ATSCs in response to low (4 %) and high (8 %) mechanical loading. Note the different scale in gene expression by PTSCs and ATSCs between the two loading conditions (*p, 0.05, with respect to nonloaded cells; #p, 0.05 with respect to 4 % stretching) (Reprinted from Zhang J, Wang JH. The effects of mechanical loading on tendons–an in vivo and in vitro model study. PLoS One. 2013 Aug 19;8(8):e71740)

adaptations is rest. In an animal model, a week of rest allowed the expression of genes to return to normal levels [123]. This demonstrates the importance of several days of rest following a bout of throwing to minimize the development of tendon degeneration and injury.

As we previously discussed, muscles can develop structural adaptations due to the stress of throwing. In addition, upper extremity muscles can also develop neuromuscular control adaptations, which can have large implications on overall shoulder function. Neuromuscular control is a complex interaction between the nervous system (motor cortex and spinal cord) and the skeletal muscles of the body to complete a specific movement or task. As we participate in sports that involve specific movements, such as throwing, we slowly create a stronger neural connection between the nervous system and our muscles [124]. However, during overuse situations, the connections can be affected by fatigue [125]. This will cause other muscles to compensate. Throughout the season, these compensatory neuromuscular strategies become "hardwired" and serve as the primary neuromuscular control pattern. This is problematic since in nonfatigued conditions, these patterns are not optimal and can increase stress on other tissues [126, 127]. In throwers, the muscles that have the greatest propensity for fatigue are often the muscles that develop neuromuscular adaptations. These muscles include the scapular stabilizers and the posterior rotator cuff [128–131]. When examining the structure and function of the scapular stabilizers, it is clear that these muscles are designed for low-load and endurance situations, such as maintaining upright posture [132]. However, the task of throwing requires high loads and endurance. During the deceleration phase of the throw, the scapular stabilizers are required to absorb the energy that was created during the acceleration phase [14]. To perform this task, the muscles perform repetitive eccentric contractions, which quickly lead to fatigue [133]. The lower trapezius and the serratus anterior are two of the scapular stabilizing muscles that have demonstrated alternated activation strategies often described as fatigue-related inhibition [96, 134–136]. These two muscles play a significant role in overhead arm function [137, 138]. One important role is to work in conjunction with the upper trapezius to produce scapular upward rotation [137]. Without the lower trapezius and serratus anterior functioning properly, the scapula will not upward rotate correctly during overhead motion and place the athlete at risk for impingement syndrome [96, 134, 135]. The serratus anterior also has an isolated function to prevent scapular internal rotation (scapular winging). Several studies have demonstrated that scapular winging decreases the subacromial space and also creates an unstable scapula [94, 99]. An unstable scapula has been hypothesized to cause the rotator cuff to act opposite of origin and insertion [139, 140]. This suggests that instead of the rotator cuff compressing the humeral head into the glenoid, the rotator cuff pulls the scapula laterally around the thoracic wall. This will decrease the dynamic restraint at the glenohumeral joint and cause instability or increased humeral head translations.

The next group of muscles that develop neuromuscular control adaptations is the posterior rotator cuff. As previously stated, the posterior rotator cuff is composed of the infraspinatus and teres minor. Relatively speaking, these muscles have a very small cross sectional area and aren't designed to resist large loads [38]. However, during throwing, these two small muscles are required to absorb a large amount of energy and assist in decelerating the shoulder. Similar to the scapular stabilizers, the large eccentric loads during the deceleration phase of the throw can quickly fatigue these muscles during a game. It has been demonstrated that these muscles can also develop fatigue-related inhibition [130]. This has also been observed and well documented in the quadriceps following an ACL injury [141]. To examine this, researchers often subject the muscle to a supramaximal burst of electrostimulation to measure the additional force production that can be produced that is beyond the voluntary activation. Since the muscle can mechanically produce higher force with a supramaximal burst of electrostimulation, it is suggested that the source of inhibition is located in the central nervous system. Improper rest and rehabilitation throughout the season will allow the inhibition to progressively worsen, diminishing the energy-absorbing properties of the posterior rotator cuff. One study examined the isometric strength of the glenohumeral IR and ER throughout the season [142]. They found that from pre- to postseason glenohumeral IR strength increased; however, glenohumeral ER strength decreased. This evidence supports the diminished neuromuscular control of the posterior rotator cuff over the season.

Pitching Mechanics

Abnormal throwing mechanics will increase stress on tissue and if not corrected will most likely lead to significant injury at either the shoulder or elbow [14, 88, 108, 143]. We have previously discussed how adaptations can alter throwing mechanics; however, there are additional mechanical alterations that are not caused by adaptations and can easily be corrected. One main area of focus is the location of lead foot contact. Normally the lead foot will stride at least 75 % of the pitchers height and be pointed directly toward home plate [1]. To examine this, high-speed cameras and expertise in throwing biomechanics are not required. The easiest way to examine this is by using the dirt on the mound. The foot prints in the dirt will easily tell you if there are alterations in lead foot location. There are two common alterations that occur. First, the lead foot does not stride to 75 % of the pitcher's height. This is an indication that the pitcher isn't fully incorporating the lower extremity into the throw. When a player strides out, momentum and passive muscular tension are being created within the hips [144]. This momentum and passive tension are essential to initiate the creation and flow of rotational energy that moves up the kinetic chain [144]. A short stride length can be caused by lower extremity fatigue or weakness. In addition, hip tightness can limit the players' ability to stride out to the optimal distance [16]. The second alteration is the lead foot not pointing toward the target. When the stride foot of a right-handed thrower lands to the left (toward first base) of the target, it causes the hips to open too early and excessively. When this alteration occurs, the throwing shoulder will be in a horizontally abducted position during the late cocking phase of the throw instead of being in the scapular plane [145, 146]. This places increased stress on the anterior capsule, places increased stress on the medial elbow, and is a position that causes internal impingement [89]. In addition, by opening the hips up early, the energy created from the lower extremity can be lost due to improper timing requiring the remaining kinetic chain to compensate for the loss [144]. This is often referred to as distal chain "catchup" and may lead to further overuse injury. When the stride foot of a right-handed thrower lands to the right (toward third base) of the target, it causes the hips to never open. This also leads to a loss of energy from the lower extremity due to passive muscular tension within the hips never being created. Again this will cause the remaining kinetic chain to compensate. In addition, the closed hip position will prevent the thorax, shoulder, and opposite hip from properly decelerating through the full range of motion, which can place additional stress on the posterior rotator cuff and scapular stabilizers [16].

Clinical Implications

The body works as a unit to achieve optimum overhead throwing function and can fail as a unit in altered performance or the "disabled throwing shoulder" (DTS). Therefore, the evaluation of the overhead athlete with DTS needs to be comprehensive and can involve evaluation of the pertinent normal mechanics, evaluation of possible pathomechanics, identification of physiological and biomechanical factors contributing to the pathomechanics, and the kinetic chain examination, as well as identification of all structural adaptations that may exist in the shoulder. Similarly, treatment should include optimization of the structural adaptations as well as restoration of the pathophysiology and pathomechanics [12].

Evaluation of mechanics and pathomechanics can be clinically accomplished by direct observation and/or video analysis of the motion. Specific methods for evaluation and criteria for determining the presence (yes) or absence (no) of the nodes have been developed for baseball [32] and tennis [13, 48] and are summarized in Tables 1.1 and 1.2. This exam can identify anatomic areas and mechanical motions that may be contributing to the symptoms and suggest areas for more detailed evaluation.

The kinetic chain exam should include a screening evaluation of the leg and core stability, observational evaluation for scapular dyskinesis, and evaluation of various elements in the shoulder. It should be supplemented by a detailed examination of the areas highlighted by the symptoms or evaluation [43] (Table 1.3).

Table 1.3 Proximal to distal kinetic chain evaluation

Examination emphasis	Normal	Abnormal	Result	Evaluation
One leg stability: stance	Negative Trendelenburg	Positive Trendelenburg	Decreased force to shoulder	Gluteus medius strength
One leg stability: squat	Control of knee varus/valgus during decent	Knee valgus or "corkscrewing" during decent	Alters arm position during task	Dynamic postural control
Hip rotation	Bilateral symmetry within known normal limits	Side-to-side asymmetry and/or not within normal limits	Decreased trunk flexibility and rotation	Internal and external rotation of the hip
Plank	Ability to maintain body position for at least 30 s	Inability to maintain body position	Decreased core stability and strength	Dynamic postural control in suspended horizontal position
Scapular dyskinesis	Bilateral symmetry with no inferior angle or medial border prominence	Side-to-side asymmetry or bilateral prominence of inferior angle and/or medial border	Decreased rotator cuff function and increased risk of internal and/or external impingement	Scapular muscle control of scapular position ("yes/no" clinical evaluation [47], [67], manual corrective maneuvers [27, 52]
Shoulder rotation	Side-to-side symmetry or internal and external rotation values less than 15° or less than 5°	Side-to-side asymmetry of 15° or more in internal and/or external rotation or 5° or more of total range of motion	Altered kinematics and increased load on the glenoid labrum	Internal and external rotation of the glenohumeral joint
Shoulder muscle flexibility	Normal mobility of pectoralis minor and latissimus dorsi	Tight pectoralis minor and/or latissimus dorsi	Scapular protraction	Palpation of pectoralis minor and latissimus dorsi
Shoulder strength	Normal resistance to testing in the anterior and posterior muscles	Weakness and/or imbalance of anterior and posterior muscles	Scapular protraction, decreased arm elevation, strength, and concavity compression	Muscle strength from a stabilized scapula
Joint internal derangement	All provocative and stress testing negative	Pop, click, slide, pain, stiffness, possible "dead arm"	Loss of concavity compression and functional stability	Labral injury, rotator cuff injury or weakness, glenohumeral instability, biceps tendinopathy

The shoulder exam should be comprehensive, emphasizing the evaluation of the anatomy (labrum, biceps, and/or rotator cuff internal derangement), physiology (muscle weakness/imbalance, flexibility), and mechanics (scapular dyskinesis, GIRD, TROMD).

Treatment should also involve a comprehensive approach, including restoration of all kinetic chain deficits, altered mechanics, and functional joint stability. Rehabilitation should address all of the physiological and mechanical factors [12, 148–150]. This would include restoration of hip range of motion and leg strength, core stability and strength, scapular control, shoulder muscle flexibility and strength, and glenohumeral rotation. Surgery should address repairing joint structures to optimize the capability for functional stability [12]. However restoration of the integrity of the kinetic chain must still be treated with reverence postoperatively.

Summary

The mechanics of throwing are truly an orchestration of motion predicated on precise muscular firing patterns acting in a coordinated fashion. Tissue breakdown due to unchecked maladaptations, kinetic chain breakdown, or improper mechanics will lead to muscle inhibition and further decompensation eventuating in potential substantial injury to the rotator cuff and labrum. Impaired performance and/or injury, the DTS, is associated with alterations in the mechanics that are called pathomechanics. They can occur at multiple locations throughout the kinetic chain. They must be evaluated and treated as part of the overall problem.

Observational analysis of the mechanics and pathomechanics using the node analysis method can be useful in highlighting areas of alteration that can be evaluated for anatomic injury or altered physiology. The comprehensive kinetic chain exam can evaluate sites of kinetic chain breakage, and a detailed shoulder exam can assess joint internal derangement of altered physiology that may contribute to the pathomechanics.

Treatment of the DTS should be comprehensive, directed toward restoring physiology and mechanics and optimizing anatomy. This will maximize the body's ability to develop normal mechanics to accomplish the overhead throwing task.

References

1. Pappas AM, Zawacki RM, Sullivan TJ. Biomechanics of baseball pitching: a preliminary report. Am J Sports Med. 1985;13:216–22.
2. Fleisig GS, Dillman CJ, Andrews JR. Biomechanics of the shoulder during throwing. In: Andrews JR, Wilk KE, editors. The athlete's shoulder. New York, NY: Churchill Livingstone; 1994.
3. Freegarde T. Introduction to the physics of waves. Cambridge: Cambridge University Press; 2012. p. 309. ISBN 9780521147163.
4. Latash ML, Scholz JP, Schoner G. Toward a new theory of motor synergies. Motor Control. 2007;11(3):276–308.
5. Hirashima M, et al. Kinetic chain of overarm throwing in terms of joint rotations revealed by induced acceleration analysis. J Biomech. 2008;41(13):2874–83.
6. Aggelousis N, et al. Modifications of neuromuscular activity and improvement in performance of a novel motor skill. Percept Mot Skills. 2001;93(1):239–48.
7. Gabriel DA, Kamen G, Frost G. Neural adaptations to resistive exercise: mechanisms and recommendations for training practices. Sports Med. 2006;36(2): 133–49.
8. Luckin KA, et al. Muscle fatigue: conduction or mechanical failure? Biochem Med Metab Biol. 1991;46(3):299–316.
9. Conwit RA, et al. Fatigue effects on motor unit activity during submaximal contractions. Arch Phys Med Rehabil. 2000;81(9):1211–6.
10. Woledge RC. Possible effects of fatigue on muscle efficiency. Acta Physiol Scand. 1998;162(3):267–73.
11. Newham DJ, et al. Ultrastructural changes after concentric and eccentric contractions of human muscle. J Neurol Sci. 1983;61(1):109–22.
12. Kibler WB, et al. The disabled throwing shoulder – spectrum of pathology: 10 year update. Arthroscopy. 2013;29(1):141–61.
13. Lintner D, Noonan TJ, Kibler WB. Injury patterns and biomechanics of the athlete's shoulder. Clin Sports Med. 2008;27(4):527–52.
14. Fleisig GS, et al. Kinetics of baseball pitching with implications about injury mechanisms. Am J Sports Med. 1995;23(2):233–9.
15. Fleisig GS, et al. Biomechanics of overhand throwing with implications for injuries. Sports Med. 1996;21:421–37.
16. Putnam CA. Sequential motions of body segments in striking and throwing skills: description and explanations. J Biomech. 1993;26:125–35.
17. Hirashima M, et al. Sequential muscle activity and its functional role in the upper extremity and trunk during overarm throwing. J Sports Sci. 2002;20: 301–10.
18. Bouisset S, Zattara M. A sequence of postural movements precedes voluntary movement. Neurosci Lett. 1981;22:263–70.
19. Zattara M, Bouisset S. Posturo-kinetic organisation during the early phase of voluntary upper limb movement. 1. Normal subjects. J Neurol Neurosurg Psychiatry. 1988;51:956–65.
20. DiGiovine NM, et al. An electromyographic analysis of the upper extremity in pitching. J Shoulder Elbow Surg. 1992;1(1):15–25.
21. Lippitt S, et al. Glenohumeral stability from concavity-compression: a quantitative analysis. J Shoulder Elbow Surg. 1993;2(1):27–35.
22. Escamilla RF, Andrews JR. Shoulder muscle recruitment patterns and related biomechanics during upper extremity sports. Sports Med. 2009;39(7):569–90.
23. Sciascia AD, et al. Kinetic chain abnormalities in the athletic shoulder. Sports Med Arthrosc Rev. 2012;20(1):16–21.
24. Davids K, et al. Movement systems as dynamical systems: the functional role of variability and its implications for sports medicine. Sports Med. 2003;33(4):245–60.
25. Sporns O, Edelman GM. Solving Bernstein's problem: a proposal for the development of coordinated movement by selection. Child Dev. 1993;64:960–81.

26. Elliott BC, Marshall R, Noffal G. Contributions of upper limb segment rotations during the power serve in tennis. J Appl Biomech. 1995;11:443–7.
27. Toyoshima S, Miyashita M. Force-velocity relation in throwing. Res Q. 1973;44(1):86–95.
28. Hirashima M, et al. Control of 3D limb dynamics in unconstrained overarm throws of different speeds performed by skilled baseball players. J Neurophysiol. 2007;97(1):680–91.
29. Young JL, et al. The influence of the spine on the shoulder in the throwing athlete. J Back Musculoskelet Rehabil. 1996;7:5–17.
30. Nieminen H, et al. Load-sharing patterns in the shoulder during isometric flexion tasks. J Biomech. 1995;28(5):555–66.
31. Fleisig GS, et al. Kinematic and kinetic comparison of baseball pitching among various levels of development. J Biomech. 1999;32(12):1371–5.
32. Davis JT, et al. The effect of pitching biomechanics on the upper extremity in youth and adolescent baseball pitchers. Am J Sports Med. 2009;37(8): 1484–91.
33. Toyoshima S, Hoshikawa T, Miyashita M. Contributions of body parts to throwing performance. In: Nelson RC, Morehouse CA, editors. Biomechanics IV. Baltimore, MD: University Park Press; 1974. p. 169–74.
34. Marshall R, Elliott BC. Long axis rotation: the missing link in proximal to distal segment sequencing. J Sports Sci. 2000;18(4):247–54.
35. Elliott B, et al. Technique effects on upper limb loading in the tennis serve. J Sci Med Sport. 2003;6(1): 76–87.
36. Meyer KE, et al. Three-dimensional scapular kinematics during the throwing motion. J Appl Biomech. 2008;24:24–34.
37. Speer KP, Garrett WE. Muscular control of motion and stability about the pectoral girdle. In: Matsen Iii FA, Fu F, Hawkins RJ, editors. The shoulder: a balance of mobility and stability. Rosemont, IL: American Academy of Orthopaedic Surgeons; 1994. p. 159–73.
38. Kibler WB. The role of the scapula in athletic function. Am J Sports Med. 1998;26:325–37.
39. Harryman II DT, et al. Translation of the humeral head on the glenoid with passive glenohumeral motion. J Bone Joint Surg (Am). 1990;72(9): 1334–43.
40. Grossman MG, et al. A cadaveric model of the throwing shoulder: a possible etiology of superior labrum anterior-to-posterior lesions. J Bone Joint Surg (Am). 2005;87(4):824–31.
41. Wilk KE, Meister K, Andrews JR. Current concepts in the rehabilitation of the overhead throwing athlete. Am J Sports Med. 2002;30(1):136–51.
42. Veeger HEJ, van der Helm FCT. Shoulder function: the perfect compromise between mobility and stability. J Biomech. 2007;40:2119–29.
43. Kibler WB, Press J, Sciascia AD. The role of core stability in athletic function. Sports Med. 2006;36(3):189–98.
44. Glazier PS, Davids K. Constraints on the complete optimization of human motion. Sports Med. 2009;39(1):16–28.
45. Bernstein N. The coordination and regulation of movement. London: Pergamon; 1967.
46. Dillman CJ, Fleisig GS, Andrews JR. Biomechanics of pitching with emphasis upon shoulder kinematics. J Orthop Sports Phys Ther. 1993;18:402–8.
47. Crockett HC, et al. Osseous adaptation and range of motion at the glenohumeral joint in professional baseball pitchers. Am J Sports Med. 2002;30(1): 20–6.
48. Kovacs M, Ellenbecker T. An 8-stage model for evaluating the tennis serve: implications for performance enhancement and injury prevention. Sports Health. 2011;3:504–13.
49. Thomas SJ, et al. Glenohumeral rotation and scapular position adaptations after a single high school female sports season. J Athl Train. 2009;44(3): 230–7.
50. Thomas SJ, et al. Internal rotation and scapular position changes following competitive high school baseball. J Sport Rehabil. 2010;19(2):125–35.
51. Thomas SJ, et al. Internal rotation and scapular position differences: a comparison of collegiate and high school baseball players. J Athl Train. 2010;45(1): 44–50.
52. Burkhart SS, Morgan CD, Kibler WB. The disabled throwing shoulder: spectrum of pathology. Part I: Pathoanatomy and biomechanics. Arthroscopy. 2003;19(4):404–20.
53. Dwelly PM, et al. Glenohumeral rotational range of motion in collegiate overhead-throwing athletes during an athletic season. J Athl Train. 2009;44(6):611–6.
54. Ellenbecker TS, et al. Glenohumeral joint total rotation range of motion in elite tennis players and baseball pitchers. Med Sci Sports Exerc. 2002;34: 2052–6.
55. Laudner KG, Lynall R, Meister K. Shoulder adaptations among pitchers and position players over the course of a competitive baseball season. Clin J Sport Med. 2013;23(3):184–9.
56. Meister K, et al. Rotational motion changes in the glenohumeral joint of the adolescent/Little League baseball player. Am J Sports Med. 2005;33(5): 693–8.
57. Myers JB, et al. Glenohumeral range of motion deficits and posterior shoulder tightness in throwers with pathologic internal impingement. Am J Sports Med. 2006;34(3):385–91.
58. Nakamizo H, et al. Loss of glenohumeral internal rotation in little league pitchers: a biomechanical study. J Shoulder Elbow Surg. 2008;17(5):795–801.
59. Wilk KE, et al. Correlation of glenohumeral internal rotation deficit and total rotational motion to shoulder injuries in professional baseball pitchers. Am J Sports Med. 2011;39(2):329–35.
60. Garrison JC, et al. Shoulder range of motion deficits in baseball players with an ulnar collateral ligament tear. Am J Sports Med. 2012;40(11):2597–603.

61. Wolff J. Das gesetz der transformation der knochen. Berlin: A. Hirshwald; 1892.
62. Krahl VE. The torsion of the humerus: its localization, cause, and duration in man. Am J Anat. 1947;80:275–319.
63. Whiteley R, et al. Indirect ultrasound measurement of humeral torsion in adolescent baseball players and non-athletic adults: reliability and significance. J Sci Med Sport. 2006;9(4):310–8.
64. Myers JB, Oyama S, Clarke JP. Ultrasonographic assessment of humeral retrotorsion in baseball players: a validation study. Am J Sports Med. 2012;40(5): 1155–60.
65. Edelson G. The development of humeral head retroversion. J Shoulder Elbow Surg. 2000;9(4):316–8.
66. Reagan KM, et al. Humeral retroversion and its relationship to glenohumeral rotation in the shoulder of college baseball players. Am J Sports Med. 2002;30(3):354–60.
67. Myers JB, et al. Humeral retrotorsion in collegiate baseball pitchers with throwing-related upper extremity injury history. Sports Health. 2011;3(4): 383–9.
68. Thomas SJ, et al. A bilateral comparison of posterior capsule thickness and its correlation with glenohumeral range of motion and scapular upward rotation in collegiate baseball players. J Shoulder Elbow Surg. 2011;20(5):708–16.
69. Neil JM, Schweitzer ME. Humeral cortical and trabecular changes in the throwing athlete: a quantitative computed tomography study of male college baseball players. J Comput Assist Tomogr. 2008;32(3):492–6.
70. Bogenschutz ED, Smith HD, Warden SJ. Midhumerus adaptation in fast-pitch softballers and the effect of throwing mechanics. Med Sci Sports Exerc. 2011;43(9):1698–706.
71. Sakurai G, et al. Morphologic changes in long head of biceps brachii in rotator cuff dysfunction. J Orthop Sci. 1998;3(3):137–42.
72. Clark JM, Harryman II DT. Tendons, ligaments, and capsule of the rotator cuff. Gross and microscopic anatomy. J Bone Joint Surg (Am). 1992;74(5): 713–25.
73. Mihata T, et al. Excessive humeral external rotation results in increased shoulder laxity. Am J Sports Med. 2004;32(5):1278–85.
74. Jobe CW, Pink MM, Jobe FW. Anterior shoulder instability, impingement, and rotator cuff tear: theories and concepts. In: Jobe FW, editor. Operative techniques in upper extremity sports injuries. St. Louis: Mosby; 1996. p. 164.
75. Borsa PA, et al. Comparison of dynamic sonography to stress radiography for assessing glenohumeral laxity in asymptomatic shoulders. Am J Sports Med. 2005;33(5):734–41.
76. Wilk KE, Arrigo CA, Andrews JR. Current concepts: the stabilizing structures of the glenohumeral joint. J Orthop Sports Phys Ther. 1997;25:364–79.
77. Gandhi J, et al. Voluntary activation deficits of the infraspinatus present as a consequence of pitching-induced fatigue. J Shoulder Elbow Surg. 2012;21(5): 625–30.
78. Huffman GR, et al. Path of glenohumeral articulation throughout the rotational range of motion in a thrower's shoulder model. Am J Sports Med. 2006;34(10):1662–9.
79. Clabbers KM, et al. Effect of posterior capsule tightness on glenohumeral translation in the late-cocking phase of pitching. J Sport Rehabil. 2007;16:41–9.
80. Rack PM, Westbury DR. The short range stiffness of active mammalian muscle. J Physiol. 1973;229(1): 16P–7.
81. Rack PM, Westbury DR. The short range stiffness of active mammalian muscle and its effect on mechanical properties. J Physiol. 1974;240(2):331–50.
82. Friden J, Sjostrom M, Ekblom B. Myofibrillar damage following intense eccentric exercise in man. Int J Sports Med. 1983;4(3):170–6.
83. Bobbert MF, Hollander AP, Huijing PA. Factors in delayed onset muscular soreness of man. Med Sci Sports Exerc. 1986;18(1):75–81.
84. Armstrong RB. Mechanisms of exercise-induced delayed onset muscular soreness: a brief review. Med Sci Sports Exerc. 1984;16(6):529–38.
85. Proske U, Morgan DL. Do cross-bridges contribute to the tension during stretch of passive muscle? J Muscle Res Cell Motil. 1999;20(5-6):433–42.
86. Rosant C, Nagel MD, Perot C. Aging affects passive stiffness and spindle function of the rat soleus muscle. Exp Gerontol. 2007;42(4):301–8.
87. Reinold MM, et al. Changes in shoulder and elbow passive range of motion after pitching in professional baseball players. Am J Sports Med. 2008;36(3): 523–7.
88. Kibler WB, Sciascia A, Moore S. An acute throwing episode decreases shoulder internal rotation. Clin Orthop Relat Res. 2012;470(6):1545–51.
89. Takagi Y, et al. Increased horizontal shoulder abduction is associated with an increase in shoulder joint load in baseball pitching. J Shoulder Elbow Surg. 2014;23(12):1757–62.
90. Mihata T, et al. Excessive glenohumeral horizontal abduction as occurs during the late cocking phase of the throwing motion can be critical for internal impingement. Am J Sports Med. 2010;38(2):369–74.
91. Park KN, et al. Comparison of the effects of local cryotherapy and passive cross-body stretch on extensibility in subjects with posterior shoulder tightness. J Sports Sci Med. 2014;13(1):84–90.
92. Laudner K, et al. Acute effects of instrument assisted soft tissue mobilization for improving posterior shoulder range of motion in collegiate baseball players. Int J Sports Phys Ther. 2014;9(1):1–7.
93. Harshbarger ND, et al. The effectiveness of shoulder stretching and joint mobilizations on posterior shoulder tightness. J Sport Rehabil. 2013;22(4): 313–9.

94. Pouliart N, Gagey O. Significance of the latissimus dorsi for shoulder instability. I. Variations in its anatomy around the humerus and scapula. Clin Anat. 2005;18(7):493–9.
95. Burkhart SS, Morgan CD, Kibler WB. The disabled throwing shoulder: spectrum of pathology. Part III: The SICK scapula, scapular dyskinesis, the kinetic chain, and rehabilitation. Arthroscopy. 2003;19(6): 641–61.
96. Cools AM, et al. Evaluation of isokinetic force production and associated muscle activity in the scapular rotators during a protraction-retraction movement in overhead athletes with impingement symptoms. Br J Sports Med. 2004;38(1):64–8.
97. Ludewig PM, Cook TM. Alterations in shoulder kinematics and associated muscle activity in people with symptoms of shoulder impingement. Phys Ther. 2000;80(3):276–91.
98. Wadsworth DJ, Bullock-Saxton JE. Recruitment patterns of the scapular rotator muscles in freestyle swimmers with subacromial impingement. Int J Sports Med. 1997;18(8):618–24.
99. Borstad JD, Ludewig PM. The effect of long versus short pectoralis minor resting length on scapular kinematics in healthy individuals. J Orthop Sports Phys Ther. 2005;35(4):227–38.
100. Solem-Bertoft E, Thuomas KA, Westerberg CE. The influence of scapular retraction and protraction on the width of the subacromial space. An MRI study. Clin Orthop Relat Res. 1993;296:99–103.
101. Weiser WM, et al. Effects of simulated scapular protraction on anterior glenohumeral stability. Am J Sports Med. 1999;27(6):801–5.
102. Borstad JD, Ludewig PM. Comparison of three stretches for the pectoralis minor muscle. J Shoulder Elbow Surg. 2006;15(3):324–30.
103. Muraki T, et al. Lengthening of the pectoralis minor muscle during passive shoulder motions and stretching techniques: a cadaveric biomechanical study. Phys Ther. 2009;89(4):333–41.
104. Proske U, Morgan DL. Muscle damage from eccentric exercise: mechanism, mechanical signs, adaptation and clinical applications. J Physiol. 2001;537(Pt 2): 333–45.
105. Norkin CC, White DJ. A guide to goniometry. Philadelphia, PA: F.A. Davis Company; 1995.
106. Ellenbecker TS, Mattalino AJ. Concentric isokinetic shoulder internal and external rotation strength in professional baseball pitchers. J Orthop Sports Phys Ther. 1997;25(5):323–8.
107. Bhatt CR, et al. Variation in the insertion of the latissimus dorsi and its clinical importance. J Orthop. 2013;10(1):25–8.
108. Nagda SH, et al. Management and outcomes of latissimus dorsi and teres major injuries in professional baseball pitchers. Am J Sports Med. 2011;39(10): 2181–6.
109. Gatton ML, et al. A three-dimensional mathematical model of the thoracolumbar fascia and an estimate of its biomechanical effect. J Biomech. 2010;43(14): 2792–7.
110. Iamsaard S, et al. Variant insertion of the teres major muscle. Anat Cell Biol. 2012;45(3):211–3.
111. Altchek DW, Dines DM. Shoulder injuries in the throwing athlete. J Am Acad Orthop Surg. 1995;3(3): 159–65.
112. Hawkins RJ, Kennedy JC. Impingement syndrome in athletes. Am J Sports Med. 1980;8(3):151–8.
113. Soslowsky LJ, et al. Neer Award 1999. Overuse activity injures the supraspinatus tendon in an animal model: a histologic and biomechanical study. J Shoulder Elbow Surg. 2000;9(2):79–84.
114. Soslowsky LJ, et al. Rotator cuff tendinosis in an animal model: role of extrinsic and overuse factors. Ann Biomed Eng. 2002;30(8):1057–63.
115. Archambault JM, et al. Rat supraspinatus tendon expresses cartilage markers with overuse. J Orthop Res. 2007;25(5):617–24.
116. Attia M, et al. Early events of overused supraspinatus tendons involve matrix metalloproteinases and EMMPRIN/CD147 in the absence of inflammation. Am J Sports Med. 2013;41(4):908–17.
117. Reuther KE, et al. Returning to overuse activity following a supraspinatus and infraspinatus tear leads to joint damage in a rat model. J Biomech. 2013;46(11):1818–24.
118. Attia M, et al. Alterations of overused supraspinatus tendon: a possible role of glycosaminoglycans and HARP/pleiotrophin in early tendon pathology. J Orthop Res. 2012;30(1):61–71.
119. Pelaez D, Huang CY, Cheung HS. Cyclic compression maintains viability and induces chondrogenesis of human mesenchymal stem cells in fibrin gel scaffolds. Stem Cells Dev. 2009;18(1):93–102.
120. Zhang J, Wang JH. The effects of mechanical loading on tendons–an in vivo and in vitro model study. PLoS One. 2013;8(8), e71740.
121. Vergari C, et al. True stress and Poisson's ratio of tendons during loading. J Biomech. 2011;44(4):719–24.
122. Lynn MD, Lee J. Periarticular tenosynovial chondrometaplasia. Report of a case at the wrist. J Bone Joint Surg (Am). 1972;54(3):650–2.
123. Rui YF, et al. Does erroneous differentiation of tendon-derived stem cells contribute to the pathogenesis of calcifying tendinopathy? Chin Med J (Engl). 2011;124(4):606–10.
124. Jelinsky SA, et al. Gene expression in rat supraspinatus tendon recovers from overuse with rest. Clin Orthop Relat Res. 2008;466(7):1612–7.
125. Pensini M, Martin A, Maffiuletti NA. Central versus peripheral adaptations following eccentric resistance training. Int J Sports Med. 2002;23(8):567–74.
126. Myers JB, et al. Proprioception and neuromuscular control of the shoulder after muscle fatigue. J Athl Train. 1999;34(4):362–7.
127. Quammen D, et al. Two different fatigue protocols and lower extremity motion patterns during a stop-jump task. J Athl Train. 2012;47(1):32–41.
128. Minshull C, et al. Effects of acute fatigue on the volitional and magnetically-evoked electromechanical delay of the knee flexors in males and females. Eur J Appl Physiol. 2007;100(4):469–78.

129. Ebaugh DD, McClure PW, Karduna AR. Scapulothoracic and glenohumeral kinematics following an external rotation fatigue protocol. J Orthop Sports Phys Ther. 2006;36(8):557–71.
130. Ebaugh DD, McClure PW, Karduna AR. Effects of shoulder muscle fatigue caused by repetitive overhead activities on scapulothoracic and glenohumeral kinematics. J Electromyogr Kinesiol. 2006;16(3):224–35.
131. Stackhouse SK, et al. Voluntary activation of the infraspinatus muscle in nonfatigued and fatigued states. J Shoulder Elbow Surg. 2010;19(2):224–9.
132. Tsai NT, McClure PW, Karduna AR. Effects of muscle fatigue on 3-dimensional scapular kinematics. Arch Phys Med Rehabil. 2003;84:1000–5.
133. Lindman R, Eriksson A, Thornell LE. Fiber type composition of the human male trapezius muscle: enzyme-histochemical characteristics. Am J Anat. 1990;189(3):236–44.
134. Moritani T, Oddson L, Thorstensson A. Electromyographic evidence of selective fatigue during the eccentric phase of stretch/shortening cycles in man. Eur J Appl Physiol Occup Physiol. 1990;60(6):425–9.
135. Cools AM, et al. Trapezius activity and intramuscular balance during isokinetic exercise in overhead athletes with impingement symptoms. Scand J Med Sci Sports. 2007;17(1):25–33.
136. Cools AM, et al. Scapular muscle recruitment patterns: trapezius muscle latency with and without impingement symptoms. Am J Sports Med. 2003; 31(4):542–9.
137. Cools AM, et al. Scapular muscle recruitment pattern: electromyographic response of the trapezius muscle to sudden shoulder movement before and after a fatiguing exercise. J Orthop Sports Phys Ther. 2002;32(5):221–9.
138. Pink M. Understanding the linkage system of the upper extremity. Sports Med Arthrosc Rev. 2001;9: 52–60.
139. Pink MM, Perry J. Biomechanics. In: Jobe FW, editor. Operative techniques in upper extremity sports injuries. St. Louis: Mosby; 1996. p. 3–14.
140. Kibler BW. Role of the scapula in the overhead throwing motion. Contemp Orthop. 1991;22: 525–32.
141. Yanagisawa O, Okumura K, Torii S. Comparison of the morphology of the rotator cuff muscles across age groups. Clin Anat. 2014;27(3):365–9.
142. Snyder-Mackler L, et al. Reflex inhibition of the quadriceps femoris muscle after injury or reconstruction of the anterior cruciate ligament. J Bone Joint Surg (Am). 1994;76(4):555–60.
143. Ramsi M, et al. Isometric shoulder rotator strength characteristics of high school swimmers over the course of a competitive season. J Sport Rehabil. 2004;13(1):9–18.
144. Fleisig G, et al. Variability in baseball pitching biomechanics among various levels of competition. Sports Biomech. 2009;8(1):10–21.
145. Robb AJ, et al. Passive ranges of motion of the hips and their relationship with pitching biomechanics and ball velocity in professional baseball pitchers. Am J Sports Med. 2010;38(12):2487–93.
146. Whiteley R. Baseball throwing mechanics as they relate to pathology and performance – a review. J Sports Sci Med. 2007;6(1):1–20.
147. Oyama S, et al. Improper trunk rotation sequence is associated with increased maximal shoulder external rotation angle and shoulder joint force in high school baseball pitchers. Am J Sports Med. 2014;42(9): 2089–94.
148. McMullen J, Uhl TL. A kinetic chain approach for shoulder rehabilitation. J Athl Train. 2000;35(3): 329–37.
149. Wilk KE, Macrina LC, Arrigo C. Passive range of motion characteristics in the overhead baseball pitcher and their implications for rehabilitation. Clin Orthop Relat Res. 2012;470:1586–94.
150. Ellenbecker TS, Cools A. Rehabilitation of shoulder impingement syndrome and rotator cuff injuries: an evidence-based review. Br J Sports Med. 2010;44: 319–27.
151. McLean J, Andrisani J. The X-factor swing. New York: Collins; 1997. ISBN 10:0062701428.

Prevention of Labral and Rotator Cuff Injuries in the Overhead Athlete

2

Nathan W. Skelley and Matthew V. Smith

The Biomechanics of Throwing

There are five main phases of the throwing motion: windup, cocking, acceleration, deceleration, and follow-through (Fig. 2.1) [1–3]. The phases of the throwing motion generate and transmit energy to the arm to create velocity [1]. Windup and follow-through compose the majority of the throwing time, but the entire process can take less than 2 s. As a result, throwing athletes require efficient and well-coordinated motion of the upper and lower extremities.

The Kinetic Chain

The kinetic chain is defined as the coordinated sequence of body movements that generate force to perform a particular action. In the throwing athlete, the kinetic chain starts when force is generated from the ground and is transmitted to the legs, the hips, torso, and the shoulder. Finally, the arm acts as the delivery mechanism of that energy [1, 4]. Coordinated movements transmit energy in a manner greater than what the individual joints could develop on their own. Using more body segments within the kinetic chain can create a greater maximum velocity to the overhead throw [5]. The goal of the athlete's kinetic chain is to develop the optimal force while applying minimal joint loads during movement [6]. When deviations in ideal body mechanics occur, individual joint loads may change with distal segments overcompensating. As a result, the athlete is prone to overuse and to injury. For example, approximately 50 % of patients with superior labral anterior posterior (SLAP) tears have signs of core weakness and deficits in hip flexibility and hip abductor and extensor strength [7–9]. The clinician should evaluate the entire kinetic chain when evaluating the at risk painful shoulder.

Evaluating the entire kinetic chain in a complex movement, like throwing, is challenging [10]. Studying individual parts of the kinetic chain in isolation, however, can provide greater understanding when put in the context of the entire kinetic chain. Coordination of the entire kinetic chain is critical to proper positioning of the arm during throwing. Sufficient power of the lower torso is essential to generate ball velocity [11]. Core and lower extremity weakness creates an unstable platform for the thrower. In fact, weakness in the gluteal region, torso, and scapular region has been postulated to contribute to injury in throwing athletes.

N.W. Skelley, MD (✉)
Department of Orthopaedic Surgery, Barnes-Jewish Hospital/Washington University in St. Louis, Saint Louis, MO, USA
e-mail: skelleyn@wudosis.wustl.edu

M.V. Smith, MD, MSc
Department of Orthopaedics, Washington University in St. Louis, Saint Louis, MO, USA

J.D. Kelly IV (ed.), *Elite Techniques in Shoulder Arthroscopy*,
DOI 10.1007/978-3-319-25103-5_2

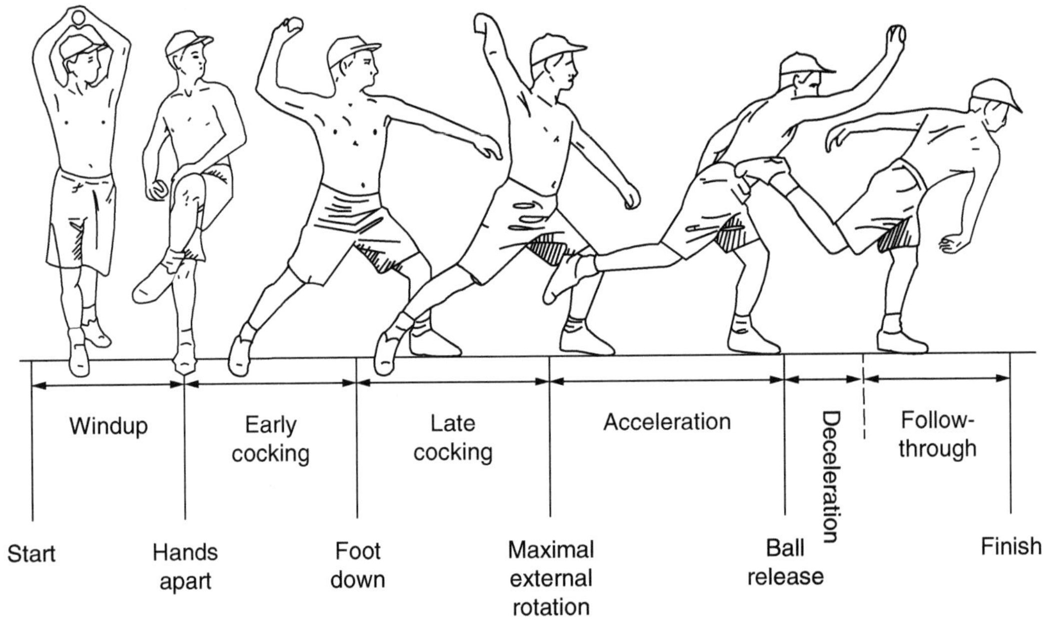

Fig. 2.1 This image demonstrates the five main phases of throwing: wind up, cocking, acceleration, deceleration, and follow-through. The stride phase is part of the lower body kinetic chain [Reprinted from DiGiovine NM, Jobe FW, Pink M, Perry J. An electromyographic analysis of the upper extremity in pitching. Journal of Shoulder and Elbow Surgery. 1992 1(1): 15–25, with permission from Elsevier]

Other areas to be inspected include lead leg internal hip rotation, lead leg quad tightness, and ankle range of motion. All "weak links" in the chain will lead to "downstream difficulties." The clinician must evaluate the *entire* kinetic chain to determine weak points that place the overhead throwing athlete at risk. Prompt care to address these abnormalities through muscle training, stretching, and improved throwing mechanics is necessary to prevent kinetic chain abnormalities that could result in shoulder injury [12].

Shoulder Mechanics

The elite overhead athlete can produce shoulder internal rotation velocity of 7000° per second. This is the fastest recorded motion by a human [1, 2]. This maximum velocity is achieved when the athlete externally rotates the arm to the maximal point of external rotation or the "set point." Seasoned athletes can obtain >130° of hyper-external rotation during the late cocking phase of throwing (Fig. 2.2). To achieve this amount of external rotation, adaptive changes in the glenohumeral mechanics are necessary. In abduction and external rotation, the inferior humeral articular surface rotates putting the anteroinferior shoulder capsule on tension. During the follow-through phase, the distraction force on the shoulder approaches 750 N or about 80 % of the pitcher's body weight [1, 4, 13]. As a result, the posterior capsular tissue hypertrophies and tightens to adapt to these high distraction forces in order to help decelerate the arm. Over time, tightness in the posterior capsule shifts the center of rotation more posterosuperior on the glenoid so that the greater tuberosity does not impinge on the posterior glenoid (Fig. 2.3). The altered center of rotation relieves tension off the anteroinferior capsule resulting in a functional "pseudolaxity" of the anterior shoulder [12]. Pseudolaxity in the anterior shoulder can also be a result of a disruption in the labral ring surrounding the glenoid. If the labrum becomes detached posteriorly, the humerus can displace to this detached area due to the loss of labral restraint. This results in pseudolaxity on the opposite (anterior) side of the detachment.

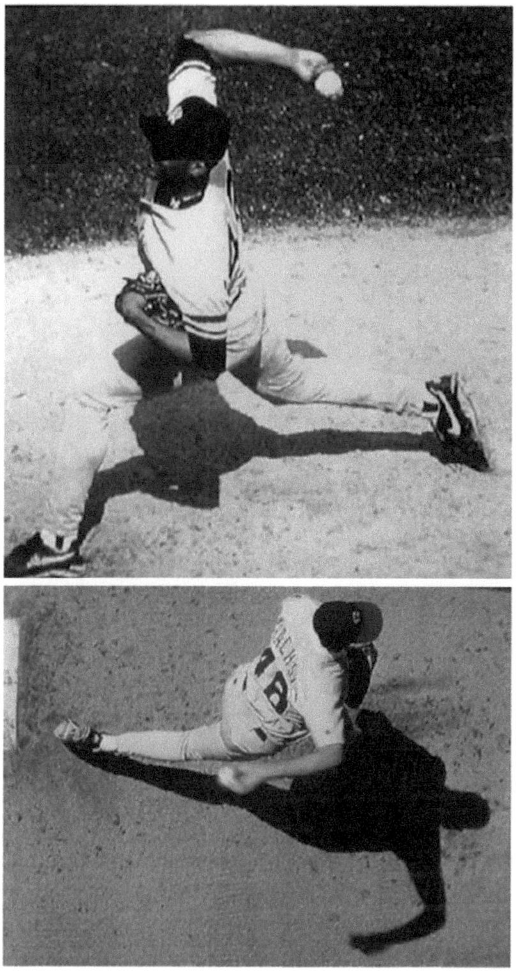

Fig. 2.2 This image demonstrates a baseball pitcher at the point of maximal external rotation or "set point" during a pitch. Notice the position of the legs and torso as elements of the kinetic chain [Reprinted from Burkhart SS, Morgan CD, Kibler WB. The disabled throwing shoulder: spectrum of pathology part I: pathoanatomy and biomechanics. Arthroscopy: The Journal of Arthroscopic & Related Surgery. 2003; 19(4): 404–420, with permission from Elsevier]

The cocking phase of the throwing motion is separated into an early stage and late stage. During the early stage, the deltoid muscle is activated and begins to place the arm and hand in the throwing position. During late cocking, the supraspinatus, infraspinatus, and teres minor are all activated to place the arm in abduction and external rotation. At this time the lower body begins shifting forward. This allows energy from the ground to be transferred through the athlete's kinetic chain resulting in a greater end force at the throwing hand [1, 2]. At the end of the late cocking phase, the shoulder reaches the "set point" [10, 12].

During the early acceleration phase, the triceps, pectoralis major, latissimus dorsi, and serratus anterior fire to maximize the energy in the kinetic chain. The deceleration phase has a high torque point as all muscles eccentrically contract to slow down the arm motion [1]. At this point, the center of gravity has shifted over the forwardly planted foot channeling the energy of the kinetic chain in the lower body. Finally, in the follow-through phase, the body rebalances forward motion, while the muscles return to a resting state.

Pathomechanics of Labral and Rotator Cuff Injury

Throwers with shoulder injury commonly describe the feeling of a "dead arm." A "dead arm" is any pathologic shoulder condition in which the thrower is unable to throw with preinjury velocity and control because of a combination of pain and subjective unease in the shoulder [7, 12]. The throwing arm is prone to injury because it requires greater abduction and external rotation to perform athletic activities compared to a non-throwing arm. Several authors have hypothesized that this greater range of motion is a result of "micro-trauma" or "micro-instability" to the anterior capsule [14]. Halbrecht studied the biomechanics of the shoulder and determined that anterior instability is not part of the pathology in the dead arm [15]. Other studies have similarly demonstrated that labral lesions are more commonly associated with dead arm syndrome instead of micro-trauma or micro-instability [12, 16].

Andrews is credited with first describing superior labral injuries. Snyder et al. further characterized SLAP injuries [17, 18]. Type II SLAP tears are defined as superior labral and biceps anchor detachment from the supraglenoid tubercle. Type II SLAP tears are common in throwing

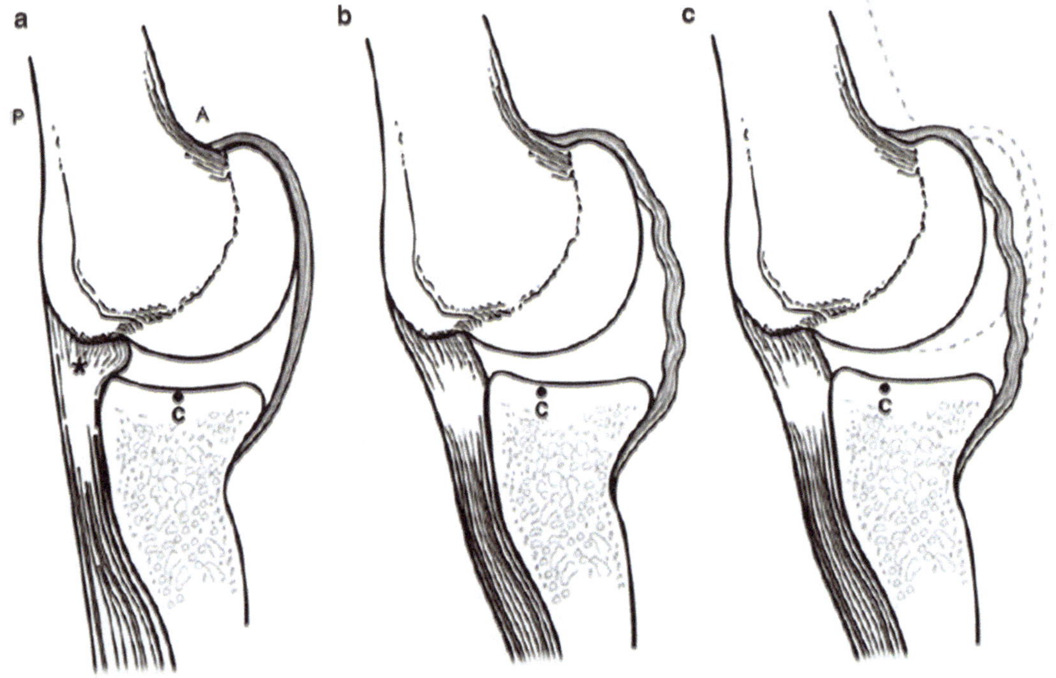

Fig. 2.3 (**a**) Normal orientation of the glenohumeral joint leads to rotator cuff impingement. (**b**) With tightening of the posterior inferior glenohumeral ligament, the humeral head moves posterior-superior and results in loss of the anterior capsule tension and a decreased cam impingement of the greater tuberosity on the posterior glenoid. This results in an anterior pseudolaxity. (**c**) Demonstrates the superimposed humeral head positions [Reprinted from Burkhart SS, Morgan CD, Kibler WB. The disabled throwing shoulder: spectrum of pathology part I: pathoanatomy and biomechanics. Arthroscopy: The Journal of Arthroscopic & Related Surgery. 2003; 19(4): 404–420, with permission from Elsevier]

athletes, particularly tears involving the posterosuperior region (Fig. 2.4) [19]. Type II SLAP repairs comprise approximately 10 % of all shoulder procedures and are the second most common shoulder arthroscopic surgery [20, 21]. The pathomechanics of labral injury are a complex interplay between activity demands and anatomy [12]. O'Brien described the inferior glenohumeral ligament (IGHL) as a two cable system [22]. Usually, the anterior and posterior cables support the humeral head like a sling while in abduction; however, if the posterior cable becomes contracted, from hypertrophy related to repetitive throwing, it can shorten and push the humeral head superiorly [23]. The hypertrophied tight posteroinferior capsule is the initial insult that shifts the humeral head allowing for hyper-external rotation, perceived pseudolaxity,

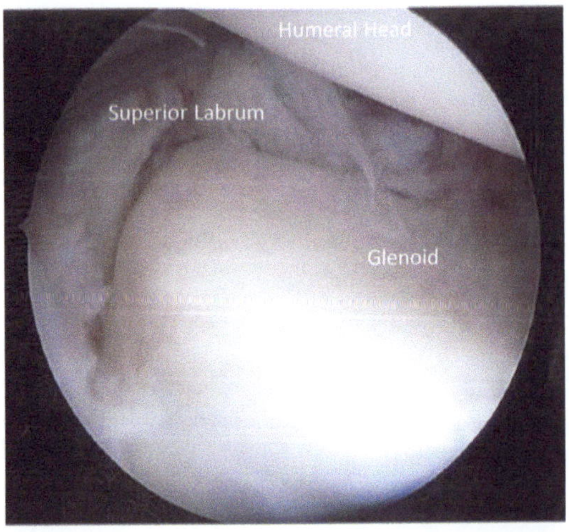

Fig. 2.4 Arthroscopic image demonstrating labral detachment from the glenoid. This disruption can allow for humeral displacement resulting in pseudolaxity on the opposite region of the glenoid

and greater ease obtaining the set point. This improved throwing mechanism is not without consequences. During the throwing motion, hyper-external rotation leads to abnormal impingement and abrasion damage to the rotator cuff [16]. The hyper-external rotation changes the vector force of the biceps tendon to a more vertical and posterior direction during abduction and external rotation [7, 12]. This vector and subsequent biceps muscle contraction create a torsional force across the posterior-superior labrum (Fig. 2.5). Abnormal twisting through the biceps origin on the glenoid leads to torsional overload and shear force injury to the labrum and rotator cuff fibers [16]. The labrum is eventually detached from its anchor as a result of this posterior-superior shift and hyper-external rotation: a "peel-back" phenomenon results.

Although Andrews et al. proposed that superior labral injuries are the result of longitudinal pull on the biceps anchor during the deceleration of the arm, others have proposed that hyper-twisting may be the mechanism causing labral injury [8, 12]. Kuhn performed a biomechanical study that supported the hyper-twisting in the acceleration phase as the mechanism recreating a labral injury [24]. This implies the biceps and superior labrum complex is "peeled off" instead of "pulled" from bone in the deceleration phase [12].

Approximately, one third of all patients with SLAP tears also have rotator cuff tears [20]. Given this association, Walch and Jobe described internal impingement as abduction and external rotation inducing a pinched posterosuperior rotator cuff between the glenoid labrum and greater tuberosity of the humerus [14, 25]. Impingement in this area may also explain the partial articular-sided rotator cuff tears commonly seen in throwing athletes. Morgan et al. reviewed arthroscopic exams and found that rotator cuff tears were also found in 31 % of throwers being treated for SLAP lesions [19]. Of these tears, 38 % were full thickness tears located in the midportion of the rotator crescent, and 62 % were partial-thickness cuff tears in labral lesion-specific anatomic locations. The superior subluxation of the humerus combined with repetitive torsional loading from hyper-external rotation has been postulated as the cause for location-specific partial-thickness cuff tears [12]. The combination of labral pathology and rotator cuff tears is a complicated multifactorial process that ultimately results in loss of shoulder function and/or athletic performance.

Burkhart et al. consolidated these factors in the development of the dead arm which have

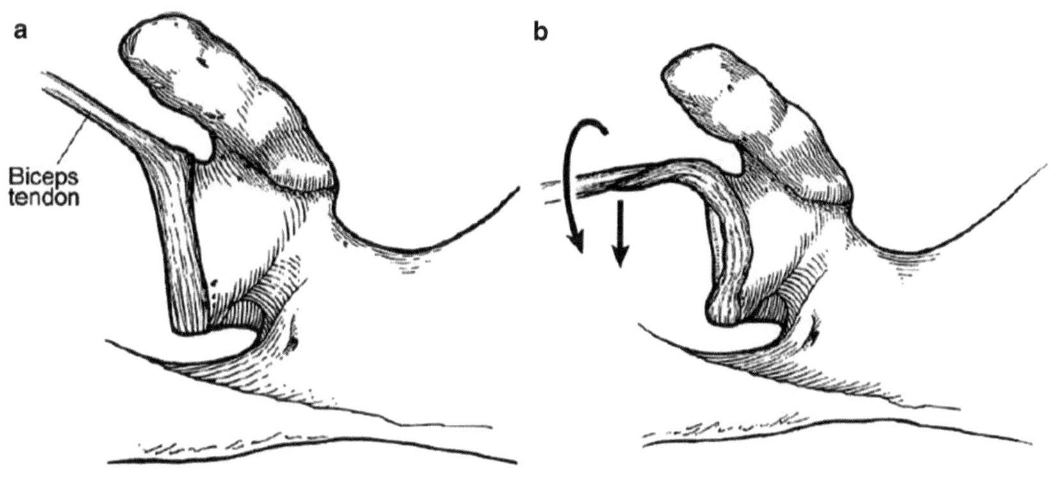

Fig. 2.5 The position of maximal external rotation results in a vector change for the biceps tendon. During overhead movement, the altered vector creates a peel-back mechanism as the biceps pulls on the labral complex [Reprinted from Burkhart SS, Morgan CD, Kibler WB. The disabled throwing shoulder: spectrum of pathology part I: pathoanatomy and biomechanics. Arthroscopy: The Journal of Arthroscopic & Related Surgery. 2003; 19(4): 404–420, with permission from Elsevier]

been supported in the literature: (1) the tight posteroinferior capsule leading to glenohumeral internal rotation deficit and a shift in the glenohumeral rotation point; (2) peel-back forces causing the SLAP injury; (3) hyper-external rotation of the humerus related to a reduction in the humeral cam effect on the anterior capsule and clearance of the greater tuberosity over the glenoid rim through a larger arc of external rotation; and (4) scapular protraction. The ultimate culprit in this series of injuries is the tight posteroinferior capsule [7, 12, 16]. Shoulder strengthening may be the best preventative measure for compensating for damaging forces in overhead activities and therefore prevent the development of shoulder pathology [16].

Glenohumeral Internal Rotation Deficient

Scapular positioning and glenohumeral rotation are key components of shoulder function. Glenohumeral internal rotation is especially important to the overhead athlete as a source of force generation. The total rotational range of motion (TROM) of the shoulder is a combination of glenohumeral internal rotation and glenohumeral external rotation with the arm abducted [6]. Maintaining the shoulder total arc of motion is important to protect the shoulder during throwing. Asymmetry of as little as 5° of TROM between shoulders is associated with increased shoulder injury risk [26]. Although studies have demonstrated a high risk of injury with a glenohumeral internal rotational deficit of 11° compared to the contralateral arm [26], most clinicians consider a glenohumeral internal rotation of 18° or greater to be diagnostic of significant glenohumeral internal rotation deficit (GIRD) (Fig. 2.6) [16, 27].

Conditioned throwers develop limitations in internal rotation from posteroinferior capsular contracture. This contracture can lead to GIRD. Prophylactic posteroinferior capsular stretching can minimize GIRD and therefore secondary pain and intra-articular symptoms [6, 12]. The sleeper stretch and cross-body stretch used

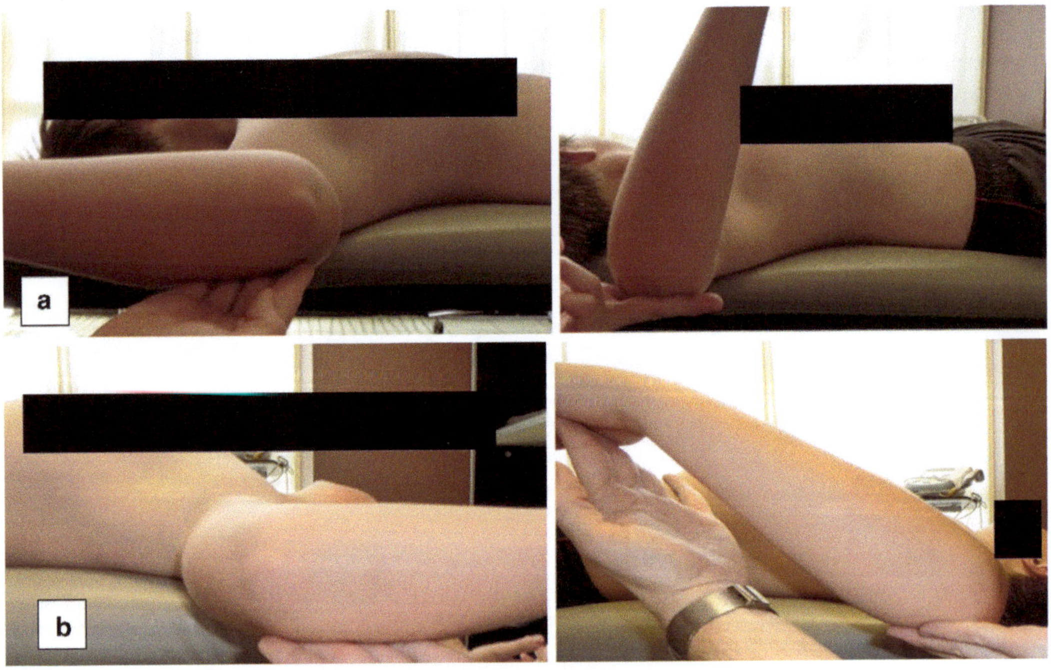

Fig. 2.6 This patient has internal rotation deficit between shoulders. (**a**) Dominant arm external rotation and internal rotation at 90° of abduction. (**b**) Nondominant arm external rotation and internal rotation at 90° of abduction

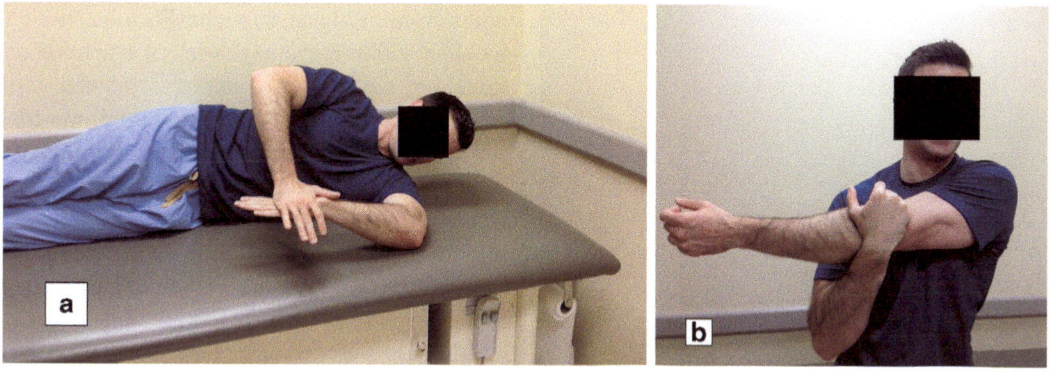

Fig. 2.7 The sleeper stretch is one of the most effective methods of stretching the posterior inferior capsule. (**a**) The athlete applies a passive internal rotation force to the abducted shoulder while lying on the side. (**b**) The cross-body stretch is also utilized to stretch the posterior capsule and shoulder musculature

over a 2-week period can frequently improve ROM to 20° or less (Fig. 2.7) [12]. The sleeper stretch is performed in a lateral decubitus position with the back against a wall to stabilize scapular motion. The shoulder is flexed to 90° and passive internal rotation is exerted by the opposite arm to stretch the posterior shoulder. The cross-body stretch is performed in a standing position by placing the non-stretched arm on the distal humerus just proximal to the elbow and passively pulling the arm across the chest. In rare cases of persistent posterior capsular tightness after a prolonged stretching program, arthroscopic release of the posteroinferior capsule followed by a stretching program can improve motion.

Scapular Dyskinesis

Scapular dyskinesis is any alteration in the normal position or motion of the scapula. The dyskinesis can be related to inflexibility, weakness, muscle activation imbalance, or a combination of these variables. The SICK scapula syndrome is a general term used to describe these presenting findings in an athlete with shoulder pain. SICK scapula syndrome is defined as scapular malposition, inferior medial border prominence, coracoid pain and malposition, and dyskinesis of scapular movement.

The thrower with SICK scapular syndrome frequently has an insidious onset of anterior shoulder pain and eventually notes a "dropped" scapula. The dropped orientation comes from anterior tilting and protraction of the scapula which also enables the pectoralis minor to contact. The coracoid is often tender to palpation and correlates with the presenting anterior shoulder pain [12]. The key finding is asymmetric scapular malposition, usually lower positioning in the dominant throwing shoulder. The associated pain should not be confused with anterior shoulder instability or a SLAP tear. Overhead athletes with existing or impending labral or rotator cuff injuries commonly note resting pain, particularly anteriorly over the coracoid. They also report pain during the late cocking and/or early acceleration phases of throwing.

Burkhart et al. have described three types of angular deformities that can be statically measured to quantify the level of scapular dyskinesis [6]. The type I is inferomedial scapular border prominence associated with pectoralis major and minor inflexibility and trapezius and serratus anterior weakness. The type II pattern demonstrates medial winging related to trapezius and rhomboid weakness (Fig. 2.8). Both conditions protract the scapular and decrease cocking ability of the shoulder. Posterosuperior labral lesions are associated with these two types of scapular dyskinesis. Type III scapular dyskinesis is associated with impingement symptoms and with rotator cuff pathology rather than labral lesions. In type III scapular dyskinesis, the superomedial border of the scapula becomes more prominent.

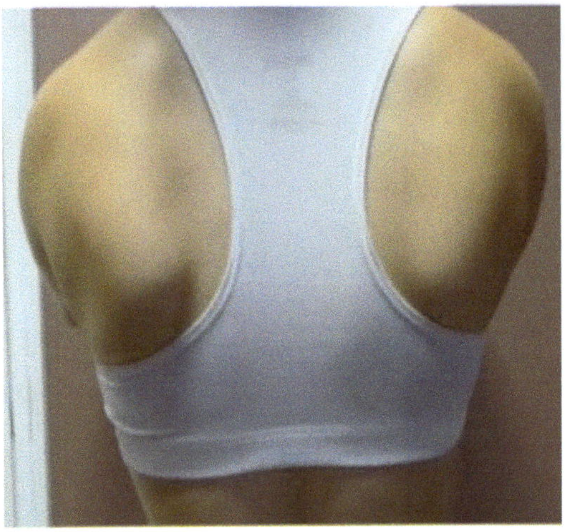

Fig. 2.8 This patient is lowering her arms from a forwardly elevated position. She has a left side type I SICK scapula with inferomedial scapular prominence from tight pectoral muscles and weak triceps and serratus anterior muscles

To appreciate the etiology of the SICK scapula, one must appreciate that the scapula is a flat bone gliding and pivoting about the ellipsoid surface of the thoracic cavity. When the scapula protracts, tilts anteriorly, and moves into abduction, it is essentially riding up and over the thorax [28]. This maneuver tilts the coracoid anteroinferiorly and moves it lateral to the midline. This heightened protraction potentiates contracture of the short head of the biceps and pectoralis minor. As the muscles tighten, they increase the static malposition and anterior tilting of the scapula. Additionally, a tight posterior shoulder capsule can exacerbate scapular malposition as the scapula is pulled anteriorly during the follow-through phase of the throwing motion.

Patients with SICK syndrome typically have difficulty performing complete forward flexion given the scapular protraction. The examiner can perform the scapular retraction test to evaluate for scapular dyskinesis. In this test, the examiner manually repositions the scapula in a retracted position allowing full forward flexion without pain. This maneuver is diagnostic for SICK scapula syndrome [6]. Treatment of throwing athletes with SICK scapular syndrome and scapular dyskinesis starts with a period of active rest and cessation from overhead activities. Focused anterior shoulder girdle stretching, with an emphasis on stretching the pectoralis minor, combined with posterior capsular stretching is started immediately. An isometric strengthening program is started for the posterior scapular muscles initially. As scapular control improves, a progressive strengthening program with closed chain isotonic exercises is initiated and lastly open chain isotonics. The goal is to restore scapular positioning and decrease pain with activities. This nonoperative treatment is typically successful after 2–3 weeks [6, 12]. The throwing athlete should be encouraged to continue these strengthening and stretching exercises to prevent recurrence of pain.

The "shoulder at risk" is an asymptomatic shoulder that demonstrates signs of GIRD, malpositioning of the scapula (SICK), or both conditions. The kinetic chain must be inspected with vigilance as something as seemingly trivial as an ankle sprain may translate to increased demand (and injury) in distal segments.

Early recognition of these conditions is crucial to prevent the natural course of pathology and avoid surgery.

References

1. Dillman CJ, Fleisig GS, Andrews JR. Biomechanics of pitching with emphasis upon shoulder kinematics. J Orthop Sports Phys Ther. 1993;18:402–8. doi:10.2519/jospt.1993.18.2.402.
2. Dun S, Kingsley D, Fleisig GS, et al. Biomechanical comparison of the fastball from wind-up and the fastball from stretch in professional baseball pitchers. Am J Sports Med. 2008;36:137–41. doi:10.1177/0363546507308938.
3. Kennedy DJ, Visco CJ, Press J. Current concepts for shoulder training in the overhead athlete. Curr Sports Med Rep. 2009;8:154–60. doi:10.1249/JSR.0b013e3181a64607.
4. Fleisig GS, Andrews JR, Dillman CJ, Escamilla RF. Kinetics of baseball pitching with implications about injury mechanisms. Am J Sports Med. 1995;23:233–9. doi:10.1177/036354659502300218.
5. Toyoshima S, Miyashita M. Force-velocity relation in throwing. Res Q. 1973;44:86–95.
6. Burkhart SS, Morgan CD, Kibler WB. The disabled throwing shoulder: spectrum of pathology. Part III: The SICK scapula, scapular dyskinesis, the kinetic

chain, and rehabilitation. Arthrosc J Arthrosc Relat Surg. 2003;19:641–61.

7. Burkhart SS, Morgan CD, Kibler WB. Shoulder injuries in overhead athletes. The "dead arm" revisited. Clin Sports Med. 2000;19:125–58.
8. Kibler WB, Press J, Sciascia A. The role of core stability in athletic function. Sports Med Auckl NZ. 2006;36:189–98.
9. Crossley KM, Zhang W-J, Schache AG, et al. Performance on the single-leg squat task indicates hip abductor muscle function. Am J Sports Med. 2011;39:866–73. doi:10.1177/0363546510395456.
10. Kibler WB. Biomechanical analysis of the shoulder during tennis activities. Clin Sports Med. 1995;14:79–85.
11. Kageyama M, Sugiyama T, Takai Y, Kanehisa H, Maeda A. Kinematic and kinetic profiles of trunk and lower limbs during baseball pitching in collegiate pitchers. J Sports Sci Med. 2014;13(4):742–50.
12. Burkhart SS, Morgan CD, Kibler WB. The disabled throwing shoulder: spectrum of pathology. Part I: Pathoanatomy and biomechanics. Arthrosc J Arthrosc Relat Surg. 2003;19:404–20. doi:10.1053/jars.2003.50128.
13. Levitz CL, Dugas J, Andrews JR. The use of arthroscopic thermal capsulorrhaphy to treat internal impingement in baseball players. Arthrosc J Arthrosc Relat Surg. 2001;17:573–7. doi:10.1053/jars.2001.24853.
14. Jobe CM. Posterior superior glenoid impingement: expanded spectrum. Arthrosc J Arthrosc Relat Surg. 1995;11:530–6.
15. Halbrecht JL, Tirman P, Atkin D. Internal impingement of the shoulder: comparison of findings between the throwing and nonthrowing shoulders of college baseball players. Arthrosc J Arthrosc Relat Surg. 1999;15:253–8.
16. Kibler WB, Kuhn JE, Wilk K, et al. The disabled throwing shoulder: spectrum of pathology-10-year update. Arthrosc J Arthrosc Relat Surg. 2013;29:141–61.e26. doi:10.1016/j.arthro.2012.10.009.
17. Andrews JR, Carson Jr WG, McLeod WD. Glenoid labrum tears related to the long head of the biceps. Am J Sports Med. 1985;13:337–41.
18. Snyder SJ, Karzel RP, Pizzo WD, et al. SLAP lesions of the shoulder. Arthrosc J Arthrosc Relat Surg. 1990;6:274–9. doi:10.1016/0749-8063(90)90056-J.
19. Morgan CD, Burkhart SS, Palmeri M, Gillespie M. Type II SLAP lesions: three subtypes and their relationships to superior instability and rotator cuff tears. Arthrosc J Arthrosc Relat Surg. 1998;14:553–65.
20. Weber SC, Martin DF, Seiler III JG, Harrast JJ. Superior labrum anterior and posterior lesions of the shoulder: incidence rates, complications, and outcomes as reported by American Board of Orthopedic Surgery. Part II candidates. Am J Sports Med. 2012;40:1538–43. doi:10.1177/0363546512447785.
21. Onyekwelu I, Khatib O, Zuckerman JD, et al. The rising incidence of arthroscopic superior labrum anterior and posterior (SLAP) repairs. J Shoulder Elbow Surg Am Shoulder Elbow Surg Al. 2012;21:728–31. doi:10.1016/j.jse.2012.02.001.
22. O'Brien SJ, Neves MC, Arnoczky SP, et al. The anatomy and histology of the inferior glenohumeral ligament complex of the shoulder. Am J Sports Med. 1990;18:449–56.
23. Clabbers KM, Kelly JD, Bader D, et al. Effect of posterior capsule tightness on glenohumeral translation in the late-cocking phase of pitching. J Sport Rehabil. 2007;16:41–9.
24. Kuhn JE, Lindholm SR, Huston LJ, et al. Failure of the biceps superior labral complex: a cadaveric biomechanical investigation comparing the late cocking and early deceleration positions of throwing. Arthrosc J Arthrosc Relat Surg. 2003;19:373–9. doi:10.1053/jars.2003.50044.
25. Walch G, Boileau P, Noel E, Donell ST. Impingement of the deep surface of the supraspinatus tendon on the posterosuperior glenoid rim: an arthroscopic study. J Shoulder Elbow Surg Am Shoulder Elbow Surg Al. 1992;1:238–45. doi:10.1016/S1058-2746(09)80065-7.
26. Wilk KE, Macrina LC, Fleisig GS, et al. Correlation of glenohumeral internal rotation deficit and total rotational motion to shoulder injuries in professional baseball pitchers. Am J Sports Med. 2011;39:329–35. doi:10.1177/0363546510384223.
27. Myers JB, Laudner KG, Pasquale MR, et al. Glenohumeral range of motion deficits and posterior shoulder tightness in throwers with pathologic internal impingement. Am J Sports Med. 2006;34:385–91. doi:10.1177/0363546505281804.
28. Matsuki K, Matsuki KO, Yamaguchi S, et al. Dynamic in vivo glenohumeral kinematics during scapular plane abduction in healthy shoulders. J Orthop Sports Phys Ther. 2012;42:96–104. doi:10.2519/jospt.2012.3584.

Keys to Successful Labral Repair

3

Dinesh Dhanaraj, Nicole S. Belkin, Miltiadis H. Zgonis, and Brian J. Sennett

Introduction

Injuries to the glenoid labrum are commonly encountered when caring for the overhead athlete [1]. Tensile forces produced during the phases of throwing predispose the superior labrum to damage and the resulting pathology is a common cause of recurrent pain and disability [2]. These injuries may prevent the overhead athlete from competing if not properly recognized and treated. Techniques in labral repair have evolved greatly with the emergence of new technology. Understanding the basic tenets of labral repair will greatly aid the surgeon when working with any subset of throwing athletes.

Evaluation and Diagnosis

Although there are several different mechanisms that cause injury to the superior labral complex, overhead athletes often have a history of pain during a throwing event. These patients may describe the "dead arm" phenomenon, which consists of acute pain with overhead activity and decreased velocity and strength during throwing [3]. Other patients may have a more gradual onset of pain, which points to a more repetitive mechanism. They may also describe the pain as anterior or superior and may have symptoms of clicking or popping within the shoulder.

The term SLAP tears (superior labrum anterior to posterior) was first coined by Snyder and colleagues in 1990 [4]. Since then, many physical exam tests have been described to diagnose SLAP tears, but no consensus currently exists on what is the single most reliable method for detecting these lesions. Most tests consist of placing stress upon the superior labral-biceps complex to elicit pain and recreate symptoms [5]. One of the more widely used is the O'Brien's active compression test [6]. This test recreates symptoms by having the patient elevate an adducted and pronated arm against resistance and then repeating the test in supination. If pain is felt in the pronated position and relieved in the supinated position, the test is said to be positive for a tear of the superior labrum. The Yergason's and Speed's tests place traction on the biceps anchor and, although nonspecific for labral pathology, are often positive in patients with SLAP lesions. In addition, the dynamic labral shear test (DLST) has also been recently described as a very effective maneuver for identifying these lesions and is the senior author's preference [7, 8].

D. Dhanaraj, MD, MSPH (✉)
Department of Orthopaedic Surgery, Princeton HealthCare System, Plainsboro, NJ, USA
e-mail: ddhanaraj@pbnj.com

N.S. Belkin, MD
Department of Orthopaedic Surgery, Hospital of the University of Pennsylvania, Philadelphia, PA, USA

M.H. Zgonis, MD • B.J. Sennett, MD
Department of Orthopaedic Surgery and Sports Medicine, University of Pennsylvania, Philadelphia, PA, USA

Penn Sports Medicine Center, Philadelphia, PA, USA

J.D. Kelly IV (ed.), *Elite Techniques in Shoulder Arthroscopy*,
DOI 10.1007/978-3-319-25103-5_3

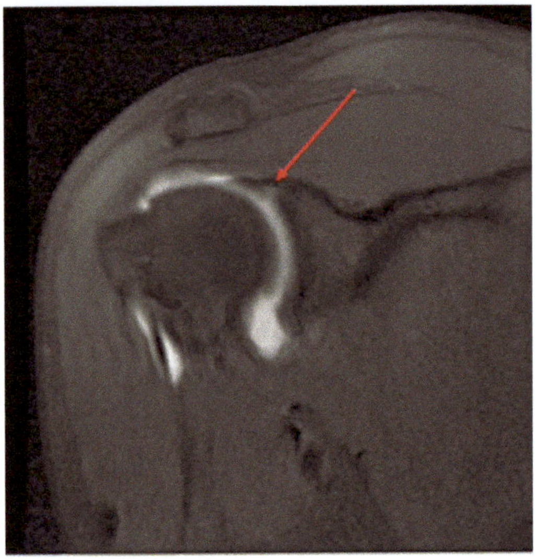

Fig. 3.1 Coronal T2 MRI showing SLAP tear in a 14 year old male [Courtesy of Dr. James L. Carey MD, MPH]

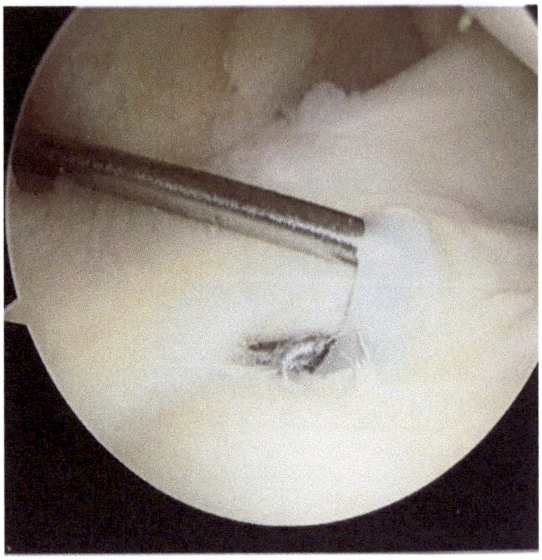

Fig. 3.2 Sublabral foramen

In regard to imaging, MRI remains the gold standard and the addition of gadolinium contrast has been shown to increase the accuracy of diagnosing these lesions [9] (Fig. 3.1).

Special Considerations

The rising incidence of superior labrum repairs as a trend has made selection of the appropriate surgical candidate equally as important as repairing the tear itself. Aside from patients with a history of trauma, most true SLAP tears are found in the dominant arm of overhead athletes who are under 40 years of age [2]. Beyond the age of 40, natural degeneration of the labrum occurs and operating in this setting may not have a beneficial effect [10]. This trend of minimizing surgical intervention for isolated SLAP tears may apply to even younger patients as well [11].

In addition to identifying proper surgical candidates, the surgeon must be aware of anatomic variations that can mimic detachment of the labrum on imaging studies and during arthroscopy. Variants, such as a meniscoid-type labrum, sublabral foramen (Fig. 3.2), or a cord-like middle glenohumeral ligament (Buford complex) [12], can often be confused for labral pathology. The surgeon must be familiar with these variations in order to avoid performing unnecessary interventions that may cause further disability.

Access to Pathology

Advancement in arthroscopic techniques and technologies has contributed significantly to the innovations made in the treatment of glenoid labrum pathology [13]. During arthroscopy, the patient may be positioned in either the lateral decubitus or beach-chair position to facilitate access. Each position offers a combination of advantages, disadvantages, and relative risks although the senior author prefers the lateral decubitus position for overall access.

The lateral decubitus position was the initially described technique for arthroscopic access to the glenohumeral joint. With the patient secured laterally, the arm can be positioned in space with variable degrees of traction and abduction via the assistance of a series of pulleys and weights. This technique facilitates access to the periphery of the glenohumeral joint without requiring an assistant to position the arm. It must be kept in mind that when utilizing traction, transient neuropraxias have been described as a complication in up to 10 % of patients in some series [14].

The beach-chair position was first described in 1988 by Skyhar in an attempt to avoid neuropathies that had been described with the lateral decubitus positioning. The patient is placed supine on an adjustable table allowing for flexion of the hips and knees and erection of the thorax [15]. Additional proposed advantages of this position include decreased surgical time, decreased risk to neurovascular structures during portal placement, and easier conversion to open procedures [16, 17]. A disadvantage of this position is the combination of the physiologic challenges to the maintenance of cerebral perfusion pressure by positioning the head above the heart combined with anesthetic-induced impedance of the sympathetic nervous system [18]. Hypotensive anesthesia has been described as a safe and effective method for minimizing blood loss during orthopedic procedures. An advantage this technique provides to arthroscopic shoulder surgery is to allow for a more bloodless surgical field optimizing visualization [19]. Additionally, arthroscopic pump pressure may be adjusted to minimize bleeding in the surgical field, but care must be taken to avoid fluid extravasation into the adjacent soft tissues which can occur with excessive pump pressure [20, 21].

Additional techniques to enhance arthroscopic visualization within the glenohumeral joint include the addition of epinephrine to the arthroscopic fluid, the utilization of electrocautery devices, and the 70° arthroscope for alternative viewing angles [22, 23].

There are a multitude of arthroscopic portal options about the shoulder. The underlying principles of the location and utilization of these include knowledge of and protection of the surrounding neurovascular structures at risk, most notably the axillary nerve, the suprascapular nerve and artery, and cephalic vein [24]. We will focus our discussion on the most relevant arthroscopic portals. The posterior portal is the safest and most commonly used portal to provide visualization of the entire joint. It is located 2–3 cm inferior to and 1–2 cm medial to the posterolateral acromion [25]. Locating it slightly lower and more lateral may provide a better trajectory for visualization for labral repairs. The anterior central portal is an essential anterior working portal in almost all arthroscopic procedures. It is located within the rotator interval, 1–2 cm inferomedial to the anterolateral acromion (Fig. 3.3). Inside-out as well as outside-in techniques have been described for the safe creation of this portal [26]. The anterolateral portal can provide an advantageous trajectory for anchor placement for SLAP repair as well as enhancing visualization of posterior lesions. This portal is made at the anterolateral corner of the acromion, entering the joint just anterior to the biceps tendon. Using a spinal needle, this portal is created with an outside-in technique. The trocar is then angulated toward the superior glenoid passing anterior to the biceps tendon. Instrumentation introduced through this portal is often combined with visualization through an anteroinferior portal, which can be formed via inside-out technique by pushing a switching stick through the anterior capsule just superior to the upper border of the subscapularis tendon. To accomplish this, the camera itself should first be driven forward from the posterior portal to the desired location along the anterior capsule until it is slightly distended. The camera is then removed,

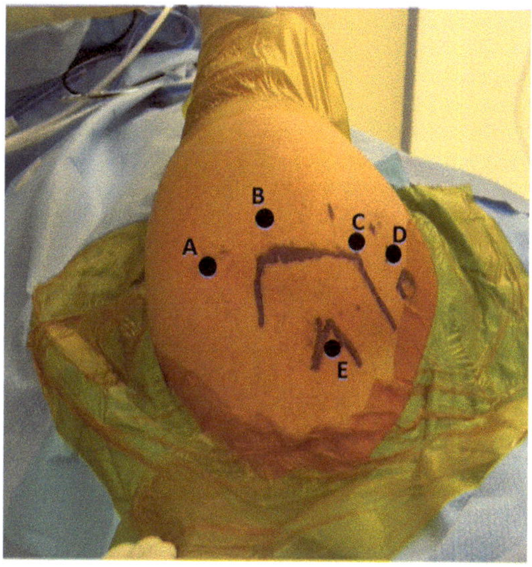

Fig. 3.3 Arthroscopic portal placement in a left shoulder. (A) Posterior portal. (B) Portal of Wilmington. (C) Anterolateral portal. (D) Anterior central portal. (E) Neviaser's portal

while the trocar is carefully held in place against the capsule. The switching stick is then introduced through the trocar to create the inside-out portal over the switching stick. The camera is then reintroduced through the trocar in the posterior portal. This combination of portals allows for ease of surgical triangulation [27]. Neviaser's portal can be created in the soft spot between the clavicle, acromion, and scapular spine. This portal provides access to the most superior aspect of the glenoid. It is important to respect the proximity of the suprascapular nerve and artery during the creation of this portal, as they are located only 3 cm medial to the supraglenoid tubercle [28, 29]. The portal of Wilmington is located 1 cm anterior and 1 cm lateral to the posterolateral edge of the acromion, passing medial to the musculotendinous junction of the rotator cuff in a vector directed toward the coracoid tip. This portal is very useful in posterior superior SLAP repairs, as it allows for anchors to be placed at a 45° angle to the glenoid surface [30].

Obtaining quality access to the pathology through meticulous surgical planning and execution of arthroscopic techniques with care taken to respect the surrounding relevant anatomy is a critical element necessary for treatment of labral pathology.

Treatment: Keys to Success

Surgical intervention is indicated in patients who have failed nonoperative methods of treatment. Successful labral repair is largely dependent upon recognition of the type of lesion and the proper choice of treatment. Actual repair of the labrum (versus debridement or biceps tenotomy) is indicated with certain types of labral pathology (e.g., type II SLAP). The remainder of this section will focus on technical tips and pearls regarding this approach.

The initial approach to superior labral repair should begin with a diagnostic arthroscopy of the shoulder. The joint should be accessed initially through the posterior portal. Normal anatomic structures should be identified and assessed, along with inspection of the labrum. Peel-back and drive-through signs can be used as additional methods of evaluating the integrity of the labrum. An anterior portal should be established to allow for placement of a probe to fully investigate the labrum and attempt to displace the biceps root from its normal attachment. Again, only true labral separation accompanied by fissuring of the chondro-labral junction will qualify for a true type 2 lesion.

Once the diagnosis of labral pathology has been confirmed and repair is indicated, the next step is to mobilize the tissue and prepare the glenoid rim for reattachment. The goal is to free up the tissue so the labrum can be repaired in a relatively tension-free manner. An elevating tool can be used to liberate the tissues, but care must be taken not to actually cut the labrum, which can greatly complicate the procedure. The senior author prefers to prepare the glenoid from a contralateral portal. For example, a type 2 posterior SLAP tear will be accessed by viewing from the anterolateral portal and working from the straight anterior portal. A rasp, shaver, or thermal device can be used to prepare the glenoid bone and create a bleeding surface to enhance the biologic healing of the torn labrum. The use of a burr is discouraged as loss of bone material increases instability. Some surgeons advocate preparation up onto the articular surface to allow for more of a bumper effect, especially in cases of instability [31]. Recent studies by Yamamoto et al. have challenged this notion, however, stating that anchor fixation on the glenoid face does not increase the translational force as compared to placement on the glenoid rim [32].

Once the tissue is mobilized and the glenoid rim prepared, stabilization of the labrum can commence. Various methods of labrum repair exist and the senior author prefers absorbable knotted fixation for several reasons (Fig. 3.4). First, the superior labrum has a large degree of native mobility and should not be over-constrained (Fig. 3.5). Secondly rigid knots and even knotless fixation composed of newer generation suture and tapes have been implicated in causing chondral injury (Fig. 3.6). Lastly, knotted (absorbable) implants can better restore labral height

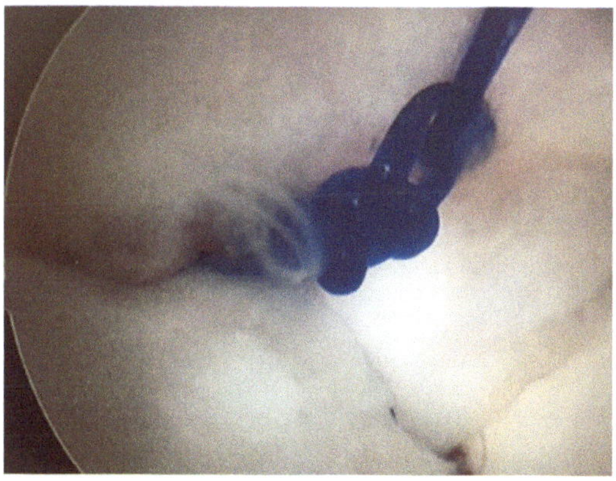

Fig. 3.4 PDS suture knot

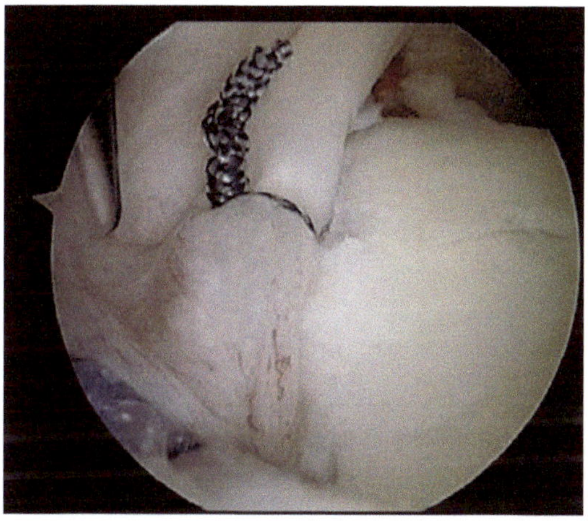

Fig. 3.5 Example of an over-constrained biceps ("hog-tied biceps")

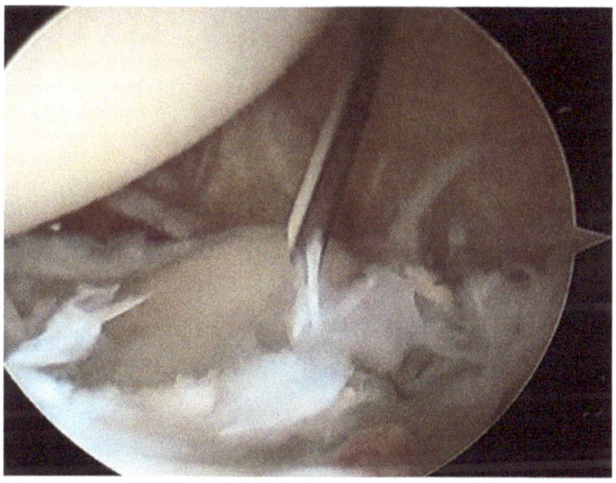

Fig. 3.6 Damage from rigid knots

which will translate to better inherent stability. Depending on the location of the lesion, additional portals or angles of approach may be needed. The ability to place suture and suture anchors percutaneously allows greater freedom that is not limited by cannula location. As mentioned before, a spinal needle is useful for establishing proper trajectory. Anchors should be placed at approximately a 45° angle to the glenoid surface to allow for sufficient bony purchase and to avoid inadvertently penetrating the articular surface. If utilizing a trans-rotator cuff portal (posterior and superior), it is wise to avoid placing a large cannula and, instead, simply insert the anchor percutaneously. Neviaser's portal may be very helpful for suture passage. The steep angle afforded by this location allows for a spinal needle to be placed directly through the cuff and capsule and underneath the superior labrum itself. Suture or wire can then be shuttled through in the appropriate site for a repair. There are many different options for suture passage instrumentation as well. Suture lassos, soft tissue penetrators, and suture shuttling devices are all options for labral repair and can be used based upon the individual surgeon's needs and preferences. The senior author prefers Neviaser's portal for posterior superior labral repairs since it is minimally invasive and facilitates suture passage *proximal* to the anchor. Proximal passage encourages the labral tissue to sit more firmly applied to the glenoid. Regardless, respect to the soft tissues and achieving the angle that works best remain the basic guiding principles. If arthroscopic knots are to be used, they should be placed away from the articular surface and against the soft tissue side of the repair to avoid abrasion of the chondral surface (Fig. 3.7). This can be achieved by making the peripheral suture limb the post when tying to ensure the knot faces away from the articular cartilage. A sliding knot or a series of half-hitches can be used depending upon the surgeon's preference (Figs. 3.8, 3.9 and 3.10).

Another challenge that may be faced is the patient with multifocal labral pathology. When tears of the superior labrum are encountered in combination with Bankart lesions or posterior

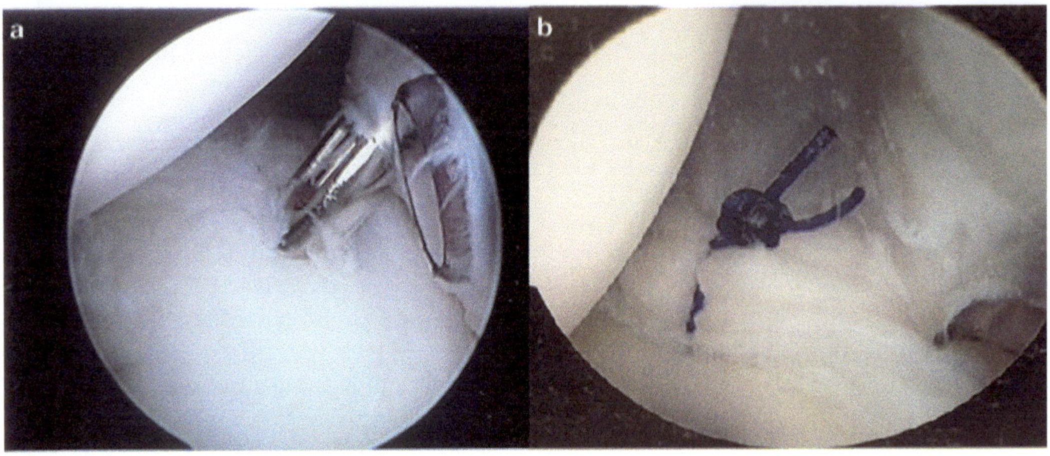

Fig. 3.7 Arthroscopic images showing percutaneous anchor placement (**a**) and fixation demonstrating absorbable knots away from articular surface (**b**)

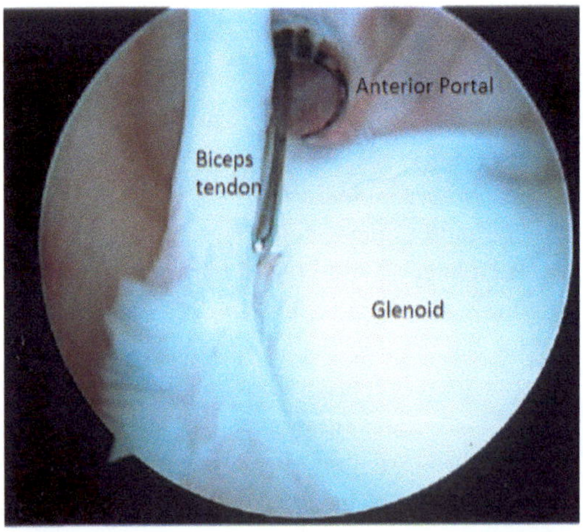

Fig. 3.8 View of the glenohumeral joint from the posterior portal (lateral decubitus position) [Courtesy of Dr. James L. Carey MD, MPH]

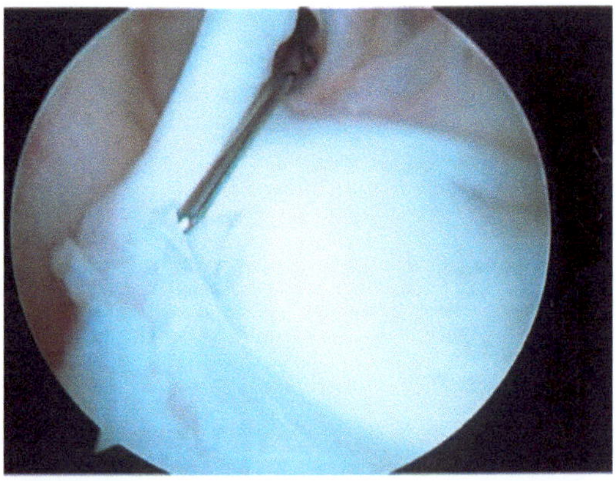

Fig. 3.9 Probe demonstrating separation of the superior labrum from the glenoid [Courtesy of Dr. James L. Carey MD, MPH]

labral tears, it is recommended to fix the superior labral tear last. This is because repair of the superior labrum will tighten up the joint somewhat, making it difficult to access the more inferior portions of the joint. However, the surgeon may consider passing the sutures in the superior labrum first, since the soft tissues in this portion of the joint tend to swell more readily and earlier than in the rest of the joint, making work here more difficult later on.

Understanding Anchor Types, Materials, Suture Options, and Insertion

Successful repair of the glenoid labrum, particularly in the arthroscopic setting, requires a thorough understanding of the glenoid rim anatomy. On average, the glenoid measures approximately 30 mm anterior to posterior and 42 mm in the superior to inferior direction. In general, the nar-

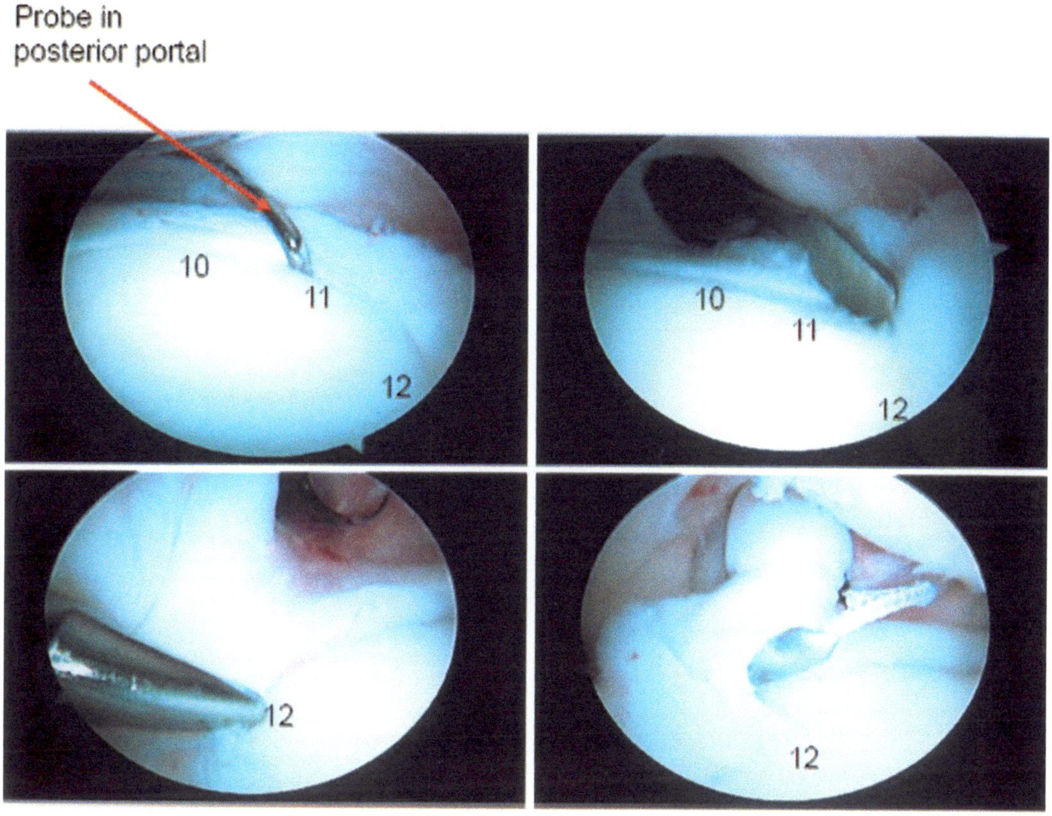

Fig. 3.10 View of the glenohumeral joint from the anterior portal. Steps showing preparation of the glenoid and labrum and suture passage [Courtesy of Dr. James L. Carey MD, MPH]

row glenoid rim can accommodate anchors with a maximal diameter of 4.1 mm [33]. Screw-in devices have been shown to provide the strongest fixation when inserted orthogonal to the glenoid rim at the point of insertion. This, however, does not specifically translate to the anterior-superior quadrant of the glenoid, which maintains its pull-out strength until anchor placement deviates greater than 20° from the orthogonal vector [34].

A multitude of suture anchor designs and materials are currently available. Biomechanical data is available for many of these devices produced over the last 20 years [35–37]. In general, anchors exist in permanent and resorbable forms and generate their purchase into the bone by interference fit. Metal anchors are very durable and their location can be easily determined radiographically but can create artifact on MRI imaging. Permanent polymers such as polyetheretherketone (PEEK) possess the benefits of permanence without negatively impacting the quality of MRI imaging. All permanent anchors also pose potential risk of becoming a permanent foreign body within the glenohumeral joint if they become dislodged or causing focal humeral head wear if they become prominent. The newest generation of permanent anchors is comprised entirely of suture material, which provides interference fixation within the bone by forming a cloverleaf shape when deployed. This has the benefits of creating smaller holes in the bone and posing no impediment to anchor placement in the revision setting. Bioabsorbable anchors such as poly-L-lactic acid (PLLA) possess the theoretical advantage of temporary existence with ultimate bone replacement, but problematic cyst formation around these devices has been described, albeit less than in the rotator cuff literature [38, 39].

Anchors are available with a wide variety of suture materials as well, including some with proprietary technology designed to prevent knot loosening. Knotless anchors are also available in which the suture is placed into the bone tunnel via an eyelet that leads the anchor device, thereby allowing for the suture to be secured in the desired amount of tension without knot placement. This technology eliminates the risk of intra-articular damage posed by the presence of a knot but, as stated earlier, compromises the formation of the labral "bumper effect."

In conclusion, the options in regard to devices available for labral fixation are numerous, but success depends mostly upon utilizing the appropriate technology for the pathology being treated and proper execution.

Outcomes

Results after labral repair in appropriately indicated patients have been shown to be favorable. One of the initial series by Snyder in 1995 demonstrated that suture anchors for labral fixation yielded favorable results [40]. Additional studies since then have continued to show this trend in younger patients with superior labral tears [41, 42]. In 2002, Kim et al. [43] published a series of 34 patients who underwent labral repair using suture anchor fixation. A total of 94 % of patients reported positive outcomes at 2 years of follow-up and beyond. In addition, the percentage of patients who showed the greatest gains in function were overhead athletes. Cordasco and colleagues [44] showed that overhead athletes with superior labral tears did not do well with simple debridement after 2 years of follow-up and that only 45 % were able to return to the previous level of sport. Other studies have shown similar findings in this particular patient population [45]. This reiterates the important notion that patients should be carefully selected when considering surgical repair. In addition, attention to the pathologic "cascade" of the throwing athlete, i.e., the kinetic chain factors which caused the initial tissue breakdown, must be addressed.

Summary Keys to Labral Repair

1) Use percutaneous portals for anchor placement.
2) Prepare labrum from contralateral portal.
3) Avoid rigid fixation material in the superior labrum.
4) Keep knots far from labrum.
5) Neviaser's portal or posterior superior labral suture passage.
6) Address kinetic chain.

References

1. Andrews JR, Carson Jr WG, McLeod WD. Glenoid labrum tears related to the long head of the biceps. Am J Sports Med. 1985;13(5):337–41.
2. Angelo RL, et al. AANA advanced arthroscopy. Shoulder. 1st ed. Philadelphia, PA: Saunders/Elsevier; 2010.
3. DeLee J, Drez D, Miller MD. DeLee & Drez's orthopaedic sports medicine: principles and practice. 3rd ed. Philadelphia, PA: Saunders/Elsevier; 2010.
4. Snyder SJ, et al. SLAP lesions of the shoulder. Arthroscopy. 1990;6(4):274–9.
5. Hegedus EJ, et al. Which physical examination tests provide clinicians with the most value when examining the shoulder? Update of a systematic review with meta-analysis of individual tests. Br J Sports Med. 2012;46(14):964–78.
6. O'Brien SJ, et al. The active compression test: a new and effective test for diagnosing labral tears and acromioclavicular joint abnormality. Am J Sports Med. 1998;26(5):610–3.
7. Ben Kibler W, et al. Clinical utility of traditional and new tests in the diagnosis of biceps tendon injuries and superior labrum anterior and posterior lesions in the shoulder. Am J Sports Med. 2009;37(9):1840–7.
8. Pandya NK, et al. Physical examination and magnetic resonance imaging in the diagnosis of superior labrum anterior-posterior lesions of the shoulder: a sensitivity analysis. Arthroscopy. 2008;24(3):311–7.
9. Major NM, et al. Evaluation of the glenoid labrum with 3-T MRI: is intraarticular contrast necessary? AJR Am J Roentgenol. 2011;196(5):1139–44.
10. Pfahler M, et al. Age-related changes of the glenoid labrum in normal shoulders. J Shoulder Elbow Surg. 2003;12(1):40–52.
11. Burns JP, Bahk M, Snyder SJ. Superior labral tears: repair versus biceps tenodesis. J Shoulder Elbow Surg. 2011;20(2 Suppl):S2–8.
12. Williams MM, Snyder SJ, Buford Jr D. The Buford complex–the "cord-like" middle glenohumeral

ligament and absent anterosuperior labrum complex: a normal anatomic capsulolabral variant. Arthroscopy. 1994;10(3):241–7.
13. Paxton ES, et al. Shoulder arthroscopy: basic principles of positioning, anesthesia, and portal anatomy. J Am Acad Orthop Surg. 2013;21(6):332–42.
14. Rains DD, Rooke GA, Wahl CJ. Pathomechanisms and complications related to patient positioning and anesthesia during shoulder arthroscopy. Arthroscopy. 2011;27(4):532–41.
15. Skyhar MJ, et al. Shoulder arthroscopy with the patient in the beach-chair position. Arthroscopy. 1988;4(4):256–9.
16. Peruto CM, Ciccotti MG, Cohen SB. Shoulder arthroscopy positioning: lateral decubitus versus beach chair. Arthroscopy. 2009;25(8):891–6.
17. Rodeo SA, Forster RA, Weiland AJ. Neurological complications due to arthroscopy. J Bone Joint Surg Am. 1993;75(6):917–26.
18. Murphy GS, Szokol JW. Blood pressure management during beach chair position shoulder surgery: what do we know? Can J Anaesth. 2011;58(11):977–82.
19. Sculco TP. Global blood management in orthopaedic surgery. Clin Orthop Relat Res. 1998;357:43–9.
20. Morrison DS, Schaefer RK, Friedman RL. The relationship between subacromial space pressure, blood pressure, and visual clarity during arthroscopic subacromial decompression. Arthroscopy. 1995;11(5):557–60.
21. Ogilvie-Harris DJ, Weisleder L. Fluid pump systems for arthroscopy: a comparison of pressure control versus pressure and flow control. Arthroscopy. 1995;11(5):591–5.
22. Jensen KH, et al. Arthroscopic shoulder surgery with epinephrine saline irrigation. Arthroscopy. 2001;17(6):578–81.
23. Bedi A, et al. Use of the 70 degrees arthroscope for improved visualization with common arthroscopic procedures. Arthroscopy. 2010;26(12):1684–96.
24. Meyer M, et al. Anatomic risks of shoulder arthroscopy portals: anatomic cadaveric study of 12 portals. Arthroscopy. 2007;23(5):529–36.
25. Andrews JR, Carson Jr WG, Ortega K. Arthroscopy of the shoulder: technique and normal anatomy. Am J Sports Med. 1984;12(1):1–7.
26. Matthews LS, et al. Anterior portal selection for shoulder arthroscopy. Arthroscopy. 1985;1(1):33–9.
27. Wolf EM. Anterior portals in shoulder arthroscopy. Arthroscopy. 1989;5(3):201–8.
28. Neviaser TJ. Arthroscopy of the shoulder. Orthop Clin North Am. 1987;18(3):361–72.
29. Bigliani LU, et al. An anatomical study of the suprascapular nerve. Arthroscopy. 1990;6(4):301–5.
30. Morgan CD, et al. Type II SLAP lesions: three subtypes and their relationships to superior instability and rotator cuff tears. Arthroscopy. 1998;14(6):553–65.
31. Burkhart SS, Lo IKY, Brady PC. Burkhart's view of the shoulder: a cowboy's guide to advanced shoulder arthroscopy. Philadelphia, PA: Lippincott Williams & Wilkins; 2006. xx, 316 p.
32. Yamamoto N, et al. Does the "bumper" created during Bankart repair contribute to shoulder stability? J Shoulder Elbow Surg. 2013;22(6):828–34.
33. Lehtinen JT, et al. Variations in glenoid rim anatomy: implications regarding anchor insertion. Arthroscopy. 2004;20(2):175–8.
34. Ilahi OA, et al. Glenoid suture anchor fixation strength: effect of insertion angle. Arthroscopy. 2004;20(6):609–13.
35. Barber FA, Herbert MA, Click JN. The ultimate strength of suture anchors. Arthroscopy. 1995;11(1):21–8.
36. Barber FA, et al. Sutures and suture anchors–update 2006. Arthroscopy. 2006;22(10):1063.e1–9.
37. Barber FA, et al. Suture anchor materials, eyelets, and designs: update 2008. Arthroscopy. 2008;24(8): 859–67.
38. Spoliti M. Glenoid osteolysis after arthroscopic labrum repair with a bioabsorbable suture anchor. Acta Orthop Belg. 2007;73(1):107–10.
39. Milewski MD, et al. Bone replacement of fast-absorbing biocomposite anchors in arthroscopic shoulder labral repairs. Am J Sports Med. 2012;40(6):1392–401.
40. Snyder SJ, Banas MP, Karzel RP. An analysis of 140 injuries to the superior glenoid labrum. J Shoulder Elbow Surg. 1995;4(4):243–8.
41. Mileski RA, Snyder SJ. Superior labral lesions in the shoulder: pathoanatomy and surgical management. J Am Acad Orthop Surg. 1998;6(2):121–31.
42. Nam EK, Snyder SJ. The diagnosis and treatment of superior labrum, anterior and posterior (SLAP) lesions. Am J Sports Med. 2003;31(5):798–810.
43. Kim S-H, et al. Results of arthroscopic treatment of superior labral lesions. J Bone Joint Surg. 2002;84(6):981–5.
44. Cordasco FA, et al. Arthroscopic treatment of glenoid labral tears. Am J Sports Med. 1993;21(3):425–30. discussion 430-1.
45. Tomlinson Jr RJ, Glousman RE. Arthroscopic debridement of glenoid labral tears in athletes. Arthroscopy. 1995;11(1):42–51.

Indications and Technique for Posterior Capsule Release

4

John G. Horneff III, G. Russell Huffman, and John D. Kelly IV

The posterior capsule of the shoulder is a complex confluence of capsule, labrum, and ligamentous structures that can often become pathologic resulting in pain and limited range of motion in some patients. Originating from the posterior capsulolabral complex of the glenoid, the superior border of the posterior capsule extends down from the posterior aspect of the long head of the biceps tendon to the inferior aspect of the glenoid [1, 2]. When visualizing the glenoid as a clockface, the posterior capsule can be thought of as extending in a counterclockwise position from 12 o'clock to 6 o'clock. At its most inferior aspect, the capsule merges into the posterior band of the inferior glenohumeral ligament (IGHL) complex. Together with the corresponding anterior band, the two bands of the IGHL serve as a hammock to support the humeral head during shoulder abduction [1, 2]. In its normal physiologic state, the posterior capsule of the shoulder works to help limit posterior translation of the humeral head when the arm is in a forward flexed, adducted, and internally rotated position. In cases of posterior capsule tightness, these motions are inhibited excessively and function may diminish as well as injury may ensue to the rotator cuff and labrum. In essence, the tightness of the posterior capsule can become so severe that it can alter the normal kinematics of the glenohumeral joint and affect the humeral head position in relation to the glenoid surface.

Cadaveric studies performed have examined isolated tightening of the posterior capsule and have demonstrated the altered kinematics that result. Harryman et al. in 1990 were the first to show that tightening of the posterior capsule resulted in limited flexion, adduction, and internal rotation of the shoulder [3]. By imbricating approximately 2 cm of the posterior capsule, the authors noted that the humeral head translated anteriorly and superiorly in relation to the glenoid surface with arm flexion and adduction compared to the unimbricated capsule. These investigators also noted that the humeral head translation was in the opposite direction of the posterior capsular tightening and referred to this phenomenon as the "capsular constraint mechanism" [3]. Many other cadaveric studies have since followed with either the use of suture plication or thermal capsulorrhaphy to shrink the posterior capsule [4–9]. The results of these various

J.G. Horneff III, MD (✉)
Rothman Institute Orthopaedics, Thomas Jefferson University, Philadelphia, PA, USA
e-mail: jghorneff3@gmail.com

G.R. Huffman, MD, MPH
Department of Orthopaedic Surgery, University of Pennsylvania, Philadelphia, PA, USA

J.D. Kelly IV, MD
Department of Orthopedics, University of Pennsylvania, Philadelphia, PA, USA

J.D. Kelly IV (ed.), *Elite Techniques in Shoulder Arthroscopy*,
DOI 10.1007/978-3-319-25103-5_4

studies have demonstrated anywhere between 23 % and 68 % reduction in glenohumeral internal rotation range of motion (ROM) with posterior capsular tightening [4, 6–9].

More importantly, posterior inferior capsular tightness causes a relative posterior superior shift in humeral head translation in the late cocking position. This change posterosuperiorly will cause obligate increased contact on the posterior rotator cuff and potentiate the occurrence of "internal impingement"—excessive contact between the posterior superior labrum and posterior rotator cuff. Furthermore, as the humeral head shifts posteriorly, "peel-back" stresses on the labrum will increase during late cocking. Clabbers et al. first noted a trend in posterior superior humeral migration in imbricated cadaveric shoulders [5]. However, Huffman et al. performed a much more sophisticated work. These investigators not only imbricated the posterior capsule but also created subtle anterior capsular laxity and applied a compressive force to mimic rotator cuff influence to more closely mimic the thrower's shoulder. They demonstrated posterior humeral head migration in late cocking and anterior inferior translation in follow-through when both posterior capsular tightness and anterior laxity were present [9]. Such changes in translation undoubtedly lead to increased cuff and labral strain in late cocking and follow-through, respectively.

Clinically, posterior capsular tightness can result from numerous causes in the orthopedic patient: idiopathic, posttraumatic, postoperative, and from repetitive throwing [1]. The discussion here is limited to the throwing athlete.

Physical exam findings reveal the extent of contracture. Perhaps the best test to assess posterior capsular contracture is performed by placing the patient in the supine position with the shoulder abducted 90° (Fig. 4.1). With the scapula stabilized, the physician is able to compare the passive internal rotation of both glenohumeral joints. The shoulder suspected of posterior capsular contracture should have a noticeable deficit of internal rotation compared to the contralateral normal shoulder. For active internal rotation, the patient may be seated and asked to reach up his/her back with the physician noting the most cephalad spinous process the patient is able to reach with the thumb (Fig. 4.2) [1, 10]. Again, a deficit should be noted on the affected side. In contrast, external rotation both passively and actively should remain fairly symmetrical bilaterally. If there is a noted deficit in passive external rotation in abduction and adduction as well, adhesive capsulitis should be suspected. Posterior capsular tightness may be responsible for "non-outlet" impingement. In classic outlet impingement, the tendon of the supraspinatus becomes impinged under a stenotic overlying acromion with forward flexion [1]. With posterior capsular tightness, obligatory anterior-superior humeral head translation occurs with forward flexion, regardless of acromial dimensions. The resulting "impingement" is remedied with posterior capsular stretching or release, not an acromioplasty.

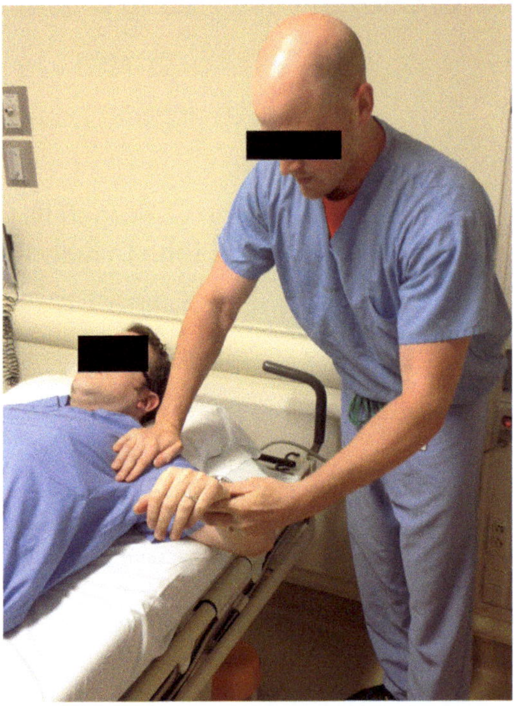

Fig. 4.1 Assessing posterior capsular contracture with patient laying supine and the affected arm abducted to 90°

The overhead throwing athlete presents with unique symptoms and findings related to posterior capsular tightness. In 1991, Verna was the first to describe a relationship between shoulder

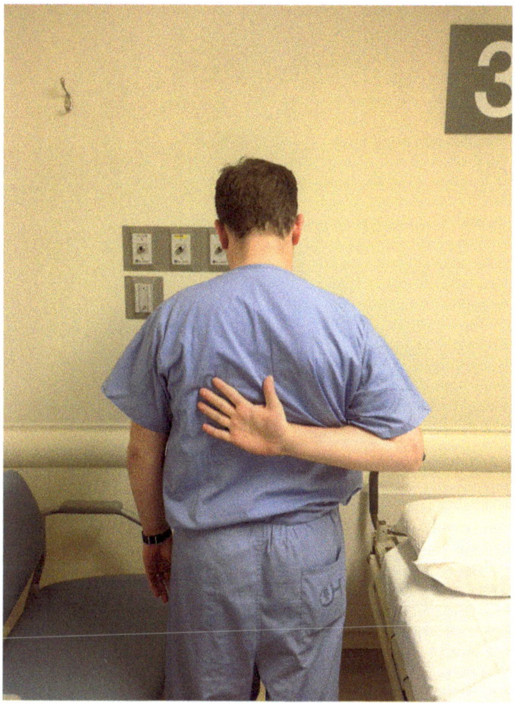

Fig. 4.2 Patient performing the active range of motion assessment of the posterior capsule by reaching up the spine to the most cephalad spinous process

dysfunction and an internal rotation range of motion deficit seen in the dominant throwing arm of overhead athletes [11]. Since that time, many authors such as Burkhart et al. have gone on to describe this phenomenon known as glenohumeral internal rotation deficit (GIRD) in which there is loss of degrees of glenohumeral internal rotation in the throwing shoulder compared to the non-throwing shoulder [12]. In Verna's initial observation, 39 professional baseball pitchers were noted to have ≤25° of internal rotation with a loss of ≥35° compared to the non-throwing shoulder [11]. These players were followed from the beginning of spring training through the entire baseball season with 60 % of them developing shoulder dysfunction that required them to stop pitching during the season [11]. Kibler, in his work with Burkhart et al., described 38 overhead athletes with arthroscopically proven Type 2 SLAP tears and found that ***all*** presented with GIRD [12]. Interestingly, throwers manifest most posterior tightness in the posteroinferior capsule [12]. As stated, this contracture can cause a posterosuperior shift of the humeral head on the glenoid fossa which can subsequently cause a shearing stress on the posterosuperior aspect of the labrum and cuff, while the biceps tendon is exerting its maximal posterior restraining force vector (peel-back phenomenon) seen in the late cocking phase of overhead throwing [12]. This increased stress leads to the higher likelihood of a SLAP lesion of the labrum. Additionally, these patients often have an increased external rotation range of motion in their throwing arm that can allow the greater tuberosity to become impinged under the posterosuperior aspect of the glenoid (posterior impingement) [1, 12].

Thomas has shown that posterior capsule tightness does correlate with increased capsular thickness as demonstrated on ultrasound [13]. Secondly, Thomas has also illustrated that increased amounts of humeral retroversion may predispose the thrower to acquire posterior inferior capsular contracture [14]. Increased humeral retroversion will cause an obligate loss of internal rotation. A diminished range of internal rotation will force the thrower to decelerate in a more confined motion arc and conceivably lead to earlier posterior cuff fatigue. Premature posterior rotator cuff fatigue may lead to increased posterior capsular strain and resultant fibrosis and thickening.

The initial approach to treating posterior capsule tightness should be nonsurgical in nature focused on stretching the tight posterior structures. The two most common and effective stretches focused on the posterior capsule are the cross-body adduction stretch and the "sleeper stretch." The former is performed with the affected arm flexed up to 90° to be even with the height of the shoulders. The unaffected arm is then used to grab the forearm of the affected arm and bring it across the body toward the unaffected shoulder. For an increased stretch, the patient may bend the involved elbow and use the uninvolved hand to grasp the involved distal humerus rather than the forearm. The patient should feel a stretching sensation at the posterosuperior aspect of the affected shoulder. This stretch can be performed with the patient sitting

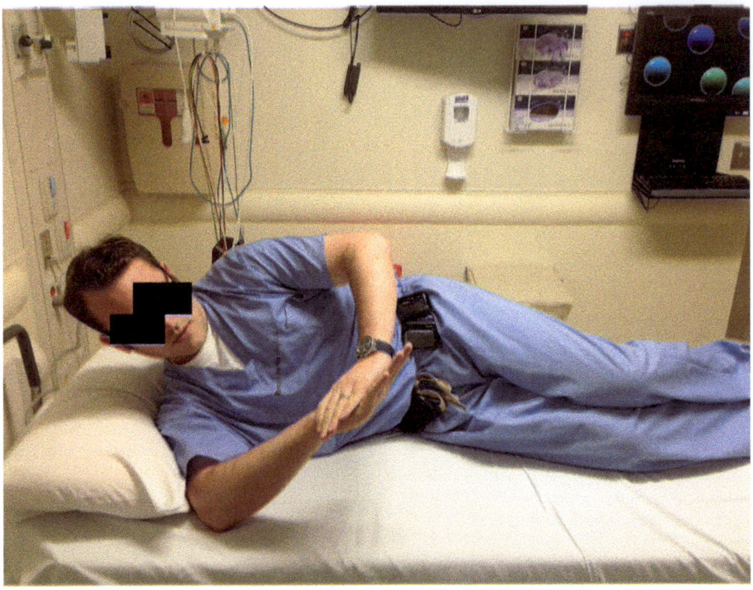

Fig. 4.3 Patient position for performing the "sleeper stretch" of the posterior capsule

upright or standing. The "sleeper stretch" is performed with the patient lying on the affected shoulder side with the arm flexed up to 90° to be even with the level of the clavicle (Fig. 4.3). The unaffected hand is then placed on the posterior aspect of the affected side forearm and placed a downward force to internally rotate the arm. The patient will sense a stretch of the posteroinferior capsule. Both of these stretches should be held for 30–60 s and be performed about five times per day. In a study looking at NCAA Division I baseball players, Aldridge et al. had players perform a daily posterior capsule stretching program centered around the "sleeper stretch" for 12 weeks [15]. The authors found that the players involved in the stretching program displayed significantly improved internal rotation and total range of motion arc in their dominant throwing arms. Other authors have suggested that the cross-body stretch is more effective than the "sleeper stretch" [16]. McClure et al. performed a randomized control trial comparing the two stretches with half of participants who displayed 10° or greater difference of internal rotation between their two shoulders placed into a 4-week cross-body stretch program with the other half placed in a 4-week "sleeper stretch" program. Both groups were compared to a control group who displayed less than 10° difference in their shoulder internal rotation arcs that performed no stretching program. Both stretching groups were found to have improvements in internal rotation compared to the control group, but only the cross-body stretching group was found to have significant gains (20.0 ± 12.9°) [16]. There was, however, no statistically significant difference in internal rotation gained between the two stretching groups [16]. Burkhart et al. have shown that nearly 90 % of throwers with symptomatic GIRD who are compliant with a focused posteroinferior stretching program will respond positively [1, 12].

Although very successful with relatively low risk, not all patients respond well to nonoperative treatment of posterior capsular contracture. Thus, surgical capsular release may be indicated. It is important for the treating physician to remember that surgical treatment should only be considered once all nonoperative modalities have been exhausted. At least a 6-week course of stretching should be instituted before considering surgery. Some patients may show slight gains with nonoperative management which eventually plateau, whereas other patients may have refractory posterior shoulder tightness that shows no improvement with stretching at all. For either of these patients, we recommend obtaining an MRI imaging study prior to proceeding to the operating room to ensure that there is not an underlying pathology being missed on clinical examination. Having a preoperative MRI allows the treating surgeon to prepare properly for the operating room should there be a concurrent issue with the labrum, rotator cuff, or other structures of the shoulder.

Once the decision to proceed to the operating room has been made, it is important to discuss the anesthesia options available to the patient for the procedure. Warner et al. have strongly recommended the use of regional anesthesia for a planned posterior capsular release as it allows for better and immediate postoperative pain control and can allow the patient to tolerate immediate postoperative range of motion exercises [10, 17]. An interscalene nerve block can be performed in either a one-time dosing that typically affords about 6–8 h of analgesia versus the placement of a catheter that allows continuous infusion of nervous blockade [10, 17]. We typically prefer a one-time interscalene nerve block as it allows the patient to have their procedure performed in the outpatient setting with no concern for an indwelling nerve catheter.

Once the patient receives the nerve block, general anesthesia may or may not be administered. In general, there are two camps regarding the positioning of a patient for shoulder arthroscopy—beach chair vs. lateral decubitus. In the technique developed by Warner et al., the authors preferred to place the patient in the beach chair position [17]. The senior authors (GRH, JDK) are proponents of lateral decubitus since it affords much better access to the posterior capsule (Fig. 4.4). Prior to prepping and incision, an examination under anesthesia is performed to assess the range of motion of the affected shoulder compared to the unaffected side. Once completed, the patient is prepped in the typical sterile fashion, and a diagnostic shoulder arthroscopy is initially performed viewing through the standard posterior portal. For the sake of this technique description, we assume that there is no other underlying pathology within the shoulder joint.

Next, the posterior capsular release is performed as initially described by Warner et al. [10, 17]. The arthroscope is placed in the anterior-superior portal with a disposable arthroscopy cannula placed in the posterior portal over a switching stick. A hook-tip electrocautery device is then introduced through the posterior cannula, and the tip is hooked around the posterior capsule just posterior to the biceps tendon [17]. Alternatively a capsular punch may be used as well. The cautery device is then pulled inferiorly until it reaches the 7 o'clock position in reference to the glenoid fossa. As the capsule is release, the muscle belly of the infraspinatus should become visible just beyond the reach of the hook-tip. As noted by Warner et al., it is important that this release is performed just adjacent to the glenoid rim as it is here that the surgeon can appreciate the muscle fibers of the infraspinatus just superficial to the capsule [10, 17]. Performing the release more laterally puts the rotator cuff tendons at risk as they become confluent with the capsule in this location, as well as maximizing space away from the axillary nerve [17, 18]. Once the release is completed, Warner et al. recommend using an arthroscopic shaver via the posterior portal to resect any additional scar in the medial and lateral directions. This opens of the gap of the release and, hopefully, prevents any recurrence of scar formation. Once this is completed, we recommend performing a thorough debridement of the subacromial space as many patients will display thickened and inflamed bursal tissue in concurrence with their posterior tightness. All instrumentation is removed from the shoulder, and a gentle manipulation is performed to encourage release of any remaining capsular tissue fibers [10, 17]. We make sure to focus our manipulation on the motions of adduction, internal rotation, and forward flexion as these are the inhibited movements seen with a tight posterior capsule and allow for the greatest stretch of any remaining fibers. At this point in time, we routinely take photos of the patient's arm at its range of motion extremes to prove to the patient what their possible arcs are with continued physical therapy postoperatively.

As described by Ticker [17], we recommend immediate postoperative range of motion therapy starting on the first day following surgery, focusing on posterior capsular stretching. We prefer the "sleeper stretch" and also emphasize scapular retraction exercises.

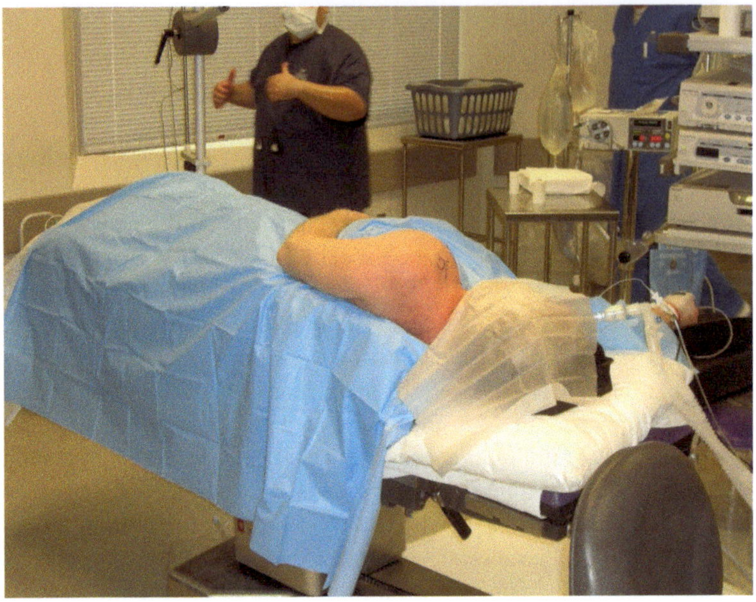

Fig. 4.4 Lateral decubitus positioning for shoulder arthroscopy

Reported results for posterior capsular release for isolated internal rotation deficit have been encouraging. Ticker et al. found that nine patients who underwent the described surgical procedure averaged a significant increase of glenohumeral internal rotation from 10° preoperatively to 47° postoperatively with the arm at 90° of abduction ($P<0.01$) [17]. Warner et al. also found an average increase in abducted internal rotation of 42° ($P<0.005$) for five patients with isolated internal rotation deficits. Constant and Murley scores improved an average of 20 points for these patients as well [10]. We have also had great success with our patient population, especially in throwers who are "non stretch responders." In accordance with the previous authors who have described the technique, we emphasize the importance of postoperative physical therapy and analgesia as a key to allowing for maximal results. We affirm that appropriate and timely postoperative therapy is essential and must be communicated to the patient both pre- and postoperatively so that they understand that the surgery itself is only one step in the multimodal approach to treating this condition.

References

1. Bach HG, Goldberg BA. Posterior capsular contracture of the shoulder. J Am Acad Orthop Surg. 2006;14(5):265–77.
2. O'Brien SJ, Neves MC, Arnoczky SP, et al. The anatomy and histology of the inferior glenohumeral ligament complex of the shoulder. Am J Sports Med. 1990;18:449–56.
3. Harryman II DT, Sidles JA, Clark JM, et al. Translation of the humeral head on the glenoid with passive glenohumeral motion. J Bone Joint Surg Am. 1990;72:1334–43.
4. Borstad JD, Dashottar A. Quantifying strain on posterior shoulder tissues during 5 simulated clinical tests: a cadaver study. J Orthop Sports Phys Ther. 2011;41:90–9.
5. Clabbers KM, Kelly JD, Bader D, et al. Effect of posterior capsule tightness on glenohumeral translation in late-cocking phase of pitching. J Sports Rehabil. 2007;16:41–9.
6. Dashottar A, Borstad J. Posterior glenohumeral joint capsule contracture. Shoulder Elbow. 2012;4(4):1–13.
7. Gerber C, Werner CML, Macy JC, Jacob HAC, Nyffeler RW. Effect of selective capsulorrhaphy on the passive range of motion of the glenohumeral joint. J Bone Joint Surg Am. 2003;48:48–55.
8. Grossman MG, Tibone JE, McGarry MH, et al. A cadaveric model of the throwing shoulder: a possible etiology of superior labrum anterior-to-posterior lesions. J Bone Joint Surg Am. 2005;87:824–31.
9. Huffman GR, Tibone JE, McGarry MH, et al. Path of glenohumeral articulation throughout the rotational

range of motion in a thrower's shoulder model. Am J Sports Med. 2006;34:1662–9.
10. Warner JJ, Allen AA, Marks PH, Wong P. Arthroscopic release of postoperative capsular contracture of the shoulder. J Bone Joint Surg Am. 1997;79:1151–8.
11. Verna C. Shoulder flexibility to reduce impingement. Presented at the 3rd Annual PBATS (Professional Baseball Athletic Trainer Society) Meeting, Mesa, Arizona. March 1991.
12. Burkhart SS, Morgan CD, Kibler WB. The disabled throwing shoulder: spectrum of pathology. I: Pathoanatomy and biomechanics. Arthroscopy. 2003;19:404–20.
13. Thomas SJ, Swanik CB, Higginson JS, Kaminski TW, Swanik KA, Bartolozzi AR, Abboud JA, Nazarian LN. A bilateral comparison of posterior capsule thickness and its correlation with glenohumeral range of motion and scapular upward rotation in collegiate baseball players. J Shoulder Elbow Surg. 2011;20(5):708–16. doi:10.1016/j.jse.2010.08.031. Epub 2010 Dec 16.
14. Thomas SJ, Swanik CB, Kaminski TW, Higginson JS, Swanik KA, Bartolozzi AR, Nazarian LN. Humeral retroversion and its association with posterior capsule thickness in collegiate baseball players. J Shoulder Elbow Surg. 2012;21(7):910–6. doi:10.1016/j.jse.2011.05.028.
15. Aldridge R, Stephen Guffey J, Whitehead MT, Head P. The effects of a daily stretching protocol on passive glenohumeral internal rotation in overhead throwing collegiate athletes. Int J Sports Phys Ther. 2012;7(4):365–71.
16. McClure P, Balaicuis J, Heiland D, et al. A randomized controlled comparison of stretching procedures for posterior shoulder tightness. J Orthop Sports Phys Ther. 2007;37(3):108–14.
17. Ticker JB, Beim GM, Warner JJP. Recognition and treatment of refractory posterior capsular contracture of the shoulder. Arthroscopy. 2000;16:27–34.
18. Clarke J, Sidles JA, Matsen FA. The relationship of the glenohumeral joint capsule to the rotator cuff. Clin Orthop. 1990;254:29–34.

5 Throwing Acquired Anterior Rotator Interval Pathology

Craig D. Morgan and Kevin J. McHale

The anatomy of the biceps soft tissue pulley outlet portion of the anterior rotator interval has been previously well described [1–3]. Despite this few understand biceps pulley function and even fewer are able to recognize and accurately diagnose pathology in this region of the shoulder. This soft tissue outlet functions like a pulley or sling which contains and stabilizes the long head of the biceps tendon through shoulder motion as it exits the joint [2, 3]. Anatomically, the pulley is comprised of three structures: (1) the coracohumeral ligament (CHL), (2) the upper reflection of the superior glenohumeral ligament (SGHL), and (3) the anterior margin of the supraspinatus tendon (SST). The pulley roof is the CHL, the anterior wall is the SGHL, and the posterior wall is the anterior margin of the SST (Fig. 5.1) [2, 3].

In an overhead throwing athlete, injury to the pulley can occur during the follow-through phase of throwing in those with improper mechanics. Throwing across the body at a high flexion angle during follow-through causes the SGHL portion of the pulley to come in contact with the anterosuperior glenoid rim, which, in turn, causes the SGHL reflection to fail—either as a frank tear or failure in continuity (Fig. 5.2) [4]. Failure of the SGHL results in a widened outlet that destabilizes the biceps through shoulder range of motion. Biceps instability due to the SGHL injury may produce biceps tendinopathy, which becomes the primary pain generator resulting in a disabled throwing shoulder in this setting [4]. This mechanism of injury was first described in trauma patients as anterosuperior glenohumeral impingement in forward flexion adduction by Werner in 2000 [3].

Clinically, throwers with isolated throwing acquired interval lesions present with very unique history and physical exam findings that are lesion specific [4]. Without exception, these throwers describe anterior superior shoulder pain in the area of the anterior rotator interval which occurs in the late cocking or early acceleration phase of the throwing cycle. Most will point with one finger to this area when asked where their pain is located. Most report pain only with throwing and deny pain with activities of daily living. With regard to the onset of symptoms, approximately 25 % reports a sudden onset of pain with one throw, whereas, about 75 % reports an insidious onset of symptoms. In addition to pain, decreased velocity and loss of command are common complaints. Mechanical symptoms are universally denied.

Four unique lesion-specific physical exam findings are usually present in throwers with isolated SGHL pulley lesions: (1) anterior superior pain in the region of the anterior rotator interval in abduction external rotation (ABER)

C.D. Morgan, MD (✉)
Morgan Kalman Clinic, Wilmington, DE, USA
e-mail: scopeshop@aol.com

K.J. McHale, MD
Department of Orthopaedic Surgery, Hospital of the University of Pennsylvania, Philadelphia, PA, USA

J.D. Kelly IV (ed.), *Elite Techniques in Shoulder Arthroscopy*,
DOI 10.1007/978-3-319-25103-5_5

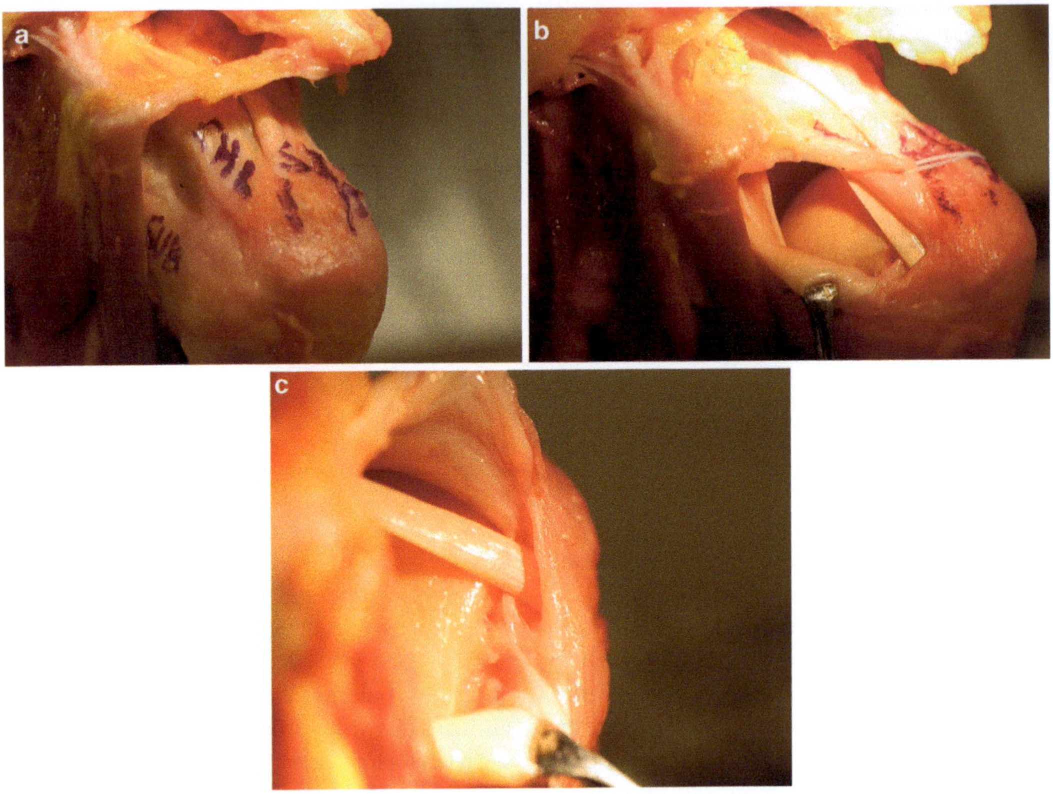

Fig. 5.1 (**a**) Left shoulder cadaveric dissection with intact anterior rotator interval. (**b**) Same shoulder as in (**a**) with CHL reflected superiorly exposing the soft tissue pulley outlet. (**c**) Same shoulder as in (**a**) and (**b**) with closeup look at the outlet: roof = CHL, anterior wall = SGHL reflection, posterior wall = anterior margin of the SST

reproducibly reduced by a posterior-directed force on the humerus (Jobe relocation maneuver), (2) pain in the upper bicipital groove to digital pressure, (3) an asymmetric increased sulcus sign in both neutral and external rotation with the arm at the side in the injured shoulder versus the uninjured shoulder, and (4) excessive abduction external rotation (ER) with the scapula stabilized and total motion arc (TMA) by approximately 25° in the injured shoulder versus the uninjured shoulder (Fig. 5.3) [4]. Anterior superior pain in ABER reduced by the Jobe relocation maneuver is explained by the following mechanism. Due to the SGHL injury with a widened outlet, in neutral, the biceps tendon is subluxed anterior-inferior out of the pulley and is free of soft tissue contact. In ABER the tendon relocates and abuts the CHL roof and the SST posterior wall, which produces pain as a result of the synovitis on the dorsum of the inflamed biceps tendon. When the Jobe relocation maneuver is applied in ABER, the tendon subluxes back out of the injured interval anterior-inferiorly into its pain-free position. Digital pain in the upper bicipital groove is caused by synovitis in the groove and biceps tendinitis produced by the destabilizing effect of the SGHL injury. The asymmetric sulcus sign is present due to laxity in the SGHL as well as laxity in the upper middle glenohumeral ligament (MGHL) and coracohumeral ligament (CHL). The MGHL laxity is the result of laxity in the entire SGHL, including the lower reflection that attaches to and suspends the upper MGHL. The excessive ER and TMA seen in these SGHL-injured shoulders are likely due to the above-mentioned laxity in the upper MGHL and CHL. Morgan [4] reported a prospective series of 32 isolated SGHL-injured throwing shoulders

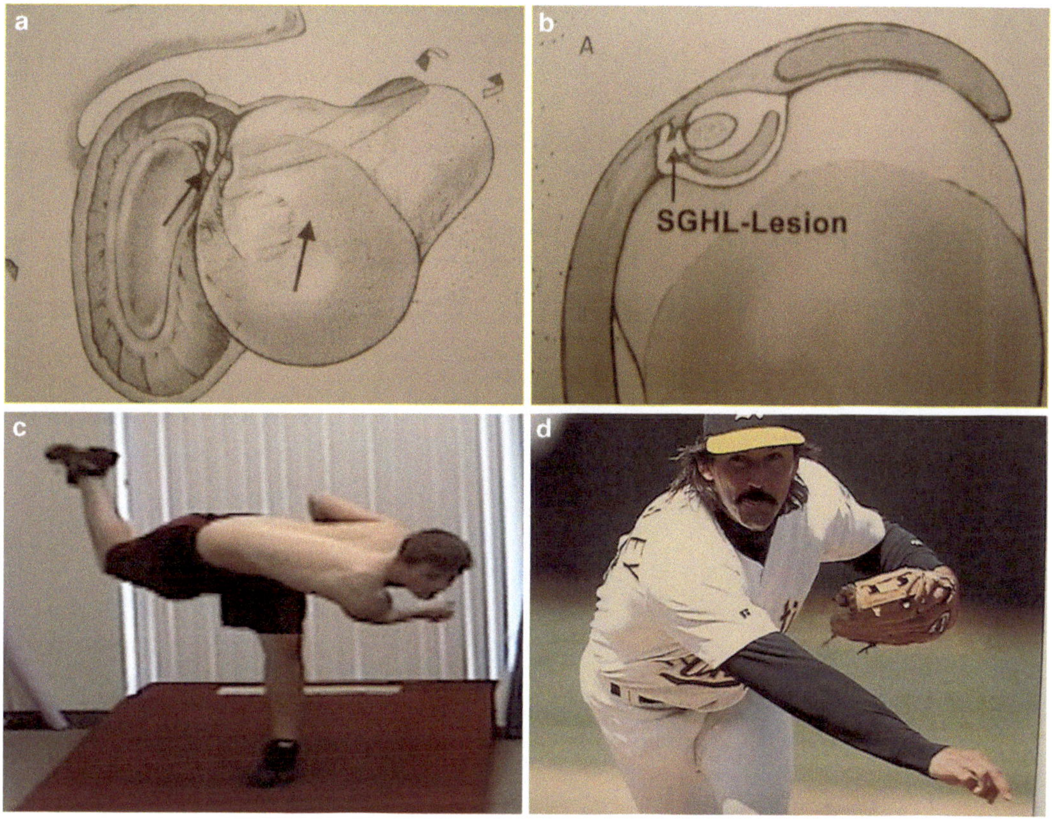

Fig. 5.2 (**a**) Line drawing illustrating the forward flexion adduction internal rotation mechanism of injury to the SGHL portion of the interval via anterosuperior glenohumeral impingement. (**b**) Line drawing illustrating the SGHL injury resulting in a widened outlet with biceps outlet instability. (**c**) Flawed mechanics of throwing across the body in follow-through at a high flexion angle, which puts the SGHL portion of the biceps outlet in jeopardy for injury. (**d**) Proper mechanics of throwing across the body in follow-through with a lower flexion angle

compared to an age-matched group of throwing shoulders without intra-articular pathology. In this series, the SGHL-injured group had excessive ER and TMA in their dominant shoulder averaging 27° with a range from 20 to 36° compared to the control group with increased ER and TMA that averaged 6° with a range from 0 to 12°. Morgan [4] first described the sagittal rotator interval angle on MRI arthrogram as a reliable diagnostic imaging tool to determine the presence or absence of anterior rotator interval pathology. On sagittal oblique cuts through the biceps outlet (where only the acromion is seen), the sagittal acromial angle is measured goniometrically by measuring the angle between two lines originating from a point central in the humeral head image: one line to the anterior margin of the SST and one line to the superior margin of the intra-articular subscapularis tendon (Fig. 5.4). In a prospective series of 32 throwing acquired SGHL-injured shoulders, the sagittal rotator interval angle averaged 58° with a range from 44 to 68° [4]. In contrast, an age-matched control group of 31 throwing shoulders with scapular dyskinesis without intra-articular pathology had an average sagittal rotator interval angle of 28° with a range from 22 to 30° [4]. In addition, Nottage independently measured the sagittal rotator interval angle in 240 shoulders without intra-articular pathology [5]. In this series, the normal sagittal rotator interval angle was 30° with a range from 28 to 33°. Sagittal oblique MRI arthrogram images through the outlet also show the subluxed biceps tendon as a biceps

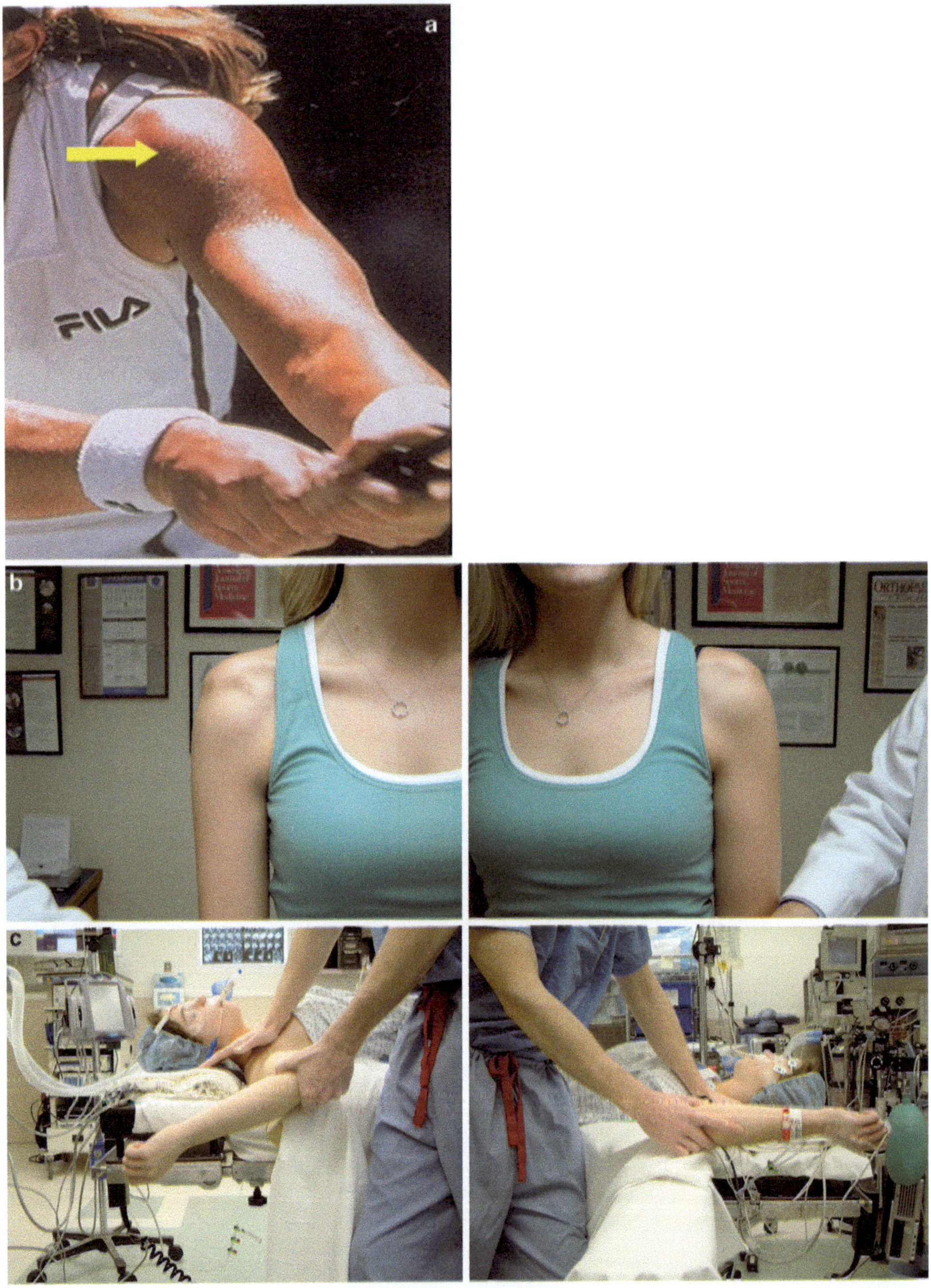

Fig. 5.3 (**a**) Anterosuperior location of interval lesion pain. (**b**) An asymmetric sulcus sign in the affected right shoulder. (**c**) Excessive scapula stabilized ER in the SGHL-injured right shoulder

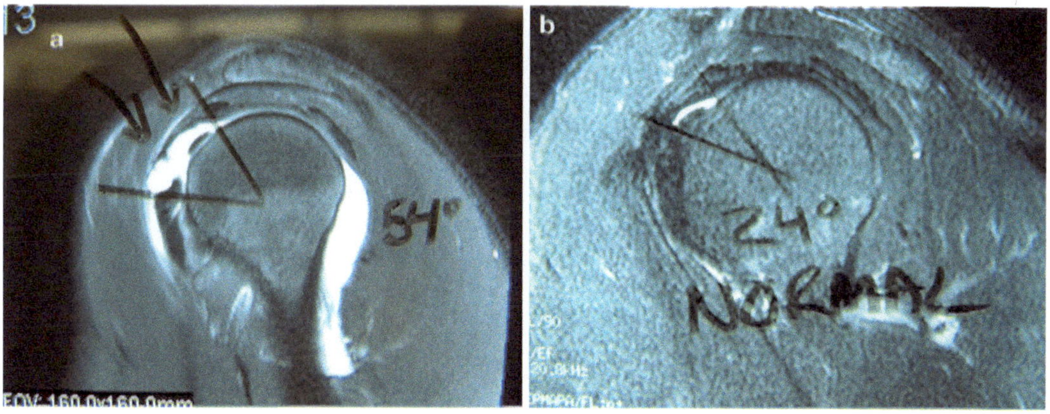

Fig. 5.4 (**a**) Sagittal oblique MRI arthrogram image of an SGHL-injured shoulder with an enlarged outlet and a pathologic 54° sagittal rotator interval angle. (**b**) Sagittal oblique MRI arthrogram image of a normal outlet with a 24° sagittal rotator interval angle

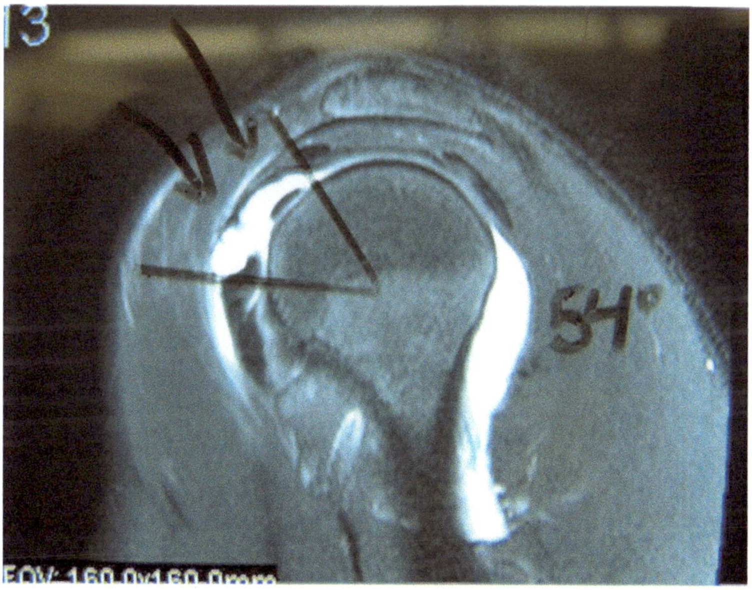

Fig. 5.5 Biceps "drop-out" sign with anterior-inferior biceps subluxation in a widened biceps outlet with a positive SGHL "chandelier" sign

"drop-out" sign and the torn SGHL hanging down as a "chandelier" sign (Figs. 5.5 and 5.6).

With regard to arthroscopic findings referable to rotator interval pathology, Walch et al. in 1994 and in 1998 reported that these lesions were "hidden" in the bony groove where they could not be seen or diagnosed with an arthroscope [6, 7]. In contrast, others have subsequently reported specific arthroscopic findings for outlet pathology associated with rotator cuff tears [8, 9]. Recently, Morgan [4] has reported four reliable arthroscopic diagnostic findings associated with isolated throwing acquired SGHL outlet lesions: (1) hyperemic synovitis in the area of the SGHL, upper MGHL, and dorsal on the intra-articular biceps tendon (Fig. 5.7); (2) a markedly widened biceps outlet (Fig. 5.8); (3) the biceps drop-out sign, biceps subluxed anterior-inferior in the widened outlet (Fig. 5.9); and (4) parallel adhesions exiting the outlet with the biceps tendon (Fig. 5.10).

Once the diagnosis is made clinically and confirmed on arthrogram MRI, the disabled

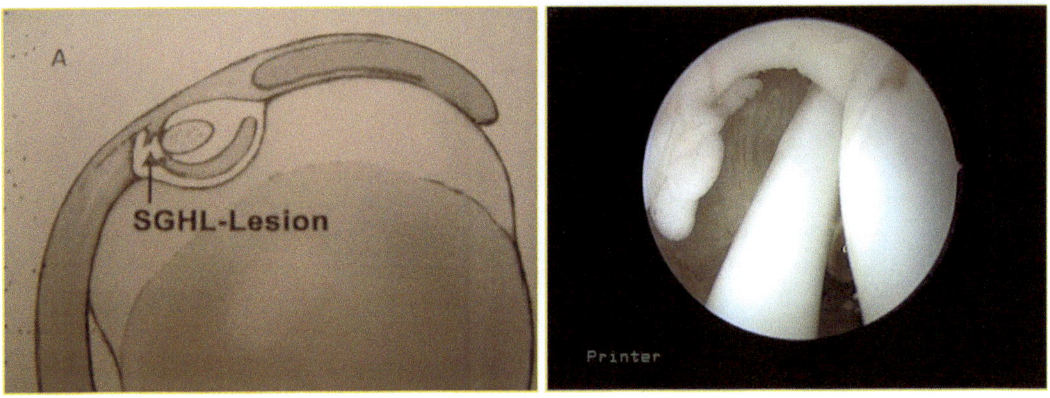

Fig. 5.6 Chandelier sign secondary to a torn SGHL

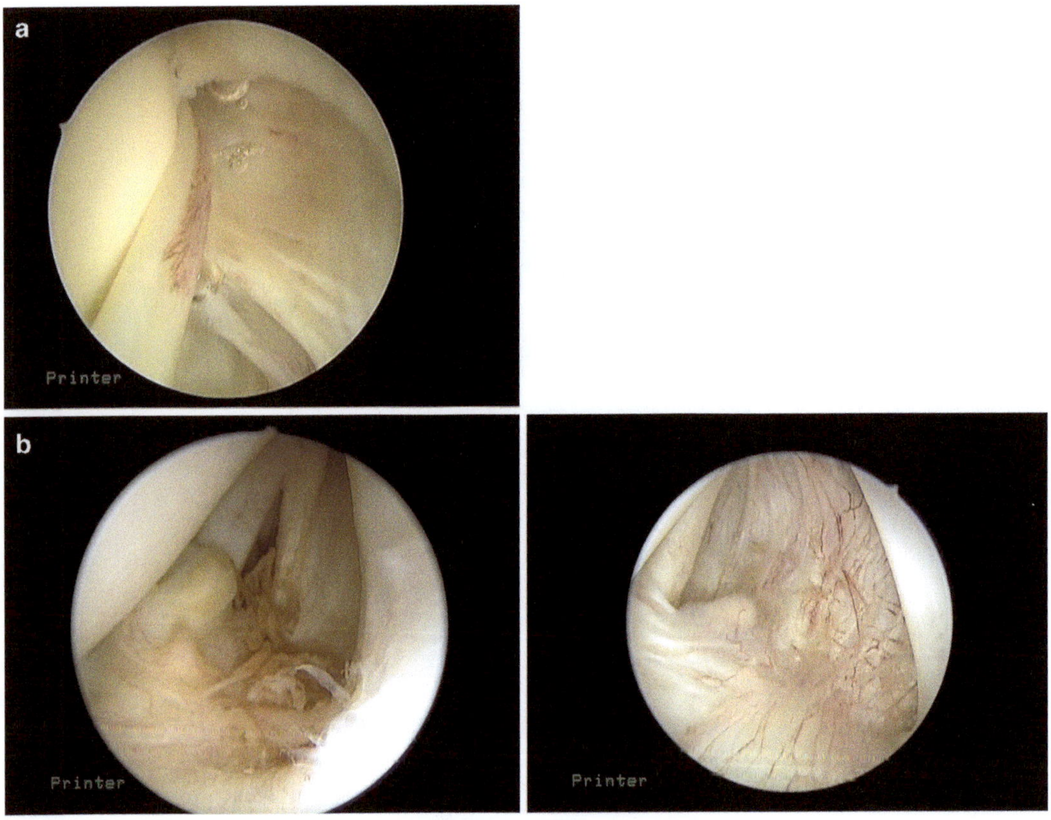

Fig. 5.7 (**a**) Dorsal "lipstick" biceps synovitic hyperemia secondary to biceps outlet instability. (**b**) Hyperemic synovitis in the lax SGHL and upper MGHL

throwing shoulder is indicated for an arthroscopic capsule-only rotator interval closure.

At the time of arthroscopy, the four rotator interval lesion-specific parameters are confirmed, and the rotator interval is closed in a manner that reduces the widened interval to a normal size and restores normal tension back to the lax upper MGHL. The operative technique is simple and

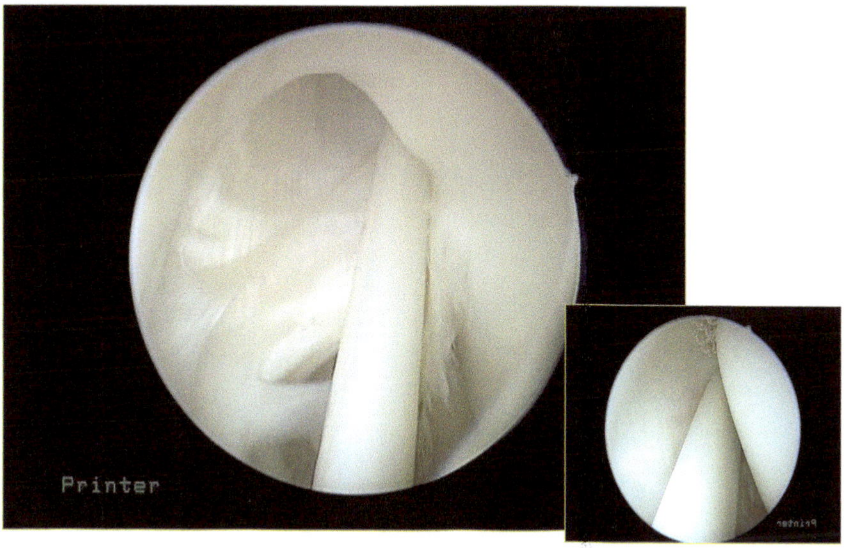

Fig. 5.8 Widened outlet with a biceps drop-out sign and an obviously torn SGHL

Fig. 5.9 Biceps drop-out sign

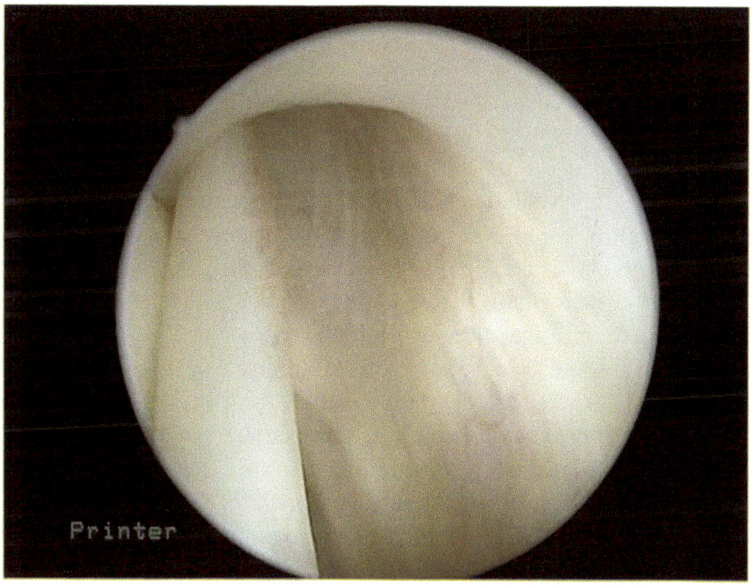

straightforward. With the arthroscope placed from a standard posterocentral approach, an operative cannula is placed central in the capsular portion of the interval. After rasping the SGHL and upper MGHL to stimulate a vascular fibroblastic response, the interval is closed north–south with #1 PDS suture (Ethicon Inc., Sommerville, NJ). Do not use permanent suture for fear of making the interval too tight! The suture is passed through the upper MGHL anterior to the labrum and then picked up with a suture retriever that penetrates the SGHL behind the

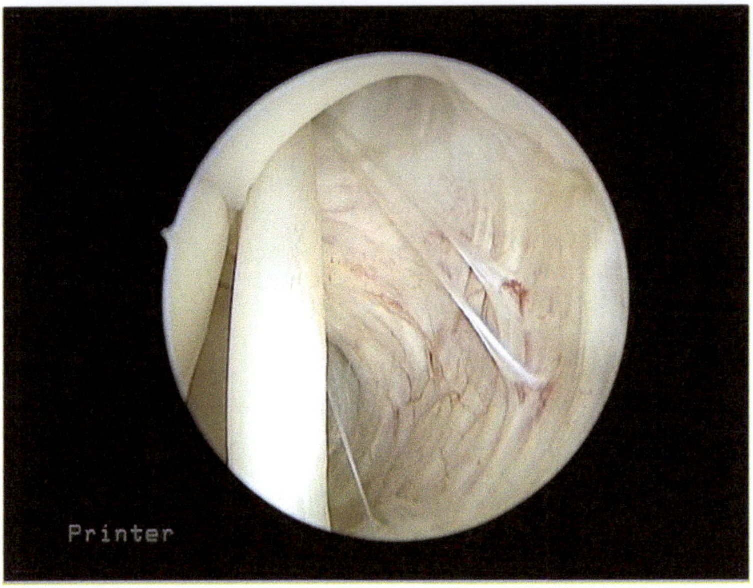

Fig. 5.10 Parallel adhesions exiting the outlet with the biceps tendon that are pathognomonic of biceps outlet instability

biceps tendon. The sutures are tied extracapsularly. Usually, a second suture is placed using similar technique ¼ inch lateral to the first suture (Fig. 5.11).

The postoperative rehabilitation protocol is as follows. The patient is maintained in sling immobilization for 4 weeks. After 4 weeks, active, active-assisted, and passive range of motion begins, avoiding ER past that of the nonoperative side. Scapular retraction exercises also begin at 4 weeks and continue indefinitely. Rotator cuff strengthening begins when the scapula is non-dyskinetic, usually at 8 weeks. A progressive distance interval throwing program on flat ground begins at 4 months postoperatively and continues for 2 months. Once throwing 220 ft on flat ground is achieved, a pitcher may begin throwing from the mound [4].

On one series [4] reported, 32 isolated SGHL-injured throwing shoulders that underwent arthroscopic anterior rotator interval closure were scored preoperatively and at 1 and 2 years postoperatively on a disabled throwing shoulder rating scale (100 points), which awarded points positive or negative for features that are unique to this problem. Clinical results at 1 and 2 years were excellent with all throwers returning to their pre-injury level of performance pain-free. During the early interval throwing portion of the rehabilitation program, two patients (6 %) developed subacromial bursitis that was treated with a cortisone injection and 1 week of rest before resuming pain-free throwing. There were no other complications.

At the time of this writing, the senior author has performed 320 rotator interval closures for throwing acquired SGHL lesions with similar results to the initial group. In this group, six patients (2 %) required repeat arthroscopies for removal of symptomatic postoperative subacromial and subcoracoid adhesions.

SGHL outlet injury can present as an isolated problem or it may present in combination with labral pathology, including Type II SLAP lesions, Bankart lesions, or posterior Bankart lesions. In this setting, successfully repairing the labrum without addressing the rotator interval lesion results in clinical failure due to persistent pain from the interval pathology. Recently, failure rates for Type II SLAP repairs have been reported between 20 % and 30 % [10–12]. Over the past 7 years, the senior author has retrospectively reviewed a case series of interval

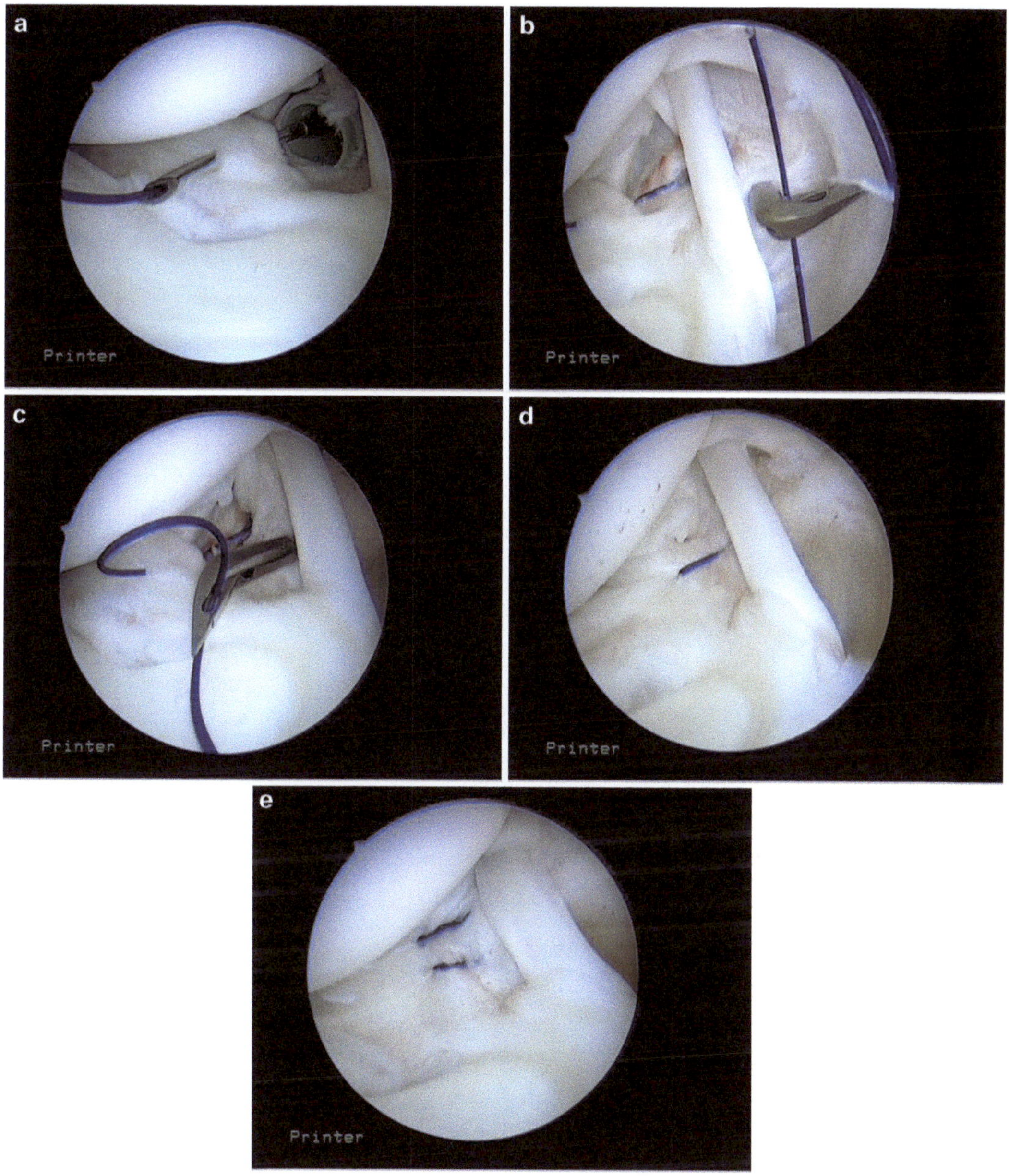

Fig. 5.11 (**a**) #1 PDS suture through the upper MGHL anterior to the labrum. (**b**) A suture retriever penetrating the upper SGHL behind the biceps tendon. (**c**) The MGHL suture being retrieved through the SGHL. (**d**) A north–south rotator interval closure tied extracapsularly. (**e**) A completed anterior rotator interval closure with two sutures closing the widened outlet and restoring normal tension back into the lax MGHL

pathology associated with labral tears. Based on these findings, if one has a Type II SLAP lesion, there is approximately a 36 % chance that a concomitant interval problem exists. If the interval is left untreated, this could explain the 20–30 % failure rates reported for SLAP repairs (Fig. 5.12). Similarly, concomitant interval lesions were noted in 46 % of those with Bankart lesions (Fig. 5.13) and 71 % of those with posterior Bankart lesions (Fig. 5.14). It is essential to address both the labral

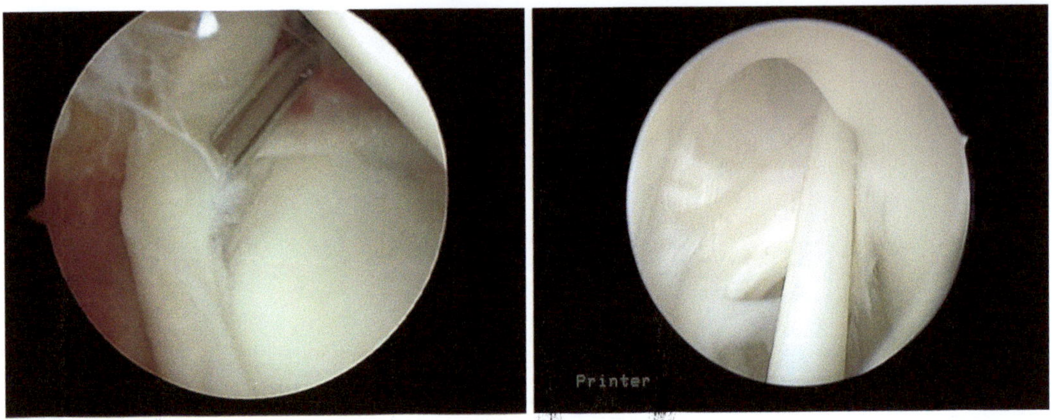

Fig. 5.12 A throwing acquired Type II SLAP lesion with an anterior rotator interval lesion

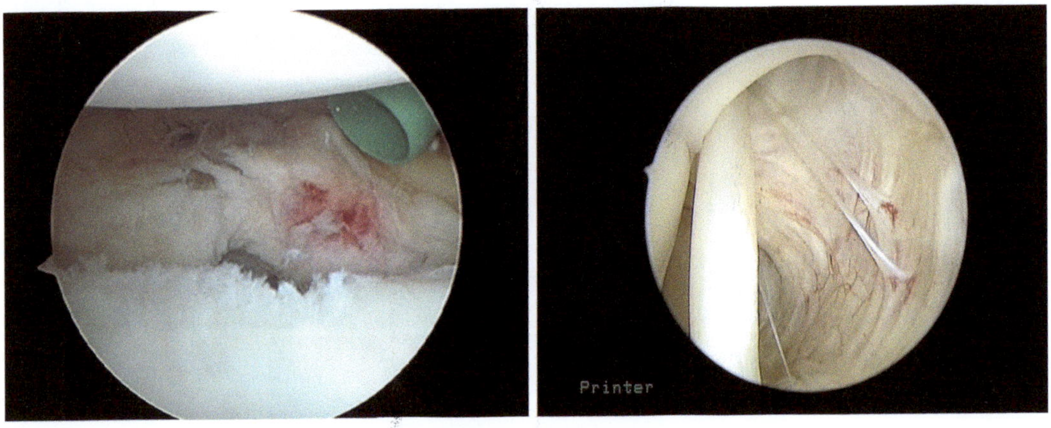

Fig. 5.13 An anterior Bankart lesion with an anterior rotator interval lesion

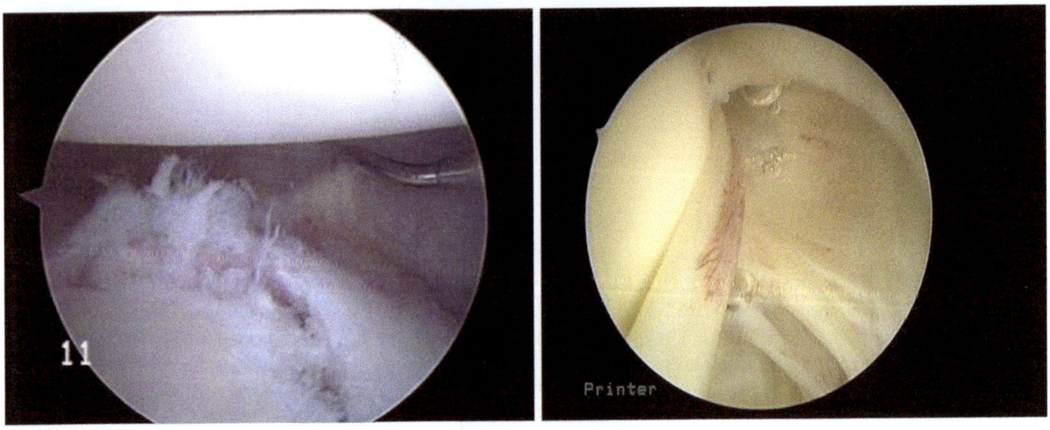

Fig. 5.14 A posterior Bankart lesion with an anterior rotator interval lesion

and rotator interval pathologies in this setting to achieve optimal clinical results.

Conclusion: Hidden interval lesions are a well-defined pathologic entity in the throwing shoulder with characteristic imaging and exam findings. Failure to treat interval laxity in the setting of shoulder instability, especially in the throwing athlete, will result in suboptimal surgical outcomes.

References

1. Gerber C, Sebesta A. Impingement of the deep surface of the subscapularis tendon and the reflection pulley on the anterosuperior glenoid rim: a preliminary report. J Shoulder Elbow Surg. 2000;9:483–90.
2. Harryman II DJ, Sidles JA, Harris SL, et al. The role of the anterior rotator interval capsule in passive range of motion and stability of the shoulder. J Bone Joint Surg Am. 1992;74(A):53–66.
3. Werner A, Mueller T, Boehm D, Gohlke F. The stabilizing sling for the long head of the biceps tendon in the rotator cuff interval. A histoanatomical study. Am J Sports Med. 2000;28:28–31.
4. Morgan CD, Boes MT, Theil JA. Arthroscopic treatment of the disabled throwing shoulder. In: Cole BJ, Sekiya JK, editors. Surgical techniques of the shoulder elbow and knee in sports medicine. 2nd ed. Amsterdam: Elsevier; 2013. p. 109–32.
5. Nottage WA. Personal Communication, 2012.
6. Walch G, Nove-Josserand L, Levigne C, et al. Tears of the supraspinatus tendon associated with "hidden" lesions of the rotator interval. J Shoulder Elbow Surg. 1994;3:353–60.
7. Walch G, Nove-Josserand L, Boileau P, et al. Subluxation and dislocation of the tendon of the long head of the biceps. J Shoulder Elbow Surg. 1998; 7:100–8.
8. Habermeyer P, Magosch P, Pritsch M, et al. Anterosuperior impingement of the shoulder as a result of pulley lesions: a prospective arthroscopic study. J Shoulder Elbow Surg. 2004;13:5–12.
9. Braun S, Horan MP, Elser F, Millett PJ. Lesions of the biceps pulley. Am J Sports Med. 2011;20:1–6.
10. Ciccotti MG, et al. Results of arthroscopic repair of Type II SLAP Lesions in overhead athletes. Am J Sports Med. 2011;39(9):1883–8.
11. Provencher MT, et al. A prospective analysis of 179 Type II SLAP repairs: outcomes and factors associated with success and failure. Am J Sports Med. 2013;41(4):880–6.
12. Weber S, et al. SLAP Lesions of the shoulder: incidence rates, complications, and outcomes. Am J Sports Med. 2012;40(7):1538–43.

Part II

Instability

6 Evaluation of Bone Loss and the Glenoid Track

Nancy A. Chauvin, Vishal Saxena, Stuart D. Kinsella, and Jose M. Morey

Biomechanics of the Glenohumeral Joint

The biomechanics of the glenohumeral joint are maintained by numerous anatomic restraints that include both the bony articulation and a complex array of dynamic and static soft tissue restraints [1]. The glenohumeral joint is provisionally constrained by osseous anatomy, which allows for a large arc of motion, but also potentiates the occurrence of instability [2, 3]. The glenoid fossa is approximately one-fourth the size of the humeral head articular surface, which allows for only about 20–30 % of the humeral head to be in contact with the glenoid at any one time [4]. In addition, the glenoid subchondral bone is relatively flat and, acting alone, does not provide an intrinsically stable socket. Due to the inherent limitations in joint surface congruity, three subsystems act in coordinated fashion to maintain glenohumeral joint stability: passive stabilizers (labrum, capsule, coracohumeral arch, and ligaments), active stabilizers (shoulder muscles), and the control system (neural) [3, 5]. The labrum acts to anchor the glenoid to the humeral head and, along with the articular cartilage, deepens the articular surface of glenoid. Cadaveric studies have demonstrated that the glenoid labrum contributes approximately 50 % of the total depth of the glenoid [6]. This osteochondral-labral composite thus plays an important role in shoulder stability.

The capsuloligamentous structures reinforce the glenohumeral joint. The glenohumeral ligaments are chiefly passive stabilizers that exert their effect by preventing glenohumeral translation when the joint is under tension. The superior glenohumeral ligament (SGHL) and coracohumeral ligament (CHL) prevent downward displacement of the humeral head and limit external

The authors have no financial disclosures.

N.A. Chauvin, MD (✉)
Department of Radiology, The Children's Hospital of Philadelphia, Philadelphia, PA, USA

Perelman School of Medicine at the University of Pennsylvania, Philadelphia, PA, USA
e-mail: chauvinn@email.chop.edu

V. Saxena, MD
Department of Orthopaedic Surgery, University of Pennsylvania, Philadelphia, PA, USA

S.D. Kinsella, MD, MTR
Department of Orthopaedic Surgery, Massachusetts General Hospital, Boston, MA, USA

J.M. Morey, MD
Department of Radiology and Biomedical Imaging, University of Virginia, Hampton, VA, USA

Department of Internal Medicine, Eastern Virginia Medical School, Hampton, VA, USA

Department of Radiology, Hampton VA Medical Center, Hampton, VA, USA

Almaden Research Lab, IBM Watson, Hampton, VA, USA

J.D. Kelly IV (ed.), *Elite Techniques in Shoulder Arthroscopy*,
DOI 10.1007/978-3-319-25103-5_6

rotation between 0 and 60° of elevation. The middle glenohumeral ligament (MGHL) is an important anterior stabilizer that limits external rotation and anterior translation from a neutral position to 90° of abduction. The inferior glenohumeral ligament (IGHL) is comprised of anterior and posterior bands. The anterior band limits elevation and anterior translation of the humeral head, especially during abduction and external rotation [7–9]. Conversely, the posterior component stabilizes the joint against posterior humeral translation during elevation and internal rotation [10]. The CHL and glenohumeral ligaments, however, become less effective at the extremes of motion [1].

Shoulder muscles contribute to shoulder stability by means of a "concavity-compression" mechanism, in which shoulder muscle activity compresses the humeral head against the concave glenoid surface, allowing for concentric rotation of the humeral head on the glenoid. Shoulder muscle forces function as powerful active stabilizers especially in positions in which the passive stabilizers are lax [1, 11]. Shoulders with weakened or deficient rotator cuff mechanisms are likely to have reduced stability from loss of concavity compression. In patients with rotator cuff tears, there is often superior migration of the humeral head due to altered compressive force of the humeral head into the glenoid cavity [1]. Wuekler et al. [12] have shown that with a 50 % reduction of rotator cuff forces, there is significant displacement of the humeral head in response to external loading at all glenohumeral joint positions. Similarly, large subscapularis tears commonly exhibit static anterior humeral translation on an axillary radiograph. The converse is true with complete tears of the infraspinatus as posterior humeral translation may be seen. Shoulder muscles play an important role in end-range positions as muscle activity protects the capsuloligamentous structures by limiting joint range of motion. Therefore, the active and passive stabilizers work in concert to maintain joint stability.

Shoulder Instability

General Considerations

Glenohumeral instability is often multifactorial and results from disruption of active and/or passive stabilizers of the shoulder. During episodes of instability, the arm is often in a "position of athletic function," which is defined as 90° of abduction and 90° of external rotation. Instability presents with anterior subluxation, posterior subluxation, or multidirectional instability (instability in two or three directions) [13]. Instability can be caused by repetitive microtrauma or a single macrotrauma. Congenital hyperlaxity and glenoid hypoplasia can predispose patients to instability. Through improved knowledge of shoulder biomechanics and the pathoanatomy of instability, the diagnosis of and surgical treatment of anterior shoulder instability has greatly improved [13].

Anterior Shoulder Dislocation

The shoulder is the most commonly dislocated large joint in the body, occurring in 1–2 % of the population [14]. Anterior dislocations represent more than 90 % of shoulder dislocations and are commonly seen in young athletes [15]. Anterior shoulder dislocations may or may not occur in the setting of an inciting traumatic event. Atraumatic dislocations are most often seen in patients with multidirectional instability and ligamentous laxity and usually lack a high-energy mechanism of injury. Traumatic dislocations occur acutely, generally after a discrete, forceful injury. The mechanism of injury, abduction and external rotation of the shoulder (position of athletic function), levers the humeral head anteriorly and out of the glenoid cavity. The relatively soft posterior humeral head impacts the harder anterior glenoid rim, often leading to a compression fracture of the posterolateral humeral head, termed a "Hill-Sachs lesion" [15]. This usually coincides with injury to the anterior glenohumeral ligaments and tearing of the labrum from the anterior, inferior aspect of the glenoid rim, known as a "Bankart lesion." In fact, a recent study investigating the association between Hill-Sachs lesions and Bankart lesions found not only a high coincidence but also a specific correlation between the size of the Bankart lesion and the grade of Hill-Sachs lesion [16]. When a glenoid osseous fragment is present, this injury is referred to as a "bony Bankart lesion." With repeated episodes of instability, attritional bone loss to the anterior glenoid may ensue. Large anterior-inferior glenoid bone loss results in what has been called *an inverted pear glenoid* because the affected glenoid en face in the sagittal oblique plane is wider superiorly than inferiorly (Fig. 6.1) [3].

The damaged anterior soft tissues generally lose integrity in cases of recurrent instability because the static glenohumeral constraints become attenuated with each dislocation episode [17]. The recurrence rate after primary anterior traumatic shoulder dislocation varies widely, with reported rates up to 90–100 % in younger athletes [18]. Established risk factors that are associated with increased anterior instability recurrence rates include young age at the time of initial dislocation, associated pathologic conditions including bone loss, immobilization in internal rotation, and athletic activity [19–21].

Posterior Shoulder Dislocation

Posterior shoulder dislocations are rare events and account for less than 2 % of all shoulder dislocations [22]. It is estimated that a reverse Hill-Sachs lesion, a bony defect of the anteromedial humeral head caused by impaction against the posterior glenoid rim [17, 23], occurs in up to 86 % of posterior dislocations. Anterior cartilage damage in reverse Hill-Sachs lesions is typically more extensive than that seen in the traditional Hill-Sachs lesion [17]. Appropriate management depends on the size of the defect, extent of the disability, as well as age and activity of the patient. Given the rarity of this lesion, further discussion will focus on anterior shoulder instability.

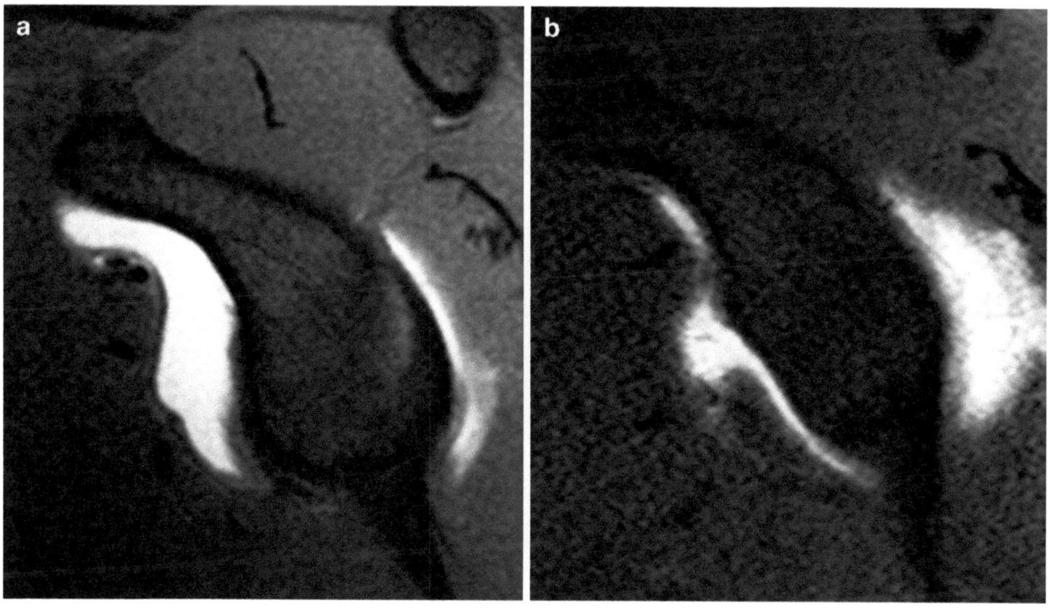

Fig. 6.1 Glenoid shape. Sagittal oblique MR arthrogram images of a 19-year-old man with shoulder instability. (**a**) Normal glenoid shape exhibiting a typical pear shape. (**b**) Follow-up imaging obtained after an anterior shoulder dislocation shows that the inferior glenoid is narrower than the superior glenoid, the "inverted pear glenoid," due to a large bony Bankart lesion

Traumatic Glenohumeral Bone Defects

Bony defects of the humeral head and glenoid are common injuries following anterior shoulder dislocation. The incidence of osseous Bankart lesions ranges from 8 % to 90 % and Hill-Sachs lesions between 77 % and 100 %, with higher rates and sizes of defects in recurrent dislocators [24–26]. Many of these bony injuries are small and do not require surgical attention; however, there is a positive correlation between the number of recurrent dislocations and the size and extent of these osseous lesions [26]. Lesions can be grouped by the bone(s) involved: humeral head, glenoid, or "bipolar lesions" (humeral plus glenoid bone loss) [27]. With profound bone loss, patients often experience frequent dislocations with various activities of daily living, even during sleep. These positions generally include activities in which the arm is in positions of much lower degrees of abduction and external rotation than are traditionally reported during primary dislocations. A significant portion of patients with significant bone loss have failed arthroscopic soft tissue repair alone, with unaddressed bone loss attributed as a cause of failure at the time of revision surgery [3, 28]. Given that treatment options for anterior shoulder instability range from nonoperative management to arthroscopic stabilization, and even open stabilization with bony augmentation, it is imperative to accurately quantify bone loss preoperatively in order to determine the appropriate treatment plan [29].

Glenoid Lesions

There are three distinct patterns of glenoid bone loss in instability: attritional bone loss of the glenoid from prior bony Bankart injury with subsequent resorption of the bony fragment, bony Bankart with rim avulsion, and frank fracture of the glenoid. The type of injury helps to dictate the most appropriate treatment plan. In the acute setting (<3 months), fracture fragments may still be present. However, resorption of the bone fragments can occur in the months following the injury. Some rim defects occur at the time of the initial anterior dislocation. Others develop in an attritional manner, related to recurrent dislocations, as up to 90 % of patients with recurrent shoulder dislocation have at least some bony component to the Bankart lesion [30].

The size of the glenoid lesion plays a critical role in determining which lesions are significant and contribute to recurrent instability. The glenoid's widest anteroposterior dimension is 23–30 mm with most adult patients falling between 24 and 26 mm [31]. Glenoid bone defects that are <3–4 mm (measured anteroposterior) from the anterior glenoid rim amount to between 0 % and 15 % of the total effective glenoid width and are less likely to materially affect recurrence. Defects that are greater than 6–10 mm correspond to 20–30% of total glenoid bone loss and are considered significant [30]. Sizeable glenoid bone lesions lead to decreased resistance to excessive anterior translation of the humeral head often with little applied force. Furthermore, the loss of the glenoid concavity decreases the ability of the concavity-compression mechanism in stabilizing the shoulder against anterior translation [26]. Furthermore, a narrower glenoid is more likely to "engage" a Hill-Sachs lesion in external rotation. Without addressing the bony glenoid defect, a firm glenoid socket cannot be maintained. Thus, it is largely accepted that an inverse relationship exists between the size of the glenoid defect and stability of the shoulder. Therefore, a critical component of the preoperative work-up is determining the amount of glenoid bone loss in order to dictate the appropriate type of repair: soft tissue Bankart repair alone versus glenoid restoration or augmentation with a Bristow or Laterjet reconstruction [32].

Hill-Sachs Lesions

As stated, compression fractures of the humeral head are very common injuries. The challenge lies in predicting which humeral lesions contribute to recurrent instability. The size, orientation, and location of the lesion should be determined on preoperative imaging and during arthroscopy, as all have implications for treatment. Assessments are based on the size of the lesion (length and depth), location along the posterolateral aspect of the humeral head, and the percent involvement of the 180° articular arc [17]. There is controversy regarding the threshold size and precise location of the defect that will materially contribute to instability; however, large Hill-Sachs are considered a risk factor for postoperative recurrence because larger humeral lesions more freely engage the glenoid rim [25]. Small Hill-Sachs lesions, less than 20 % of the humeral head curvature, are generally not considered significant sources of recurrent instability [33], though some authors report lesions as little as 12.5 % of the humeral head may prove consequential to shoulder instability [34]. Regardless, most authors agree that Hill-Sachs lesions greater than 40 % of the humeral head curvature are significant enough to warrant surgical treatment [2, 20, 21]. Lesions that are 20–40 % may be significant depending on their location, orientation, engagement, and coexistence with a glenoid bone lesion. The combination of a Hill-Sachs lesion and glenoid defect substantially reduces the normal arc of shoulder movement [33]. If a Hill-Sachs lesion is present, a dynamic examination should be performed at arthroscopy in which the shoulder is brought through full range of motion in order to discern "engagement" of the humeral head defect with the anterior glenoid rim [3].

The Engaging Lesion

Burkart and De Beer [35] were the first to report that one of the factors responsible for failure of arthroscopic soft tissue stabilization was traumatic bone deficiency, introducing the concept of "significant bone loss of the humeral head and glenoid." Significant bone loss of the glenoid was defined at arthroscopy if the glenoid had the appearance of an inverted pear. A significant humeral head bone defect was defined at arthroscopy as an "engaging" Hill-Sachs lesion: a lesion that presents parallel to the anterior glenoid when the shoulder is placed in a functional position of abduction and external rotation. The location of the defect allows the lesion to engage or "hook" the corner of the anterior glenoid due to an articular-arc deficit (Fig. 6.2).

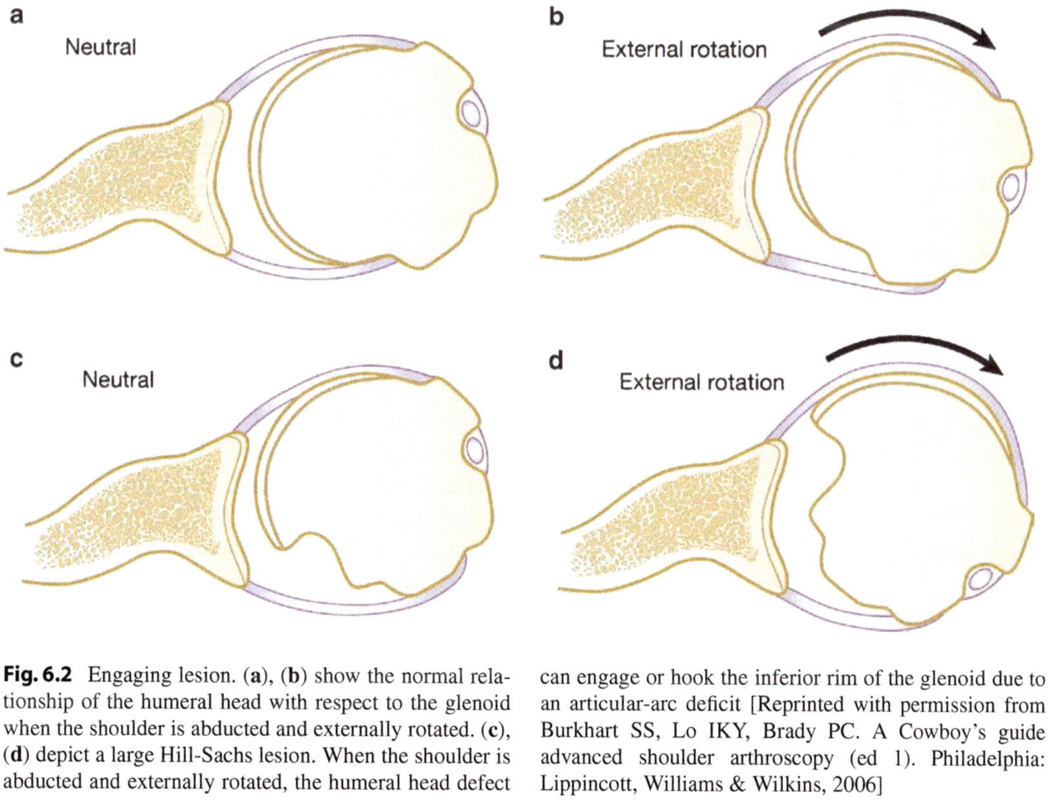

Fig. 6.2 Engaging lesion. (**a**), (**b**) show the normal relationship of the humeral head with respect to the glenoid when the shoulder is abducted and externally rotated. (**c**), (**d**) depict a large Hill-Sachs lesion. When the shoulder is abducted and externally rotated, the humeral head defect can engage or hook the inferior rim of the glenoid due to an articular-arc deficit [Reprinted with permission from Burkhart SS, Lo IKY, Brady PC. A Cowboy's guide advanced shoulder arthroscopy (ed 1). Philadelphia: Lippincott, Williams & Wilkins, 2006]

Conversely, a nonengaging Hill-Sachs lesion was defined as a defect that is presented in a nonparallel angle to the anterior glenoid in a functional position (abducted and externally rotated) or one in which engagement occurs in a nonfunctional position of shoulder extension or of low shoulder abduction (<70° abduction). This study emphasized the role of arthroscopy as a dynamic diagnostic tool. The authors advocated for not only repair of the soft tissue Bankart lesion but also an operative measure to address significant bony lesions in order to prevent the Hill-Sachs lesion from engaging. In addition, the authors confirmed the higher likelihood of substantial glenoid bone loss in patients with recurrent dislocations. Though the sizes of the lesions were not defined, other studies have shown that larger volume lesions are more strongly associated with recurrent shoulder dislocation [36, 37].

Itoi et al. [38] supported the importance of bone loss in a three-dimensional (3D) CT imaging study, reporting that a glenoid defect with a width that is at least 21 % of the total glenoid length may materially affect recurrence after instability surgery. As a result, restoring the width of the glenoid may be beneficial in limiting recurrence. Other authors focused on the size of the Hill-Sachs lesions as a predictor of instability. Rowe et al. [39] classified Hill-Sachs lesions into three sizes and demonstrated that there was an increasing rate of recurrent dislocation with larger bone defects. Several authors have reported positive results of small case series in which patients with Hill-Sachs lesions greater than 20 % of the humeral head underwent reconstruction with allograft [40–42]. The confusion and continued debate in the literature regarding which bony lesions truly need to be addressed operatively laid the ground work for the critically important concept of the "glenoid track."

The Glenoid Track

Yamamoto et al. [24] introduced the concept of the "glenoid track" to determine which Hill-Sachs lesions have the potential to engage with the glenoid. Using cadaveric shoulders and 3D CT imaging, the authors demonstrated that as the arm is elevated, the glenoid contact area with the humeral head traveled from the inferomedial to the superolateral portion of the articular surface of the posterior humeral head, creating a zone of contact which the authors referred to as the "glenoid track." If the Hill-Sachs lesion falls lateral to the glenoid track, there is minimal likelihood of engagement. On the contrary, if the margin of a Hill-Sachs lesion falls medial to the glenoid track, there is significant risk that the humeral head will override the glenoid rim and engage. The authors computed that the width of the glenoid track (medial margin of the contact area to the medial margin of the rotator cuff attachment) is 84 % of the width of the glenoid. With glenoid bone loss, as the width of the glenoid track decreases, the probability that the Hill-Sachs lesion will fall medial to the "track" increases and thus "engagement" is more likely to occur. This concept has been very useful because the authors introduced the notion that not only the size of the Hill-Sachs lesion but also its location impacts engagement. Furthermore, the glenoid track concept highlights the interdependence of both glenoid and humeral bone loss in predicting recurrence. The width of the glenoid track and the size and location of the Hill-Sachs lesion are closely linked factors that need to be considered when addressing anterior instability.

All bipolar (glenoid and humerus) lesions can be considered "engaging," as the initial insult led to the glenoid rim-humeral contact necessary for the formation of bone loss. While Burkhart and DeBeer initially applied the term "engagement" to refer to the abduction and external rotation position, in truth, bone loss can only occur when the glenoid rim and humeral head contact. If the initial insult is repeated, bipolar lesions become increasingly more likely to engage. While dynamic intraoperative arthroscopic assessment of engagement is performed during Bankart repair, this diagnostic technique may lead to overestimation of whether a Hill-Sachs engages because concomitant ligament insufficiency is commonly present. Such laxity may permit excessive anterior translation or external rotation of the humeral head and facilitate engagement that would not be present when ligamentous integrity was present [27]. The prevalence of engaging Hill-Sachs lesions has been reported to be between 1.5 % [23] and 33 % [43]; however, the term "engagement" needs to be more precisely defined.

Further work by Kurokawa et al. using the glenoid track concept [25] sought to determine the prevalence of Hill-Sachs lesions that need to be addressed surgically. Using CT images, the authors observed that 7 % of 100 shoulders which demonstrated recurrent anterior instability had Hill-Sachs lesions that extended medially over the glenoid track. The authors divided the seven engaging lesions into two subtypes: a wide and large Hill-Sachs lesion (three cases) and a narrow but medially located Hill-Sachs lesion (four cases). This study supports the notion that not only the size of the Hill-Sachs lesion predicts engagement but also the medial extent of the lesion. All seven engaging Hill-Sachs lesions also demonstrated large (20 %) glenoid defects, supporting the increased risk of engagement from decreased width of the glenoid track secondary to the bony glenoid defect itself.

Arthroscopic Assessment of Glenoid Bone Loss

Glenoid bone loss can be measured directly arthroscopically by referencing the glenoid bare area, as first described by Burkhart et al. [44]. The etiology and development of the bare area are unclear, but it is thought that the bare area is a region of attenuated cartilage that arises due to repetitive stress loading over the subchondral tubercle of Assaki [45]. The normal glenoid is shaped like a pear; Burkhart measured the distance from the bare area to the anterior, posterior, and inferior glenoid margins in 56 patients without instability and found that the bare area was approximately equidistant from the anterior, posterior, and inferior margins. Since the majority of bone loss in anterior instability is anterior and inferior, the amount of bone loss can be calculated by factoring in the distance from the bare area to the posterior margin and assuming this distance is roughly the same from the bare area to the anterior rim in a normal shoulder.

Subsequent studies have questioned the utility of the bare area as a consistent reference point in glenoid bone loss determination. The main criticism of this technique is that the bare area is absent or eccentrically located in a large percentage of patients [31, 46]. Barcia et al. [47] recently showed that in a series of 52 patients undergoing arthroscopy without a diagnosis of instability, the bare area was present in only 48 % of patients. In patients in whom the bare area was found, it was centrally located in only 37 % [47]. Thus, an anterior bare area would lead to overestimation of bone loss and potential unnecessary glenoid augmentation procedures. Conversely, a posterior bare area would lead to underestimation of bone loss, and those patients may not undergo glenoid augmentation when it is indicated. Due to the limitation in intraoperative arthroscopic measurements, preoperative imaging is therefore required to accurately and reliably calculate glenoid bone loss.

Imaging Techniques

Radiographic Evaluation

The initial evaluation of shoulder instability should begin with a conventional radiograph series: a true anteroposterior (Grashey) view, internal and external rotation views, a scapular Y-view, an axillary lateral view, and an apical oblique (Garth) view [3]. These projections demonstrate the relationship of the humeral head to the glenoid and allow for assessment of bone defects, joint space narrowing, and osteophytes. Each projection plane offers unique information in the assessment of instability. The Garth view is optimal for evaluating bony Bankart fractures and Hill-Sachs lesions [30]. Additional views such as the West Point axillary and Stryker notch views may provide additional detail about the size of the bony Bankart and Hill-Sachs lesions, respectively. The West Point axillary view is designed to assess defects within the anterior-inferior glenoid rim [26]. The Stryker notch view, obtained by placing the hand on top of the head and X-ray beam angled 10° cephalad, can be used to evaluate the presence, size, and orientation of the Hill-Sachs lesion, as the internal rotation of the humeral head brings the defect into direct view [17]. Radiographic measurements are typically performed by measuring the defect or notch width and the depth with respect to a tangent line. Cross-sectional imaging has become increasingly popular in assessment, and its usefulness is discussed later in this chapter.

In many cases, additional cross-sectional imaging is required for a complete evaluation, as half of all bony lesions may be missed by conventional radiographs, and it is difficult to discern lesion size on plain films alone [48]. Therefore, those patients with a negative plain film evaluation, but a history and physical examination concerning for bony defects, should undergo additional cross-sectional imaging with either CT, MRI, or both, in order to accurately quantify bone loss. Arthrography should be used to increase the sensitivities of these examinations unless there is a contraindication to joint injection. Patients with evidence of glenoid boss loss on conventional radiographs will still benefit from additional cross-sectional imaging in order to better characterize the size, location, and extent of the bony lesion, as well as to evaluate for concomitant soft tissue injury such as rotator cuff tears and bicep tendon injuries, labrocartilaginous injuries, and capsuloligamentous disruptions [3].

Computed Tomography

CT imaging combined with 3D reformatting is a superior, noninvasive option for evaluating bone loss due to superb contrast between bone and soft tissues. The usefulness of CT scanning to define the morphological characteristics of glenoid defects and Hill-Sachs lesions and quantify the amount of bone loss has been well documented [2, 17, 49, 50]. Reasonable indications for CT scanning include multiple dislocations, bilateral shoulder dislocations, failed stabilization procedures, dislocations after trivial trauma with little or no provocation, radiographs or MRI demonstrating significant bone loss, and instability in midranges of motion [30].

As noted above, accurate assessment of glenohumeral bone loss is imperative in guiding surgical management. There are various methods to assess the size of the bony glenoid defect: defect length, width to length ratio, glenoid index (defect width/circle diameter), Pico method (defect area/circle area), and glenoid arc angle [27, 29, 51]. These measurements can all be performed after the acquisition of a standard CT scan of the shoulder. A standard shoulder CT protocol is performed with acquisition of both shoulders simultaneously in the axial plane, scanning from the superior aspect of the acromion to the inferior aspect of the glenoid fossa. The arm should be kept down in a neutral position. General parameters include field of view (FOV) 48 cm, pitch 0.9, collimation 1 mm, 120 kV, 200 mA (or dose modulation) with 1 mm image reconstruction. Image reformations are generated in the coronal oblique and sagittal oblique (with the glenoid en face) planes. In addition, 3D reconstructions should be created. After digital subtraction of the humeral head from the glenohumeral complex, the scapula and glenoid fossa can be optimally visualized as they are no longer obscured by the humerus, and glenoid bone loss can be precisely quantified. Due to the convention of CT imaging, the contralateral shoulder is imaged at no additional cost and can be used for comparison. In healthy subjects, there has been no significant difference in right-sided and left-sided glenoid measurements [49]. It is important to stress that thresholds for "critical" bone loss need to be determined specifically for the measurement technique being used.

Various techniques have been described to quantify glenoid bone loss, and the three most common techniques will be described. The "circle method" technique described by Sugaya et al. [51] computes the percentage of bone loss by evaluating the surface area of both the glenoid and the osseous fragment with the glenoid viewed en face. A "best-fit circle" can be drawn on the glenoid which estimates what the uninjured glenoid size would be and can be used to determine the size of the defect in order to guide management. Using specialized computer software, the surface area of the glenoid proper as well as the osseous fragment can be measured. The percent bone loss is calculated as the [surface area of the osseous fragment/surface area of the "true-fit" circle] × 100 %.

Another quantification of glenoid bone loss is based on glenoid rim distances. This technique can be used at arthroscopy, CT scan reformations, or 3D images in the sagittal oblique plane with the glenoid en face. The bare area is approximated on the glenoid fossa, and a "best-fit" circle is drawn by using the bare area approximation as the center. The glenoid is bisected along the longitudinal axis. A horizontal axis is then constructed perpendicular to the longitudinal axis. The distances of the anterior and posterior glenoid rims to the center are measured (Fig. 6.3). The percent bone loss is calculated: [distance from the posterior glenoid rim to center – distance from the anterior glenoid rim to center]/distance from the posterior glenoid rim to center × 2.

Nofsinger et al. [52] evaluated normal shoulders and defined the anatomic glenoid index (AGI), which supported the notion that the normal inferior glenoid is a near perfect circle and, in turn, validated methods of calculation that use a best-fit circle. Based on this premise, Dumont et al. [29] proposed an area-based determination of bone loss using the glenoid arc angle. Using the en face projection of the glenoid, a best-fit circle is drawn on the inferior aspect of the glenoid. An arc angle is constructed based on the area of bone loss along the anterior glenoid (Fig. 6.4). Using an established equation, the percentage area of glenoid defect = $[(\alpha - \sin(\alpha))/2\pi] \times 100$ %. Alternatively, a reference chart is available for conversion [29]. In this method, measurements require only a circle-shaped tool and angle measurement tool which are available on most imaging systems. An arc angle of 120° represents 19.6 % surface area bone loss, which can serve as a critical angle when using the arc angle method.

Though there are many studies that establish the usefulness of CT imaging for evaluating glenoid bone loss, the literature for the evaluation of Hill-Sachs lesion is considerably less voluminous. Accuracy of measuring Hill-Sachs lesions with CT by using 2D imaging has been established and is best calculated in axial and sagittal planes [53]. Hill-Sachs size is obtained by measuring the edge to edge width of the defect in order to obtain a length. A best-fit circle is created, and the depth is calculated by measuring

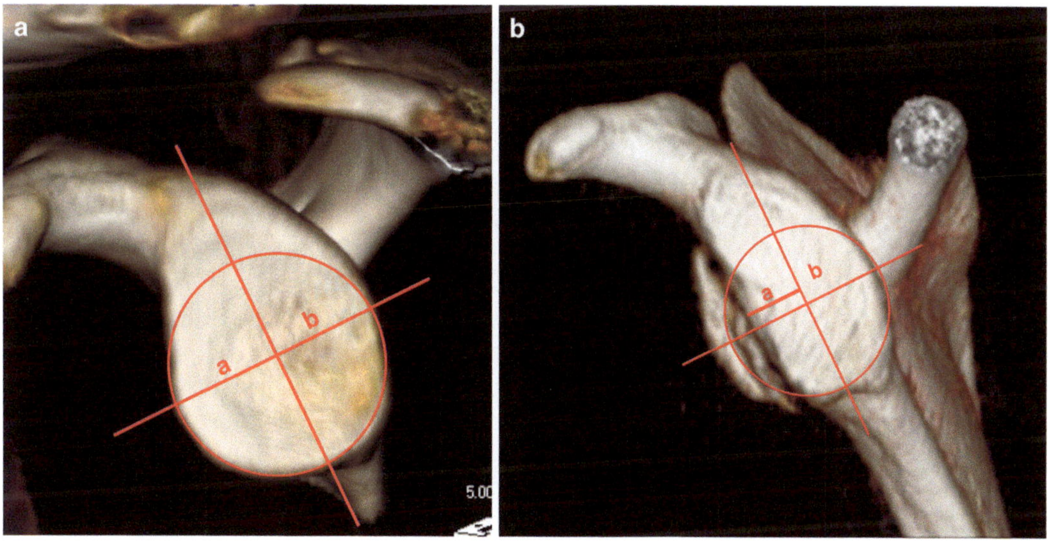

Fig. 6.3 Glenoid rim distances. (A) 3D CT sagittal oblique reformatted image with the glenoid en face of a normal shoulder. A best-fit circle is drawn within the inferior aspect of the glenoid. Based on the longitudinal and horizontal axes, the center to posterior rim (b) and center to anterior rim (a) can be estimated. (B) 3D CT sagittal oblique reformatted image of a 24-year-old man with recent shoulder dislocation and glenoid fracture. Percent bone loss is calculated as [b–a]/2b

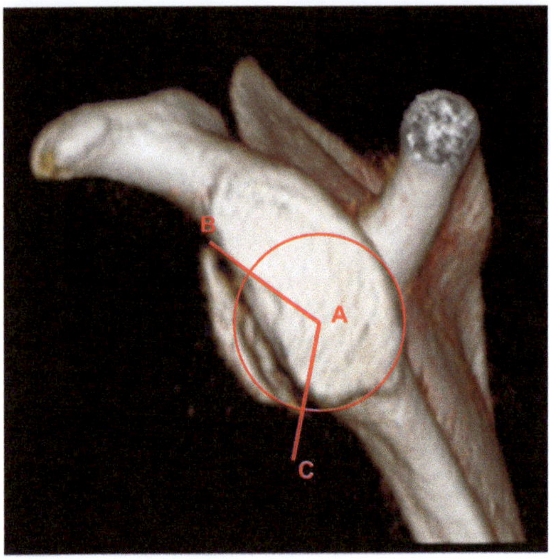

Fig. 6.4 Anatomic glenoid index (AGI). 3D CT reconstruction with the glenoid en face of a 24-year-old patient with large osseous Bankart lesion. The glenoid arc angle (BAC) can be used to determine the percentage of the glenoid surface area with bone loss

the distance from the circle to the deepest aspect of the defect. Cho et al. [43] retrospectively evaluated Hill-Sachs lesions in 104 shoulders on 3D CT imaging and compared measurements with findings of engagement on dynamic arthroscopic evaluation. The authors determined that engaging Hill-Sachs lesions were larger in size and more horizontally oriented to the humeral shaft compared with nonengaging lesions. The size of the lesion was measured on axial and coronal imaging and expressed as a percentage of the diameter of the humeral head, as measured by a best-fit circle. On 3D imaging, the orientation of the lesion can be assessed using a Hill-Sachs angle, which is the angle formed by the axis of the deepest groove of the Hill-Sachs lesion and the longitudinal axis of the humeral shaft. Thus, preoperative imaging may aid in depicting those humeral head lesions that should be addressed.

There are some inherent limitations to CT imaging. The plane of the CT image or the angle of the reconstructed image is important in assessing glenoid anatomy and is not always optimal. Reconstructions are usually made along the long axis of the scapular body. Curvature of the scapular body may lead to variability up to 10° from the true en face view, imposing a degree of measurement error. Measurements of bone fragments are prone to error if they are situated in a different plane from the glenoid fossa. In patients with chronic attritional bone loss or in cases of bone resorption, the size of the fragment may be underestimated [52]. Thus, the size of the glenoid deficiency can be inaccurate, particularly if the circle method measurement is used. In addition, measurements obtained at arthroscopy may be different compared with preoperative CT, as CT measurements are based on bone morphology solely and do not take into account labral integrity.

Finally, CT scans do subject patients to appreciable levels of ionizing radiation which may have future implications in the occurrence of thyroid and breast neoplasia.

Magnetic Resonance Imaging

Magnetic resonance imaging (MRI) with or without arthrography optimally evaluates the soft tissues of the shoulder, adding information on the status of the labroligamentous complex that is suboptimally evaluated by CT. Often, MRI and CT are concomitantly performed in order to optimally evaluate both the soft tissue and osseous structures. MRI of the shoulder is best performed with the patient in the supine position and with a proper shoulder coil. Three Tesla imaging is optimal. The MRI protocol should consist of imaging in the axial, coronal, and sagittal planes (with respect to the scapular body) with FOV of 12 × 12 cm, matrix 256 × 200, and slice thickness 2–3 mm without interslice gap.

MRI with arthrography has shown high sensitivity and specificity for the presence of labroligamentous injuries [54, 55]. More recently, MRI has played a promising role in the detection of glenoid bone defects [56, 57]. Huijsmans et al. [58] first demonstrated the accuracy of MRI in the estimation of glenoid bone loss. Their findings were further supported in a more recent cadaveric study by Gyftopoulos et al. [57], in which MRI was used to measure glenoid bone loss by means of the circle method and compared to measurements achieved using CT and 3D CT.

The authors concluded that MRI is an effective modality for calculating glenoid bone loss. However, accuracy greatly depends on the level of familiarity and experience with the circle technique. MRI can also be used to diagnose humeral head lesions. Hayes et al. [59] recently demonstrated high sensitivity (96.3 %) and specificity (90.6 %) of MRI in detecting Hill-Sachs lesions. Currently, MRI is considered superior for evaluation of soft tissue injury related to shoulder dislocation, but further refinements are needed in order to optimize MRI measurement techniques for glenohumeral bone deficiency in order to supplant the need for CT scanning, replete with the aforementioned radiation risks.

Impact on Management

Surgical intervention is usually indicated with significant glenoid bone loss, particularly in those patients who fail conservative treatment. Surgery is generally recommended to reestablish quality of life for patients who are young (<25–30 years of age) and highly athletic (especially overhead or contact athletes) and have had multiple episodes of instability. In addition, patients with an acute bony Bankart which comprises more than 25–30 % of the glenoid surface area may benefit from earlier operative bony repair [30]. For athletes with recurrent shoulder instability and small osseous lesions (<15 % glenoid bone loss), bone restoration of the glenoid is generally not essential, and these patients may be treated with soft tissue stabilization alone. While it is generally accepted that glenoid injuries with 25 % or more bone loss of the inferior glenoid diameter must be addressed by glenoid bone augmentation, no clear guidelines exist on how to address patients with bipolar lesions and varying degrees of glenohumeral bone loss [27]. The evolution of the glenoid track concept will likely lend innumerable insights regarding what constitutes critical bone loss. Our labs are endeavoring to create 3D MRI reconstructions which will afford the surgeon the ability to precisely quantify bone loss as well as predict engagement of head defects.

Future Directions

The importance of glenohumeral bone loss as an element of shoulder stability has been well established. A thorough evaluation to determine the percentage of glenoid bone loss as well as the location and size of the Hill-Sachs is critical. It is imperative to continue to improve preoperative imaging techniques in order to help predict which lesions will engage. The refinement of the glenoid track concept will clearly aid surgical decision making. In addition, further research and experience in MR imaging, including 3D reconstructions, is vital to expand its ability to accurately assess bone loss so that we can obviate the use of CT and avoid additional radiation.

References

1. Lippitt S, Matsen F. Mechanisms of glenohumeral joint stability. Clin Orthop Relat Res. 1993;291:20–8.
2. Skendzel JG, Sekiya JK. Diagnosis and management of humeral head bone loss in shoulder instability. Am J Sports Med. 2012;40(11):2633–44.
3. Bushnell BD, Creighton RA, Herring MM. Bony instability of the shoulder. Arthroscopy. 2008;24(9):1061–73.
4. Weisel SW. Operative techniques in orthopaedic surgery. vol. III, 1st ed. Lippincott Williams & Wilkins; 2012.
5. Panjabi MM. The stabilizing system of the spine. Part I. Function, dysfunction, adaptation, and enhancement. J Spinal Disord. 1992;5(4):383–9. discussion 397.
6. Howell SM, Galinat BJ. The glenoid-labral socket. A constrained articular surface. Clin Orthop Relat Res. 1989;243:122–5.
7. O'Connell PW, Nuber GW, Mileski RA, Lautenschlager E. The contribution of the glenohumeral ligaments to anterior stability of the shoulder joint. Am J Sports Med. 1990;18:579–84.
8. O'Brien SJ, Schwartz RS, Warren RF, Torzilli PA. Capsular restraints to anterior-posterior motion of the abducted shoulder: a biomechanical study. J Shoulder Elbow Surg. 1995;4:298–308.
9. McMahon PJ, Tibone JE, Cawley PW, et al. The anterior band of the inferior glenohumeral ligament: biomechanical properties from tensile testing in the position of apprehension. J Shoulder Elbow Surg. 1998;7:467–71.
10. Hess SA. Functional stability of the glenohumeral joint. Man Ther. 2000;5(2):63–71.
11. Labriola JE, Lee TQ, Debski RE, McMahon PJ. Stability and instability of the glenohumeral joint: the role of shoulder muscles. J Shoulder Elbow Surg. 2005;14(1 Suppl S):32S–8.

12. Wuelker N, Korell M, Thren K. Dynamic glenohumeral joint stability. J Shoulder Elbow Surg. 1998;7(1):43–52.
13. Gaskill TR, Taylor DC, Millett PJ. Management of multidirectional instability of the shoulder. J Am Acad Orthop Surg. 2011;19(12):758–67.
14. Kirkley A, Litchfield R, Thain L, Spouge A. Agreement between magnetic resonance imaging and arthroscopic evaluation of the shoulder joint in primary anterior dislocation of the shoulder. Clin J Sport Med. 2003;13: 148–51.
15. Good CR, MacGillivray JD. Traumatic shoulder dislocation in the adolescent athlete: advances in surgical treatment. Curr Opin Pediatr. 2005;17(1):25–9.
16. Horst K, Von Harten R, Weber C, Andruszkow H, Pfeifer R, Dienstknecht T, Pape HC. Assessment of coincidence and defect sizes in Bankart and Hill-Sachs lesions after anterior shoulder dislocation: a radiological study. Br J Radiol. 2014;87(1034):20130673.
17. Provencher MT, Frank RM, Leclere LE, Metzger PD, Ryu JJ, Bernhardson A, Romeo AA. The Hill-Sachs lesion: diagnosis, classification, and management. J Am Acad Orthop Surg. 2012;20(4):242–52.
18. Arciero RA, Wheeler JH, Ryan JB, et al. Arthroscopic Bankart repair versus nonoperative treatment for acute, initial anterior shoulder dislocation. Am J Sports Med. 1994;22:589–94.
19. Law BK, Yung PS, Ho EP, Chang JJ, Chan KM. The surgical outcome of immediate arthroscopic Bankart repair for first time anterior shoulder dislocation in young active patients. Knee Surg Sports Traumatol Arthrosc. 2008;16:188–93.
20. Flinkkila T, Hyvonen P, Ohtonen P, Leppilahti J. Arthroscopic Bankart repair: results and risk factors of recurrence of instability. Knee Surg Sports Traumatol Arthrosc. 2010;18:1752–8.
21. Ahmed I, Ashton F, Robinson CM. Arthroscopic Bankart repair and capsular shift for recurrent anterior shoulder instability: functional outcomes and identification of risk factors for recurrence. J Bone Joint Surg Am. 2012;94:1308–15.
22. Cicak N. Posterior dislocation of the shoulder. J Bone Joint Surg Br. 2004;86(3):324–32.
23. Saupe N, White LM, Bleakney R, Schweitzer ME, Recht MP, Jost B, Zanetti M. Acute traumatic posterior shoulder dislocation: MR findings. Radiology. 2008;248(1):185–93.
24. Yamamoto N, Itoi E, Hidekazu A, Minagawa H, Seki N, Shimada Y, Okada K. Contact between the glenoid and the humeral head in abduction, external rotation, and horizontal extension: a new concept of glenoid track. J Shoulder Elbow Surg. 2007;16(5):649–56.
25. Kurokawa D, Yamamoto N, Nagamoto H, Omori Y, Tanaka M, Sano H, Itoi E. The prevalence of a large Hill-Sachs lesion that needs to be treated. J Shoulder Elbow Surg. 2013;22(9):1285–9.
26. Lynch JR, Clinton JM, Dewing CB, Warme WJ, Matsen III FA. Treatment of osseous defects associated with anterior shoulder instability. J Shoulder Elbow Surg. 2009;18(2):317–28.
27. Di Giacomo G, Itoi E, Burkhart SS. Evolving concept of bipolar bone loss and the Hill-Sachs lesion: from "engaging/non-engaging" lesion to "on-track/off-track" lesion. Arthroscopy. 2014;30(1):90–8.
28. Balg F, Boileau P. The instability severity index score. A simple pre-operative score to select patients for arthroscopic or open shoulder stabilisation. J Bone Joint Surg Br. 2007;89(11):1470–7.
29. Dumont GD, Russell RD, Browne MG, Robertson WJ. Area-based determination of bone loss using the glenoid arc angle. Arthroscopy. 2012;28(7):1030–5.
30. Bhatia S, Ghodadra NS, Romeo AA, Bach BR, Verma NN, Vo ST, Provencher MT. The importance of the recognition and treatment of glenoid bone loss in an athletic population. Sports Health. 2011;3(5):435–40.
31. Huysmans PE, Haen PS, Kidd M, Dhert WJ, Willems JW. The shape of the inferior part of the glenoid: a cadaveric study. J Shoulder Elbow Surg. 2006;15:759–63.
32. Itoi E, Lee SB, Amrami KK, Wenger DE, An KN. Quantitative assessment of classic anteroinferior bony Bankart lesions by radiography and computed tomography. Am J Sports Med. 2003;31(1):112–8.
33. Bollier MJ, Arciero R. Management of glenoid and humeral bone loss. Sports Med Arthrosc. 2010; 18(3):140–8.
34. Sekiya JK, Wickwire AC, Stehle JH, Debski RE. Hill-Sachs defects and repair using osteoarticular allograft transplantation: biomechanical analysis using a joint compression model. Am J Sports Med. 2009;37: 2459–66.
35. Burkhart SS, De Beer JF. Traumatic glenohumeral bone defects and their relationship to failure of arthroscopic Bankart repairs: significance of the inverted-pear glenoid and the humeral engaging Hill-Sachs lesion. Arthroscopy. 2000;16(7):677–94.
36. Kralinger FS, Golser K, Wischatta R, Wambacher M, Sperner G. Predicting recurrence after primary anterior shoulder dislocation. Am J Sports Med. 2002;30: 116–20.
37. Voos JE, Livermore RW, Feeley BT, et al. Prospective evaluation of arthroscopic bankart repairs for anterior instability. Am J Sports Med. 2010;38:302–7.
38. Itoi E, Lee SB, Berglund L, Berge L, An KN. The effect of a glenoid defect on anteroinferior stability of the shoulder after bankart repair: a cadaveric study. J Bone Joint Surg. 2000;82A(1):35–46.
39. Rowe CR, Zarins B, Ciullo JV. Recurrent anterior dislocation of the shoulder after surgical repair. J Bone Joint Surg Am. 1984;66(2):159–63.
40. Buhler M, Gerber C. Shoulder instability related to epileptic seizures. J Bone Joint Surg. 2002;11(4):339–44.
41. Diklic ID, Ganic ZD, Blagojevic ZD, Nho SJ, Romeo AA. Treatment of locked chronic posterior dislocation of the shoulder by reconstruction of the defect in the humeral head with an allograft. J Bone Joint Surg Br. 2010;92(1):71–6.
42. Miniaci A, Gish MW. Management of anterior glenohumeral instability associated with large Hill–Sachs defects. Techniques Shoulder Elbow Surg. 2004;5(3):170–5.

43. Cho SH, Cho NS, Rhee YG. Preoperative analysis of the Hill-Sachs lesion in anterior shoulder instability: how to predict engagement of the lesion. Am J Sports Med. 2011;39(11):2389–95.
44. Burkhart SS, Debeer JF, Tehrany AM, Parten PM. Quantifying glenoid bone loss arthroscopically in shoulder instability. Arthrosc J Arthrosc Relat Surg. 2002;18:488–91.
45. Warner JJ, Bowen MK, Deng XH, Hannafin JA, Arnoczky SP, Warren RF. Articular contact patterns of the normal glenohumeral joint. J Shoulder Elbow Surg. 1998;7:381–8.
46. Kralinger F, Aigner F, Longato S, Rieger M, Wambacher M. Is the bare spot a consistent landmark for shoulder arthroscopy? A study of 20 embalmed glenoids with 3-dimensional computed tomographic reconstruction. Arthroscopy. 2006;22:428–32.
47. Barcia AM, Rowles DJ, Bottoni CR, Dekker TJ, Tokish JM. Glenoid bare area: arthroscopic characterization and its implications on measurement of bone loss. Arthrosc J Arthrosc Relat Surg. 2013;2:1671–5.
48. Bushnell BD, Creighton RA, Herring MM. The bony apprehension test for instability of the shoulder: a prospective pilot analysis. Arthroscopy. 2008;24(9):974–82.
49. Griffith JF, Antonio GE, Tong CW, Ming CK. Anterior shoulder dislocation: quantification of glenoid bone loss with CT. Am J Roentgenol. 2003;180(5):1423–30.
50. Griffith JF, Antonio GE, Yung PS, Wong EM, Yu AB, Ahuja AT, Chan KM. Prevalence, pattern, and spectrum of glenoid bone loss in anterior shoulder dislocation: CT analysis of 218 patients. Am J Roentgenol. 2008;190(5):1247–54.
51. Sugaya H, Moriishi J, Dohi M, Kon Y, Tsuchiya A. Glenoid rim morphology in recurrent anterior glenohumeral instability. J Bone Joint Surg Am. 2003;85A(5):878–84.
52. Nofsinger C, Browning B, Burkhart SS, Pedowitz RA. Objective preoperative measurement of anterior glenoid bone loss: a pilot study of a computer-based method using unilateral 3-dimensional computed tomography. Arthroscopy. 2011;27(3):322–9.
53. Kodali P, Jones MH, Polster J, Minaici A, Fening SD. Accuracy of measurement of Hill-Sachs lesion with computed tomography. J Shoulder Elbow Surg. 2011;20:1328–34.
54. Bencardino JT, Beltran J, Rosenberg ZS, Rokito A, Schmahmann S, Mota J, Mellado JM, Zuckerman J, Cuomo F, Rose D. Superior labrum anterior-posterior lesions: diagnosis with MR arthrography of the shoulder. Radiology. 2000;214(1):267–71.
55. Waldt S, Burkart A, Imhoff AB, Bruegel M, Rummeny EJ, Woertler K. Anterior shoulder instability: accuracy of MR arthrography in the classification of anteroinferior labroligamentous injuries. Radiology. 2005;237(2):578–83.
56. Probyn LJ, White LM, Salonen DC, Tomlinson G, Boynton EL. Recurrent symptoms after shoulder instability repair: direct MR arthrographic assessment--correlation with second-look surgical evaluation. Radiology. 2007;245(3):814–23.
57. Gyftopoulos S, Hasan S, Bencardino J, Mayo J, Nayyar S, Babb J, Jazrawi L. Diagnostic accuracy of MRI in the measurement of glenoid bone loss. Am J Roentgenol. 2012;199(4):873–8.
58. Huijsmans PE, Haen PS, Kidd M, Dhert WJ, Ven der Hulst V, Willems WJ. Quantification of a glenoid defect with three-dimensional computed tomography and magnetic resonance imaging: a cadaveric study. J Bone Joint Surg. 2007;16:803–9.
59. Hayes ML, Collins MS, Morgan JA, Wenger DE, Dahm DL. Efficacy of diagnostic magnetic resonance imaging for articular cartilage lesions of the glenohumeral joint in patients with instability. Skeletal Radiol. 2010;39:1199–204.

Management of Capsular Laxity

7

C. Edward Hoffler II , Fotios P. Tjoumakaris, and Luke Austin

Introduction

Glenohumeral instability is classified into static and dynamic subtypes [1]. In static instability, the humeral head is displaced at rest, and subluxation or dislocation is visible radiographically. Dynamic instability is labeled as unidirectional or multidirectional with or without hyperlaxity [1]. In both cases, capsular tension is deficient and may or may not be accompanied by labral injury. Instability related solely to capsular laxity can be described as multidirectional instability (MDI) with hyperlaxity. MDI has been estimated to occur in 5 % of glenohumeral instability patients [1]. Neer and Foster classified symptomatic capsular laxity as atraumatic multidirectional instability with involuntary inferior subluxation or dislocation associated with both anterior and posterior dislocations/subluxations of the shoulder [2]. Capsular laxity is not always equivalent with MDI. MDI has inconsistent definitions, which affects the reported incidence [1, 3–5].

Despite the confusion, capsular instability occurs when the glenohumeral joint capsule becomes so mechanically compromised that the remaining static and dynamic joint stabilizers cannot prevent symptomatic glenohumeral subluxation and/or dislocation. If the joint capsule and its contained glenohumeral ligaments are the only lax structures, then there is isolated capsular instability. Isolated capsular instability may result from the capsule experiencing repetitive microtrauma or may be from a single trauma, which stretches the glenohumeral ligaments, increasing the capsular volume and widening the rotator interval. By definition, these micro or macro traumatic events are not significant enough to create a frank labral tear, rotator cuff tear, or fracture. A generalized hyperlaxity secondary to a connective tissue disorder or focal glenohumeral hyperlaxity may be risk factors for capsular instability [2].

Capsular pathology may occur in the presence of other glenohumeral pathology and contribute to joint instability. The most common example is traumatic anteroinferior instability secondary to significant stretching of the inferior glenohumeral ligament with accompanied labral avulsion and/or a glenoid rim fracture. These combined pathologies are discussed in other chapters.

The glenohumeral joint is a highly mobile articulation capable of movement in multiple planes. There is minimal bony constraint, and

C.E. Hoffler II , PhD, MD
The Miami Hand and Upper Extremity Institute, Miami, FL, USA

F.P. Tjoumakaris, MD (✉)
Department of Orthopaedic Surgery, The Rothman Institute, Thomas Jefferson University Hospital, Egg Harbor Township, NJ, USA
e-mail: Fotios.tjoumakaris@rothmaninstitute.com

L. Austin, MD
Department of Orthopaedic Surgery, Thomas Jefferson University Hospital, Sewell, NJ, USA

J.D. Kelly IV (ed.), *Elite Techniques in Shoulder Arthroscopy*, DOI 10.1007/978-3-319-25103-5_7

stability is chiefly dictated by static and dynamic soft tissue structures. Static stabilizers include bony and soft tissue restraints. The glenoid has inherent osseous concavity covered with articular cartilage, which is slightly thicker at the periphery. The glenoid labrum improves the contact surface with the humeral head and provides 50 % of the total glenoid concavity depth, in addition to providing a "suction seal" to the joint [6–8].

Ligamentous restraints are primarily thickenings of the joint capsule and enhance stability at the extremes of motion as they become taut. The origin and insertion of the ligaments dictates the glenohumeral position in which they limit motion of the humeral head [9]. The superior glenohumeral ligament (SGHL) limits inferior translation in adduction. The SGHL also limits posterior translation in forward flexion, adduction, and internal rotation. The middle glenohumeral ligament (MGHL) limits external rotation in adduction and anterior/posterior translation in partial abduction and external rotation. The inferior glenohumeral ligament (IGHL) limits anterior, posterior, and inferior translation at 45–90° of elevation. The coracohumeral ligament does not significantly limit inferior humeral migration in the adducted position when the SGHL is intact. The coracohumeral ligament limits external rotation significantly and is likely compromised in higher degrees of anterior shoulder instability. Additional stabilizers include the coracoacromial ligament restraint to anterior and superior humeral head migration and the concavity compressive effect of the glenoid labrum and cartilage working in concert with the rotator cuff [3, 10].

Dynamic stability is conveyed by several muscles of the shoulder girdle. As discussed, the rotator cuff muscles, especially the supraspinatus, compress the humeral head into the glenoid. The subscapularis and teres minor are more predominantly humeral head depressors, yet they confer appreciable anterior and posterior glenohumeral stability respectively. In addition, the deltoid acts at 90° of elevation to compress the humeral head into the glenoid as well. The latissimus dorsi, teres major, and pectoralis major may also contribute to "concavity compression." The biceps tendon is a humeral head depressor of debated significance. However, the biceps does work synergistically with the IGHL in restricting external rotation [3, 11]. The rhomboids, serratus anterior, and other scapulothoracic muscles stabilize the scapula against the thorax, which allows the humeral head to articulate with a stable glenoid [12, 13].

Proper control of the scapulothoracic and glenohumeral musculature requires normal neuromuscular proprioceptive function. Several studies have identified abnormal shoulder girdle muscle function and glenohumeral kinetics in patients with atraumatic MDI. Barden and colleagues used an isokinetic dynamometer to demonstrate that neuromuscular dysfunction of the rotator cuff, posterior deltoid, and pectoralis major exists in shoulders with MDI [14]. Differential electromyographic deltoid activity between normal and MDI shoulders was found in a prior investigation by Morris et al. [15], but rotator cuff function was similar. Muscle dysfunction can lead to noncon-centric alignment of the humeral head on the glenoid. Three-dimensional magnetic resonance reconstructions of extended MDI shoulders demonstrated more posterior humeral head translation than normal controls [16].

No single structure is responsible for stability in all glenohumeral positions [8]. Depending on humeral abduction and translation, the capsular ligaments provide a significant percentage of the passive restraint to glenohumeral translation [17]. Therefore, addressing capsular laxity goes a long way in helping to address shoulder instability in symptomatic patients. The following chapter will discuss techniques to evaluate and effectively address capsular laxity in the unstable shoulder.

Evaluation

Most patients with symptomatic capsular laxity do not have a history of trauma and complain of activity-related pain. Athletes may admit to increasing weakness and declining performance. Multidirectional instability patients may have difficulty with activities of daily living and bilateral symptoms. Patients with more advanced symptoms may describe diffuse upper extremity paresthesias. The vague collection of symptoms can hamper early diagnosis. Clarifying which activities exacerbate symptoms and which shoulder positions are routinely avoided can be instructive. Functional limitations should be reviewed in detail. Repetitive overhead athletes have a higher prevalence of MDI. The presence of a connective tissue disorder also increases the risk of developing MDI. Younger patients, by virtue of increased tissue elasticity, are more at risk of MDI or unidirectional traumatic instability [18]. Patients approaching middle age are more likely to sustain rotator cuff tears and may not have the capsule as the primary source of their pain or subjective instability complaints. It is important to have patients clearly define their symptoms. Is the primary complaint pain, indicating rotator cuff overload, or is it painful subluxation and dislocation? For the former, is it strenuous use of the arm that precipitates symptoms? Routine use of the arm at the extremes of motion, such as reaching in the back seat of the car for an object while driving, may provoke instability related pain. In vague cases where the symptoms are less clear, a mild reduction in the velocity of a pitch or failure to "throw the deep ball" may be the first signs of an instability problem.

The physical examination, in addition to exploring instability, should also probe for other intrinsic shoulder disease, cervical pathology, and connective tissue disorders. Comparison with the contralateral side is mandatory. The shoulder examination begins with inspection, assessing symmetry, atrophy, and surgical incisions. Palpation should include at least the acromion, acromioclavicular joint, and bicipital groove. Range of motion, strength, and scapular coordination should be assessed. Positions of apprehension should be noted and confirmed with relocation tests. Diffuse capsular tenderness is not uncommon in these patients.

The load and shift test can be used to assess glenohumeral translation [18]. Passive glenohumeral abduction beyond 105° indicates laxity of the IGHL [19]. The jerk test is used to assess posterior instability [20]. The Kim test can be used to identify posteroinferior labral lesions, which may be a cause of instability [21]. Of note, both the

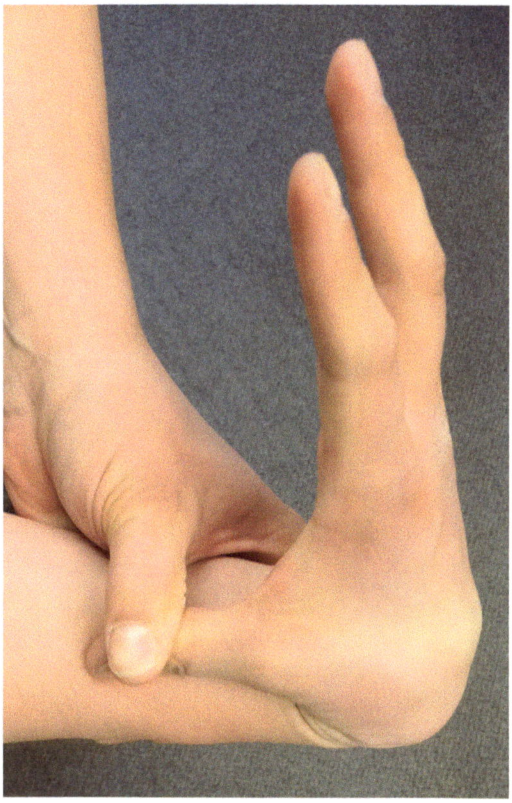

Fig. 7.1 Contact between the thumb and forearm during passive wrist flexion may indicate generalized ligamentous laxity

Jerk test and Kim test require pain on reduction to indicate associated labral tears.

Generalized ligamentous laxity should be evaluated by assessing elbow and knee hyperextension beyond 10°, passive little finger dorsiflexion beyond 90°, passive thumb contact on the forearm with wrist flexion (Fig. 7.1), forward trunk flexion such that palms rest easily on the floor [22], and the anterolateral acromial sulcus sign. Hypermobility can be scored from 0 to 9 using the Beighton scale [23], which has good-to-excellent interobserver reliability [24]. A sulcus sign greater than 2 cm that persists with external rotation may indicate laxity of SGH/CHL complex of the rotator interval in symptomatic patients [9, 10] (Fig. 7.2). Physical examination identifies laxity, which should not be confused with instability. The clinician must distinguish between multidirectional instability with or

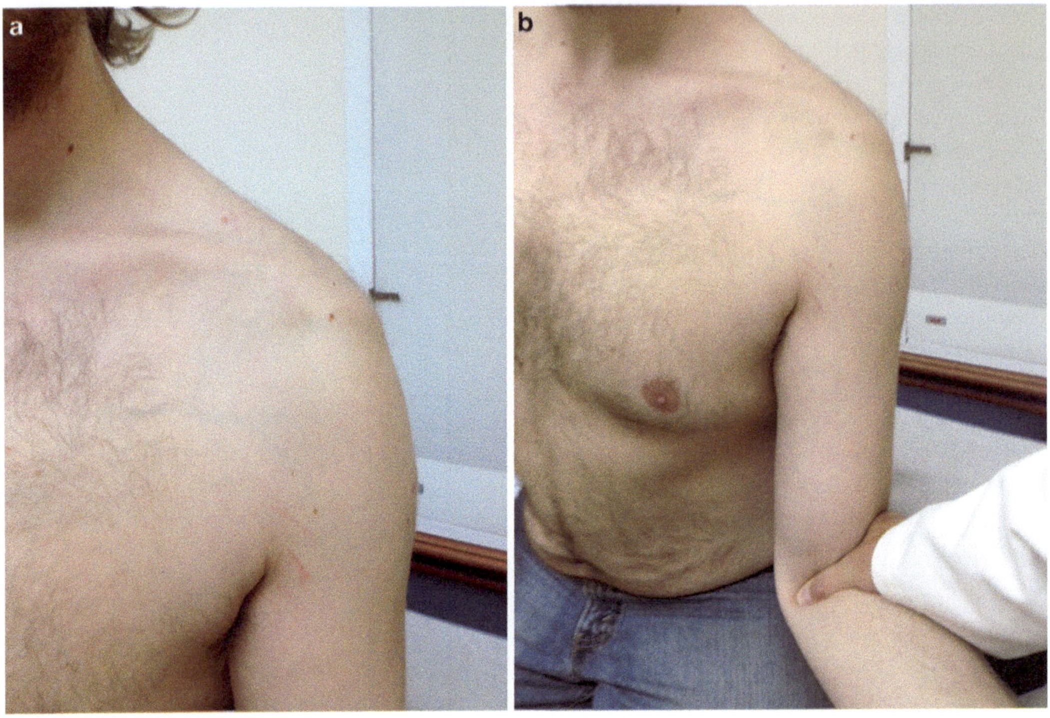

Fig. 7.2 (**a**) Sulcus sign. (**b**) Sulcus sign persisting in external rotation

without hyperlaxity, unidirectional instability with hyperlaxity, and glenohumeral hyperlaxity [4, 9, 18, 25]. The discerning feature for *instability* is provocation of symptoms.

Radiographic evaluation begins with plain radiographs. We routinely obtain internal and external rotation AP views, a scapular "Y" and an axillary view. Glenoid pathology may include bone loss, dysplasia with a shallow concavity, or abnormal version. The humeral head may have a posterolateral impaction fracture consistent with prior dislocations. Computed tomography is used to guide surgical planning or for diagnostic support when plain film bony detail is inadequate.

Magnetic resonance imaging or arthrography may be used to evaluate the glenohumeral soft tissue envelope. Its primary role is to rule out the presence of other pathology that may contribute to glenohumeral instability. Arthrography can distend the capsule and potentially improve visualization of the labrum, rotator interval, and capsular ligaments [26, 27]. While not diagnostic, a patulous glenohumeral capsule [5, 28, 29], increased glenohumeral volume, or labral pathology may be identified. Provencher and colleagues noted that rotator interval dimensions were the same in normal shoulders as well as those with anterior instability, posterior instability, or MDI [30]. Kim et al. did not study shoulders with MDI, but found increased rotator interval dimensions in patients with anterior instability [31]. Both investigators used MRA measurements to evaluate rotator interval widening as a pathologic feature of instability. However, Kuhn et al. did demonstrate that sectioning of the CHL increased external humeral rotation appreciably [32].

The evaluation of glenoid morphology in conjunction with the labrum should be taken into account. Relative glenoid hypoplasia or retroversion may contribute to posterior instability; in addition, the labrum contribution to version should be assessed. Chondrolabral retroversion can greatly contribute to posterior instability in the absence of bony deformity secondary to a blunted or atrophic posterior labrum [33].

Treatment Considerations

Glenohumeral instability occurs when the static and dynamic joint stabilizers cannot prevent symptomatic subluxation and/or dislocation. The objective of any rehabilitation, repair, or reconstruction is to impart sufficient stability to static and/or dynamic stabilizers to eliminate symptomatic subluxation and dislocation. The initial treatment of MDI patients is proprioceptive and strengthening physiotherapy. Rotator cuff strengthening and coordination may improve humeral head centering and compression while increasing resistance to subluxating shear forces. Scapulothoracic coordination may enhance glenoid positioning. Most investigators recommend a minimum of 6 months of physiotherapy before considering surgical management for symptomatic capsular laxity. When or if physical therapy fails, the majority of patients will respond favorably to arthroscopic capsular plication. It is imperative, however, that the patient is educated regarding the outcome of the procedure. A successful outcome typically results in a pain-free shoulder that has diminished range of motion or near normal when compared to the preoperative state. Patients that engage in overhead sports should be counseled that it may be difficult to continue that sport postoperatively due to loss of external rotation. Switching positions (for throwers) or modifying technique may be necessary in the absence of full cessation of overhead sports.

Rehabilitation

In their landmark study, Burkhead and Rockwood reported that muscle strengthening exercises yielded good or excellent results in 35 of 39 patients with MDI [34]. In contrast, Misamore et al. found that only 8 of 38 young athletic patients remained pain-free and instability-free after 8 years of follow-up [35]. There are also reports that shoulder kinematics and electromyographic function return to normalcy more closely in patients treated with capsular shift and physiotherapy when compared to physiotherapy alone [36, 37]. Despite these findings, the possibility of successful symptomatic management followed by a maintenance program remains attractive as it may obviate the need for surgical intervention.

Arthroscopic Techniques for Capsular Instability

Improvements in arthroscopic techniques and instrumentation have advanced arthroscopic procedures as the dominant modality to address MDI and capsular laxity. When compared with open treatment, arthroscopy offers the advantages of improved visualization and direct confirmation of capsular laxity or other glenohumeral pathology. There is decreased surgical morbidity as the subscapularis need not be compromised. Also, anterior and posterior pathology can be addressed through the same approach. Whether treatment is open or arthroscopic, an examination under anesthesia (EUA) is mandatory as a final preoperative assessment. The magnitudes and directions of glenohumeral translation are established. Cofield and colleagues reported 100 % sensitivity and 93 % specificity in diagnosing shoulder instability-based intraoperative EUA comparing the surgical and normal sides [38]. It should be noted, however, that other studies have demonstrated a consistent ability to subluxate the humeral head over the glenoid rim under anesthesia in patients without a diagnosis of instability [39]. It is paramount, therefore, that correlation to the patient's history, examination findings both under and out of anesthesia, and imaging findings are used concurrently to arrive at an accurate diagnosis.

The earliest technique described for arthroscopic management of capsular instability was a glenoid-based inferior capsular shift, which was conceptually similar to the humerus-based open inferior shifts [40]. Capsular plication and capsulolabral augmentation (capsular plication which incorporates the labrum) were introduced later [41, 42]. The common threads of all surgical techniques for decreasing capsular instability are shortening and reinforcing the capsule while reducing capsular volume [2]. Several cadaveric models have sought to demonstrate changes in capsular volume with specific surgical techniques. Wiater and coworkers reported that progressive humerus-based open inferior capsular shifts decreased capsular volume in a linear fashion [43]. Lubowitz et al. also demonstrated decreased capsular volume with open inferior shift, but the amount of change varied when measured with MRI, ultrasound, and saline injection [44].

Several investigators have quantified capsular volume reduction in cadaveric models. Flanigan and coworkers reported that 10 mm of capsular plication decreased capsular volume by 33.7 % [45]. Volume can be reduced incrementally with sequential plications. Karas and colleagues found that four capsulolabral plications from 4 to 8 o'clock decreased capsular volume 19 % [46]. Incremental capsular plication has also been shown to reduce capsular volume but in a nonlinear fashion [47]. After 4 cm of total plication, additional plication becomes less effective. Volume reduction was not affected by the use of suture anchors or suture alone [47]. Suture anchor-based capsular plication has been demonstrated to reduce capsular volume at least as well as traditional open capsular shift techniques in cadavers [48].

Capsulolabral augmentation involves incorporating intact labrum into the plication. It has analogous effects on the capsule, but is also hypothesized to enhance stability via increased glenoid depth and labral width. Cadaveric models demonstrate decreased humeral head displacement following capsulolabral augmentation [41].

Inferior Shift

Arthroscopic glenoid-based inferior capsular shifts secured to the glenoid via a bone anchor have been described by several authors [40, 49]. In one series of 25 patients, 3 had recurrent instability at an average 5-year follow-up [40, 49]. Fleega and El Shewey described an arthroscopic inferior shift technique for isolated anteroinferior capsular instability with lower recurrence [50]. At a minimum of 7 years follow-up, 3 of the 75 patients had dislocations after significant trauma.

Capsular Plication and Capsulolabral Augmentation

Successful capsular plication for patients with multidirectional instability and capsular redundancy has been reported by Wichman [42], and Whitehurst [51]. Gartsman and colleagues described a similar technique, but his patients did not have isolated capsular instability [52]. In 47 shoulders, 28 labral tears requiring repair were identified. When treating traumatic or atraumatic instability in two directions in the absence of structural lesions, arthroscopic capsular plication and open capsular shift have comparable recurrent instability, return to sport, loss of external rotation, and complications [53].

Baker et al. described an approach for young athletic patients, where each direction of instability was addressed sequentially. Shoulders with isolated patulous capsules received capsulolabral plication with or without suture anchors. All patients with labral tears received a capsulolabral plication with suture anchors. Two patients had failures based on low ASES score (American Shoulder and Elbow Surgeons standardized shoulder assessment score). Two more had failures based on WOSI scores (University of Western Ontario shoulder instability index percentage) [54]. It is not clear if the failures had isolated capsular or capsulolabral pathology.

Ma and colleagues reported on 23 overhead athletes with multidirectional instability and isolated capsular laxity who were treated with pancapsular plication and interval closure. At a minimum 2-year follow-up, all patients were satisfied with stability, but only five returned to the same level of competitive sport [28].

Capsulolabral augmentation with suture anchors has been shown to be at least as strong and as stiff as using suture alone [55, 56]. While capsulolabral repair is distinct from capsulolabral augmentation, many of the repair techniques, like the multiple pleated plication method [57], can easily be adapted for augmentation.

Interval Closure

Since Harryman and colleagues demonstrated that imbrication of the rotator interval capsule increased resistance to posterior and inferior humeral translation in an open surgery cadaveric model [58], investigators have debated the clinical importance of interval closure in glenohumeral instability. An arthroscopic cadaveric model suggested that interval closure reduces anterior humeral translation and external rotation at 90° of abduction [59], but the impact on stability in other directions is unclear. Furthermore, the preponderance of arthroscopic studies employs a "north-south" interval closure which does not mimic the "east-west" course of the CHL. Gartsman recommended interval closure if laxity remained after arthroscopic capsular shift [52]. Several arthroscopic techniques for interval closure have been described [60–63]. Almazan and coworkers suggested that interval closure may address laxity created by the placement of arthroscopic cannulas during capsular plication or labral repair surgery [60]. While no clear clinical benefit has been demonstrated, some investigators believe interval closure may be appropriate when capsular plication does not produce adequate stability in MDI patients [28, 54]. Similar to plication, interval closure can result in loss of external rotation [59]. The closure should be tensioned with the humerus in 30° of external rotation to minimize loss of motion.

Thermal Capsulorrhaphy

Thermal capsulorrhaphy offered the possibility of speed, simplicity, and direct visual assessment of capsular shrinkage. Early reports suggested that it was viable alternative to capsular shift techniques [29, 64], but long-term results were plagued by chondrolysis, thermal nerve injury, and high rates of recurrent instability [65–68]. We mention this technique for historical completeness, but it is not recommended for the treatment of MDI.

Author's Preferred Technique

A preoperative interscalene anesthetic block is used for analgesia and muscle relaxation. In addition, we use general endotracheal anesthesia for definitive airway control because patients are placed in the lateral decubitus position. The lateral decubitus position affords greatly enhanced access to the inferior and posterior joint recesses.

We employ a systemic sequential approach, similar to that described by Bradley [54]. All patients receive an EUA, and directions and magnitudes of humeral head translation are recorded. We prefer the lateral decubitus position with an upper extremity traction boom for glenohumeral instability procedures. Lateral decubitus position is maintained with a bean bag. An axillary roll is placed to improve thoracic excursion and to relieve pressure on the brachial plexus and axillary neurovascular structures. All nonoperative extremities are padded to protect bony prominences and superficial nerves. The traction boom is attached anterior to the patient at the foot of the operating table. The arm covered with a stockinette that has a distal strap to connect with the traction boom. We usually apply 15 lbs of in-line traction. The shoulder is placed in slight flexion (20–30°) and abduction (45°), which helps to open the posterior capsule and axillary recess respectively (Fig. 7.3). Diagnostic arthroscopy identifies redundant capsule, labral abnormalities, and any other intra-articular pathology. For the majority of patients, a balanced plication is in order. The shoulder joint appearance also lends clues to principal directions of instability. Labral fraying, fissuring, and chondral changes of the glenoid and humerus indicate directions of increased translations. In essence, a surgical goal is to effect a balanced plication with the humeral head resting in a neutral position with traction released. Based on the degree of sulcus sign, the rotator interval is closed in a medial to lateral direction (to effectively shorten the CHL) if the sulcus sign does not diminish with external rotation. Prior to plication, the IGHL, posterior band of the IGHL, and capsule are gently debrided

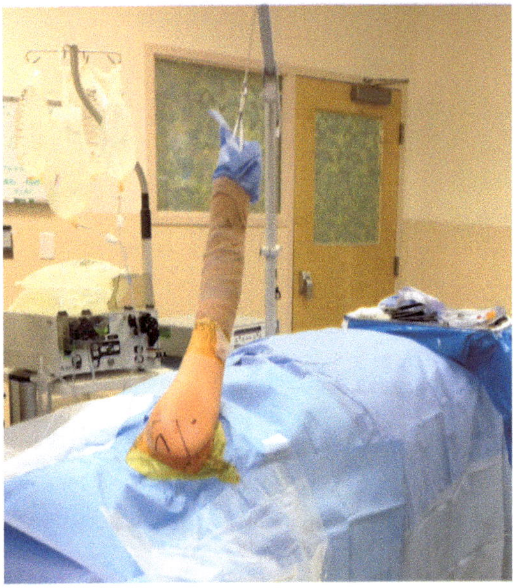

Fig. 7.3 Lateral decubitus position with traction boom placed anteriorly at the foot of the operating table. Shoulder is abducted 45° and forward flexed 20°. The posterior superior shoulder is visible and the surface anatomy has been marked

with an arthroscopic rasp to promote healing. Plication begins in the direction of the largest translation. Gerber et al. have demonstrated predictable patterns of motion decrease with selective glenohumeral capsule plication in cadavers [69]. We typically begin inferior and work superior, since each plication decreases capsular volume and working space. This avoids the inconvenience of working in the distant inferior pouch through a narrow superior glenohumeral interval. We prefer to secure the capsular plication with suture anchors to prevent loosening of the plication in patients who may not be as compliant postoperatively. If possible, two working portals are usually established for the arthroscopic technique. The less puncture holes that are placed in the glenohumeral joint capsule for working, the better able we are to restore capsular stability. The anterior portal and 7 mm cannula are placed in the rotator interval, while the posterior portal and cannula are placed in line with the lateral edge of the acromion at the level of the posterior "soft spot" to facilitate anchor placement along the posterior glenoid rim.

The labrum is only gently debrided and single-threaded anchors (typically size 2.3 mm) are placed along the glenoid margin with nonabsorbable #2 suture. The sutures are shuttled through the capsule and labrum using a suture hook shuttle device and tied down individually after passage (Fig. 7.4). Each suture limb can be passed multiple times for a pleated plication to titrate the repair based on the degree of laxity as described by Sekiya (45°). After each stage of plication is complete, a repeat EUA is performed to confirm adequate stability in the treated direction and to determine the direction of maximum residual stability. For patients with primarily posterior and global laxity, the posterior portal is closed using standard suture passage techniques with the cannula backed just beyond the capsule. For those patients with significant rotator interval laxity (as described prior), the rotator interval portal is closed instead. The goal of capsular plication is to restore glenohumeral alignment and prevent subluxation of the humeral head beyond the glenoid margin. This must be confirmed before completing the procedure. Aggressive plication can result in a preferential loss of external rotation.

Postoperative Management

The rehabilitation protocol following arthroscopic management of MDI must be tailored to the directions of instability and the quality of the stabilization procedure. Following stabilization, we routinely place patients in an abduction sling for 4 weeks. Pendulum exercises are begun at 2 weeks along with active wrist and elbow motion. A passive range of motion protocol is initiated at 4 weeks and continued until near full range of motion is achieved. Active-assisted range of motion is initiated at 6 weeks, and full active motion of the shoulder is advanced by 6–8 weeks. Gentle strengthening begins at 10 weeks or when 80 % of range of motion has been attained. For athletes, sport-specific training begins at 4 months. We restrict full participation in sports until nearly 80 % of strength has been achieved with near-normal glenohumeral range of motion.

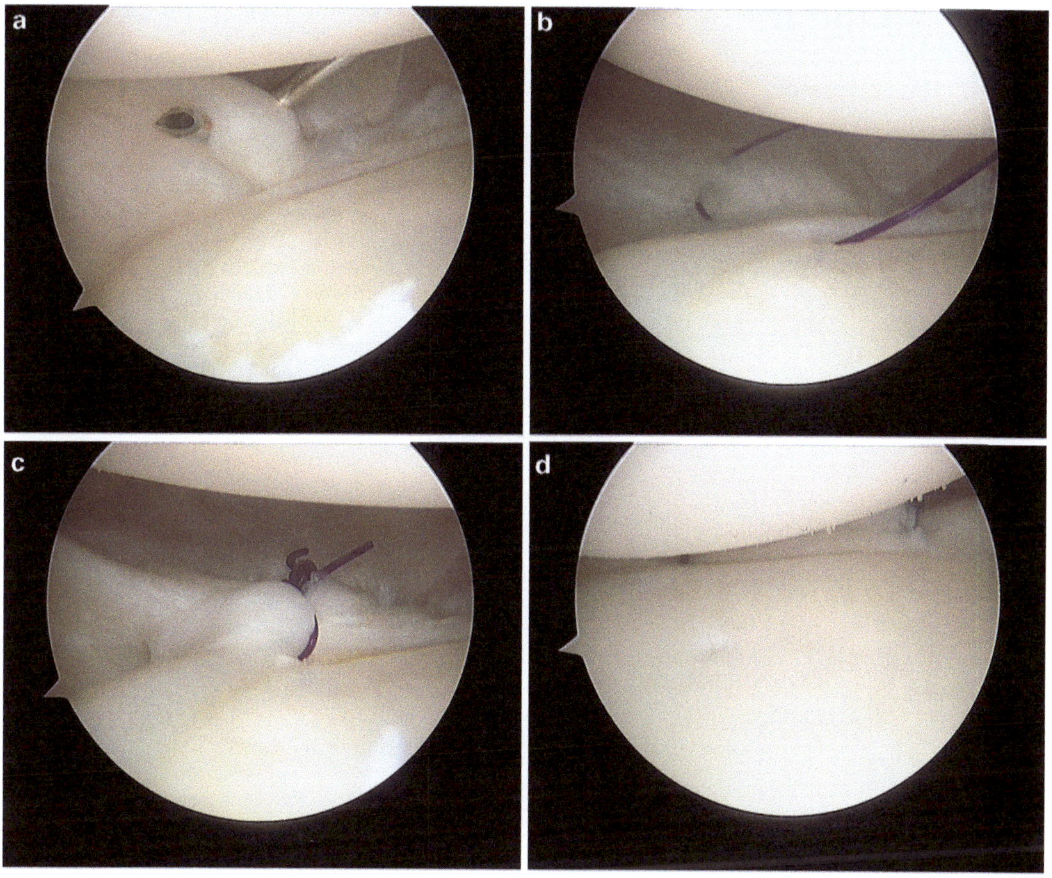

Fig. 7.4 (**a**) Suture hook through inferior glenohumeral ligament. (**b**) PDS plication stitch through inferior glenohumeral ligament and labrum. (**c**) Capsulolabral plication. (**d**) Two anterior capsulolabral plication sutures with humeral head reduced to glenoid fossa

Complications

Recurrent instability following arthroscopic management of capsular instability has been reported to be 0–21 % [28, 42, 49, 53, 54, 70]. These studies are challenging to interpret as they include some patients with unidirectional capsular instability [42] and labral lesions requiring repair [54]. The surgical techniques also vary. Treacy and colleagues [49] described a glenoid-based inferior shift secured through a transglenoid tunnel, while Hewitt et al. [70] and Ma et al. [28] used a capsular plication secured around the labrum with suture only. Treacy [49] and Ma [28] routinely closed the rotator interval, while Hewitt [70] reserved closure for patients with a persistent sulcus following stabilization. Treacy [49] reported 2 failures of 11 patients with 60 months follow-up. Hewitt [70] had 3 recurrent instabilities in 30 shoulders with follow-up of 57 months. Ma's [28] series reported that they did not have recurrent instability in 23 patients with 36 months of follow-up. Of these five collective episodes of recurrent instability, four were traumatic and one patient had previous surgery. While these are not large samples, the data suggest that trauma is the major risk factor for recurrent instability.

Ma et al. did not find any difference in pre- and postoperative external rotation following arthroscopic stabilization with capsulolabral augmentation and interval closure in athletes [28].

However, the group of patient who returned to sport averaged 10° more of preoperative external rotation. This difference was not compared statistically. Treacy and colleagues [49] reported that no patients lost external rotation. Hewitt [70] found a mean loss of 8.5°.

No neurologic or postoperative complications were reported [28, 70]. Treacy noted similar results with the exception of two patients who had their posterior suture knot removed for persistent pain [49].

Summary

Diagnosing capsular instability can be challenging. A careful history and examination are aimed at distinguishing multidirectional instability with or without hyperlaxity, unidirectional instability with hyperlaxity, and glenohumeral hyperlaxity. Plain radiographs and MR arthrography are primarily used to rule out causes other than capsular laxity for glenohumeral instability. Rehabilitation may be successful and is the mainstay of nonoperative treatment, especially in patients who do not sustain significant trauma. Essentially physiotherapy only improves symptoms in a small fraction of athletes and does not recreate kinematics or muscle function in the absence of surgical stabilization. Arthroscopy offers improved visualization when compared with open treatment and allows direct confirmation of capsular laxity or other glenohumeral pathology. All arthroscopic techniques for decreasing capsular instability shorten and reinforce the capsule while decreasing capsular volume. EUA is mandatory to document preoperative laxity and confirm postoperative stability. Rehabilitation following arthroscopic management of capsular instability is dictated by the directions of instability and the quality of the repair. Sport-specific training usually begins 4 months postoperatively. Postoperative trauma is a major risk factor for failed arthroscopic instability surgery. While recurrent instability is a significant concern, the surgeon must avoid overzealous stabilization, which may result in unacceptable postoperative stiffness and loss of function.

References

1. Gerber C, Nyffeler RW. Classification of glenohumeral joint instability. Clin Orthop Relat Res. 2002;400:65–76. Available at: http://eutils.ncbi.nlm.nih.gov/entrez/eutils/elink.fcgi?dbfrom=pubmed&id=12072747&retmode=ref&cmd=prlinks.
2. Neer CS. Involuntary inferior and multidirectional instability of the shoulder: etiology, recognition, and treatment. Instr Course Lect. 1985;34:232–8.
3. Matsen FA, Chebli C, Lippitt S, American Academy of Orthopaedic Surgeons. Principles for the evaluation and management of shoulder instability. J Bone Joint Surg Am. 2006;88(3):647–59.
4. McFarland EG, Kim TK, Park HB, Neira CA, Gutierrez MI. The effect of variation in definition on the diagnosis of multidirectional instability of the shoulder. J Bone Joint Surg Am. 2003;85-A(11):2138–44.
5. Neer CS, Foster CR. Inferior capsular shift for involuntary inferior and multidirectional instability of the shoulder. A preliminary report. J Bone Joint Surg Am. 1980;62(6):897–908.
6. Howell SM, Galinat BJ. The glenoid-labral socket. A constrained articular surface. Clin Orthop Relat Res. 1989;243:122–5.
7. Lippitt S, Matsen F. Mechanisms of glenohumeral joint stability. Clin Orthop Relat Res. 1993;291:20–8.
8. Curl LA, Warren RF. Glenohumeral joint stability. Selective cutting studies on the static capsular restraints. Clin Orthop Relat Res. 1996;330:54–65.
9. Bahk M, Keyurapan E, Tasaki A, Sauers EL, McFarland EG. Laxity testing of the shoulder: a review. Am J Sports Med. 2006;35(1):131–44. doi:10.1177/0363546506294570.
10. Warner JJ, Deng XH, Warren RF, Torzilli PA. Static capsuloligamentous restraints to superior-inferior translation of the glenohumeral joint. Am J Sports Med. 1992;20(6):675–85.
11. Rodosky MW, Harner CD, Fu FH. The role of the long head of the biceps muscle and superior glenoid labrum in anterior stability of the shoulder. Am J Sports Med. 1994;22(1):121–30.
12. Veeger HEJ, van der Helm FCT. Shoulder function: the perfect compromise between mobility and stability. J Biomech. 2007;40(10):2119–29. doi:10.1016/j.jbiomech.2006.10.016.
13. Labriola JE, Lee TQ, Debski RE, McMahon PJ. Stability and instability of the glenohumeral joint: the role of shoulder muscles. J Shoulder Elbow Surg. 2005;14(1):S32–8. doi:10.1016/j.jse.2004.09.014.
14. Barden JM, Balyk R, Raso VJ, Moreau M, Bagnall K. Atypical shoulder muscle activation in multidirectional instability. Clin Neurophysiol. 2005;116(8):1846–57. doi:10.1016/j.clinph.2005.04.019.
15. Morris AD, Kemp GJ, Frostick SP. Shoulder electromyography in multidirectional instability. J Shoulder

Elbow Surg. 2004;13(1):24–9. doi:10.1016/S1058274603002489.
16. Inui H, Sugamoto K, Miyamoto T, et al. Three-dimensional relationship of the glenohumeral joint in the elevated position in shoulders with multidirectional instability. J Shoulder Elbow Surg. 2002; 11(5):510–5. doi:10.1067/mse.2002.126768.
17. Debski RE, Sakone M, Woo SL, Wong EK, Fu FH, Warner JJ. Contribution of the passive properties of the rotator cuff to glenohumeral stability during anterior-posterior loading. J Shoulder Elbow Surg. 1999;8(4):324–9.
18. Silliman JF, Hawkins RJ. Classification and physical diagnosis of instability of the shoulder. Clin Orthop Relat Res. 1993;291:7–19.
19. Gagey OJ, Gagey N. The hyperabduction test. J Bone Joint Surg Br. 2001;83(1):69–74.
20. Matsen FA, Harryman DT, Sidles JA. Mechanics of glenohumeral instability. Clin Sports Med. 1991;10(4):783–8.
21. Kim SH, Park J-S, Jeong W-K, Shin S-K. The Kim test: a novel test for posteroinferior labral lesion of the shoulder–a comparison to the Jerk test. Am J Sports Med. 2005;33(8):1188–92. doi:10.1177/0363546504272687.
22. Beighton P, Horan F. Orthopaedic aspects of the Ehlers-Danlos syndrome. J Bone Joint Surg Br. 1969;51(3):444–53.
23. Beighton P, Solomon L, Soskolne CL. Articular mobility in an African population. Ann Rheum Dis. 1973;32(5):413–8.
24. Juul-Kristensen B, Røgind H, Jensen DV, Remvig L. Inter-examiner reproducibility of tests and criteria for generalized joint hypermobility and benign joint hypermobility syndrome. Rheumatology. 2007;46(12):1835–41. doi:10.1093/rheumatology/kem290.
25. Wilk KE, Andrews JR, Arrigo CA. The physical examination of the glenohumeral joint: emphasis on the stabilizing structures. J Orthop Sports Phys Ther. 1997;25(6):380–9. doi:10.2519/jospt.1997.25.6.380.
26. Lee JC, Guy S, Connell D, Saifuddin A, Lambert S. MRI of the rotator interval of the shoulder. Clin Radiol. 2007;62(5):416–23. doi:10.1016/j.crad.2006.11.017.
27. Nobuhara K, Ikeda H. Rotator interval lesion. Clin Orthop Relat Res. 1987;223:44–50.
28. Ma H-L, Huang H-K, Chiang E-R, Wang S-T, Hung S-C, Liu C-L. Arthroscopic pancapsular plication for multidirectional shoulder instability in overhead athletes. Orthopedics. 2012;35(4):e497–502. doi:10.3928/01477447-20120327-15.
29. Savoie FH, Field LD. Thermal versus suture treatment of symptomatic capsular laxity. Clin Sports Med. 2000;19(1):63–75. vi.
30. Provencher MT, Dewing CB, Bell SJ, et al. An analysis of the rotator interval in patients with anterior, posterior, and multidirectional shoulder instability. Arthroscopy. 2008;24(8):921–9. doi:10.1016/j.arthro.2008.03.005.
31. Kim K-C. Estimating the dimensions of the rotator interval with use of magnetic resonance arthrography. J Bone Joint Surg Am. 2007;89(11):2450. doi:10.2106/JBJS.F.01262.
32. Kuhn JE, Bey MJ, Huston LJ, Blasier RB, Soslowsky LJ. Ligamentous restraints to external rotation of the humerus in the late-cocking phase of throwing. A cadaveric biomechanical investigation. Am J Sports Med. 2000;28(2):200–5.
33. Kim S-H, Noh K-C, Park J-S, Ryu B-D, Oh I. Loss of chondrolabral containment of the glenohumeral joint in atraumatic posteroinferior multidirectional instability. J Bone Joint Surg Am. 2005;87(1):92–8. doi:10.2106/JBJS.C.01448.
34. Burkhead WZ, Rockwood CA. Treatment of instability of the shoulder with an exercise program. J Bone Joint Surg Am. 1992;74(6):890–6.
35. Misamore GW, Sallay PI, Didelot W. A longitudinal study of patients with multidirectional instability of the shoulder with seven- to ten-year follow-up. J Shoulder Elbow Surg. 2005;14(5):466–70. doi:10.1016/j.jse.2004.11.006.
36. Illyés A, Kiss J, Kiss RM. Electromyographic analysis during pull, forward punch, elevation and overhead throw after conservative treatment or capsular shift at patient with multidirectional shoulder joint instability. J Electromyogr Kinesiol. 2009;19(6):e438–47. doi:10.1016/j.jelekin.2008.09.008.
37. Nyiri P, Illyés A, Kiss R, Kiss J. Intermediate biomechanical analysis of the effect of physiotherapy only compared with capsular shift and physiotherapy in multidirectional shoulder instability. J Shoulder Elbow Surg. 2010;19(6):802–13. doi:10.1016/j.jse.2010.05.008.
38. Cofield RH, Nessler JP, Weinstabl R. Diagnosis of shoulder instability by examination under anesthesia. Clin Orthop Relat Res. 1993;291:45–53.
39. Jia X. An analysis of shoulder laxity in patients undergoing shoulder surgery. J Bone Joint Surg Am. 2009;91(9):2144. doi:10.2106/JBJS.H.00744.
40. McIntyre LF, Caspari RB, Savoie FH. The arthroscopic treatment of multidirectional shoulder instability: two-year results of a multiple suture technique. Arthroscopy. 1997;13(4):418–25.
41. Metcalf MH, Pon JD, Harryman II DT, Loutzenheiser T, Sidles JA. Capsulolabral augmentation increases glenohumeral stability in the cadaver shoulder. J Shoulder Elbow Surg. 2001;10(6):532–8. doi:10.1067/mse.2001.118411.
42. Wichman MT, Snyder SJ. Arthroscopic capsular plication for multidirectional instability of the shoulder. Oper Techniques Sports Med. 1997;5(4):238–43.
43. Wiater JM, Vibert BT. Glenohumeral joint volume reduction with progressive release and shifting of the inferior shoulder capsule. J Shoulder Elbow Surg. 2007;16(6):810–4. doi:10.1016/j.jse.2007.02.117.
44. Lubowitz J, Bartolozzi A, Rubinstein D, et al. How much does inferior capsular shift reduce shoulder volume? Clin Orthop Relat Res. 2004;328:86–90.

45. Flanigan DC, Forsythe T, Orwin J, Kaplan L. Volume analysis of arthroscopic capsular shift. Arthroscopy. 2006;22(5):528–33. doi:10.1016/j.arthro.2006.01.010.
46. Karas SG, Creighton RA, DeMorat GJ. Glenohumeral volume reduction in arthroscopic shoulder reconstruction: a cadaveric analysis of suture plication and thermal capsulorrhaphy. Arthroscopy. 2004;20(2):179–84. doi:10.1016/j.arthro.2003.11.004.
47. Ponce BA, Rosenzweig SD, Thompson KJ, Tokish J. Sequential volume reduction with capsular plications: relationship between cumulative size of plications and volumetric reduction for multidirectional instability of the shoulder. Am J Sports Med. 2011;39(3): 526–31. doi:10.1177/0363546510391634.
48. Sekiya JK, Willobee JA, Miller MD, Hickman AJ, Willobee A. Arthroscopic multi-pleated capsular plication compared with open inferior capsular shift for reduction of shoulder volume in a cadaveric model. Arthroscopy. 2007;23(11):1145–51. doi:10.1016/j.arthro.2007.05.019.
49. Treacy SH, Savoie FH, Field LD. Arthroscopic treatment of multidirectional instability. J Shoulder Elbow Surg. 1999;8(4):345–50.
50. Fleega BA, El Shewy MT. Arthroscopic inferior capsular shift: long-term follow-up. Am J Sports Med. 2012;40(5):1126–32. doi:10.1177/0363546512438509.
51. Whitehurst JB, Snyder SJ, Karzel RP, Loren GJ. Arthroscopic pan-capsular plication for glenohumeral multidirectional instability (SS-43). Arthroscopy. 2003;19(5):74–5. doi:10.1016/S0749-8063(07)60122-4.
52. Gartsman GM, Roddey TS, Hammerman SM. Arthroscopic treatment of multidirectional glenohumeral instability. Arthroscopy. 2001;17(3):236–43. doi:10.1053/jars.2001.21529.
53. Jacobson ME, Riggenbach M, Wooldridge AN, Bishop JY. Open capsular shift and arthroscopic capsular plication for treatment of multidirectional instability. Arthroscopy. 2012;28(7):1010–7. doi:10.1016/j.arthro.2011.12.006.
54. Baker CL, Mascarenhas R, Kline AJ, Chhabra A, Pombo MW, Bradley JP. Arthroscopic treatment of multidirectional shoulder instability in athletes: a retrospective analysis of 2- to 5-year clinical outcomes. Am J Sports Med. 2009;37(9):1712–20. doi:10.1177/0363546509335464.
55. Gillis RC, Donaldson CT, Kim H, Love JM, Dreese JC. Arthroscopic suture anchor capsulorrhaphy versus labral-based suture capsulorrhaphy in a cadaveric model. Arthroscopy. 2012;28(11):1615–21. doi:10.1016/j.arthro.2012.04.149.
56. Provencher MT, Verma N, Obopilwe E, et al. A biomechanical analysis of capsular plication versus anchor repair of the shoulder: can the labrum be used as a suture anchor? Arthroscopy. 2008;24(2):210–6. doi:10.1016/j.arthro.2007.08.013.
57. Sekiya JK. Arthroscopic labral repair and capsular shift of the glenohumeral joint: technical pearls for a multiple pleated plication through a single working portal. Arthroscopy. 2005;21(6):766.e1–7. doi:10.1016/j.arthro.2005.03.024.
58. Harryman DT, Sidles JA, Harris SL, Matsen FA. The role of the rotator interval capsule in passive motion and stability of the shoulder. J Bone Joint Surg Am. 1992;74(1):53–66.
59. Provencher MT, Mologne TS, Hongo M, Zhao K, Tasto JP, An K-N. Arthroscopic versus open rotator interval closure: biomechanical evaluation of stability and motion. Arthroscopy. 2007;23(6):583–92. doi:10.1016/j.arthro.2007.01.010.
60. Almazán A, Ruiz M, Cruz F, Pérez FX, Ibarra C. Simple arthroscopic technique for rotator interval closure. Arthroscopy. 2006;22(2):230.e1–4. doi:10.1016/j.arthro.2005.11.009.
61. Gartsman GM, Taverna E, Hammerman SM. Arthroscopic rotator interval repair in glenohumeral instability: description of an operative technique. Arthroscopy. 1999;15(3):330–2.
62. Karas SG. Arthroscopic rotator interval repair and anterior portal closure. Arthroscopy. 2002;18(4):436–9. doi:10.1053/jars.2002.32165.
63. Treacy SH, Field LD, Savoie FH. Rotator interval capsule closure: an arthroscopic technique. Arthroscopy. 1997;13(1):103–6.
64. Frostick SP, Sinopidis C, Maskari Al S, Gibson J, Kemp GJ, Richmond JC. Arthroscopic capsular shrinkage of the shoulder for the treatment of patients with multidirectional instability: minimum 2-year follow-up. Arthroscopy. 2003;19(3):227–33. doi:10.1053/jars.2003.50034.
65. Good CR, Shindle MK, Kelly BT, Wanich T, Warren RF. Glenohumeral chondrolysis after shoulder arthroscopy with thermal capsulorrhaphy. Arthroscopy. 2007;23(7):797.e1–5. doi:10.1016/j.arthro.2007.03.092.
66. Hawkins RJ, Krishnan SG, Karas SG, Noonan TJ, Horan MP. Electrothermal arthroscopic shoulder capsulorrhaphy: a minimum 2-year follow-up. Am J Sports Med. 2007;35(9):1484–8. doi:10.1177/0363546507301082.
67. Levine WN, Clark AM, D'Alessandro DF, Yamaguchi K. Chondrolysis following arthroscopic thermal capsulorrhaphy to treat shoulder instability. A report of two cases. J Bone Joint Surg Am. 2005;87(3):616–21. doi:10.2106/JBJS.D.02158.
68. Miniaci A, McBirnie J. Thermal capsular shrinkage for treatment of multidirectional instability of the shoulder. J Bone Joint Surg Am. 2003;85-A(12): 2283–7.
69. Gerber C, Werner C, Macy JC, Jacob H, Nyffeler RW. Effect of selective capsulorrhaphy on the passive range of motion of the glenohumeral joint. J Bone Joint Surg Am. 2003;85(1):48–55.
70. Hewitt M, Getelman MH, Snyder SJ. Arthroscopic management of multidirectional instability: pancapsular plication. Orthop Clin N Am. 2003;34(4):549–57. doi:10.1016/S0030-5898(03)00094-4.

8 Remplissage: Technique and Results

Christos D. Photopoulos, Min Jung Park, and John D. Kelly IV

Introduction

The association of humeral head defects with glenohumeral instability has been described since the nineteenth century [1, 2]. In 1940, Dr. Harold Hill and Dr. Maurice Sachs described the eponymous Hill-Sachs lesion—a "line of condensation" in the posterolateral aspect of the humeral head frequently visualized in patients with a previous dislocation event [3]. This lesion was postulated to occur as a direct consequence of compressive contact forces between the humeral head and the anterior glenoid during dislocation.

Much has been studied regarding the association of glenoid bone loss and instability. However, the contributing role of humeral head defects cannot be overlooked. The notion of an engaging Hill-Sachs was first popularized by Palmer and Widen in 1948, where the authors exposed the inherent failure of capsulolabral repair to stabilize dislocators with sizable humeral head defects [3]. This was further corroborated by Burkhart and De Beer in 2000, who further defined an engaging Hill-Sachs lesion as a "defect parallel to the anterior glenoid with the shoulder in a functional position of abduction and external rotation" [3, 4]. Recently, studies have revealed that Hill-Sachs defects are found in 65–71 % of first-time dislocators and up to 100 % of recurrent dislocators [5].

Surgical Options and Remplissage

Surgical management of glenohumeral instability usually addresses glenoid pathology, whether in repair of a torn labrum and capsule or in repair or augmentation of deficient glenoid bone [6]. However, in the setting of engaging humeral head defects, separate options must be considered. These include capsular shift, glenoid bone augmentation, humeral head disimpaction, humeral head resurfacing, humeral allograft, and tissue filling [7]. The effectiveness of each of these options has been well described in the literature but deserve some mention.

Capsular shift as a means of treating Hill-Sachs lesions is predicated on the notion that enough restriction of external rotation of the humerus will prevent engagement. While effective in preventing anterior instability episodes, restriction of external rotation can increase joint reactive forces, potentiate posterior humeral head

C.D. Photopoulos, MD (✉)
Department of Orthopaedic Surgery, Hospital of the University of Pennsylvania, Philadelphia, PA, USA
e-mail: christos.photopoulos@uphs.upenn.edu

M.J. Park, MD, MMSc
Department of Orthopaedic Surgery, Southern California Permanente Medical Group, Lancaster, CA, USA

J.D. Kelly IV, MD
Department of Orthopaedics, University of Pennsylvania, Philadelphia, PA, USA

J.D. Kelly IV (ed.), *Elite Techniques in Shoulder Arthroscopy*,
DOI 10.1007/978-3-319-25103-5_8

subluxation, and promote premature degenerative changes [8].

Glenoid bone augmentation (Bristow, Latarjet) has gained much favor and clearly has merit in the presence of appreciable glenoid bone loss. However, when used to treat Hill-Sachs lesions, in the absence of substantial glenoid bone loss (less than 15 %), bone resorption may manifest in the coracoid graft [9]. This is a consequence of Wolf's law, which states that bone applied to a region with minimal mechanical transduction would be expected to atrophy.

Humeral head disimpaction requires an open delto-pectoral approach and is most effective in the acute setting [10]. Humeral resurfacing, while a reasonable option for elderly patients, lacks long-term follow-up, is not physiologic, is not suited for larger lesions, and may potentiate early wear [11].

Humeral allograft is expensive and invasive, creates an opportunity for disease transmission, and has been associated with long-term resorption [12].

The concept of tissue filling was first popularized in 1972 by the Connolly technique—a procedure that involves the open transfer of the infraspinatus as well as part of the greater tuberosity into the humeral head defect [13]. By tenodesing the infraspinatus into the Hill-Sachs void, intra-articular lesions are made extra-articular, and engagement of the humeral head upon the glenoid is effectively prevented [13]. Modifications of this came about with the advent of arthroscopy. The remplissage procedure (from the French word *remplir, to fill*) was first described by Wolf et al. in 2007 and further modified by Koo et al. in 2009 as a method of arthroscopically tenodesing the infraspinatus into humeral head defects [1, 14, 15]. By both filling an engaging humeral head defect and functioning as a check-rein to prevent anterior motion of the humeral head, arthroscopic remplissage has shown to be an effective method to treat glenohumeral instability [7]. Arthroscopic remplissage has gained widespread popularity as an effective and safe option for the treatment of the engaging Hill-Sachs lesion.

Indications

The evaluation of patients with glenohumeral instability always begins with a thorough history and physical examination. Of note, a positive apprehension test in lesser degrees of abduction suggests appreciable bone loss. Supplemental imaging should include radiographs as well as magnetic resonance imaging, so that both osseous and soft-tissue pathology becomes maximally visualized. The degree of both glenoid and humeral head bone loss is a large determinant of the degree of a patient's instability. In the setting of recurrent instability with large glenoid defects (>25 % of the glenoid surface), studies have consistently proven that glenoid augmentation options, such as a Latarjet reconstruction with coracoid autograft, are most suitable [16, 17]. However, in the setting of recurrent instability with glenoid bone loss less than 25 % of the glenoid width and concomitantly large (>30 % humeral head) Hill-Sachs defects, the humeral head lesions must be addressed. It is in this situation that the role of arthroscopic remplissage may prove most useful, which, in combination with capsulolabral repair, has been shown to be an effective means to limit humeral head engagement and consequent instability. In addition, since Sekiya [18] has shown that humeral head lesions as small as 12.5 % have potential implications in affecting stability, it is the senior author's practice (JDK) to treat all lesions greater than 1 cm in width.

Technique

After the patient is placed on the surgical room table and anesthesia is administered, a bilateral shoulder examination is performed. The patient's shoulders are taken through full range of motion, and a modified "load-shift" exam is performed in the lateral position in order to discern which positions make the glenohumeral joint most unstable. The patient is carefully positioned in the lateral decubitus position on a beanbag with a slight posterior tilt so that the glenoid of the affected shoulder remains parallel to the floor. The affected extremity is held in 30–45° of abduction and 15° of forward flexion. Initially, 5 pounds of traction is applied, though this can be up to 15 pounds if required [17].

Three arthroscopic portals are typically required to complete this procedure. The posterolateral portal is made 2 cm inferior and 2 cm medial to the posterolateral edge of the acromion and is used as the primary viewing portal as well as the working portal during anchor passage. The anterosuperolateral portal is localized just off the lateral edge of the anterolateral acromion, and it utilized as a viewing portal during the remplissage component of the procedure. The anterior portal is made 1 cm lateral to the coracoid and is utilized as a working portal during the initial diagnostic arthroscopy as well as during a possible capsulolabral repair.

After the posterolateral portal is made, the diagnostic glenohumeral arthroscopy is performed. From this posterior vantage point, the labrum is examined circumferentially to look for any pathology. Likewise, the Hill-Sachs lesion on the posterosuperolateral humeral head is examined.

Upon completion of the initial diagnostic arthroscopy and confirmation of the Hill-Sachs lesion, the anterosuperolateral portal is created. The arthroscope in this portal affords a "bird's-eye" view of both the humeral head and the labrum. It also provides for dynamic visualization of possible Hill-Sachs engagement upon the anteroinferior glenoid if the arm is to be taken into abduction and external rotation (Figs. 8.1 and 8.2). This portal is also used to evaluate the adequacy of the posterior portal—it is important that this posterior portal is placed directly superior to the humeral head in order for anchor placement in subsequent steps. If remplissage is undertaken, the senior author feels strongly that the Bankart lesion is prepared first and then repaired after completion of remplissage. Since the posterior infraspinatus tenodesis reduces the humeral head posteriorly, it is easier to tension the anterior capsule after the remplissage. Thus, the labrum is liberated, and the glenoid is rasped before the humeral head is addressed.

While viewing from above, the shaver is inserted posteriorly. In preparation for the remplissage, the Hill-Sachs defect is gently debrided down to its bleeding base.

After preparation of the Hill-Sachs, a cannula is placed through the posterior portal. Using this cannula, a double-loaded anchor is inserted just lateral to the myotendinous junction of the infraspinatus, and it is inserted into the Hill-Sachs defect, making sure that the trajectory remains perpendicular to the bone. If the initial portal is

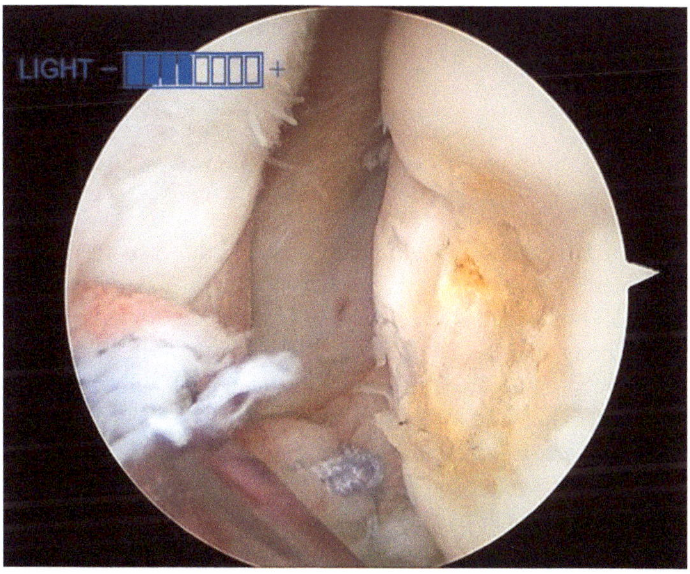

Fig. 8.1 Smaller but medial Hill-Sachs lesion which will "engage"

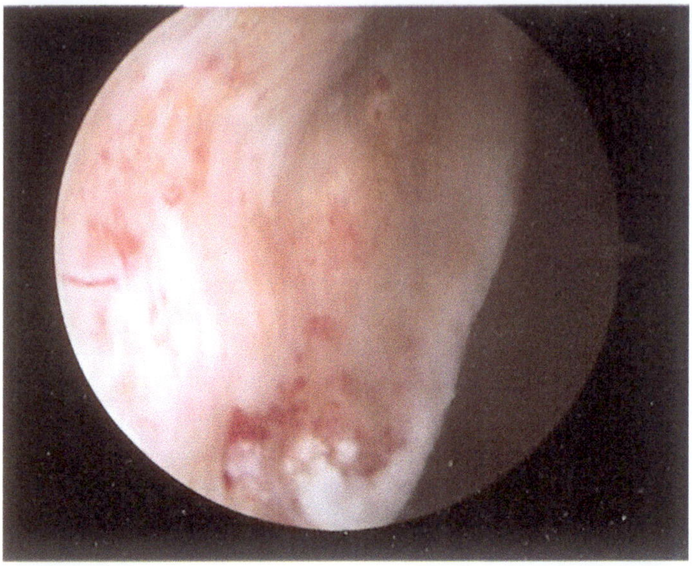

Fig. 8.2 Large, engaging, Hill-Sachs lesion

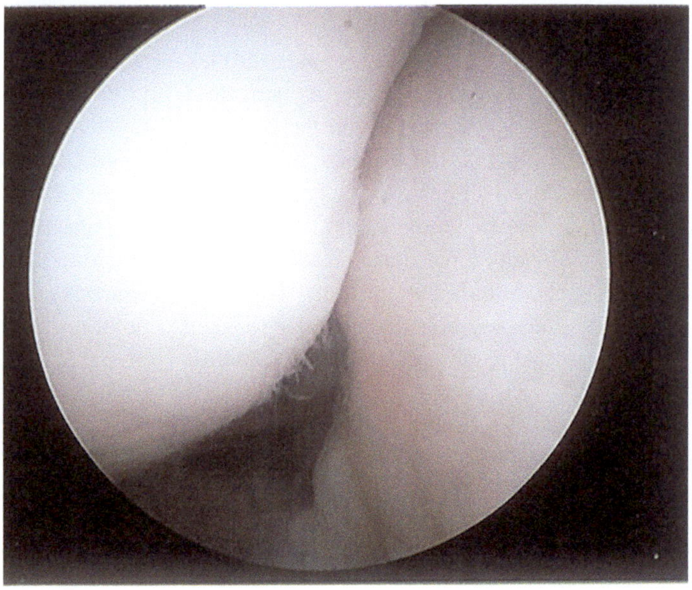

Fig. 8.3 Post-remplissage: arthroscopic view of infraspinatus tenodesis into Hill-Sachs lesion

deemed too medial, an additional, more distal, and lateral portal is created. After anchor placement, all four suture limbs are withdrawn outside of the body, and the cannula is pulled from the joint and into the sub-deltoid space, just external to the infraspinatus muscle. A penetrating grasper is then inserted into the cannula and across the infraspinatus tendon, superior to the site of the tendon where the anchor was passed. One suture limb from the first pair is grabbed and retrieved. This step is performed again, this time with another suture limb from the other suture pair. This time, the penetrating grasper is inserted inferiorly, in order to effect a stronger tenodesis. In the presence of good tissue, only two suture limbs will suffice. Once all four sutures are outside the body, the inferior pair is tied first within the sub-deltoid space. The superior suture limb pair is subsequently tied. The infraspinatus is thus tenodesed within the Hill-Sachs lesion, and the remplissage is complete (Fig. 8.3). If an additional anchor is necessary, it is important to proceed with the distal most aspect of the lesion first. The senior author prefers to complete the tenodesis first in the distal anchor before proceeding to the more proximal region. Often an additional more proximal portal is necessary for the second anchor. The capsulolabral repair can then be performed, and a sharp obturator is used to reestablish a new posterior portal which will be used for suture shuttling during the Bankart repair.

Results

Overall, arthroscopic remplissage has proven to be safe in the treatment of recurrent anterior glenohumeral instability. Compared to other methods of addressing humeral head defects, remplissage provides several distinct advantages. The procedure can be performed entirely arthroscopically, thus avoiding the morbidity and the prolonged recovery often encountered with open procedures. Likewise, it is a procedure that can be performed in conjunction with other arthroscopic procedures, such as Bankart repair, without adding substantial operative time [17]. The infraspinatus does appear to integrate well into the defect as Park [19] has shown at least 75 % fill of the lesion on post-op magnetic resonance imaging (Fig. 8.4). Likewise, the presence of fibrocartilaginous-like signal on postoperative magnetic resonance imaging scans suggests the potential for the infraspinatus tissue to have more bony properties in time [19] (Fig. 8.5).

Several biomechanical studies have been performed to evaluate the effectiveness of remplissage. In 2012, Giles et al. evaluated cadaveric specimens with Hill-Sachs lesions on a shoulder simulator and found that remplissage was effective in preventing engagement and dislocation of humeral heads with Hill-Sachs defect sizes of both 30 % and 45 % [20]. A separate cadaveric analysis by Elkinson et al. in 2012 helped further elucidate this. In their investigations, the authors evaluated Hill-Sachs lesions sized at 15 % and 30 % and treated with a combination of Bankart repair with remplissage. They found that when treated with Bankart alone, none of the 15 % Hill-Sachs lesions engaged and dislocated, whereas all of the 30 % lesions did. However, the dislocation rate of the 30 % Hill-Sachs lesions was significantly reduced if remplissage was added in conjunction to Bankart repair—thus helping to corroborate the notion that remplissage is most effective in the setting on minimal glenoid bone loss and sizable engaging Hill-Sachs defects [21].

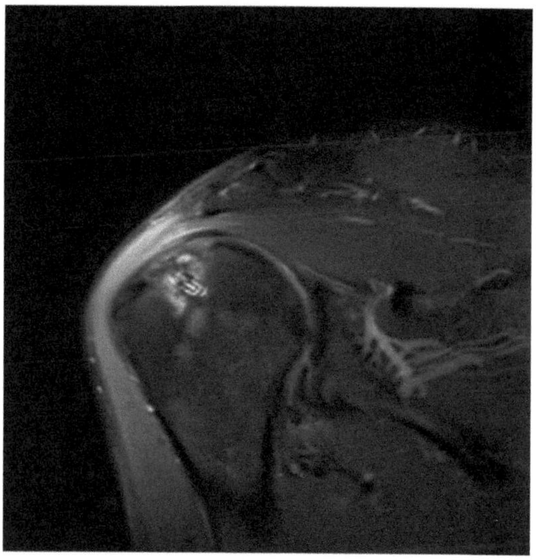

Fig. 8.4 Postoperative magnetic resonance imaging demonstrating healing of remplissage into defect

Clinically, several studies have been performed highlighting the effectiveness of remplissage with both good clinical and functional outcome scores [7, 14, 22, 23]. In 2001, Park et al. examined a series of 20 patients who underwent the procedure and concluded that remplissage was an effective procedure to help restore function, alleviation, and patient satisfaction [23]. Complications, such as posterosuperior shoulder pain as well as loss of shoulder motion, particularly external rotation, have been described [24, 25]. Despite this, several investigations have revealed that arthroscopic remplissage is well tolerated without postoperative shoulder pain or loss of motion [1, 14, 22, 23, 26]. In a systematic review, Buza et al. concluded that the results of remplissage compared favorably to those of Bankart repair performed in the absence of appreciable bone loss [7].

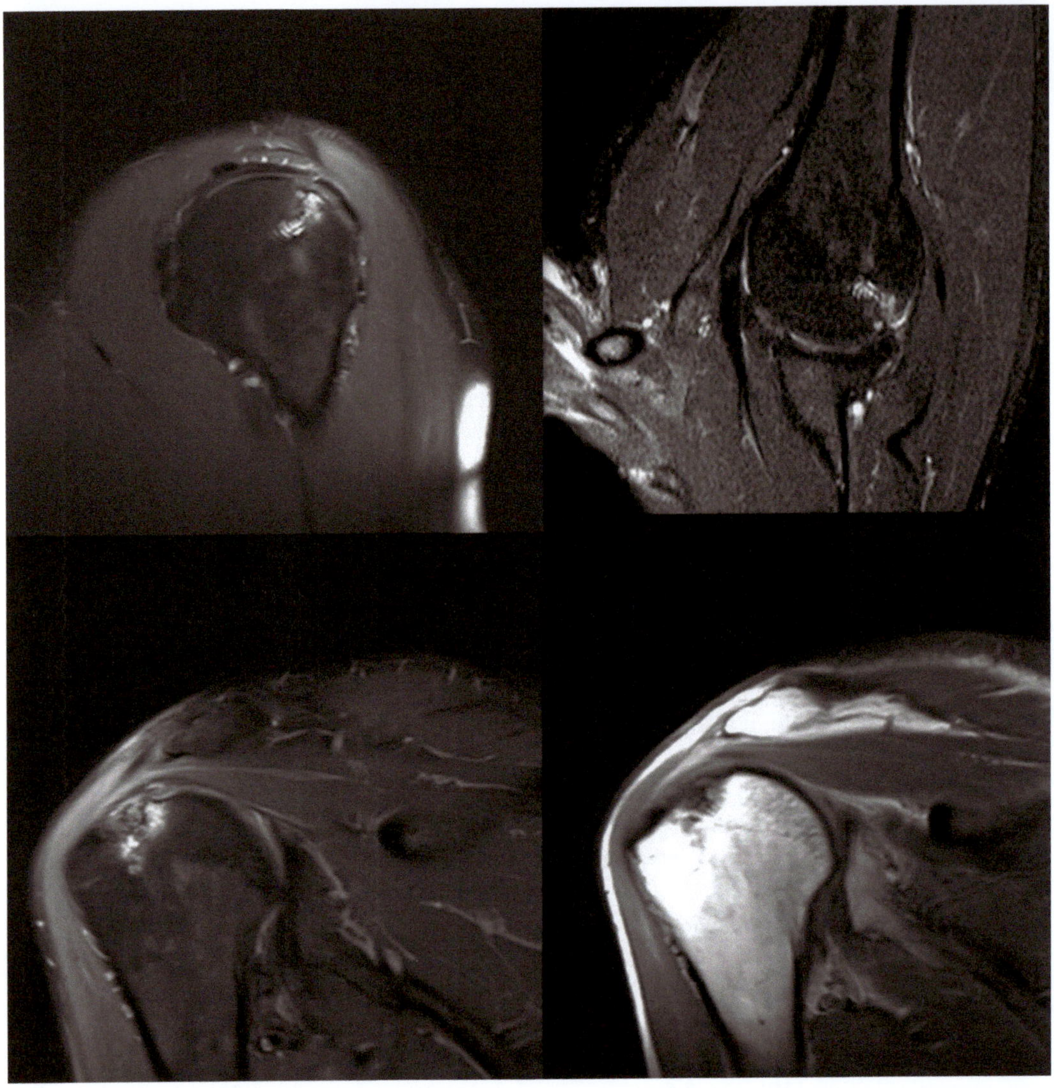

Fig. 8.5 5.5 months status post-remplissage demonstrating infraspinatus integration into bone

Conclusion

Several treatment options exist for the management of recurrent anterior shoulder instability. Defining the pathogenesis of this instability is an important first step in helping to guide these options. It is generally accepted that management of large glenoid defects (greater than 25 % width) typically demands bony augmentation techniques, such as coracoid transfer. However, management of the engaging Hill-Sachs lesion is likely best served with a biologic and focal solution. The premise of "tissue filling" was initially described in the 1970s. Since that time, the field of orthopedic surgery has witnessed the maturation of this method into today's arthroscopic remplissage procedure. The indications for remplissage have become better defined, but as the pathogenesis and the pathomechanics of shoulder instability continue to become more elucidated, they will surely continue to evolve. Both safe and effective, arthroscopic remplissage continues to gain widespread acceptance as a treatment option for shoulder in the setting of humeral head defects. Is has proven effective in minimizing recurrence, has been shown to incorporate, and has not been shown to appreciably affect motion. Remplissage will undoubtedly continue to remain an important part of a surgeon's armamentarium in the treatment of shoulder instability.

References

1. Koo SS, Burkhart SS, Ochoa E. Arthroscopic double-pulley remplissage technique for engaging Hill-Sachs lesions in anterior shoulder instability repairs. Arthroscopy. 2009;25(11):1343–8.
2. Saha AK. Recurrent dislocation of the shoulder: physiopathology and operative corrections. Stuttgart: Georg Thieme Verlag; 1981.
3. Palmer I, Widen A. The bone block method for recurrent dislocation of the shoulder joint. J Bone Joint Surg Br. 1948;30B(1):53–8.
4. Burkhart SS, De Beer JF. Traumatic glenohumeral bone defects and their relationship to failure of arthroscopic Bankart repairs: significance of the inverted-pear glenoid and the humeral engaging Hill-Sachs lesion. Arthroscopy. 2000;16(7):677–94.
5. Longo UG, et al. Remplissage, humeral osteochondral grafts, weber osteotomy, and shoulder arthroplasty for the management of humeral bone defects in shoulder instability: systematic review and quantitative synthesis of the literature. Arthroscopy. 2014;30(12):1650–66.
6. Provencher MT, et al. The Hill-Sachs lesion: diagnosis, classification, and management. J Am Acad Orthop Surg. 2012;20(4):242–52.
7. Buza III JA, et al. Arthroscopic Hill-Sachs remplissage: a systematic review. J Bone Joint Surg Am. 2014;96(7):549–55.
8. Hawkins RJ, Angelo RL. Glenohumeral osteoarthrosis. A late complication of the Putti-Platt repair. J Bone Joint Surg Am. 1990;72(8):1193–7.
9. Di Giacomo G, et al. Does the presence of glenoid bone loss influence coracoid bone graft osteolysis after the Latarjet procedure? A computed tomography scan study in 2 groups of patients with and without glenoid bone loss (vol 23, pg 514, 2014). J Shoulder Elbow Surg. 2014;23(9):1415.
10. Re P, Gallo RA, Richmond JC. Transhumeral head plasty for large Hill-Sachs lesions. Arthroscopy. 2006;22(7):798a-U69.
11. Dawson CK, Rolf RH, Holovacs TF. The management of localized articular cartilage lesions of the humeral head in the athlete. Oper Techniques Sports Med. 2008;16(1):14–20.
12. Minjaci A, Gish M. Management of anterior glenohumeral instability associated with large Hill-Sachs defects. Tech Shoulder Elbow Surg. 2004;5:170–5.
13. Connolly C. Humeral head defects associated with shoulder dislocation: their diagnostic and surgical significance. Instr Course Lect. 1972;21:42–54.
14. Purchase RJ, et al. Hill-Sachs "remplissage": an arthroscopic solution for the engaging Hill-Sachs lesion. Arthroscopy. 2008;24(6):723–6.
15. Wolf EM, Pollack M, Smalley C. Hill-Sachs "Remplissag": an arthroscopic solution for the engaging Hill-Sachs lesion. Arthroscopy. 2007;23:e1–2.
16. Burkhart SS, et al. Results of modified Latarjet reconstruction in patients with anteroinferior instability and significant bone loss. Arthroscopy. 2007;23(10): 1033–41.
17. McHale KJ, Park MJ, Kelly JDI. Arthroscopic remplissage for humeral head defects. Techniques Orthop. 2015;30(1):39–41.
18. Sekiya JK, et al. Hill-Sachs defects and repair using osteoarticular allograft transplantation: biomechanical analysis using a joint compression model. Am J Sports Med. 2009;37(12):2459–66.
19. Park MJ, et al. The evaluation of arthroscopic remplissage by high-resolution magnetic resonance imaging. Am J Sports Med. 2012;40(10):2331–6.
20. Giles JW, et al. Moderate to large engaging Hill-Sachs defects: an in vitro biomechanical comparison of the remplissage procedure, allograft humeral head reconstruction, and partial resurfacing arthroplasty. J Shoulder Elbow Surg. 2012;21(9):1142–51.
21. Elkinson I, et al. The effect of the remplissage procedure on shoulder stability and range of motion: an in vitro biomechanical assessment. J Bone Joint Surg Am. 2012;94(11):1003–12.
22. Zhu YM, et al. Arthroscopic Bankart repair combined with remplissage technique for the treatment of anterior shoulder instability with engaging Hill-Sachs lesion: a report of 49 cases with a minimum 2-year follow-up. Am J Sports Med. 2011;39(8):1640–7.
23. Park MJ, et al. Arthroscopic remplissage with Bankart repair for the treatment of glenohumeral instability with Hill-Sachs defects. Arthroscopy. 2011;27(9):1187–94.
24. Nourissat G, et al. A prospective, comparative, radiological, and clinical study of the influence of the "remplissage" procedure on shoulder range of motion after stabilization by arthroscopic Bankart repair. Am J Sports Med. 2011;39(10):2147–52.
25. Deutsch AA, Kroll DG. Decreased range of motion following arthroscopic remplissage. Orthopedics. 2008;31(5):492.
26. Haviv B, Mayo L, Biggs D. Outcomes of arthroscopic "remplissage": capsulotenodesis of the engaging large Hill-Sachs lesion. J Orthop Surg Res. 2011;6:29.

9 Arthroscopic Latarjet

Sohale Sadeghpour, Michael J. O'Brien, and Felix H. Savoie III

Introduction

Anterior shoulder instability associated with significant (>20 %) glenoid bone loss can be disabling. This loss of normal glenoid architecture limits its ability to withstand shear stresses and significantly increases glenohumeral contact stresses [1, 2]. The importance of glenoid bone loss as a contributor to recurrent glenohumeral instability has been illustrated by various authors [2–5].

Burkhart and De Beer highlighted the consequences of bone loss in their classic paper, demonstrating a much higher failure rate in patients with engaging Hill-Sachs lesions [3]. Since then, further research by Itoi et al. has enhanced our understanding of the glenoid track and its importance in instability [4]. Determination of the degree of bone loss necessary to create "off-track" engaging bone lesions is evolving. As a result, numerous surgical techniques have been developed to address this bone loss/defect [6–8].

One of the most commonly performed procedures for significant glenoid bone loss is the Latarjet procedure. The Latarjet procedure was originally described by Latarjet in 1954 as a modification of the Trillat procedure, an incomplete osteotomy of the coracoid process, for the treatment of recurrent anterior glenohumeral instability. The procedure involved transferring the horizontal portion of the coracoid, along with the conjoined tendon, to the deficient anterior glenoid rim. In 1958, Helfet described a similar technique designed by his mentor Rowley Bristow [6]. The Bristow procedure involved suturing of the harvested coracoid tip to an abraded region on the anterior scapular neck. Modifications to both the Bristow and the Latarjet procedure over the years eventually led to the procedures being almost identical [9]. The original success of the Latarjet procedure was attributed to augmentation of glenoid surface area, which increases the stable arc of motion. It was not until 1985 when Patte et al. described the so-called triple blocking effect [10] of the coracoid transfer that we began to fully understand the biomechanics of the bony, muscular, and capsular contributions of the coracoid transfer to stability of the shoulder. The success of the "triple blocking effect" relies on three principles. First, the transferred coracoid augments the bony arc of glenohumeral motion. Second, the transferred conjoined tendon creates a sling effect and tensions the subscapularis muscle, resulting in reinforcement of the anterior capsule. This effect becomes more crucial as the joint moves into abduction and external rotation. Lastly, the anterior capsule and/or remaining coracoacromial ligament is reattached to the anterior glenoid. This final portion creates a "bumper effect," bolstering construct stability further.

S. Sadeghpour, MD (✉) • M.J. O'Brien, MD
F.H. Savoie III, MD
Department of Orthopaedics, Tulane University School of Medicine, New Orleans, LA, USA
e-mail: ssadeghp@tulane.edu

J.D. Kelly IV (ed.), *Elite Techniques in Shoulder Arthroscopy*,
DOI 10.1007/978-3-319-25103-5_9

The Latarjet procedure was classically described as an open procedure and has shown excellent results in recent studies [9, 11–15]. With advancements in technology and arthroscopy, there has been an expansion in surgical options for bone restoration in glenohumeral instability. Arthroscopy allows for more advanced intra-articular visualization, more versatility when treating concomitant intra-articular pathology, more accurate graft placement, and less adhesion formation. As is the case in other joints, arthroscopy offers postoperative advantages of less pain, earlier mobility, quicker rehabilitation, faster return to sport, and improved cosmetic result [7]. It is only natural that with these advances, the Latarjet procedure has evolved from an open procedure to an all arthroscopic one. Lafosse and Boyle are credited with the inception of the all-arthroscopic technique which he began performing in 2003 [7]. His technique showed excellent results at short- to mid-term follow-up with minimal complications.

While studies of both open and arthroscopic techniques have shown good results, many of them continue to report arthritis as a concern [9, 13, 16–18]. It is postulated that nonanatomic repair of the glenoid arc, extra-articular nonanatomic repair of the capsulolabral tissues, and insufficient chondral surface reconstitution may lead to degenerative arthritis after stabilization procedures [19, 20]. Arthroscopy provides enhanced visualization during graft placement, thus helping to minimize overhang and recreate a more anatomic glenoid arc. Ideally, an anatomic arc would diminish risk of arthritis progression. It is important to recognize the considerable learning curve and excellent knowledge of anatomy required to successfully perform the arthroscopic Latarjet procedure. The procedure is indicated after appropriate preoperative assessment; however, it may not be indicated until after diagnostic arthroscopy.

Patient History and Physical Examination

While a thorough preoperative history and physical exam is necessary when assessing all patients with shoulder pathology, it is of paramount importance in patients with symptoms of traumatic anterior shoulder instability. A detailed history and physical can provide information regarding risk of recurrence, degree of functional impairment, potential success of surgical interventions, and indications for operative versus nonoperative treatment. It is important to note the patient's age, hand dominance, profession, pre-injury activity level, and, more importantly, the patient's expectations from treatment particularly with respect to pain [21–23].

The history should include both the patient's age and mechanism of injury at time of original dislocation. The most significant risk factor for predicting recurrent instability has shown to be younger age at initial dislocation [9, 13, 24–26]. Also, a high-energy mechanism of injury and time spent dislocated before reduction should raise suspicion for glenoid bone loss [3]. Inquiries should be made about the site of pain, number of recurrent episodes, reduction maneuvers, and any other concomitant injuries. A history of frequent dislocations during activities of daily living or instability symptoms while sleeping is highly suggestive for osseous glenoid defect [27, 28]. Any history of sudden strength or sensation loss in the affected extremity (dead arm) may also guide diagnosis. While the diagnosis of recurrent anterior shoulder instability may be made easily on the basis of a traumatic event, recurrence, and positive apprehension test, it must be noted that the diagnosis may be difficult in select patient populations [28]. Collision athletes such as rugby players may present without a clear history of a dislocation event and may only complain of pain and weakness with abduction/external rotation [29]. In addition, many patients become accustomed to recurrent subluxations episodes. As a result, they only report mild pain and crepitus. Finally, much of recurrent instability population will have had surgical intervention prior to presentation. It is imperative to obtain and review operative reports and medical records before surgical consideration.

The physical examination is performed with the patient in the standing, sitting, and supine positions. The exam begins with visual inspection of the patient to assess for posture, any asymmetry, scapular winging, and muscle atrophy. Next, examination of the cervical spine including a Spurling's and Adson's test should be performed to rule out any neck pathology. Both active and passive range of shoulder motion should be assessed, taking care to also note any signs of scapulothoracic dysfunction/asymmetry. Compare motion with that of the contralateral side during the exam.

The next portion of the exam should include evaluation of the rotator cuff. While traumatic instability patients younger than 40 years of age tend to have concomitant labral and biceps pathology, patients older than 40 often have rotator cuff tears. Preferred tests of the rotator cuff include the Whipple, supraspinatus stress, supraspinatus isolation, external rotation, and belly press. The presence of generalized ligamentous laxity should also be assessed, taking care to note any and all joints that may exhibit hypermobility.

The presence of instability is then assessed. This is performed in both the sitting and supine positions. With the patient sitting, the proximal humerus is stabilized, and a gentle load from the elbow is applied in the anterior, posterior, and inferior directions. This circumduction maneuver may demonstrate subtle instability [30]. During the apprehension test, the shoulder is moved into 90° abduction with increasing external rotation, causing apprehension and often pain in patients with anterior shoulder instability. Additionally, in patients with significant bone loss, apprehension is noted during external rotation in lower levels (45°) of abduction. Relocation with a posteriorly directed force on the proximal humerus alleviates the discomfort.

The examiner should also check for a sulcus sign during this portion of the exam. Next, with the patient supine, both load and shift and Jobe's apprehension/relocation tests are performed [31].

Diagnostic Imaging

Diagnostic imaging begins with plain radiographs of the shoulder including anteroposterior, scapular Y, and axillary views. Supplemental views may be obtained to better identify any osseous defects. A West Point axillary view may be helpful for visualizing bony Bankart lesions, and the Stryker notch view is helpful for assessing Hill-Sachs lesions. At our institution, we routinely perform Bernageau [15, 32] views to assess for glenoid defects. The Bernageau view reveals flattening of the anterior-inferior glenoid in cases of bone loss (Fig. 9.1a, b). If there is 10 % or larger loss on the Bernageau radiograph, we obtain a computed tomography (CT) scan with three-dimensional (3-D) reconstruction to further delineate bone loss. As shown by Sugaya [29]

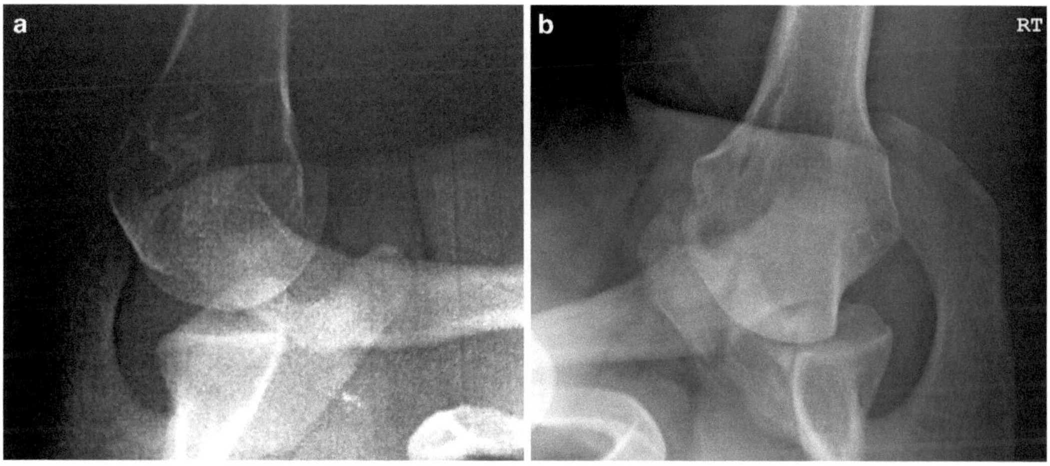

Fig. 9.1 (**a**) Bernageau view illustrating glenoid without bone loss. *Published with kind permission of © Dr. Felix H. Savoie, III 2015. All Rights Reserved.* (**b**) Bernageau view illustrating glenoid with bone loss. *Published with kind permission of © Dr. Felix H. Savoie, III 2015. All Rights Reserved*

three-dimensional CT scan is the most important imaging study for accurately assessing glenoid morphology and quantifying the percentage of bone loss [29].

There has been considerable attention paid to the concept of the "inverted pear" glenoid, which represents a great risk for failure after soft tissue stabilization and the method to accurately quantify this bone loss [1–4, 27, 29, 33–35]. Itoi et al. has shown that as little as 6 mm of glenoid bone loss leads to significantly increased instability of the glenohumeral joint. [4] Percentage of bone loss based on 3-D CT scan measurements and during arthroscopy have both been described [2, 3, 29, 36]. Anywhere from as little as 19–30 % glenoid bone loss has been shown to lead to significant increases in instability. Treatment based on percentage of glenoid bone loss has not been fully defined as of yet. We can, however, guide treatment based on several of these prior studies. In general, recurrent instability patients with <20 % bone loss may be considered for soft tissue stabilization procedures alone, whereas those with >25 % should be considered for bony augmentation.

We do not routinely perform MRI or MR arthrography as part of the workup for recurrent anterior shoulder instability. While these are helpful for assessing soft tissue lesions such as humeral avulsion of the glenohumeral ligament (HAGLs), Bankart lesions, and capsular injuries, these injuries may be better visualized during diagnostic arthroscopy.

The goal of a thorough clinical exam and radiographic workup is to identify clinical situations in which a soft tissue Bankart repair alone would be inadequate for stability and when a Latarjet procedure would be indicated. It is important to note that even with full preoperative radiographic workup, the decision to perform an arthroscopic Latarjet procedure sometimes is made after arthroscopic examination.

Indications and Contraindications

The arthroscopic Latarjet procedure is indicated in symptomatic patients with recurrent anterior shoulder instability and significant (>20 %) glenoid bone loss. An engaging or "on-track" humeral head defect is often present. Patients at high risk of redislocation secondary to increased activity levels such as rugby players and baseball pitchers are ideal candidates for the arthroscopic Latarjet procedure. The procedure allows for quicker rehabilitation time and return to sport for this population. Patients with epilepsy, voluntary dislocators, high-risk surgical candidates, and those unable to comply with postoperative rehabilitation protocols are not ideal candidates for surgery.

Conservative Treatment

Conservative treatment in this population is reserved for those patients not suitable for operative intervention as mentioned previously and/or elderly low-demand patients. Treatment is primarily based on strengthening periscapular and rotator cuff musculature. Ideal patients for conservative treatment have less than 20 % glenoid bone loss and are low demand. Successful conservative treatment entails maintenance of a stable shoulder with activities of daily living.

Arthroscopic Treatment

As stated, arthroscopic Latarjet procedure is indicated after appropriate preoperative workup has identified patients with significant (>20 %) glenoid bone loss and symptoms of instability. It is imperative to recognize scenarios where isolated soft tissue procedures are likely to fail. A surgeon's personal experience and comfort level should dictate the surgical treatment performed.

The preference at our institution is to harvest the coracoid via a mini-open approach, harvest iliac crest, or use fresh osteochondral distal tibial articular surface [19] to reconstruct the glenoid, depending on age of patient, ligamentous laxity, and prior surgical history. If coracoid transfer or iliac crest is the source, the capsule is repaired arthroscopically to the native glenoid, making the graft extra-articular. Theoretically, this could reduce odds of developing arthritis. When the distal tibial articular surface is the bone source, we repair the capsule to the perimeter of the graft, making the bone transfer intra-articular. This combined technique of mini-open/arthroscopic bone grafting with capsule preservation and repair has been termed the "Tulane Technique."

Technique

The patient is placed in the lateral decubitus position, rolled back approximately 30°. A standard posterior portal is made, and a diagnostic arthroscopy performed to confirm the amount of bone loss as well as evaluate the entire glenohumeral joint (Fig. 9.2).

An incision is made from the tip of the coracoid distally for approximately 3–5 cm (Fig. 9.3a). The coracoid is exposed and harvested using a standard Latarjet technique. We prefer to use a guide to ensure proper placement of the drill holes in the coracoid, but the harvest can certainly be performed free hand. The pectoralis minor is released, and the coracoid is attached to the Lafosse Latarjet holding device (Fig. 9.3b). The posterior concave surface of the coracoid is lightly abraded using a high-speed spur. The portion that will be the articular side (lateral) is also evaluated and burred to a smooth surface. The edge of the graft that will lie adjacent to the glenoid is marked to allow easier visualization once it is placed in the joint.

The arthroscope is then inserted back into the joint, and an anterior-superior viewing portal established just anterior to the supraspinatus tendon (not through the tendon). Utilizing the anterior incision, a cannula is inserted over the subscapularis and the capsule elevated completely from the glenoid neck and retracted. It is important that the capsule elevation from the glenoid continue to the attachment of the posterior-inferior glenohumeral ligament (PIGHL) on the posterior glenoid in order to allow later repair

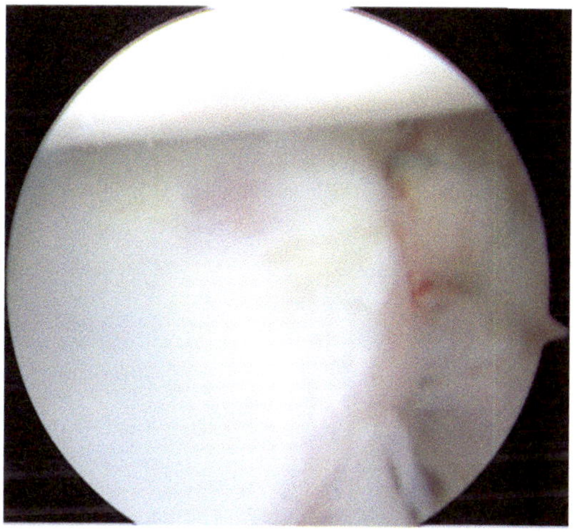

Fig. 9.2 Anterior superior viewing portal in a left shoulder demonstrating anterior glenoid bone loss. *Published with kind permission of © Dr. Felix H. Savoie, III 2015. All Rights Reserved*

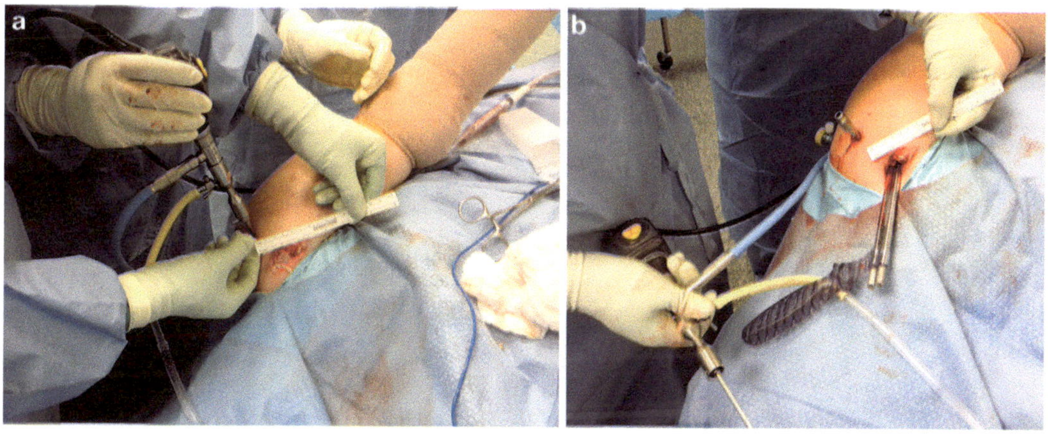

Fig. 9.3 (**a**) Anterior incision for coracoid graft harvest. *Published with kind permission of © Dr. Felix H. Savoie, III 2015. All Rights Reserved.* (**b**) Anterior incision with coracoid graft holder in place. *Published with kind permission of © Dr. Felix H. Savoie, III 2015. All Rights Reserved*

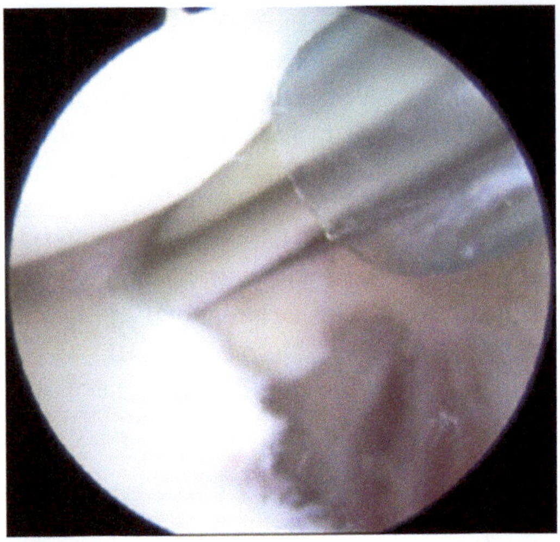

Fig. 9.4 The capsule is elevated to the level of the PIGHL attachment so that external rotation is not limited after repair. *Published with kind permission of © Dr. Felix H. Savoie, III 2015. All Rights Reserved*

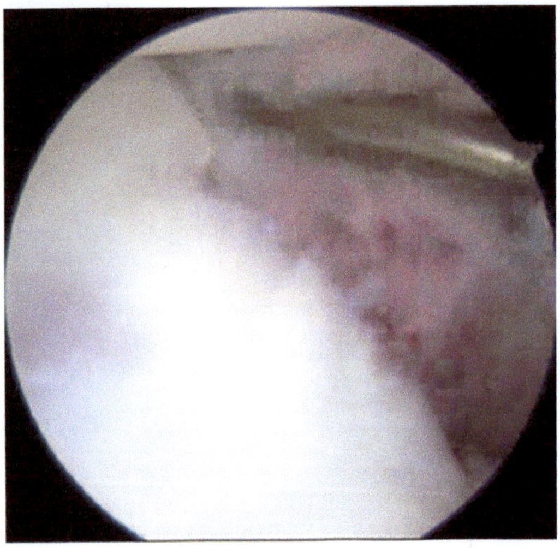

Fig. 9.5 Crochet hook inserted to keep capsule retracted. *Published with kind permission of © Dr. Felix H. Savoie, III 2015. All Rights Reserved*

without limiting external rotation (Fig. 9.4). A crochet hook is inserted percutaneously to retract the capsule during the next step of the surgery (Fig. 9.5).

A switching stick is inserted via the posterior portal and passed across the glenoid, through the muscle belly of the subscapularis and out the small anterior incision. A series of dilators used to facilitate cannula passage are then inserted over the switching stick to create an atraumatic path through the subscapularis muscle. The graft, still attached to the holder, is slid along the switching stick into the joint under arthroscopic visualization through this dilated path. The graft is positioned with its center in the center of the defect, usually 4 O'clock, and it is fixated in this position by two Kirschner wires that are drilled across the glenoid neck exiting out the posterior aspect of the shoulder. Each wire is clamped to prevent accidental removal; the inferior hole is drilled, measured and the screw inserted. The length of the screw is usually 36–38 mm. The more superior hole is managed the same way. The anterior aspect of the bone block can be visualized with the arthroscope to confirm full seating of the screws into the bone graft (Fig. 9.6a, b). Any malalignment or protuberances on the bone graft can be burred at this time.

The retractor holding the capsule is then removed, allowing the capsule to fall back toward the glenoid. A double-loaded suture anchor is placed into the native glenoid via the anterior-inferior portal (that had been made through the small incision). The arthroscope may be placed posteriorly, and the superior portal used to shift the anterior/inferior capsule in a superior direction. A retrograde retriever is then utilized to create two double, oblique vertical mattress sutures so that the capsule can be repaired over the bone block and back to the native glenoid. This is performed with the arm externally rotated 90° and completes the reconstruction (Fig. 9.7).

Fluoroscopy can be used to confirm screw placement. Radiographs are taken in recovery room (Fig. 9.8).

Postoperative Rehabilitation

The patient is placed in an abduction sling for the early postoperative phase. Scapular retraction is started immediately. Limited active isometric exercises are also started week 1. Once the shoulder "settles down," usually 3–4 weeks, the immobilization device is discontinued and active exercise initiated. There is no stretching allowed in physical

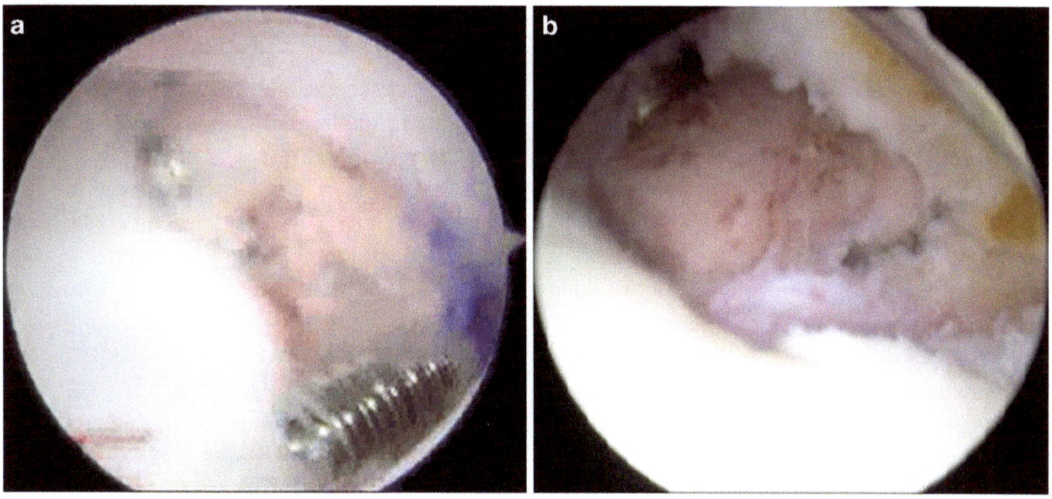

Fig. 9.6 (**a**) Graft being placed through subscapularis onto glenoid. *Published with kind permission of © Dr. Felix H. Savoie, III 2015. All Rights Reserved*. (**b**) Bone block position on glenoid. *Published with kind permission of © Dr. Felix H. Savoie, III 2015. All Rights Reserved*

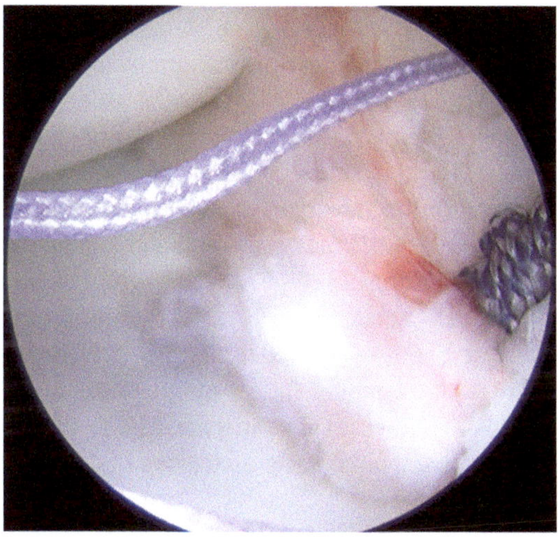

Fig. 9.7 Capsule repaired over bone block. *Published with kind permission of © Dr. Felix H. Savoie, III 2015. All Rights Reserved*

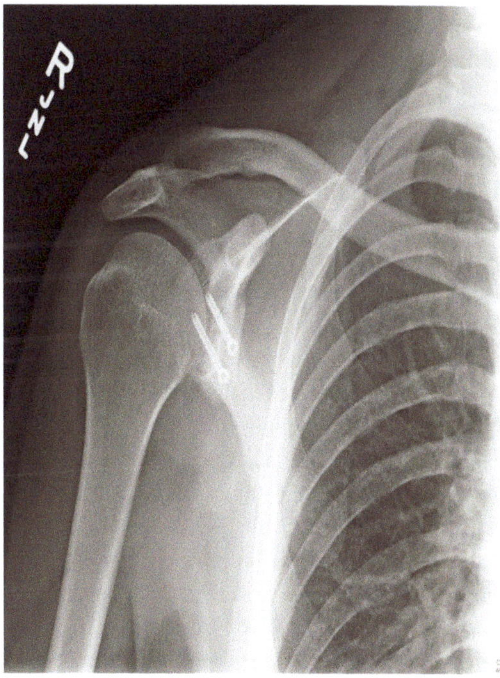

Fig. 9.8 Postoperative radiograph illustrating proper placement of screws. *Published with kind permission of © Dr. Felix H. Savoie, III 2015. All Rights Reserved*

therapy. X-rays are taken at 3 and 6 weeks, and we attempt to obtain a computed tomography (CT) scan at the 6–8 week mark.

Complications

Over time, multiple studies have established the Latarjet as a viable option for treating glenoid bone loss; however, more recent reports have uncovered associated technical difficulties [7, 20, 22, 37–39]. While the Latarjet procedure can reliably stabilize the chronically unstable shoulder, it is not without potential setbacks.

Complications may consist of hematoma, infection, neurovascular injury, hardware impediments (broken, migrated), coracoid/glenoid fracture, coracoid lysis, osteoarthritis, decreased external rotation, and recurrent instability/reoperations.

In the most recent systematic review to date, Bhatia et al. [20] examined five studies which dealt with postoperative complications in open and arthroscopic cases [3, 7, 11, 22, 39]. Burkhart and De Beer [3] reported a 5 % complication rate in a cohort of 102 patients (2 hematomas, 2 asymptomatic screw loosenings, 1 asymptomatic fibrous union). Lafosse and Boyle [7] reported 2 hematomas, 1 intraoperative graft fracture, 1 transient musculocutaneous nerve palsy, 4 cases of nonunion, and 3 cases of screw osteolysis in their first 100 patients. Scmhid et al. [22] documented a 12 % complication rate (6/49 patients) that included 4 delayed wound healing cases, 1 case of adhesive capsulitis, and 1 malunion of the coracoid graft.

Shah et al. [39] noted an overall short-term complication rate of 25 % in their study (6 % infection, 8 % recurrent instability, 10 % neurologic injury). Griesser et al. [38] discovered a similar overall complication rate of 30 % in their systematic review of both the open and arthroscopic Latarjet procedures. This study also found a statistically significant decrease in reoperation rates within the arthroscopic Latarjet group (2.7 %) compared to the open group (7.5 %). It is important to recognize that these studies consist of higher volume surgeons with expertise in the area of shoulder instability. In another recent study, Castricini et al. [40] looked at the first 30 patients in which an arthroscopic Latarjet procedure was performed to analyze the associated learning curve. This study resulted in a 10 % complication rate (three graft fractures) and found that age >40 was associated with complications. The operative time decreased from 132 min in the first 15 patients to 99 min in the last 15 patients with no significant differences in terms of clinical score or patient satisfaction between the two groups.

Gracitelli et al. [37] aimed to determine the safety and practicality of the arthroscopic Latarjet through a cadaveric study. The procedure was performed on cadavers by orthopedic surgeons new to the technique. Their results revealed a 33 % (4/12) success rate. The study illustrated the high rate of failure due to the complex technical objectives required of the arthroscopic Latarjet. Ultimately, it is imperative to recognize the substantial learning curve and technical difficulty associated with the Latarjet procedure.

Outcomes

An arthroscopic Latarjet is a promising procedure with some distinct advantages over the traditional open technique. Recent primary data has shown favorable outcomes. Lafosse and Boyle reported no recurrent dislocations in their first set of 98 patients [7]. Patients in this series at 18-month follow-up felt the procedure outcome deserved an excellent or good grade in 98 % of cases (80 % excellent, 18 % good) with all returning to work at an average of 2 months. At 26 months, satisfaction remained high at 91 % excellent scores in patient reports. Complications consisted of one intraoperative graft fracture, one temporary musculocutaneous nerve palsy, four graft nonunions, and three sets of prominent screws.

Boileau later described an arthroscopic Bankart-Bristow-Latarjet technique. [41] At an average of 16-month follow-up, none of the 47 patients in this case series sustained a dislocation. One graft fractured early and seven grafts went on to nonunion.

With the "Tulane Technique," there have been no recurrent dislocations in a group of 30 patients. American Shoulder and Elbow Surgeons (ASES) scores in 24 patients were excellent, 3 scores were good, 2 were fair, and 1 was poor. One patient, who underwent four previous surgeries, sustained a transient musculocutaneous nerve palsy (resolved in 8 weeks). Other complications noted were one screw erosion due to superficial placement near articular surface and two delayed coracoid unions.

Overall, these variants of an arthroscopic Latarjet have demonstrated encouraging short-term data. Longer-term data collected in the coming years will allow for a more thorough comparison to their open counterparts.

References

1. Greis PE, Scuderi MG, Mohr A, Bachus KN, Burks RT. Glenohumeral articular contact areas and pressures following labral and osseous injury to the anteroinferior quadrant of the glenoid. J Shoulder Elbow Surg. 2002;11(5):442–51. doi:10.1067/mse.2002.124526.
2. Lo IK, Parten PM, Burkhart SS. The inverted pear glenoid: an indicator of significant glenoid bone loss. Arthroscopy. 2004;20(2):169–74. doi:10.1016/j.arthro.2003.11.036.
3. Burkhart SS, De Beer JF. Traumatic glenohumeral bone defects and their relationship to failure of arthroscopic Bankart repairs: significance of the inverted-pear glenoid and the engaging Hill-Sachs lesion. Arthroscopy. 2000;16(7):677–94. doi:10.1053/jars.2000.17715.
4. Itoi E, Lee SB, Berglund LJ, An KN. The effect of a glenoid defect on anterior stability of the shoulder after Bankart repair, a cadaveric study. J Bone Joint Surg Am. 2000;82(1):35–46.
5. Warner JJ, Gill TJ, O'Hollerhan JD, Pathare N, Millett PJ. Anatomical glenoid reconstruction for recurrent anterior glenohumeral instability with glenoid deficiency using an autogenous tricortical iliac crest bone graft. Am J Sports Med. 2006;34(2):205–12. doi:10.1177/0363546505281798.
6. Helfet AJ. Coracoid transplantation for recurring dislocation of the shoulder. J Bone Joint Surg Br. 1958;40-B:198–202.
7. Lafosse L, Boyle S. Arthroscopic Laterjet procedure. J Shoulder Elbow Surg. 2010;19:2–12. doi:10.1016/j.jse.2009.12.010.
8. Latarjet M. Treatment of recurrent dislocation of the shoulder. Lyon Chir. 1954;49:994–7. French.
9. Hovelius LK, Sandstrom BC, Rosmark DL, Saebo M, Sundgren KH, Malmqvist BG. Long-term results with the Bankart and Bristow-Latarjet procedures: recurrent shoulder instability and arthropathy. J Shoulder Elbow Surg. 2001;10:445–52. doi:10.1067/mse.2001.117128.
10. Patte D, Debeyre J. Luxations recidivantes de l'epaule. Encycl Med Chir. Technique Chirurgicales. Orthopedie-Traumatologie. Paris: Elsevier; 1980. p. 44–265. 4-02.
11. Allain J, Goutallier D, Glorion C. Long-term results of the Latarjet procedure for the treatment of anterior instability of the shoulder. J Bone Joint Surg Am. 1998;80:841–52.
12. Collin P, Rochcongar P, Thomazeau H. Treatment of chronic anterior shoulder instability using a coracoid bone block (Latarjet procedure): 74 cases. Rev Chir Orthop Reparatrice Appar Mot. 2007;93:126–32. doi:RCO-04-2007-93-2-0035-1040-101019-200520004.
13. Hovelius L, Sandstrom B, Sundgren K, Saebo M. One hundred eighteen Bristow-Latarjet repairs for recurrent anterior dislocation of the shoulder prospectively followed for fifteen years: study Idclinical results. J Shoulder Elbow Surg. 2004;13:509–16. doi:10.1016/j.jse.2004.02.013.
14. Spoor AB, de Waal Malefijt J. Long-term results and arthropathy following the modified Bristow-Latarjet procedure. Int Orthop. 2005;29:265–7. doi:10.1007/s00264-005-0634-x.
15. Walch G. Chronic anterior glenohumeral instability. J Bone Joint Surg Br. 1996;78:670–7.
16. Ghodadra N, Gupta A, Romeo AA, et al. Normalization of glenohumeral articular contact pressures after Latarjet or iliac crest bone grafting. J Bone Joint Surg Am. 2010;92(6):1478–89. doi:10.2106/JBJS.I.00220.
17. Hindmarsh J, Lindberg A. Eden-Hybbinette's operation for recurrent dislocation of the humero-scapular joint. Acta Orthop Scand. 1967;38(4):459–78.
18. Oster A. Recurrent anterior dislocation of the shoulder treated by the Eden-Hybinette operation: follow-up on 78 cases. Acta Orthop Scand. 1969;40(1):43–52.
19. Bhatia S, Van Thiel GS, Ghodadra N, Cole BJ, Bach BR, Shewman E, Wang VM, Romeo AA, Verma NN, Provencher MT. Comparison of glenohumeral contact pressures and contact areas after glenoid reconstruction with Latarjet or distal tibia osteochondral allografts. Am J Sports Med. 2013;41(8). doi:10.1177/0363546513490644
20. Bhatia S, Frank RM, Ghodadra NS, Hsu AR, Romeo AA, Bach BR, Boileau P, Provencher MT. The outcomes and surgical techniques of the Latarjet procedure. Arthroscopy. 2014;30(2):227–35. doi:10.1016/j.arthro.2013.10.013.
21. Provencher MT, Bhatia S, Ghodadra NS, et al. Recurrent shoulder instability: current concepts for evaluation and management of glenoid bone loss. J Bone Joint Surg Am. 2010;92 Suppl 2:133–51. doi:10.2106/JBJS.J.00906.
22. Schmid SL, Farshad M, Catanzaro S, Gerber C. The Latarjet procedure for the treatment of recurrence of anterior instability of the shoulder after operative repair: a retrospective case series of forty-nine patients. J Bone Joint Surg Am. 2012;94(11):e75. doi:10.2106/JBJS.K.00380.
23. Silliman JF, Hawkins RJ. Classification and physical diagnosis of instability of the shoulder. Clin Orthop. 1993;291:7–19.
24. Arciero RA, Taylor DC. Primary anterior dislocation of the shoulder in young patients. A ten-year prospective study. J Bone Joint Surg Am. 1998;80:299–300.
25. Cofield RH, Simonet WT. The shoulder in sports. Mayo Clinic Proc. 1984;59:157–64.
26. Rowe CR. Prognosis in dislocations of the shoulder. J Bone Joint Surg Am. 1956;38:957–77.
27. Montgomery Jr WH, Wahl M, Hettrich C, Itoi E, Lippitt SB, Matsen FA. Anteroinferior bone-grafting can restore stability in osseous glenoid defects. J Bone Joint Am. 2005;87(9):1972–7. doi:10.2106/JBJS.D.02573.
28. Piasecki DP, Verma NN, Romeo AA, Levine WN, Bach Jr BR, Provencher MT. Glenoid bone deficiency in recurrent anterior shoulder instability: diagnosis

and management. J Am Acad Orthop Surg. 2009;17(8):482–93.
29. Sugaya H. Instability with bone loss. AANA Advanced Arthroscopy: The Shoulder. 2010. p. 136–46.
30. Savoie FH. Multidirectional instability of the shoulder joint. AANA Advanced Arthroscopy: The Shoulder. 2010. p. 124–35.
31. Jobe FW, Tibone JE, Jobe CM, Kvitner RS. The shoulder in sports. In: Rockwood CA, Matsen III FA, editors. The shoulder, vol. 2. Philadelphia, PA: Saunders; 1990.
32. Edwards TB, Boulahia A, Walch G. Radiographic analysis of bone defects in chronic anterior shoulder instability. Arthroscopy. 2003;19(7):732–9. doi:10.1016/S0749-8063(03)00684-4.
33. Bigliani LU, Newton PM, Steinmann SP, Connor PM, MvIlveen SJ. Glenoid rim lesions associated with recurrent anterior dislocation of the shoulder. Am J Sports Med. 1998;26:41–45.6.
34. Cassagnaud X, Maynou C, Mestdagh H. Clinical and computed tomography results of 106 Latarjet-Patte procedures at mean 7.5 year follow-up [in French]. Rev Chir Orthop Reparatrice Appar Mot. 2003;89:683–92.doi:RCO-12-2003-89-8-0035-1040-101019-ART3.
35. Mologne TS, Provencher MT, Menzel KA, Vachon TA, Dewing CB. Arthroscopic stabilization in patients with an inverted pear glenoid: results of patients with a loss of the anterior glenoid. Am J Sports Med. 2007;35(8):1276–83. doi:10.1177/0363546507300262.
36. Huysmans PE, Haen PS, Kidd M, Dhert WJ, Willems JW. The shape of the inferior part of the glenoid: a cadaveric study. J Shoulder Elbow Surg. 2006;15:759–63. doi:10.1016/j.jse.2005.09.001.
37. Gracitelli MEC, Neto AAF, Benegas E, Malavolta EA, Sunada EE, Assuncao JH. Arthroscopic Latarjet procedures: safety evaluation in cadavers. Acta Orthop Bras. 2013;21(3):139–43. doi:10.1590/S1413-78522013000300002.
38. Griesser MJ, Harris JD, McCoy BW, Hussain WM, Jones MH, Bishop JY, Miniaci A. Complications and re-operations after Bristow-Latarjet shoulder stabilization: a systematic review. J Shoulder Elbow Surg. 2013;22:286–92. doi:10.1016/j.jse.2012.09.009.
39. Shah AA, Butler RB, Romanowski J, Goel D, Karadagli D, Warner JJ. Short-term complications of the Latarjet procedure. J Bone Joint Surg Am. 2012;94:495–501. doi:10.2106/JBJS.J.01830.
40. Castricini R, Benedetto MD, Orlando N, Rocchi M, Zini R, Pirani P. Arthroscopic Latarjet procedure: analysis of the learning curve. Musculoskelet Surg. 2013;97 Suppl 1:S93–8. doi:10.1007/s12306-013-0262-3.
41. Boileau P, Mercier N, Roussanne Y, Thélu CÉ, Old J. Arthroscopic Bankart-Bristow-Latarjet procedure: the development and early results of a safe and reproducible technique. Arthroscopy. 2010;26(11):1434–50. doi:10.1016/j.arthro.2010.07.011.

Posterior Instability

10

Pramod B. Voleti, Fotios P. Tjoumakaris, Brian J. Sennett, and James P. Bradley

Introduction

Posterior shoulder instability is a relatively rare condition that accounts for approximately 5 % of cases of glenohumeral joint instability [1]. The reported incidence is 1.1 per 100,000 population per year [2]; however, this incidence may be greater in patient populations that routinely engage in activities that are likely to provoke posterior shoulder injury, such as football players, weight lifters, throwing athletes, and rock climbers [3]. Excessive retroversion of the glenoid cavity is another risk factor for posterior instability [4]. With increased awareness, posterior instability is being diagnosed more frequently [5]. However, accurate assessment of the true prevalence of this condition is difficult due to the lack of concrete diagnostic criteria.

The most commonly affected individuals are men between 20 and 30 years of age who are recreational or competitive athletes, typically in overhead or contact sports. While approximately 50 % of patients report a discrete injury to the shoulder that immediately preceded the symptoms, a documented episode of posterior dislocation requiring relocation is relatively less common (23 %) [1, 6]. Of those patients with a known history of dislocation, the most common etiology is trauma, but other potential causes include seizures and electrical shock [7]. The patients with no confirmed dislocation usually have a history of a substantial injury that did not result in dislocation ("macrotrauma") or a history of repetitive minor injuries with the shoulder in the provocative position of flexion, adduction, and internal rotation ("microtrauma") [8–10].

The stability of the glenohumeral joint relies on static restraints (capsule, labrum, humeral head, glenoid fossa) and dynamic stabilizers (rotator cuff, scapular and thoracic musculature, neuromuscular control). Pathology within any of these structures can predispose toward recurrent posterior instability. In particular, pathologies of the posterior capsulolabral complex are believed to be the main contributors toward posterior instability.

P.B. Voleti, MD
Department of Orthopaedic Surgery, Hospital of the University of Pennsylvania, Philadelphia, PA, USA
e-mail: Pramod.Voleti@uphs.upenn.edu

F.P. Tjoumakaris, MD (✉)
Department of Orthopaedic Surgery, The Rothman Institute, Thomas Jefferson University Hospital, Egg Harbor Township, NJ, USA
e-mail: Fotios.tjoumakaris@rothmaninstitute.com

B.J. Sennett, MD
Department of Orthopaedic Surgery, University of Pennsylvania, Philadelphia, PA, USA

Penn Sports Medicine Center, Philadelphia, PA, USA

J.P. Bradley, MD
Department of Orthopaedic Surgery, University of Pittsburgh School of Medicine, Pittsburgh, PA, USA

J.D. Kelly IV (ed.), *Elite Techniques in Shoulder Arthroscopy*,
DOI 10.1007/978-3-319-25103-5_10

Evaluation

A meticulous patient history is critical for diagnosis of posterior shoulder instability. Affected individuals may report a history of dislocation, shoulder trauma, seizure disorder, or electrical shock. Patients with an acute posterior dislocation complain of pain with attempted range of motion, are most comfortable with their arm resting in a sling in internal rotation, and have difficulty with external rotation of the shoulder. A pathognomonic sign is the inability to supinate the forearm with the elbow fully extended. These patients require emergent closed reduction of the glenohumeral joint. In contrast, patients with posterior instability without dislocation have less well-defined symptoms. They may have increased pain with certain positions or motions, such as cross-body adduction or overhead throwing. They may also report numbness, paresthesias, weakness, or fatigue in the affected extremity.

The physical examination should include assessment of the cervical spine, as this may contribute to the shoulder pain. The shoulder exam must include palpation for tenderness, strength testing, assessment for atrophy, passive and active range of motion, impingement signs, and scapular rhythm. Provocative measures, such as the jerk, Kim, and circumduction tests, are useful in assessing for posterior instability and resulting pain, whereas load-and-shift testing can elucidate the extent of glenohumeral laxity. The Kim test is especially useful in detecting posterior inferior labral tears (also known as Kim lesions), while the jerk test is more specific for straight posterior labral injuries. The apprehension sign and relocation test can be used to evaluate for anterior instability, and the sulcus sign suggests multidirectional instability. As always, a careful neurovascular examination of both upper extremities is necessary. Ligamentous laxity of other joints, such as the knee, elbow, and metacarpophalangeal joints, should also be evaluated.

Plain radiographs, including anteroposterior, scapular Y, and axillary views, should be performed in all patients with suspected posterior instability. In a patient with an acute posterior dislocation, the true anteroposterior radiograph (Grashey view) may reveal the "lightbulb sign" when the proximal humerus takes on the shape of a lightbulb secondary to internal rotation of the shoulder and the "empty glenoid sign" when the glenoid fossa appears relatively empty (Fig. 10.1a). The axillary view is necessary to confirm a posterior dislocation (Fig. 10.1b). If a traditional axillary view cannot be obtained due to obligate internal rotation of the shoulder, a Velpeau axillary view may be helpful. The axillary view should never be forgone, as the remaining views may fail to diagnose a posterior dislocation. The scapular Y view is simply insufficient to absolutely rule out posterior instability. Plain radiographs may also reveal a reverse Hill-Sachs lesion on the anterior humeral head, a bone defect in the posterior glenoid rim, and associated fractures of the proximal humerus. A CT scan may be a helpful adjunct for further defining associated fractures, determining the size of the reverse Hill-Sachs lesion, evaluating the extent of posterior glenoid rim bone deficiencies, and determining the degree of glenoid retroversion. MRA or MRI may aid in identifying posterior capsulolabral complex lesions, rotator cuff tears, impaction fractures, and articular cartilage defects. MRI findings that are suggestive of posterior instability include posterior labral injury, posterior labrocapsular avulsion, posterior glenoid bone defects, posterior humeral head translation, humeral avulsion of the posterior band of the inferior glenohumeral ligament, and anterior humeral head bone defects (Fig. 10.2).

Treatment Considerations

Nonoperative treatment should be considered in most cases of posterior shoulder instability. Conservative treatment consists of physical therapy to regain full and symmetric shoulder range of motion, with subsequent emphasis on strengthening of the rotator cuff and the scapular stabilizing muscles. Strengthening the dynamic stabilizers of the glenohumeral joint, such as the rotator cuff and the periscapular musculature, may permit compensation for deficient static stabilizers, such as the labrum and the capsule.

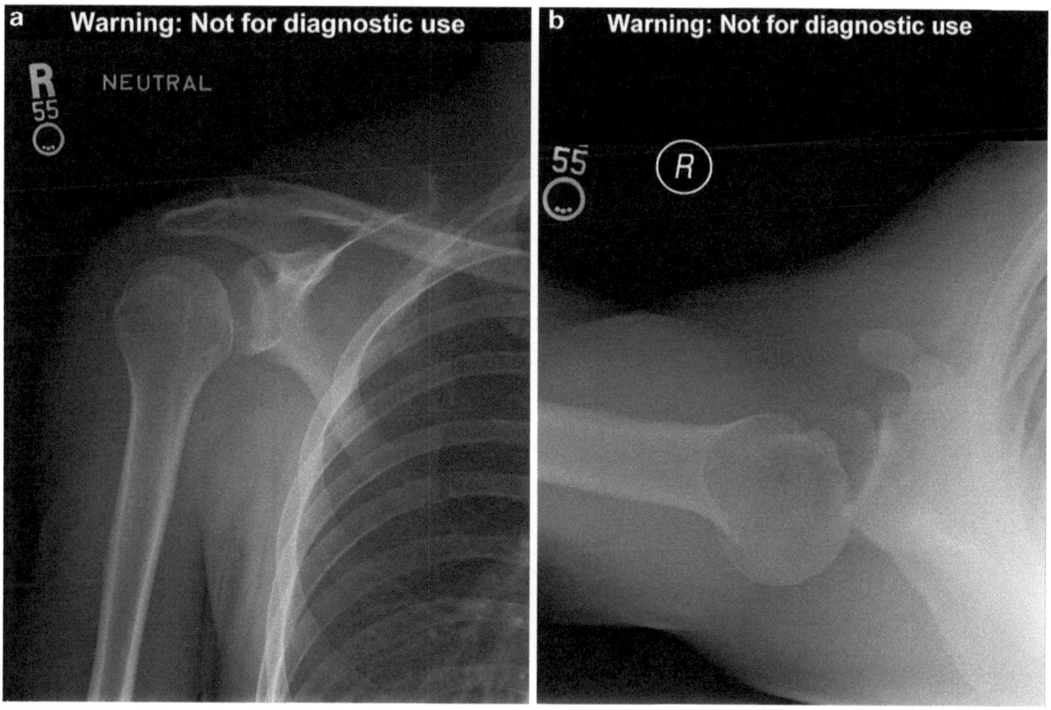

Fig. 10.1 (a) Anteroposterior (Grashey view) and (b) axillary radiographs demonstrating a posterior shoulder dislocation. Note the positive "lightbulb sign" and "empty glenoid sign" on the Grashey view

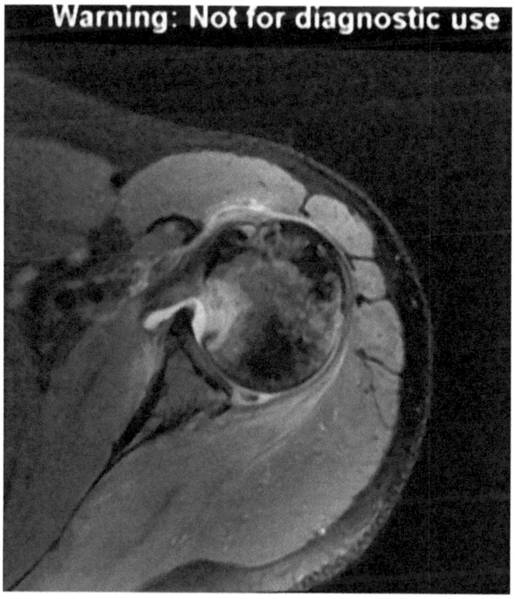

Fig. 10.2 Axial T2-weighted shoulder MRI demonstrating sequelae of prior posterior shoulder dislocation: posterior labral tear, posterior glenoid bone defect, and reverse Hill-Sachs lesion

If nonoperative treatment is successful in restoring full range of motion without recurrent instability, gradual return to sport may be initiated.

Surgical treatment of posterior instability is indicated when conservative management fails to alleviate pain or prevent recurrent instability. Historically, these patients were treated with open posterior stabilization procedures. These techniques had high recurrence rates (as high as 40 %), and few patients treated with these open procedures returned to their previous and desired level of activity [5, 8, 9, 11–14]. With the advent of advanced arthroscopic techniques, the mean recurrence rate following surgical treatment for posterior shoulder instability has decreased to 5 %, with a range of 0–10 % in most recent series. Furthermore, a greater percentage of patients have returned to their previous level of activity or sport (89–100 %) [15–17]. When comparing open versus arthroscopic stabilization procedures, the latter has been shown to result in superior functional outcomes [18]. Arthroscopic procedures are generally more successful because they are more effective at restoring native anatomy. Cadaver biomechanics studies have shown that open bone block procedures, which involve creating a buttress against posterior humeral translation, over-constrain the joint and do not restore inferior stability as effectively as arthroscopic posterior Bankart repairs [19].

Arthroscopic Technique for Posterior Instability

In the majority of patients with posterior shoulder instability, arthroscopic surgery can result in excellent functional outcomes with low rates of recurrence and complications. The authors' preferred technique is described below.

Prior to surgical intervention, patient history, physical examination, and imaging studies should be reviewed. Concomitant pathology, such as rotator cuff tears, SLAP tears, bone defects, and loose bodies, should be identified in advance. General anesthesia with an interscalene block is most effective at achieving complete muscle relaxation. Prior to positioning, an examination under anesthesia is performed to confirm the diagnosis and to assess the degree of instability. The examination may include the sulcus test, load-and-shift test, jerk test, Kim test, and/or circumduction test. We prefer lateral decubitus positioning as it allows greater exposure of the posterior labrum and capsule when compared to beach-chair positioning. An inflatable beanbag should be utilized to restrain the patient, with appropriate cushioning of the axilla and bony prominences. The operative extremity is placed in balanced arm traction in 45° of abduction and 20° of forward flexion using 10–15 pounds of weight.

We prefer an all-arthroscopic repair technique. A single posterior portal in line with the lateral edge of the acromion and through the deltoid is created first. This portal is utilized for anchor placement and suture management. It should permit an anchor placement trajectory of 45° relative to the glenoid face. Placement of this portal slightly lateral to the standard posterior portal may allow superior access to the posterior glenoid rim for lateral anchor placement. Alternatively, if the anchor placement trajectory is less than ideal through the posterior portal, an accessory lateral portal may provide better access, particularly to the 7-o'clock position of the glenoid margin. The anterior portal is then created through the rotator interval just inferior to the biceps tendon via either an inside-out technique with a switching stick or an outside-in technique with a spinal needle. Clear cannulas are placed through both portals: a 5.75-mm cannula anteriorly for arthroscopic visualization and an 8.25-mm cannula posteriorly for the working portal.

With the arthroscope in the posterior portal, a diagnostic arthroscopy is performed. The articular surfaces of the glenohumeral joint are inspected for chondral damage, the humeral head is evaluated for Hill-Sachs lesions, and the glenoid rim is assessed for bone defects. The anterior and inferior labrum and the glenohumeral ligaments are visualized and inspected. The biceps tendon and superior labrum should be probed through the anterior portal to detect concomitant pathology, such as a SLAP tear. Finally, the rotator cuff should be inspected, including the subscapularis tendon. The arthroscope is then placed into the anterior portal where it remains for the rest of the operation. Through the anterior portal, the posterior labrum and capsule are inspected and probed. In addition, the anterior humeral head is evaluated for a reverse Hill-Sachs lesion.

Following a thorough diagnostic arthroscopy, a periosteal elevator is used to elevate the labrum off the posterior glenoid rim. Alternatively, the labrum may be mobilized with an arthroscopic rasp or chisel. The posterior margin of the glenoid is then débrided using a motorized burr or shaver device. The elevator, rasp, chisel, burr, and/or shaver may be introduced through an accessory anterior portal for ease of access.

Once the labrum has been elevated and the glenoid rim débrided, the arthroscope remains in the anterior portal. A 70° arthroscope may provide superior visualization of the posterior and inferior glenoid margins. Using the posterior portal as the working portal, anchors are placed along the posterior glenoid margin, starting inferiorly and progressing superiorly as needed (Fig. 10.3).

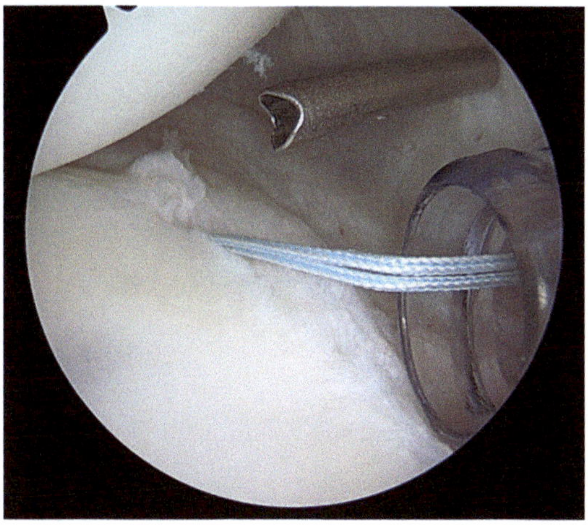

Fig. 10.3 Arthroscopic photograph demonstrating placement of the first anchor along the posterior glenoid margin

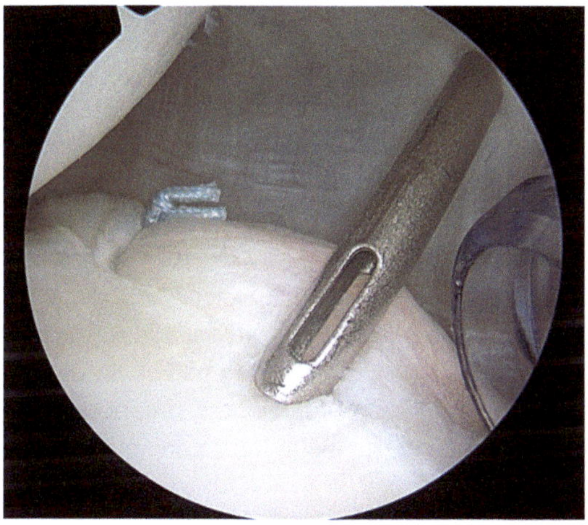

Fig. 10.4 Arthroscopic photograph demonstrating typical anchor spacing (3–5 mm) so as to avoid fragmentation or fracture of the posterior glenoid

Alternatively, anchors may be placed through small stab incisions if the posterior portal does not afford sufficient access to the glenoid. We recommend biocomposite anchors with a 2- to 2.4-mm diameter, spaced 3–5 mm apart, so as to avoid fragmentation or fracture of the posterior glenoid (Fig. 10.4). The anchor pilot holes are predrilled, and the anchor is inserted with a mallet. The anchors should be placed such that the sutures are perpendicular to the glenoid rim.

Next, the posterior suture limb of the inferiormost anchor is shuttled around the labrum and capsule (Fig. 10.5). In order to achieve capsular plication, the capsular bite should extend inferior and lateral to the anchor. The direction of suture passage is aimed at restoring tension to the posterior band of the inferior glenohumeral ligament. Patients with significant posterior instability may require a more aggressive plication than those with isolated pathology to the glenoid labrum. Capsular plication should be avoided in high-level throwing athletes who would be impaired by excessive tightening of the posterior capsule: in these cases, the suture can be shuttled around the labrum at the location of anchor placement. Suture passage may be achieved with a suture hook, taking care not to cross the suture. The two limbs of the suture are then tied: the limb that has been passed through the capsule and the labrum should be used as the post limb so as to ensure that the knot is placed away from the glenohumeral joint. The suture limbs of the remaining anchors are then tied in an inferior to superior direction (Fig. 10.6). The tension achieved with each advancing stitch should be assessed. For labral tears that extend to the superior margin of the labrum, care must be taken to avoid abrasion of the knot against the posterosuperior rotator cuff during shoulder motion. To accomplish this, we prefer using either 2-mm anchors loaded with No. 1 suture or a knotless 2.9-mm anchor (Fig. 10.7).

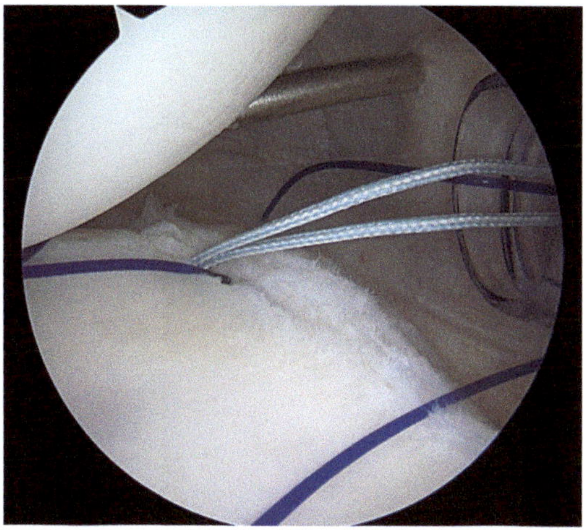

Fig. 10.5 Arthroscopic photograph demonstrating shuttling of the posterior suture limb around the labrum and capsule

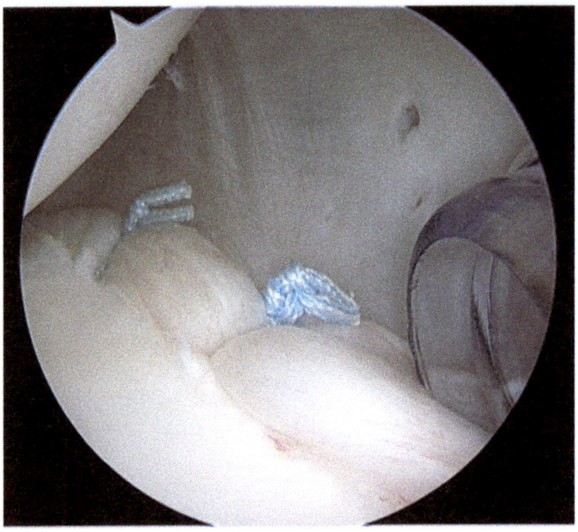

Fig. 10.6 Arthroscopic photograph demonstrating tied suture limbs securing the posterior labrum and capsule to their anatomic position

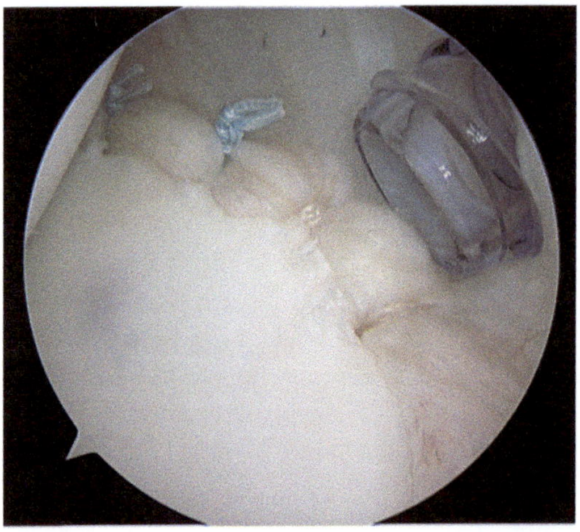

Fig. 10.7 Arthroscopic photograph demonstrating use of 2-mm anchors loaded with No. 1 suture at the superior margin of the labrum to avoid abrasion of the knot against the posterosuperior rotator cuff during shoulder motion

Once all the sutures have been tied, the posterior capsule is closed (Fig. 10.8). First, an arthroscopic awl is used to penetrate the posterior bare area of the humerus so as to augment the healing response. The posterior cannula is then withdrawn to a level just posterior to the capsule. A crescent suture hook loaded with suture is used to penetrate one side of the posterior capsular rent, and the suture is retrieved through the opposite side of the rent with a penetrating grasper.

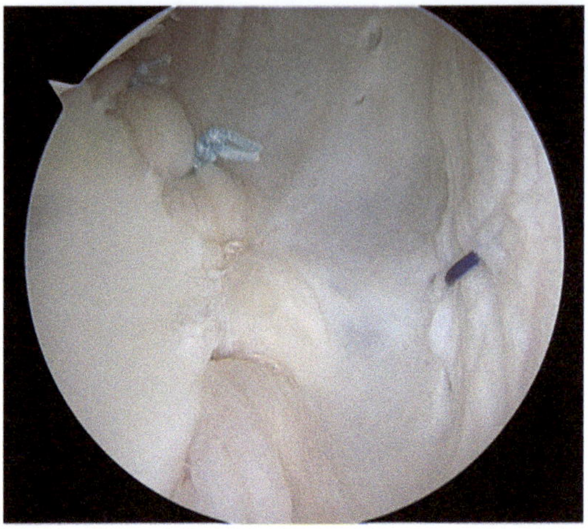

Fig. 10.8 Arthroscopic photograph demonstrating closure of the posterior capsule

The suture is then tied blindly just beyond the posterior capsule. Additional tension may be applied to the posterior capsule by varying the distance of the suture from the capsular rent on either side. If further plication is warranted (such as in cases of multidirectional instability), additional sutures may be placed in the rotator interval or anterior capsule as needed. The rotator interval is not routinely addressed as interval closure has not been shown to potentiate results. Once the repair is complete, the skin portals are closed with interrupted nylon suture and a sterile dressing is applied.

Postoperatively, we recommend use of an abduction sling. Passive range of motion may be initiated on postoperative day 1. At 4 weeks, external rotation to 0° and forward elevation to 90° are permitted. At 6 weeks, the sling is discontinued and active-assisted range-of-motion exercises and gentle passive range-of-motion exercises are initiated. The patient then progresses gradually to active motion without any constraints. The shoulder is typically pain-free with near-normal range of motion at 4 months; at this time, rotator cuff strengthening and conditioning may be initiated. Isotonic and isokinetic exercises are advanced at 5 months. At 6 months, patients are assessed for return to play. Non-throwing athletes may be released to a sport-specific program once 80 % of their strength and endurance relative to the contralateral extremity has been achieved. Overhead athletes may begin a throwing program at this stage of rehabilitation, provided they have achieved 80 % of their strength and endurance. Full, competitive throwing is typically not attained until 12 months after surgery.

Summary

Posterior shoulder instability presents a surgical challenge. Of critical importance is a meticulous preoperative evaluation, including a thorough patient history, focused physical examination, and appropriate imaging studies. If nonoperative management is unsuccessful in restoring full range of motion without recurrent instability, surgical treatment should be considered. Arthroscopic techniques have revolutionized our ability to treat posterior instability, affording decreased recurrence rates, greater likelihood of return to activity, superior functional outcomes, and improved satisfaction.

References

1. Wolf EM, Eakin CL. Arthroscopic capsular plication for posterior shoulder instability. Arthroscopy. 1998;14: 153–63. doi:10.1016/S0749-8063(98)70034-9.
2. Robinson CM, Seah M, Akhtar MA. The epidemiology, risk of recurrence, and functional outcome after an acute traumatic posterior dislocation of the shoulder. J Bone Joint Surg Am. 2011;93:1605–13. doi:10.2106/JBJS.J.00973.
3. Antoniou J, Duckworth DT, Harryman DT. Capsulolabral augmentation for the management of posteroinferior instability of the shoulder. J Bone Joint Surg Am. 2000;82:1220–30.
4. Brewer BJ, Wubben RC, Carrera GF. Excessive retroversion of the glenoid cavity. A cause of non-traumatic posterior instability of the shoulder. J Bone Joint Surg Am. 1986;68:724–31.
5. Tibone JE, Bradley JP. The treatment of posterior subluxation in athletes. Clin Orthop Relat Res. 1993;124–37. doi:10.1097/00003086-199306000-00014.
6. McIntyre LF, Caspari RB, Savoie FH. The arthroscopic treatment of posterior shoulder instability: two-year results of a multiple suture technique. Arthroscopy. 1997;13:426–32. doi:10.1016/S0749-8063(97)90119-5.
7. Millett PJ, Clavert P, Hatch GFR, Warner JJP. Recurrent posterior shoulder instability. J Am Acad Orthop Surg. 2006;14:464–76. doi:10.2106/JBJS.D.02906.
8. Hawkins RJ, Koppert G, Johnston G. Recurrent posterior instability (subluxation) of the shoulder. J Bone Joint Surg Am. 1984;66:169–74.
9. Fronek J, Warren RF, Bowen M. Posterior subluxation of the glenohumeral joint. J Bone Joint Surg Am. 1989;71:205–16.
10. Pollock R, Bigliani L. Glenohumeral instability: evaluation and treatment. J Am Acad Orthop Surg. 1993;1:24–32. Available at: http://www.ncbi.nlm.nih.gov/pubmed/10675853.
11. Bigliani LU, Pollock RG, McIlveen SJ, Endrizzi DP, Flatow EL. Shift of the posteroinferior aspect of the capsule for recurrent posterior glenohumeral instability. J Bone Joint Surg Am. 1995;77:1011–20.
12. Misamore GW, Facibene WA. Posterior capsulorrhaphy for the treatment of traumatic recurrent posterior subluxations of the shoulder in athletes. J Shoulder Elbow Surg. 2000;9:403–8. doi:10.1067/mse.2000.108963.
13. Meuffels DE, Schuit H, van Biezen FC, Reijman M, Verhaar JAN. The posterior bone block procedure in posterior shoulder instability: a long-term follow-up study. J Bone Joint Surg Br. 2010;92:651–5. doi:10.1302/0301-620X.92B5.23529.
14. Yong GR, Dong HL, Chan TL. Posterior capsulolabral reconstruction in posterior shoulder instability: deltoid saving. J Shoulder Elbow Surg. 2005;14:355–60. doi:10.1016/j.jse.2004.10.014.
15. Bahk MS, Karzel RP, Snyder SJ. Arthroscopic posterior stabilization and anterior capsular plication for recurrent posterior glenohumeral instability. Arthroscopy. 2010;26:1172–80. doi:10.1016/j.arthro.2010.06.016.
16. Bradley JP, Baker CL, Kline AJ, Armfield DR, Chhabra A. Arthroscopic capsulolabral reconstruction for posterior instability of the shoulder: a prospective study of 100 shoulders. Am J Sports Med. 2006;34:1061–71. doi:10.1177/0363546505285585.
17. Kim S-H, Ha K-I, Park J-H, et al. Arthroscopic posterior labral repair and capsular shift for traumatic unidirectional recurrent posterior subluxation of the shoulder. J Bone Joint Surg Am. 2003;85-A:1479–87. doi:10.1016/S0749-8063(07)60138-8.
18. Bottoni CR, Franks BR, Moore JH, DeBerardino TM, Taylor DC, Arciero RA. Operative stabilization of posterior shoulder instability. Am J Sports Med. 2005;33:996–1002. doi:10.1177/0363546504271509.
19. Wellmann M, Bobrowitsch E, Khan N, et al. Biomechanical effectiveness of an arthroscopic posterior bankart repair versus an open bone block procedure for posterior shoulder instability. Am J Sports Med. 2011;39:796–803. doi:10.1177/0363546510389991.

Part III

Glenohumeral Arthritis

Pearls for Thorough Debridement, Capsular Release, and Role of Microfracture

11

Brian C. Domby, Brian J. Cole, and Eric C. McCarty

Introduction

There has been increasing interest in arthroscopic treatment of glenohumeral arthritis over the last 10–15 years. While total shoulder arthroplasty is considered a reliable procedure for treatment of glenohumeral arthritis, concerns for glenoid loosening especially in a young and active population have led to increased interest in alternative treatments [1]. Sperling et al. reported a 38 % incidence of glenoid component failure in a series of 33 patients with a mean age of 46 years that underwent total shoulder arthroplasty for arthritis following instability surgery [1]. The early failure of arthroplasty in younger, more active patients has prompted attention to arthroscopic approaches to glenohumeral arthritis. Numerous studies have reported improved function, pain relief, and range of motion after arthroscopic treatment [2–7].

Nonoperative management for symptomatic osteoarthritis of the shoulder includes activity modification, corticosteroid injections, off-label use of viscosupplementation, and physical therapy [8]. When nonoperative treatment fails to provide a level of desired symptomatic relief, operative treatment is indicated. Arthroscopic treatment of the glenohumeral joint may include debridement, chondroplasty, capsular release, removal of loose bodies, microfracture, autologous chondrocyte implantation, osteochondral grafting, biceps tenotomy or tenodesis, and removal of osteophytes [9]. Other sources of pain such as the subacromial space, distal clavicle, and suprascapular nerve entrapment should also be addressed when relevant. Millet et al. have also advocated axillary nerve neurolysis and debridement of inferior humeral head osteophyte, and this approach is elucidated further in another chapter [7].

The goal of this chapter is to review the role of debridement, microfracture, and capsular release in addressing glenohumeral arthritis. The authors' preferred operative technique will be discussed along with technical pearls.

Debridement

Arthroscopic debridement of the glenohumeral joint is a palliative treatment strategy that can stabilize cartilage lesions (chondroplasty), reduce mechanical symptoms, and reduce the biologic burden that the synovium is subjected to. Addressing concomitant pathology such as the

B.C. Domby, MD (✉)
Orthopaedic Sports Medicine and Spine Center, Florida Medical Clinic, Tampa, FL, USA
e-mail: bdomby@gmail.com

B.J. Cole, MD, MBA
Department of Orthopaedics, Rush University Medical Center, Chicago, IL, USA

E.C. McCarty, MD
Department of Orthopaedic Surgery, University of Colorado School of Medicine, Aurora, CO, USA

J.D. Kelly IV (ed.), *Elite Techniques in Shoulder Arthroscopy*,
DOI 10.1007/978-3-319-25103-5_11

biceps, acromioclavicular (AC) joint, subacromial space, rotator cuff, and suprascapular nerve should be performed when indicated as this strategy is associated with improved surgical outcomes [2–7]. Arthroscopic capsular release should be considered if range of motion is limited [4, 7].

Ogilvie-Harris et al. first reported on successful arthroscopic treatment of mild glenohumeral arthritis in the shoulder in 1986 [10]. Since then, multiple authors have reported improved outcomes with arthroscopic debridement [2–7].

Van Thiel et al. from one of the senior author's (BJC) institution reported significant improvements in pain, Simple Shoulder Test, American Shoulder and Elbow Surgeon (ASES) score, and rage of motion at short-term follow-up in 71 patients that underwent arthroscopic debridement of glenohumeral cartilage lesions [6]. Sixteen shoulders (22 %) underwent arthroplasty at mean 10.1 months after debridement. A higher failure rate was observed in those with grade IV bipolar diseases, joint space less than 2 mm, and large osteophytes [6].

Cameron et al. reported significant improvements in pain, patient satisfaction, and function at 28 months in 54 of 61 (88 %) in patients with grade IV osteochondral lesions that underwent arthroscopic debridement with or without capsular release [3]. Concomitant procedures such as acromioplasty, distal clavicle resection, labral debridement, and labral repair did not have a negative impact on functional results. Lesions greater than 2 cm^2 were associated with failure [3].

Weinstein et al. performed arthroscopic lavage, debridement of labral tears and chondral lesions, loose body removal, partial synovectomy, and subacromial bursectomy in 25 patients. At average follow-up of 34 months, they concluded that arthroscopic debridement is a reasonable approach for treating early glenohumeral osteoarthritis that has failed to respond to nonoperative treatment in which the humeral head and glenoid remain concentric, and there is visible joint space on an axillary radiograph [2].

Kerr et al. from one of the senior author's (ECM) institution reported on 19 shoulders younger than 55 years with grade II–IV changes in the glenohumeral joint that underwent arthroscopic debridement with minimum 12-month follow-up. The grade of the lesion did not influence outcomes, but bipolar lesions were associated with inferior outcomes [5].

Millet et al. recently reported on their results of the "Comprehensive Arthroscopic Management (CAM) procedure" for 30 shoulders in active patients with glenohumeral arthritis. They performed chondroplasty; removal of loose bodies if present; humeral osteoplasty and osteophyte resection; anterior, posterior, and inferior capsular release; subacromial decompression; axillary nerve neurolysis; and biceps tenodesis. There was a 92 % survival rate at 1 year and 85 % at 2 years. Patients with larger osteophytes had greater improvements in range of motion but were less satisfied. Patients with joint space less than 2 mm had significantly higher failure rate [7].

In summary, arthroscopic debridement is a valuable treatment option for patients with focal cartilage lesions found incidentally at the time of another shoulder procedure and for treatment of early glenohumeral arthritis. Debridement can be combined with other procedures such as capsular release, biceps tenotomy or tenodesis, and distal clavicle excision in patients with concomitant symptoms. Bipolar lesions and a joint space less than 2 mm on preoperative radiographs have been shown to be associated with inferior outcomes.

Capsular Release

Capsular tightness restricts range of motion of the shoulder and increases contact pressures in the glenohumeral joint. Active motion applied to a contracted joint increases joint reactive forces. A more supple joint requires less compression to effect active motion. Releasing the capsule decreases the contact pressure and allows increased range of motion [4]. Richards et al. reported improved range of motion in a series of eight patients and mean symptom-free period of 9 months in patients that underwent arthroscopic debridement and capsular release for glenohumeral osteoarthritis. They reported mean improvement of

21.4° forward flexion, 16.6° external rotation, and 31.1° of internal rotation. Cameron et al. performed capsular release in 22 of 61 patients with stiff shoulders in addition to debridement in there series. They reported significant improvement in forward elevation, external rotation, and internal rotation [3].

Millet et al. recently reported on their results of "Comprehensive Arthroscopic Management (CAM) procedure" for 30 shoulders in active patients with glenohumeral arthritis. They performed chondroplasty; removal of loose bodies if present; humeral osteoplasty and osteophyte resection; anterior, posterior, and inferior capsular release; subacromial decompression; axillary nerve neurolysis; and biceps tenodesis. Capsular release was performed in all patients, and they reported significant improvement in range or motion [7].

Arthroscopic capsular release should be considered in patients undergoing arthroscopic treatment of glenohumeral arthritis with limited range of motion. It may be combined with other procedures to treat glenohumeral arthritis as indicated.

Microfracture

Microfracture was first popularized by Steadman et al. in treating chondral defects in the knee [11]. Microfracture is a marrow-stimulation procedure that produces a fibrocartilaginous hyalinelike tissue [12]. More recently, microfracture has been used to treat isolated full-thickness cartilage defects in the shoulder with encouraging results [13–16]. However, the articular cartilage anatomy of the shoulder varies significantly from the knee. The articular cartilage on the glenoid is thicker at the periphery than it is centrally. In contrast, the cartilage on the humeral head is thickest centrally (1.2–1.3 mm) and is thinner peripherally (approximately 1 mm) [17].

Millet et al. reported on 31 shoulders with full-thickness chondral defects of the glenohumeral joint treated with microfracture with minimum 2-year follow-up. Concomitant procedures with the exception of rotator cuff repair were performed when indicated. At a mean follow-up of 47 months, they reported improvement in ASES score, decreased pain, and improved ability to work and to perform sports activities. There was 19 % failure rate. A negative correlation was found between size of the lesion and ASES score improvement. Bipolar lesions were also associated with worse results [13].

Frank et al. also from one of the senior (BJC) author's institution reported on 17 shoulders with full-thickness chondral defects in the glenohumeral joint treated with microfracture. Concomitant procedures with the exception of labral and rotator cuff repair were also performed. At average follow-up of 27.8 months (range 12.1–89.2months), they reported significantly improved visual analogue scale ratings, ASES score, and Simple Shoulder Test (SST) [14].

Siebold et al. reported decreased pain and improved function in patients that underwent open microfracture and periosteal-flap insertion. A significant reduction of the repaired cartilage lesion was seen in three patients that underwent second-look arthroscopy [15].

Microfracture is indicated to treat focal contained cartilage defects in the shoulder and focal degenerative lesions. Bipolar lesions are not a contraindication; however, they are associated with inferior outcomes. While the procedure itself is not technically difficult, there are several technical pearls that are important for success.

Authors' Operative Technique

The patient is positioned in beach chair position (Fig. 11.1a). Examination under anesthesia is performed prior to draping to assess for loss of motion in forward elevation, abduction, internal rotation and external rotation with the arm at the side, and internal and external rotation with the arm in 90° abduction. A mechanical arm holder is used and adjusted as needed to hold the arm in the optimal position during the procedure. Standard posterior and anterosuperior portals are established and adjusted as needed based on procedure being performed. A standard diagnostic arthroscopy is always performed.

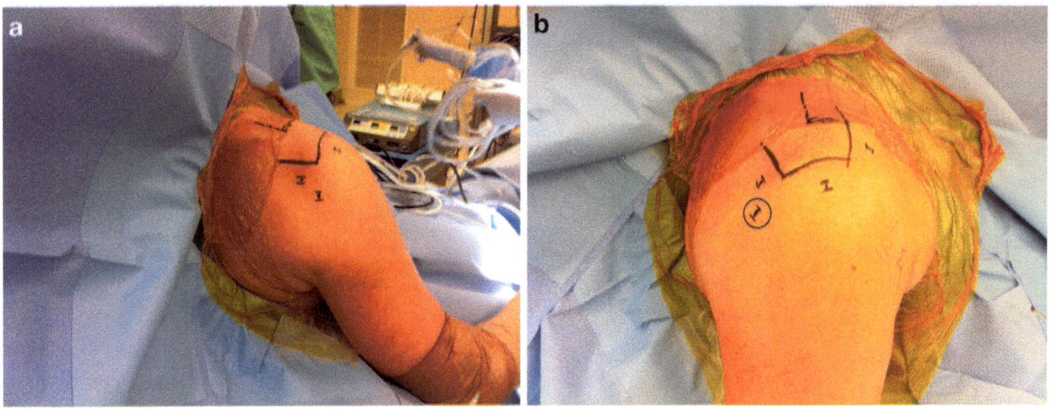

Fig. 11.1 (**a**) The patient is positioned in a beach chair position. Anatomic landmarks and portals are drawn. (**b**) The posterior portal is placed more superiorly and an accessory posteroinferior portal (*circled*) is also drawn; however, this is localized with a spinal needle under direct visualization

Debridement Technique

Standard posterior, lateral, and anterior portals are used and a standard diagnostic arthroscopy is performed. The posterior portal is typically positioned more superiorly to allow improved visualization for debridement (Fig. 11.1b). A 4.0-mm arthroscopic shaver is used to debride the labrum and the cartilage lesion to stable vertical walls. A curette is use as needed to create stable walls. A posteroinferior accessory portal is used to access the axillary pouch, remove loose bodies, and debride inferior humeral bone spur (Figs. 11.2 and 11.3a). A subacromial decompression, distal clavicle excision, and biceps tenodesis are performed as indicated.

Capsular Release Technique

Examination under anesthesia is performed to assess for loss of motion in forward elevation, abduction, internal rotation and external rotation with the arm at the side, and internal and external rotation with the arm in 90° abduction. Standard posterior and anterosuperior portals are established with an anterior working cannula. A standard diagnostic arthroscopy is performed. A posteroinferior portal is then established under direct visualization to allow access to axillary pouch and inferior capsule (Fig. 11.2). A spinal needle is used to localize this portal. A hooked electrocautery probe is introduced through the posteroinferior portal and the inferior capsular release is

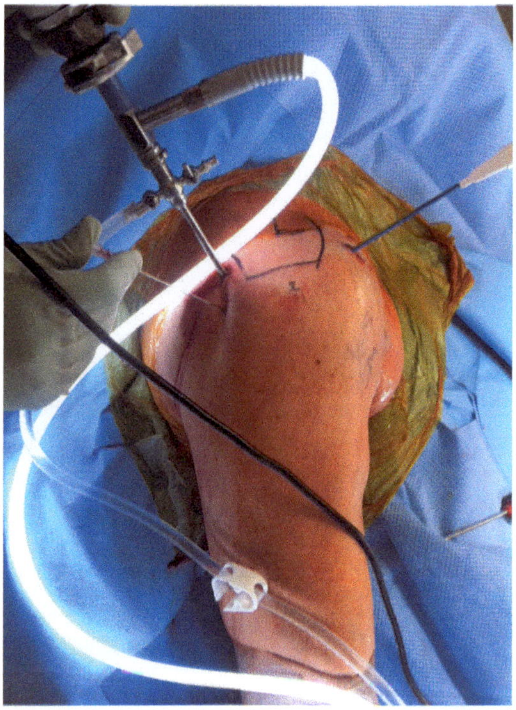

Fig. 11.2 The arthroscope is in the posterior portal and a spinal needle is used to localize the accessory posteroinferior portal in the axillary pouch. This allows access for debridement in the axillary pouch and inferior capsular release

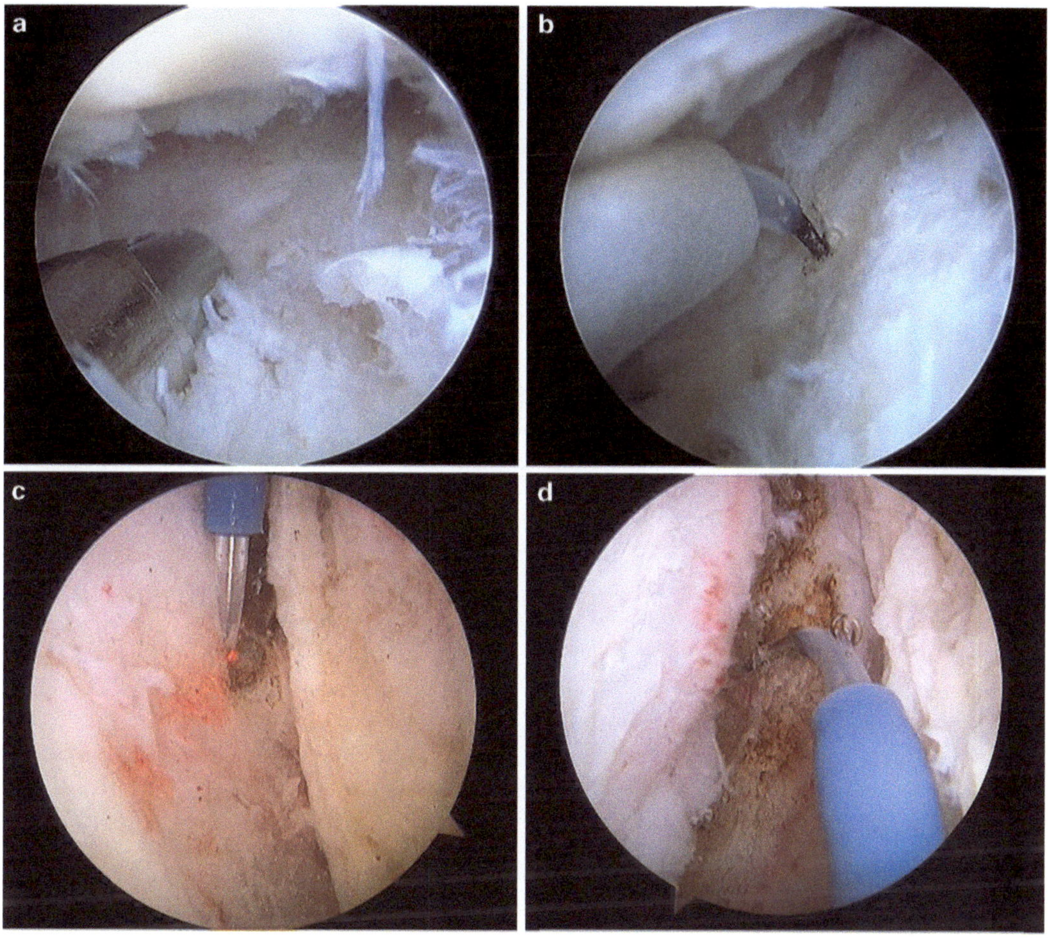

Fig. 11.3 (**a**) The shaver is introduced through the posteroinferior portal into the axillary pouch to remove loose bodies. (**b**) The hooked electrocautery probe is introduced through the posteroinferior portal to perform inferior capsular release. Release is performed at the capsulolabral junction and the probe is angled toward the glenoid neck. (**c**) The probe is introduced through the anterior portal and anterior capsular release is performed at the capsulolabral junction. The rotator interval is also released. Care is taken not to damage the subscapularis. (**d**) The scope is placed through the anterior portal and the probe through the posterior portal to perform posterior capsular release. This is connected with the inferior capsular release

performed under direct visualization (Fig. 11.3b). The arm is placed in abduction to increase the distance of the axillary nerve away from the glenoid and thus away from the area of release. The capsular release is performed just off the capsulolabral junction with the hook aimed at the glenoid neck. Care must be taken not to injure the axillary nerve and adherence close to the labrum will minimize this risk. Anterior capsular release is then performed through the anterosuperior portal (Fig. 11.3c). A combination of a shaver and electrocautery device is used to release the rotator interval to the coracoid. Care must be taken not to damage the coracoacromial ligament. The anterior capsule is then released at the capsulolabral junction to connect with the inferior capsular release. Care must be taken not to damage the subscapularis.

A switching stick is then introduced into the anterior portal under direct visualization and another through the posterior portal. The scope is switched to the anterosuperior portal and the working cannula is placed in the posterior portal. A combination of electrocautery device and

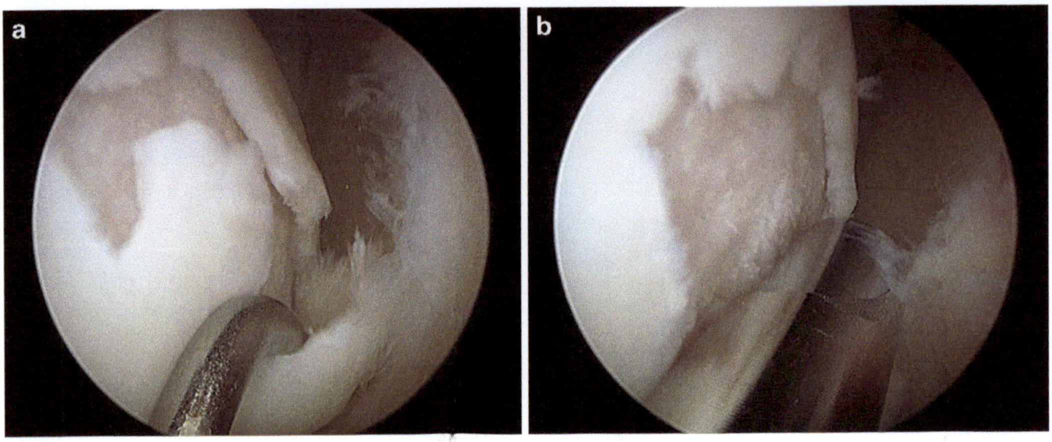

Fig. 11.4 Arthroscopic view through the posterior portal. (**a**) Grade IV lesion with unstable cartilage flaps is demonstrated with a probe. (**b**) A combination of a 4.0-mm arthroscopic shaver and curettes is used to debride the unstable cartilage flaps

shaver is then used to perform the posterior capsular release just off the capsulolabral junction (Fig. 11.3d). The release is started at the posterior extension of the inferior capsular release and extended superiorly at the capsulolabral junction. Care must be taken not to inadvertently injure the posterior rotator cuff. Following extensive release of the capsule, the arthroscope is taken out and the shoulder is manipulated in all directions.

Microfracture Technique

If there are isolated cartilage defects, then a microfracture of the defect is indicated. After a standard diagnostic arthroscopy is performed, the arm should be positioned to allow optimal access to the lesion. A mechanical arm holder is very helpful to hold the arm with the lesion rotated into optimal position. Accessory portals can be used in addition to standard anterior and posterior portals as needed to achieve optimal trajectory to access the lesion. A combination of an arthroscopic shaver and curette is used to debride unstable flaps and create stable vertical walls (Fig. 11.4a, b). The calcified cartilage layer should be removed with a curette. This layer is thinner in the shoulder than it is in the knee, so care must be taken to not remove subchondral bone. A sharp microfracture awl is then used to penetrate the subchondral bone as perpendicular as possible to a depth of 3–4 mm (Fig. 11.5a). This is started in the periphery of the lesion, and they should be spaced approximately 3 mm apart. It is critical that the pump or inflow is turned off and bleeding is confirmed from the subchondral bone (Fig. 11.5b).

Postoperative Rehabilitation

A sling is typically worn for a few days for comfort. Pendulum exercises are started immediately along with full passive range of motion. Early range of motion is important to prevent stiffness and to stimulate healing of the microfracture. If microfracture is performed, active range of motion and weight bearing is typically avoided for 6–8 weeks. If microfracture is not performed, active range of motion is allowed immediately. Strengthening is typically started around 8 weeks. Return to full activities and sports is usually allowed at 4–6 months.

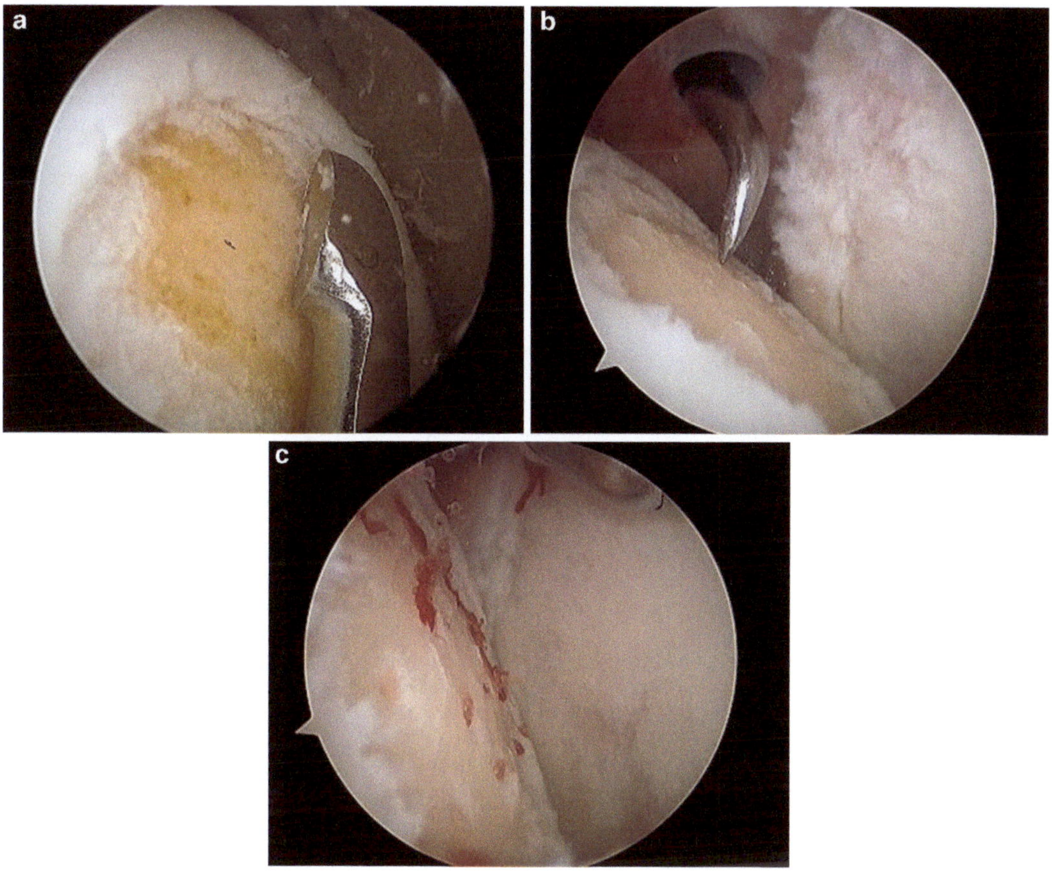

Fig. 11.5 (**a**) Stable vertical walls are obtained at the periphery and the calcified cartilage layer is debrided with a curette. (**b**) A microfracture awl is used to perform microfracture of this focal grade IV cartilage lesion on the humeral head and spaced approximately 3 mm apart. (**c**) The inflow is turned off and bleeding is confirmed from the microfracture holes

Conclusion

Arthroscopic treatment of glenohumeral osteoarthritis should be tailored to meet each patient's needs. Chondroplasty should be performed to stabilize the borders of focal cartilage lesions and for incidental lesions found during another procedure. Debridement can be combined with other procedures such as biceps tenotomy or tenodesis and distal clavicle excision in patients with concomitant symptoms. Bipolar lesions and a joint space less than 2 mm on preoperative radiographs have been shown to portend an inferior outcome. Microfracture is a valuable tool in treating focal contained cartilage defects and focal DJD lesions; however, bipolar lesions are associated with poorer outcomes. Arthroscopic capsular release should be considered in patients undergoing arthroscopic treatment of glenohumeral arthritis with limited range of motion. Capsular release decreases joint contact pressure and reliably increases range of motion.

Pearls

- Bipolar lesions and a joint space less than 2 mm are associated with worse outcomes.
- Concomitant symptomatic pathology such as biceps tendinopathy, subacromial bursitis, and AC joint arthrosis should be addressed.
- Using a mechanical arm holder is helpful to hold arm in optimal position for capsular release and/or microfracture of isolated cartilage defects.

- Placing the posterior portal more superior aids in visualization for capsular release and extensive debridement.
- A posteroinferior accessory portal should be used to access axillary recess for removal of loose bodies, inferior capsular release, and removal of inferior osteophyte if indicated.
- Abduct the arm during inferior capsular release to increase distance to axillary nerve.
- Early physical therapy is critical to maintain motion gained during surgery.

References

1. Sperling JW, Antuna SA, Sanchez-Sotelo J, Schleck C, Cofield RH. Shoulder arthroplasty for arthritis after instability surgery. J Bone Joint Surg Am. 2002; 84-A(10):1775–81.
2. Weinstein DM, Bucchieri JS, Pollock RG, Flatow EL, Bigliani LU. Arthroscopic debridement of the shoulder for osteoarthritis. Arthroscopy. 2000;16(5): 471–6.
3. Cameron BD, Galatz LM, Ramsey ML, Williams GR, Iannotti JP. Non-prosthetic management of grade IV osteochondral lesions of the glenohumeral joint. J Shoulder Elbow Surg. 2002;11(1):25–32.
4. Richards DP, Burkhart SS. Arthroscopic debridement and capsular release for glenohumeral osteoarthritis. Arthroscopy. 2007;23(9):1019–22.
5. Kerr BJ, McCarty EC. Outcome of arthroscopic débridement is worse for patients with glenohumeral arthritis of both sides of the joint. Clin Orthop Relat Res. 2008;466(3):634–8.
6. Van Thiel GS, Sheehan S, Frank RM, Slabaugh M, Cole BJ, Nicholson GP, Romeo AA, Verma NN. Retrospective analysis of arthroscopic management of glenohumeral degenerative disease. Arthroscopy. 2010;26(11):1451–5.
7. Millett PJ, Horan MP, Pennock AT, Rios D. Comprehensive Arthroscopic Management (CAM) procedure: clinical results of a joint-preserving arthroscopic treatment for young, active patients with advanced shoulder osteoarthritis. Arthroscopy. 2013; 29(3):440–8.
8. Denard PJ, Wirth MA, Orfaly RM. Management of glenohumeral arthritis in the young adult. J Bone Joint Surg Am. 2011;93(9):885–92.
9. Bhatia S, Hsu A, Lin EC, Chalmers P, Ellman M, Cole BJ, Verma NN. Surgical treatment options for the young and active middle-aged patient with glenohumeral arthritis. Adv Orthop. 2012;2012:846843.
10. Ogilvie-Harris DJ, Wiley AM. Arthroscopic surgery of the shoulder. A general appraisal. J Bone Joint Surg Br. 1986;68(2):201–7.
11. Steadman JR, Rodkey WG, Briggs KK. Microfracture to treat full-thickness chondral defects: surgical technique, rehabilitation, and outcomes. J Knee Surg. 2002;15:170–6.
12. Bae DK, Yoon KH, Song SJ. Cartilage healing after microfracture in osteoarthritic knees. Arthroscopy. 2006;22:367–74.
13. Millett P, Huffard BH, Horan MP, Hawkins RJ, Steadman JR. Outcomes of full-thickness articular cartilage injuries of the shoulder treated with microfracture. Arthroscopy. 2009;25(8):856–63.
14. Frank RM, Van Thiel GS, Slabaugh MA, Romeo AA, Cole BJ, Verma NN. Clinical outcomes after microfracture of the glenohumeral joint. Am J Sports Med. 2010;38(4):772–81.
15. Siebold R, Lichtenberg S, Habermeyer P. Combination of microfracture and periostal-flap for the treatment of focal full thickness articular cartilage lesions of the shoulder: a prospective study. Knee Surg Sports Traumatol Arthrosc. 2003;11(3):183–9.
16. Snow M, Funk L. Microfracture of chondral lesions of the glenohumeral joint. Int J Shoulder Surg. 2008; 2(4):72–6.
17. Fox JA, Cole BJ, Romeo AA, Meininger AK, Williams JM, Glenn Jr RE, Bicos J, Hayden JK, Dorow CB. Articular cartilage thickness of the humeral head: an anatomic study. Orthopedics. 2008;31(3):216.

12 The Comprehensive Arthroscopic Management (CAM) Procedure for Young Patients with Glenohumeral Osteoarthritis

Peter J. Millett, Joshua A. Greenspoon, and Ryan J. Warth

Introduction

Glenohumeral osteoarthritis (OA) is a common condition typically associated with increasing age and often previous trauma. Patients typically present in later stages with generalized shoulder pain due to degeneration of articular cartilage with limited active and passive range of motion as a result of capsular contractures. There are many *potential* causes of glenohumeral OA (e.g., posttraumatic or iatrogenic); however, the majority of cases are idiopathic in nature.

Although glenohumeral OA is most commonly observed in the aging population, younger patients can still be afflicted with the condition. As a referral practice, we have seen a particularly large number of younger patients (e.g., <60 years of age) with glenohumeral OA who prefer to either avoid or delay arthroplasty using a joint-preserving approach.

The rationale to pursue joint preservation is based upon the limitations and risks currently associated with total shoulder arthroplasty (TSA) in young patients. Specifically, it is well known that the clinical outcomes and patient satisfaction following TSA are less favorable in patients younger than 50 years of age [1–8]. This effect is perhaps due to the fact that younger patients are more likely to engage in higher-demand activities and are generally more active. Due to limited implant longevity, TSA in younger patients may necessitate revision TSA which, in itself, is also known to produce less optimal outcomes when compared to primary TSA [9–11]. Thus, the risk for failure after TSA is particularly elevated in those who participate in higher-demand activities which may accelerate polyethylene wear and lead to implant loosening.

Arthroscopic joint preservation is considered a palliative measure designed to address known and treatable pain generators in the shoulder in order to alleviate symptoms and either delay or prevent the need for future arthroplasty. The comprehensive arthroscopic management (CAM) procedure involves glenohumeral debridement and chondroplasty, humeral head osteoplasty, capsular releases, and axillary nerve neurolysis. Microfracture, subacromial decompression with or without acromioplasty, and biceps tenodesis are also performed when necessary. Preliminary results

Research Performed at the Steadman Philippon Research Institute, Vail, CO.

P.J. Millett, MD, MSc (✉)
Vail Valley Medical Center, The Steadman Clinic, Vail, CO, USA
e-mail: drmillett@thesteadmanclinic.com

J.A. Greenspoon, BSc
Vail Valley Medical Center, Steadman Philippon Research Institute, Vail, CO, USA

R.J. Warth, MD
Department of Orthopaedic Surgery, University of Texas Health Sciences Center, Houston, TX, USA

J.D. Kelly IV (ed.), *Elite Techniques in Shoulder Arthroscopy*,
DOI 10.1007/978-3-319-25103-5_12

of this procedure have been encouraging [12]. The purpose of this chapter is to describe and illustrate the CAM procedure in detail and to review the clinical results following arthroscopic joint-preserving approaches for glenohumeral OA.

The Comprehensive Arthroscopic Management Procedure

Patient Selection

Appropriate patient selection is critical to achieve a successful outcome following the CAM procedure. The procedure is generally indicated for young, active patients with glenohumeral OA who wish to delay arthroplasty. The precise age at which the CAM procedure may be most appropriate and beneficial has not been clearly defined; however, Spiegl et al. found that arthroscopic management was the preferred treatment strategy for patients younger than 47 years who had glenohumeral OA, TSA was the preferred treatment strategy for patients older than 66 years, and either procedure was reasonable for patients between the ages of 47 and 66 years [13]. Millett et al. also noted that patients who presented with <2.0 mm of joint space preoperatively were eight times more likely to progress to arthroplasty [12]. In addition, patients with greater range of motion limitations preoperatively, particularly regarding internal rotation, were more satisfied with the procedure. Of importance, it is always necessary to ensure that patient and physician expectations coincide before undertaking operative management [14].

Surgical Technique

Following the decision to pursue arthroscopic joint preservation, the patient is brought to the surgical suite and placed supine on the operating table. An interscalene catheter is placed which provides analgesia during the initial phases of postoperative rehabilitation. General anesthesia is then administered, and the patient is placed in the modified beach chair position. This positioning allows for intraoperative manipulation of the arm which improves visualization of the inferior "goat's beard" osteophyte both fluoroscopically and arthroscopically. This technique is also helpful to ensure the lack of axillary nerve impingement. A fluoroscopic C-arm is also draped into the surgical field using sterile techniques to assist with visualization and resection of the inferior osteophyte (Fig. 12.1).

Examination under anesthesia is then performed bilaterally, specifically evaluating any

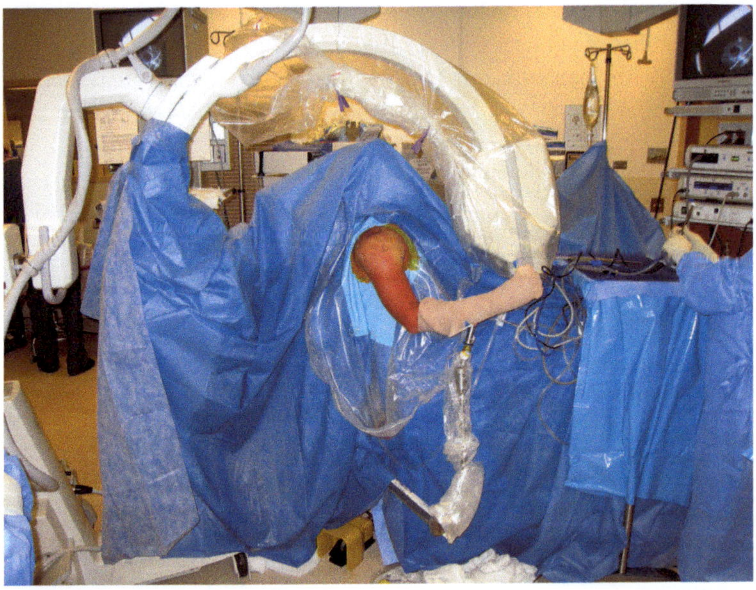

Fig. 12.1 Preoperative photograph of the surgical setup in a patient who eventually underwent the CAM procedure. Note that the C-arm is draped into the surgical field to allow for dynamic fluoroscopic examination intraoperatively

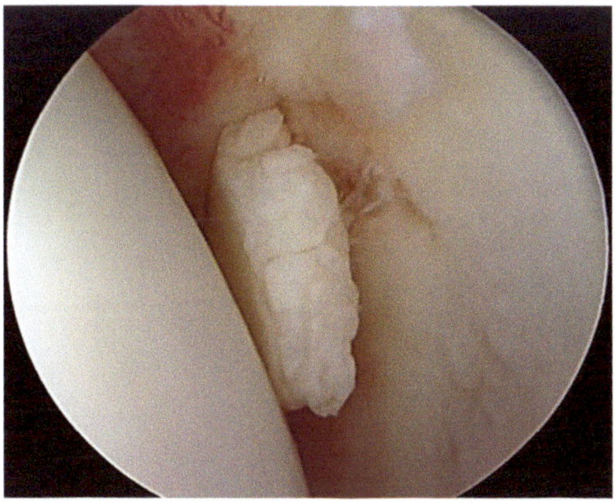

Fig. 12.2 Arthroscopic image of a loose body found upon diagnostic arthroscopy in a young patient with glenohumeral OA

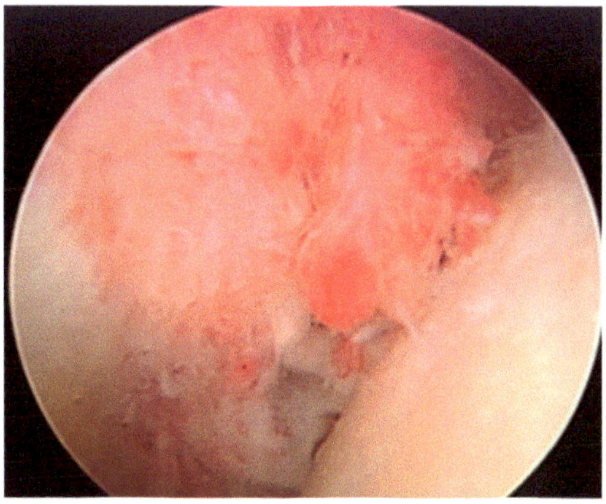

Fig. 12.3 Arthroscopic image demonstrating the typical appearance of significant synovitis that ultimately underwent debridement and resection

range of motion limitations. In general, range of motion loss of >15° in any plane is consistent with capsular contracture. The affected motion planes are noted to aid in the planning of arthroscopic contracture releases.

The glenohumeral joint is localized with a spinal needle, and a standard posterior portal is established approximately 2 cm medial and 2 cm inferior to the posterolateral corner of the acromion. An anterosuperior portal is then created through the rotator interval and a 5-mm cannula is inserted. Diagnostic arthroscopy is then performed using a combination of 30° and 70° arthroscopes.

Glenohumeral Debridement and Chondroplasty

Following an evaluation of both the glenoid and humeral joint surfaces, an arthroscopic shaver is used for the debridement of unstable articular cartilage and degenerative labral tissues to stable borders to prevent the production of a stress riser which may lead to mechanical irritation and acceleration of joint degeneration. Microfracture is performed for focal, full-thickness chondral defects with stable borders. Loose bodies are removed using standard methods (Fig. 12.2). Particular attention is paid to the subscapularis recess, where loose bodies tend to localize. This area is best accessed with an anterior superior viewing portal and straight anterior working portal. Areas of synovial hypertrophy (Fig. 12.3) are resected using radiofrequency ablation or an arthroscopic shaver. In addition, scar tissue is removed from the rotator interval to restore the coracohumeral motion interface. The capsule is otherwise preserved at this time.

Humeral Head Osteoplasty

Using an 18-gauge spinal needle, an accessory posteroinferior portal (i.e., low 7-o'clock portal) is established under direct visualization to allow access to the inferior axillary recess, humeral neck, and axillary nerve. The spinal needle should always enter the inferior recess near the junction of the medial and central thirds of the inferior capsule just anterior to the margin of the posterior band of the inferior glenohumeral ligament (IGHL). A small skin incision is made, and a switching stick is placed into the axillary pouch following the path of the previously placed spinal needle. Tissue dilators are inserted over the switching stick and a 5- or 6-mm cannula is inserted bluntly to avoid iatrogenic injury to the axillary nerve which runs from anteromedial to posterolateral through the inferior recess. The capsule of the axillary pouch is preserved at this point to protect the axillary nerve. When present, the intra-articular inferior osteophyte (Fig. 12.4) is then removed using a shielded, high-speed 4- or 5-mm arthroscopic bur, arthroscopic shavers, and handheld curettes. The arm is extended and internally and externally rotated during the procedure

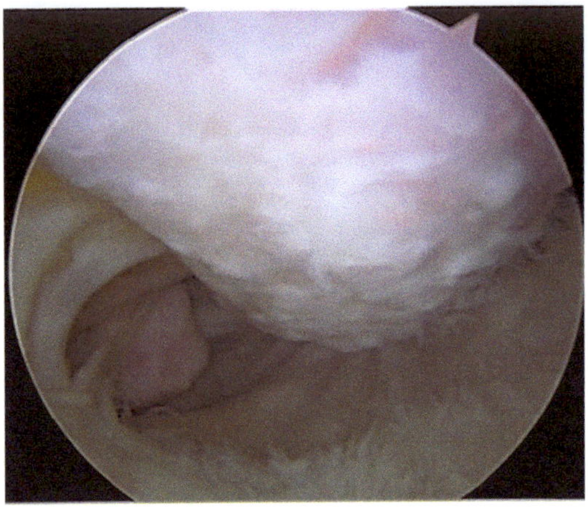

Fig. 12.4 Arthroscopic image showing a large osteophyte located on the inferior aspect of the humeral head

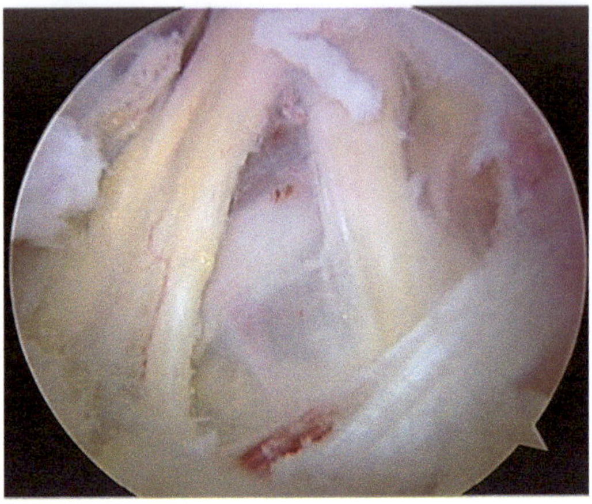

Fig. 12.5 Arthroscopic image showing the bifurcation of the axillary nerve. Neurolysis should always be performed from proximal to distal in order to mitigate the risk of iatrogenic injury to small, distal branches of the axillary nerve

to bring all areas of the osteophyte into view or within the plane of the fluoroscope to ensure adequate bony resection. Curettes can also be used to remove hypertrophic bone from the anteroinferior areas that are more difficult to access with motorized instruments. While complete removal of hypertrophic bone is desired, this may not be possible in some cases. It is always the goal to remove enough bone to decompress the axillary nerve throughout the range of shoulder motion.

Inferior Capsular Release and Axillary Neurolysis

Large inferior humeral head osteophytes almost always occur in the presence of a thickened, contracted inferior capsule which limits both active and passive glenohumeral abduction capacity. Release of the inferior capsule is always performed after humeral head osteoplasty, as the intact capsular tissue can help protect the axillary nerve from iatrogenic injury [15]. Arthroscopic scissors, an arthroscopic punch, and a monopolar radiofrequency probe are used to complete this portion of the procedure. The inferior capsular release is begun posteriorly near the insertion site of the posteroinferior cannula, and the capsule is transected from proximal to distal. A blunt trocar is also helpful to establish tissue planes between the capsule and surrounding soft tissues. Once the axillary nerve is identified, dissection is carried out from proximal to distal to avoid damage to any branches of the axillary nerve. While the nerve classically has two main branches, it is not uncommon to find multiple arborations. Working from proximal to distal helps prevent damage to small distal branches of the axillary nerve as they course beneath the axillary pouch.

Axillary neurolysis is performed in patients who present with posterior or lateral shoulder pain (following the distribution of the axillary nerve) or those with evidence of nerve impingement on diagnostic images or direct arthroscopic visualization [16]. Isolated atrophy of the teres minor, best seen on T1 sagittal MRI images, suggests axillary nerve compression.

Following the inferior capsular release, the axillary nerve is identified just inferior to the junction between the middle and anterior thirds of the axillary pouch. Release of adherent tissues around the axillary nerve is performed from proximal to distal and from medial to lateral using blunt dissection to avoid inadvertent injury or irritation of the small distal branches of the axillary nerve (Fig. 12.5). It is important to maintain hemostasis during neurolysis in order to improve visualization, prevent postoperative hematoma formation, and reduce the risk of scar tissue postoperatively. Neurolysis is complete when the axillary nerve is clearly visible along its entire course between the subscapularis and teres

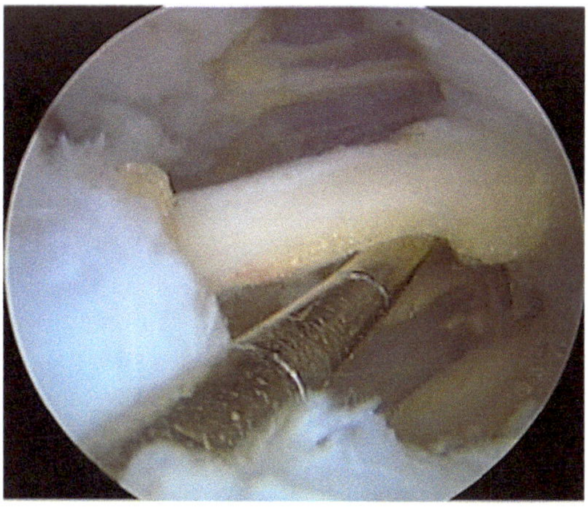

Fig. 12.6 Arthroscopic image of the axillary nerve following neurolysis

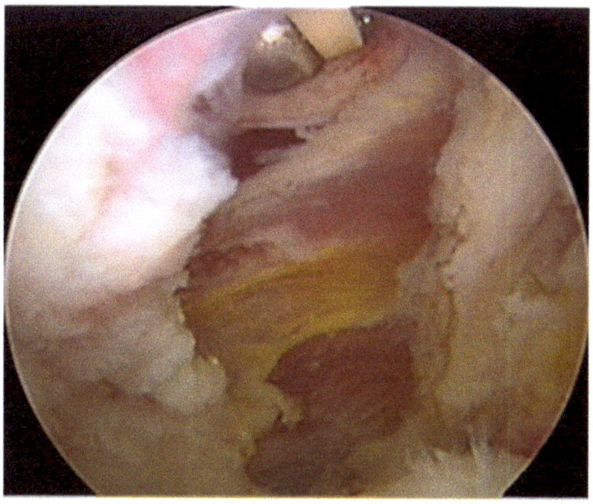

Fig. 12.7 Arthroscopic image showing the fibers of the subscapularis muscle following anterior capsular release

minor muscles without soft tissue adherence or osseous impingement (Fig. 12.6). Adequate clearance is directly visualized arthroscopically during dynamic examination.

Anterior and Posterior Capsular Releases

Anterior and posterior capsular releases should always be performed after osteophyte resection and axillary neurolysis to prevent fluid extravasation into the axillary space, which may limit visualization during these delicate procedures. Soft tissue releases are first performed within the rotator interval (medial to the biceps reflection pulley and inferior to the superior glenohumeral ligament) using electrocautery and a motorized shaver. The anterior capsule is released medially from superiorly to approximately the 5-o'clock position (in a right shoulder) along the capsulolabral junction. The fibers of the subscapularis muscle are then visualized. Care should be taken to avoid injury to the fibers of the subscapularis muscle (Fig. 12.7). Anterior capsular tissue is also released through the rotator interval from superior to inferior until the coracoid and coracoacromial (CA) ligament are clearly visible from within the joint.

The arthroscope is then placed into the anterosuperior portal to allow visualization of the posterior capsule and capsulolabral junction. Using the posterior portal for instrumentation, the posterior capsule is released from inferior (approximately 7-o'clock position in a right shoulder) to superior (approximately 11-o'clock in a right shoulder) medially along the capsulolabral junction to avoid damaging the posterior cuff tendons which are situated more laterally. The posterior release is typically connected to the inferior release which was performed earlier in the procedure. Dynamic examination is then performed under both arthroscopic and fluoroscopic visualization to evaluate shoulder range of motion following capsular releases. Range of motion capacity is then compared to the contralateral shoulder. Manipulation of the shoulder can be performed at this point in the procedure to maximize functional range of motion of the shoulder.

Additional Procedures

1. Subacromial Decompression/Acromioplasty

   The arthroscope is then placed back into the posterior portal to access the subacromial space. Bursectomy is always performed to allow for visualization of the rotator cuff tendons and to restore the scapulohumeral motion interface. Acromioplasty is performed using an arthroscopic bur through the lateral portal for cases in which visible fraying or scuffing of the CA ligament (i.e., impingement lesion), a Bigliani type III acromion, or a large anterolateral acromial spur is present

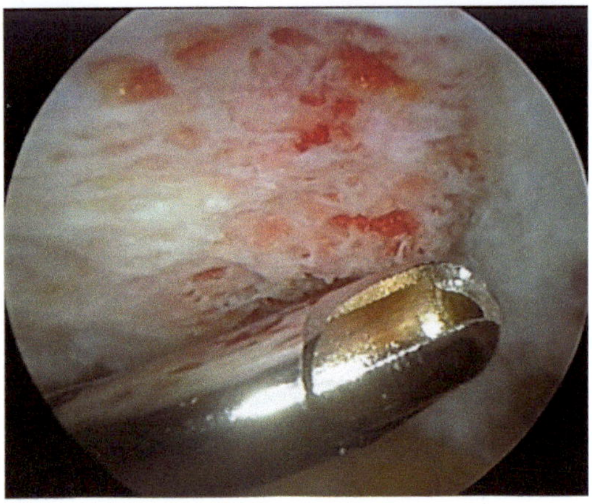

Fig. 12.8 Arthroscopic image of the inferior acromion following subacromial decompression and acromioplasty

(Fig. 12.8). Otherwise, acromioplasty is not routinely performed.

2. Long Head of the Biceps Tenodesis

   When injured or inflamed, the long head of the biceps (LHB) tendon can be a significant pain generator. The LHB tendon may also restrict forward elevation in some cases (e.g., hourglass deformity) [17]. Therefore, arthroscopic release of the LHB tendon with subsequent open subpectoral tenodesis is commonly performed in patients with a degenerative shoulder. LHB tendon release and tenodesis are typically indicated for patients with LHB tendonitis, bicipital groove tenderness, degenerative SLAP tears, or any condition that may compromise the ability of the LHB tendon to glide freely and painlessly within the bicipital groove. The procedural details for open subpectoral LHB tenodesis have been described elsewhere [18, 19].

Postoperative Rehabilitation

The primary goals of postoperative rehabilitation are to maintain joint motion and to improve overall shoulder kinematics. Nonsteroidal anti-inflammatory drugs (NSAID) are used liberally to help decrease inflammation and pain during the postoperative period. Postoperative rehabilitation follows a phasic approach where individual customization may be necessary depending on concomitant pathologies and procedures. The first phase of rehabilitation begins immediately postoperatively and focuses on passive range of motion, active-assisted range of motion, and cautious stretching (to avoid further pain and inflammation). At approximately 6 weeks postoperatively, functional strengthening is begun, particularly implementing elastic resistance bands. At approximately 3 months postoperatively, more advanced strengthening exercises are begun followed by a return to normal activities and sports between 4 and 6 months postoperatively.

Risks and Complications

There are several surgical risks and potential complications that can be avoided when the procedure is performed systematically using meticulous surgical technique. Small branches of the axillary nerve are particularly susceptible to iatrogenic injury during inferior capsular release and axillary neurolysis because they are typically difficult to appreciate arthroscopically. In all cases, it is important to work from proximal to distal during axillary neurolysis to help visualize distal arborization. Anterior and posterior capsular releases should always be performed after addressing the axillary nerve to prevent fluid excursion or leakage into the axillary space. This fluid egress may decrease visualization during the delicate neurolysis procedure and may produce increased postoperative pain as a result of increased compartment pressure. Expeditious inferior capsular release and neurolysis while also using lower fluid pump pressures may help decrease the risk for this complication. Although uncommon, the inferior capsular scar tissue that often develops postoperatively may involve the axillary nerve, potentially resulting in recurrent posterior and lateral shoulder pain. Recurrent positional symptoms may also be caused by incomplete humeral osteoplasty. While concern about postoperative instability exists due to the extent of the capsular release, we have not seen this complication likely due to the overall stiff soft tissue envelope associated with the underlying glenohumeral OA.

Clinical Results

For patients with glenohumeral OA, the goals of arthroscopic management are to relieve symptoms related to mechanical impingement (through stabilization of chondral defects and labral tears), to improve functional range of motion (through capsular releases), and to delay the need for joint arthroplasty. Several studies have evaluated the results of arthroscopic management for glenohumeral OA (Table 12.1). Most of these studies reported significant pain relief where improved postoperative range of motion was demonstrated in those patients who underwent capsular releases.

Recent evidence suggests that axillary nerve impingement may be produced by the large

Table 12.1 Summary of studies that evaluated the clinical outcomes following arthroscopic management for glenohumeral OA in young patients

Authors	Year	*N*	Mean age	Technique	Revisions and complications	Preoperative status	Postoperative outcomes
Weinstein et al. [19]	2000	25	46	Debridement	None	NR	Improved pain in all
Cameron et al. [20]	2002	70	50	Debridement ± capsular releases	NR	Functional score (0–60): 24 Satisfaction: 0.67 FE: 119° IR: L2	Functional score (0–60): 38.7 Satisfaction: 6/10 FE: 157° IR: T11
Richards and Burkhart [21]	2007	8	55	Debridement ± capsular releases	NR	FE: 131.9° IR: 17.2° ER: 42.8°	FE: 153.3° IR: 48.3° ER: 59.4°
Kerr and McCarty [22]	2008	20	38	Debridement ± tenotomy, microfracture	NR	NR	ASES: 75.3 Marx: 12.6 SANE: 63 % WOOS: 0.64
de Beer et al. [23]	2010	31	Median 57.5	Debridement, glenoid resurfacing, tenotomy	Axillary paresis (1) Material failure (2) Synovitis (1) Contusion from MUA (1)	Median constant: 40	Median constant: 64.5
Van Thiel et al. [24]	2010	81	47	Debridement ± capsular releases, tenotomy, microfracture, acromioplasty	Arthroplasty (16) at mean 10.1 months	ASES: 51.8 SST: 6.1 VAS: 4.8 SF-12: 35.9	ASES: 72.7 SST: 9.0 VAS: 2.7 SF-12: 36.1 Constant: 72.0 UCLA: 28.3 SANE: 71.1 FE: 137° Abduction: 129° ER: 48°
Millett et al. [25]	2013	30	52	Debridement ± capsular releases, humeral osteoplasty, axillary neurolysis, acromioplasty	Arthroplasty (6) at mean 1.9 years	ASES: 58 SF-12 PCS: 42.8 FE: 98.2° ER: 13.4° ER at 90° abduction: 27.3° IR: 23.8°	ASES: 83 SF-12 PCS: 49.4 FE: 152.9° ER: 62.2° ER at 90° abduction: 75.4° IR: 60.8°

Abbreviations: *ASES* American Shoulder and Elbow Surgeons' score, *ER* external rotation, *FE* forward elevation, *IR* internal rotation, *MUA* manipulation under anesthesia, *NR* not reported, *SANE* Single Assessment Numeric Evaluation score, *SF-12* short form-12, *SF-12 PCS* short form-12 physical component summary, *SST* simple shoulder test, *UCLA* University of California Los Angeles shoulder score, *VAS* Visual Analog Scale for pain, *WOOS* Western Ontario Osteoarthritis score inferior humeral head osteophyte that is common in patients with glenohumeral OA [20]. As noted, Millett et al. found that larger humeral head osteophytes were significantly correlated with increased fatty infiltration of the teres minor muscle. Impingement of the axillary nerve may also serve as a stimulus for scar tissue formation which can further entrap the axillary nerve. As a result of this research, the senior surgeon began to perform humeral osteoplasty and axillary neurolysis in patients with evidence of axillary nerve impingement to enhance pain relief and further delay the need for arthroplasty. In a series of 30 shoulders, Millett et al. performed debridement and capsular releases with additional humeral osteoplasty and axillary neurolysis (CAM procedure) [12]. In that study, 6 of 30 patients underwent TSA at a mean of 1.9 years following this arthroscopic treatment regimen. In the remaining shoulders, American Shoulder and Elbow Surgeons' (ASES) scores improved from 58 preoperatively to 83 postoperatively after a mean 2.6-year follow-up period. In an unpublished study from our institution with over 100 patients, predictors of a poor outcome after the CAM procedure included a narrowed joint space and a Walch types B2 or C glenoid (biconcave). Although further study is needed to define the longevity of this joint-preserving technique, preliminary data suggests that the CAM procedure can be an effective treatment option to help decrease pain, improve function, and delay arthroplasty in younger patients with glenohumeral OA.

Conclusion

Arthroscopic joint preservation strategies can reduce pain and improve function while also helping to delay the need for future shoulder arthroplasty in young patients with glenohumeral OA. The CAM procedure is a safe technique that utilizes additional humeral osteoplasty and axillary neurolysis to further reduce pain and enhance postoperative function in these patients.

References

1. Bartelt R, Sperling JW, Schleck CD, Cofield RH. Shoulder arthroplasty in patients aged fifty-five years or younger with osteoarthritis. J Shoulder Elbow Surg. 2011;20(1):123–30.
2. Cheung EV, Sperling JW, Cofield RH. Revision shoulder arthroplasty for glenoid component loosening. J Shoulder Elbow Surg. 2008;17(3):371–5.
3. Denard PJ, Raiss P, Sowa B, Walch G. Mid- to long-term follow-up of total shoulder arthroplasty using a keeled glenoid in young adults with primary glenohumeral arthritis. J Shoulder Elbow Surg. 2013;22(7):894–900.
4. Deutsch A, Abboud JA, Kelly J, Mody M, Norris T, Ramsey ML, Iannotti JP, Williams GR. Clinical results of revision shoulder arthroplasty for glenoid component loosening. J Shoulder Elbow Surg. 2007;16(6):706–16.
5. Papadonikolakis A, Neradilek MB, Matsen III FA. Failure of the glenoid component in anatomic total shoulder arthroplasty: a systematic review of the English-language literature between 2006 and 2012. J Bone Joint Surg Am. 2013;95(24):2205–12.
6. Raiss P, Aldinger PR, Kasten P, Rickert M, Loew M. Total shoulder replacement in young and middle-aged patients with glenohumeral osteoarthritis. J Bone Joint Surg Br. 2008;90(6):764–9.
7. Rasmussen JV. Outcome and risk of revision following shoulder replacement in patients with glenohumeral osteoarthritis. Acta Orthop Suppl. 2014;85(355):1–23.
8. Sperling JW, Cofield RH, Rowland CM. Minimum fifteen-year follow-up of Neer hemiarthroplasty and total shoulder arthroplasty in patients aged fifty years or younger. J Shoulder Elbow Surg. 2004;13(6):604–13.
9. Em B, Roberts SM, Siegel E, Yannopoulos P, Higgins LD, Warner JJ. Reverse shoulder arthroplasty as salvage for failed prior arthroplasty in patients 65 years of age or younger. J Shoulder Elbow Surg. 2014;23(7):1036–42.
10. Dines JS, Fealy S, Strauss EJ, Allen A, Craig EV, Warren RF, Dines DM. Outcomes analysis of revision total shoulder replacement. J Bone Joint Surg Am. 2006;88(7):1494–500.
11. Walker M, Willis MP, Brooks JP, Pupello D, Mulieri PJ, Frankle MA. The use of the reverse shoulder arthroplasty for treatment of failed total shoulder arthroplasty. J Shoulder Elbow Surg. 2012;21(4):514–22.
12. Millett PJ, Horan MP, Pennock AT, Rios D. Comprehensive Arthroscopic Management (CAM) procedure: clinical results of a joint-preserving arthroscopic treatment for young, active patients with advanced shoulder osteoarthritis. Arthroscopy. 2013;29(3):440–8.
13. Spiegl UJ, Faucett SC, Horan MP, Warth RJ, Millett PJ. The role of arthroscopy in the management of

glenohumeral osteoarthritis: a Markov decision model. Arthroscopy. 2014;30(11):1392–9.
14. Warth RJ, Briggs KK, Dornan GJ, Horan MP, Millett PJ. Patient expectations before arthroscopic shoulder surgery: correlation with patients' reasons for seeking treatment. J Shoulder Elbow Surg. 2013;22(12): 1676–81.
15. de Beer JF, Bhatia DN, van Rooyen KS, Du Toit DF. Arthroscopic debridement and biological resurfacing of the glenoid in glenohumeral arthritis. Knee Surg Sports Traumatol Arthrosc. 2010;18(12):1767–73.
16. Elser F, Dewing CB, Millett PJ. Chondral and osteochondral lesions of the humerus: diagnosis and management. Oper Tech Sports Med. 2008;16(4):178–86.
17. Boileau P, Ahrens PM, Hatzidakis AM. Entrapment of the long head of the biceps tendon: the hourglass biceps – a cause of pain and locking of the shoulder. J Shoulder Elbow Surg. 2004;13(3):249–57.
18. Mazzocca AD, Rios CG, Romeo AA, Arciero RA. Subpectoral biceps tenodesis with interference screw fixation. Arthroscopy. 2005;21(7):896.
19. Millett PJ, Sanders B, Gobezie R, Braun S, Warner JJ. Interference screw vs. suture anchor fixation for open subpectoral biceps tenodesis: does it matter? BMC Musculoskelet Disord. 2008;9:121.
20. Millett PJ, Schoenahl JY, Allen MJ, Motta T, Gaskill TR. An association between the inferior humeral head osteophyte and teres minor fatty infiltration: evidence for axillary nerve entrapment in glenohumeral osteoarthritis. J Shoulder Elbow Surg. 2013;22(2):215–21.
21. Weinstein DM, Bucchieri JS, Pollock RG, Flatow EL, Bigliani LU. Arthroscopic debridement of the shoulder for osteoarthritis. Arthroscopy. 2000;16(5): 471–6.
22. Cameron BD, Galatz LM, Ramsey ML, Williams GR, Iannotti JP. Non-prosthetic management of grade IV osteochondral lesions of the glenohumeral joint. J Shoulder Elbow Surg. 2002;11(1):25–32.
23. Richards DP, Burkhart SS. Arthroscopic debridement and capsular release for glenohumeral osteoarthritis. Arthroscopy. 2007;23(9):1019–22.
24. Kerr BJ, McCarty EC. Outcome of arthroscopic debridement is worse for patients with glenohumeral arthritis of both sides of the joint. Clin Orthop Relat Res. 2008;466(3):634–8.
25. Van Thiel GS, Sheehan S, Frank RM, Slabaugh M, Cole BJ, Nicholson GP, Romeo AA, Verma NN. Retrospective analysis of arthroscopic management of glenohumeral degenerative disease. Arthroscopy. 2010;26(11):1451–5.

Graft Interposition Arthroplasty 13

Michael J. O'Brien and Felix H. Savoie III

Introduction

Treatment of glenohumeral arthritis in the young patient under 50 years of age remains challenging. When conservative treatment options fail to provide relief to worsening pain and function, then arthroplasty usually is considered. While total shoulder arthroplasty (TSA) remains the gold standard for most patients with shoulder arthritis to alleviate pain and improve function [1], not all patients are ideal candidates because of age, activity level, or associated pathology. Sperling et al. [1, 2] studied shoulder arthroplasty in patients under 50 years of age and reported a high rate of glenoid lucency following TSA and glenoid erosions following hemiarthroplasty. Biologic resurfacing of the glenoid emerged as a potential surgical option to decrease pain and preserve bone stock in the young, active patient with arthritis. As arthroscopic techniques and instrumentation have improved, arthroscopic biologic resurfacing of the glenoid has developed as a temporary, intermediate step in the surgical treatment of arthritis in these young patients [3, 4].

When arthroplasty is considered, the choice of shoulder replacement is controversial. Studies in older patients have shown better results after total shoulder arthroplasty when compared to hemiarthroplasty with regard to motion, pain relief, and the need for early revision surgery [3, 5–9]. However, total shoulder replacement necessitates certain lifelong restrictions in lifting and activity level. Polyethylene wear and glenoid component loosening and joint failure [1, 2] are worrisome problems for the very active patient, as well as laborers that must repetitively lift heavy loads. Thus, placement of a glenoid component is not a viable long-term solution in a young, active patient. Humeral head resurfacing is an option, which will improve patient's pain and range of motion. However, this does not address glenoid sided wear.

Interposition arthroplasty may be an option in the young patient with concentric glenohumeral arthritis in which a majority of the wear is on the glenoid side. This procedure aims to resurface the glenoid with a soft tissue patch to create a permanent, durable, biologically active surface to decrease friction, decrease pain, and improve range of motion and function. In the best scenarios, it may even produce hyaline-like tissue [4]. The procedure preserves glenoid bone, avoids the potential problems of glenoid component loosening, and leaves open the possibility for later conversion to TSA.

First proposed by Burkhead and Hutton [10] in 1988, biologic resurfacing of the glenoid combined with hemiarthroplasty has been used in the treatment of glenohumeral arthritis in young, active patients but with variable results.

M.J. O'Brien, MD (✉) • F.H. Savoie III, MD
Department of Orthopaedics, Tulane University
School of Medicine, New Orleans, LA, USA
e-mail: mobrien@tulane.edu

J.D. Kelly IV (ed.), *Elite Techniques in Shoulder Arthroscopy*,
DOI 10.1007/978-3-319-25103-5_13

The durability of the procedure was reported by Krishnan et al. [11] in their 2- to 15-year follow-up of 36 patients. These authors reported 86 % good and excellent results. Glenoid erosions did occur but seemed to stabilize at 5 years. Conversely, more recent studies have found a failure rate as high as 50 % at 3 years postoperative [8, 12].

The primary indication for biologic glenoid resurfacing is pain and functional impairment due to arthritis in an active patient that has failed to respond to nonoperative management. These patients have failed trials of rest, activity modification, nonsteroidal anti-inflammatory medication, intra-articular cortisone injections, and physical therapy. The surgery may also be considered in patients who have undergone previous arthroscopic debridement or capsular release and have not attained adequate pain relief. This patient population is often laborers or patients whose work and sporting activities would not allow them to comply with the restrictions of placing a polyethylene glenoid component. While chronological age is an important factor, physiologic age and patient expectations are perhaps more important decision-making variables [9]. Contraindications include advanced glenoid bone loss, advanced rheumatoid arthritis, failed prior glenoid resurfacing, and active infection. There is no "gold standard" for soft tissue interposition, and various techniques have been described, including autograft capsule, autograft fascia lata, Achilles tendon allograft, lateral meniscal allograft, and a variety of commercially available grafts and scaffolds [3–5, 8–15].

Resurfacing of the glenoid with an interposition soft tissue graft may be performed arthroscopically or in conjunction with humeral head arthroplasty. It has been proposed as an option to improve outcomes and avoid the potential complications associated with TSA, such as glenoid component loosening and polyethylene wear [4, 10]. It is important to note that soft tissue glenoid resurfacing should always be considered a temporary, time-buying solution until the patient reaches the age for total shoulder arthroplasty.

Surgical Technique

The operative technique has been previously described by Savoie [4] and de Beer [3]. Surgery is performed arthroscopically with the patient in the lateral decubitus position. This position offers the advantages of full access to both anterior and posterior compartments of the shoulder, access to the inferior humeral head for possible osteophyte resection, and 360° access to the glenoid rim and labrum. The operative arm is suspended with an arm suspensory device with ten pounds of traction to provide distraction across the glenohumeral joint.

Standard arthroscopic portals are utilized. The arthroscope is first placed through a standard posterior portal. Diagnostic arthroscopy is performed, and the presence of glenohumeral arthritis is confirmed (Fig. 13.1). An anterior-inferior portal is established just above the subscapularis as the primary working portal. An accessory

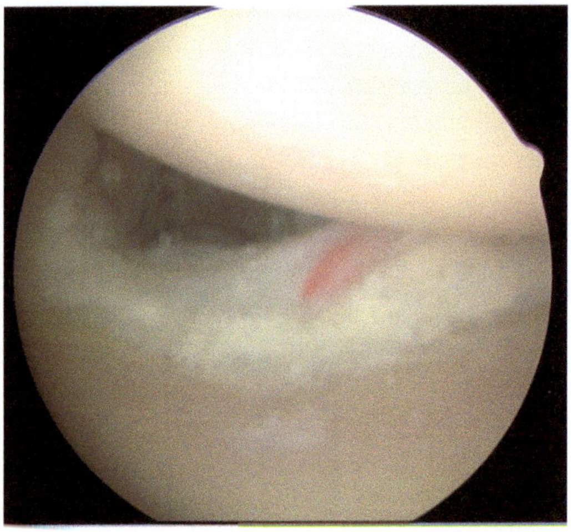

Fig. 13.1 This image shows the arthroscopic view through a posterior portal of the glenohumeral joint in a right shoulder. The patient is in the lateral decubitus position with the humeral head at the *top* of the image and the glenoid at the *bottom* of the image. Note the complete loss of cartilage on the glenoid and humeral head with a concentric glenohumeral joint. An 8.5 mm cannula has been placed in the anterior-inferior portal just above the subscapularis [Published with permission of © Michael J. O'Brien 2015]

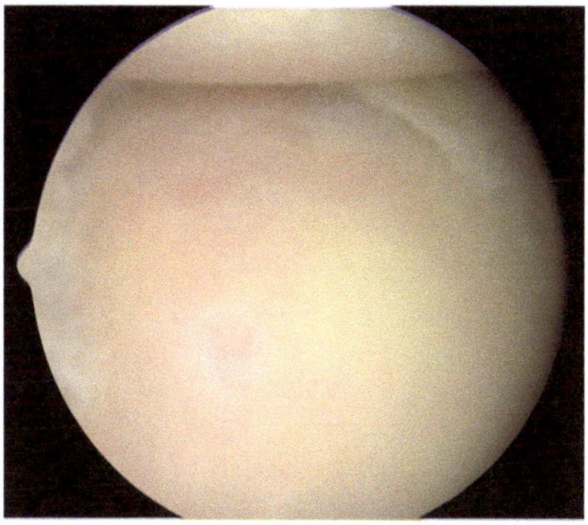

Fig. 13.2 This image of the same right shoulder viewed through the anterior-superior portal again demonstrates complete loss of articular cartilage on the humeral head and glenoid with a concentric glenohumeral joint. The anterior-superior viewing portal allows full access to both anterior and posterior compartments of the joint [Published with permission of © Michael J. O'Brien 2015]

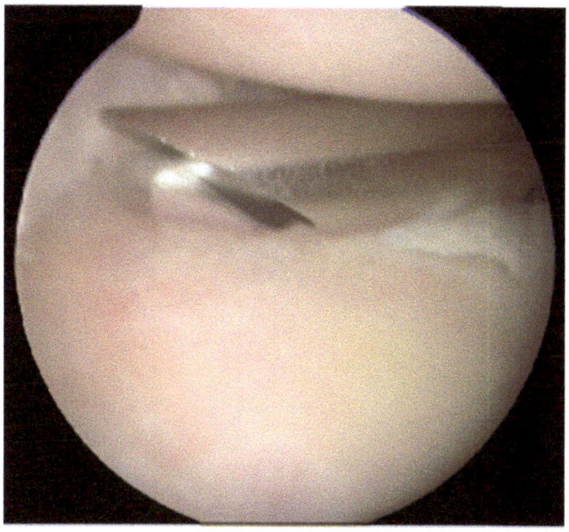

Fig. 13.3 A motorized burr introduced through the posterior portal allows the surgeon to burr the glenoid to a smooth, flat surface, removing all remnants of articular cartilage. The arthroscope is in the anterior-superior viewing portal [Published with permission of © Michael J. O'Brien 2015]

anterior-superior portal is established as the viewing portal for the arthroscope. It is important to keep a wide skin bridge between the two anterior portals to create adequate working space for the passage of instruments in and out of the anterior-inferior cannula.

The arthroscope is then placed in the anterior-superior viewing portal; this allows full visualization of the glenohumeral joint in both anterior and posterior compartments (Fig. 13.2). An 8.5 mm cannula is placed in the anterior-inferior portal. The larger cannula is necessary here to allow for later graft passage. A 5 mm cannula is placed in the posterior portal. Hypertrophic synovium can be resected with the shaver and all degenerative fraying of the labrum, rotator cuff, and biceps is debrided. Loose bodies can be removed when identified. If significant stiffness is present, a complete capsular release just off the labrum is performed.

A flat, concentric surface must be created for placement of the graft. A motorized burr is introduced through the posterior portal while viewing from the anterior-superior portal, and the glenoid face is burred to a smooth uniform surface (Fig. 13.3). Occasionally, it may be necessary to alternate the burr between the anterior and posterior portals so that the entire glenoid surface can be burred smooth and flat. Bony ridges can be removed and limited biconcavity can be planed to a flat surface. It is important to remove any residual cartilage.

Next, a microfracture of the glenoid face is performed. This can be accomplished most readily with Steadman microfracture awls. It is important to penetrate deep enough with the microfracture to allow the release of marrow contents (Fig. 13.4). The marrow cells help the biologic interposition graft heal to the native glenoid.

One single-loaded, bioabsorbable suture anchor is then placed anteroinferiorly and one anterosuperiorly, and the posterior labrum, which is usually hypertrophic, is used for posterior-inferior and posterior-superior sutures (Fig. 13.5). These are typically placed at 1, 4, 8, and 11 o'clock with respect to the glenoid face. Alternatively, if inadequate posterior labral tissue is deficient, suture anchors may be placed posteriorly as well. The anterior anchors may be placed through the anterior-inferior cannula. The posterior anchors are usually placed percutaneously using a small posterolateral portal. As each anchor is placed, the sutures are retrieved without tangling

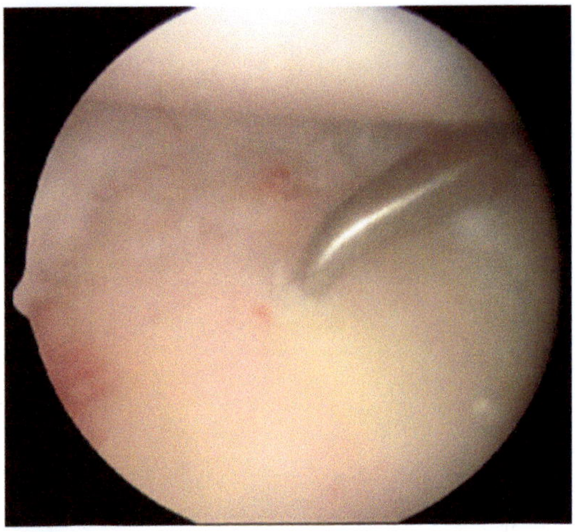

Fig. 13.4 A Steadman awl introduced through the posterior portal is used to perform a microfracture to the entire glenoid face. It is important to penetrate deep enough with the awl to allow the release of marrow contents into the joint [Published with permission of © Michael J. O'Brien 2015]

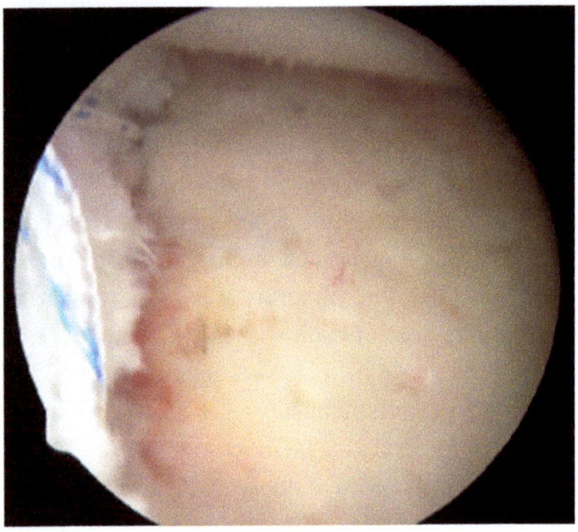

Fig. 13.5 This view from the anterior superior portal shows the glenoid after microfracture and placement of two single-loaded suture anchors. The anterior-superior anchor is placed at the 1 o'clock position and the anterior-inferior anchor placed at the 4 o'clock position [Published with permission of © Michael J. O'Brien 2015]

and maintained in a separate "quadrant" of the cannula. Suture management is paramount for the remainder of the procedure. Using a hemostat, each suture can be secured to the drapes in the corresponding position inside the shoulder

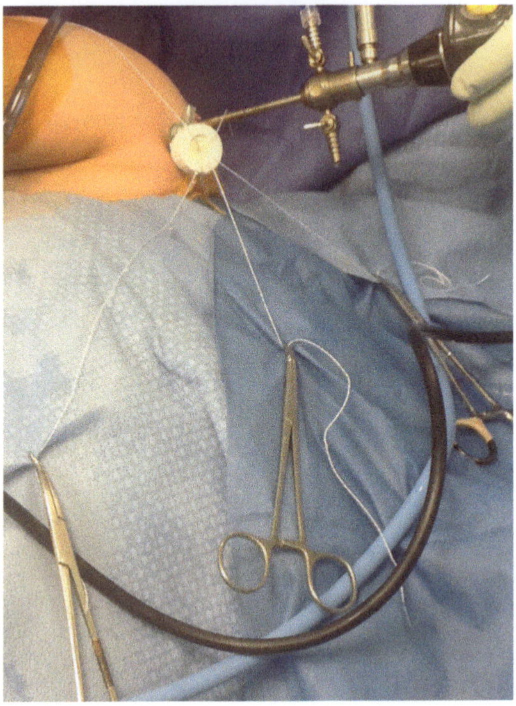

Fig. 13.6 This external photograph of a right shoulder in the lateral decubitus position demonstrates how the sutures can be secured to the drapes using hemostats to keep the sutures in the correct "quadrants" of the glenohumeral joint. The sutures are secured under tension to prevent tangles. Suture management and attention to detail are paramount for successful graft passage into the shoulder joint [Published with permission of © Michael J. O'Brien 2015]

joint (Fig. 13.6). The sutures should be secured under tension. A grasper may be run down and up the sutures individually to confirm the absence of any tangles.

At this stage, the interposition graft can be prepared. At our institution, the surgeons currently prefer to use human acellular dermal matrix. Two common techniques can be used to measure the dimensions of the native glenoid. A calibrated probe can be placed across the face of the glenoid from the posterior portal. The anterior-posterior width is measured at the widest portion of the glenoid. The authors' preferred technique is to directly measure the glenoid width with a free suture (Fig. 13.7). A knot is tied in a free suture, and then the suture is placed through the anterior cannula across the face of the glenoid

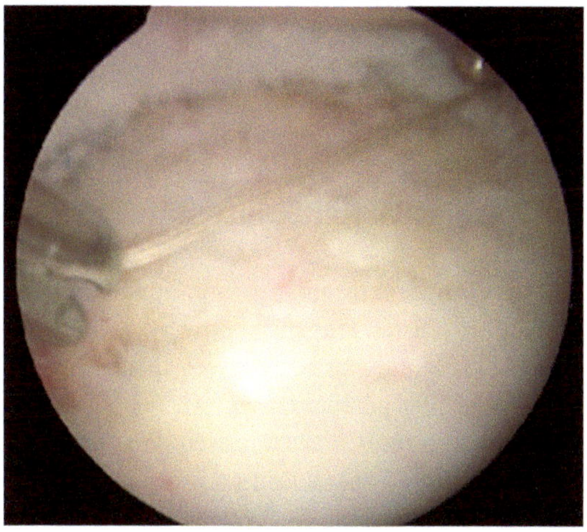

Fig. 13.7 The anterior-posterior width is measured using a free suture at the widest portion of the glenoid. The length of suture can be measured with a ruler on the back table, and the graft dimensions calculated using a 3:2 ratio of height to width [Published with permission of © Michael J. O'Brien 2015]

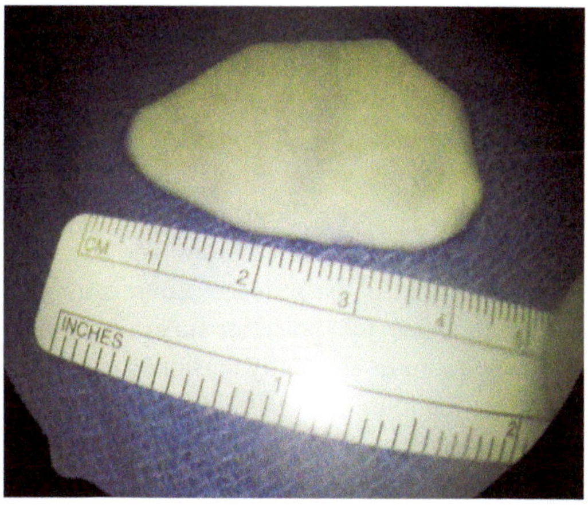

Fig. 13.8 Once the glenoid dimensions have been calculated, the dimensions are drawn onto the graft, and an oval-shaped graft is cut to approximate the shape of the native glenoid [Published with permission of © Michael J. O'Brien 2015]

and out the posterior cannula. An assistant holds the suture taught so the tied knot lies at the posterior glenoid rim. A suture grasper is placed through the anterior cannula, and the free suture is secured with the grasper at the anterior glenoid rim. The suture is removed from the anterior cannula with the grasper in place. The glenoid width is then measured between the tip of the grasper and the tied knot.

The average glenoid dimension has a 3:2 ratio of height to width. The width measurement is used to calculate the height from superior to inferior. The graft is marked on the back table, and an oval is drawn onto the graft to match the native glenoid. The appropriate size graft is then cut out of the human dermal matrix with scissors (Fig. 13.8). It is important to mark the subcutaneous side of the graft, which should be placed against the native glenoid bone. The dermal side should face upward.

Using a free needle, one limb of each suture is passed through the graft corresponding with the anchor location on the glenoid. A mulberry knot or short-tailed interference knot (STIK) as described by Wong [16] can be tied and pulled to sit flush against the graft (Fig. 13.9). Suture management is essential to avoid crossing or twisting of the sutures.

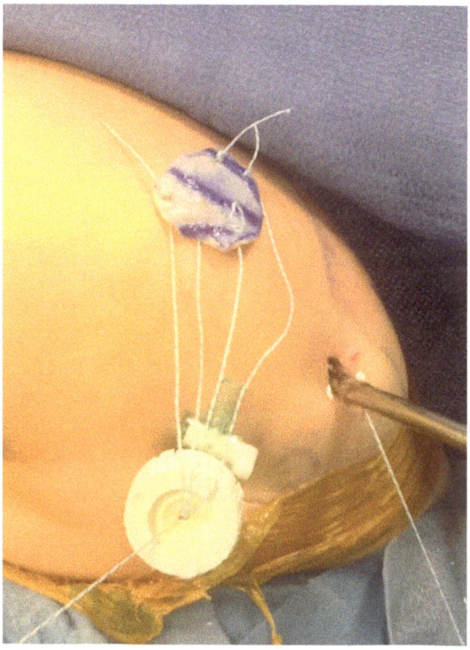

Fig. 13.9 This photograph shows the prepared graft prior to passage into the glenohumeral joint. Using a free needle, one limb of each suture is placed through the graft corresponding to the suture location in the glenoid. A mulberry knot or STIK can be tied and pulled flush with the graft to facilitate passing the graft into the joint [Published with permission of © Michael J. O'Brien 2015]

The graft is now ready for passage into the shoulder joint. The graft is rolled up and placed into the anterior-inferior cannula. A large 8.5 mm cannula is necessary to allow passage of the graft into the shoulder joint. The posterior-inferior suture is passed down the cannula and retrieved under the posterior-inferior labrum. The posterior-superior stitch is passed the same way and retrieved under the posterior-superior labrum. These two sutures are gently tensioned to pull the graft into the joint. An assistant holds the posterior sutures tight while the anterior sutures are individually tensioned. Carefully pulling on all four sutures will lay the graft flat on the glenoid. A probe can be used to assist with the position of the graft, ensuring it is flush with glenoid (Fig. 13.10). Next, the four individual sutures are tied sequentially. We tie the anterior-inferior suture first and then the anterior-superior stitch. When a STIK has been used, the posterior sutures can be retrieved through the posterior cannula and each suture sequentially tied. Alternatively, the posterior sutures may be tied to each other on the outside of the posterior labrum. The compression of the humeral head on the glenoid will hold the graft flush against the glenoid. The microfracture allows the marrow contents from the glenoid to pool between the glenoid and graft, facilitating healing of the graft to the bony glenoid.

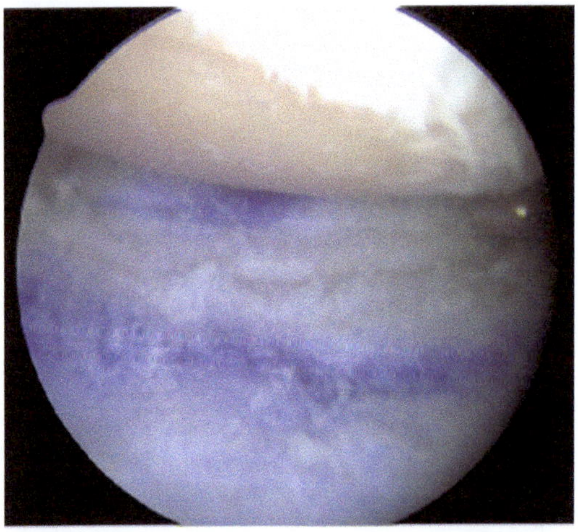

Fig. 13.10 This final image shows the biologic graft sitting flush with the glenoid surface. A probe may be used to smooth the graft flush. The four sutures are sequentially tied to secure the graft to the glenoid, and the humeral head provides compression of the graft against the glenoid while incorporation occurs [Published with permission of © Michael J. O'Brien 2015]

Postoperative Rehabilitation

The operative extremity is immobilized in an abduction pillow sling in neutral rotation for 6 weeks. The sling can be removed to shower and dress. The first postoperative visit occurs at 5–7 days, and the sutures are removed. Passive range of motion using distraction on the joint is instituted early followed by active-assisted range-of-motion exercises at 4 weeks post-surgery. At 6 weeks, the sling is removed and active range of motion is initiated. Rotator cuff and periscapular strengthening are commenced at 12 weeks post-operative. Physical therapy is continued until 5–6 months postoperative at which time the patient is transitioned to a home exercise program.

Results

Only two published studies report on arthroscopic biologic resurfacing of the glenoid with a success rate of approximately 75 %. Savoie et al. [4] reviewed 20 consecutive patients who underwent all-arthroscopic resurfacing of the glenoid with a biologic patch (Restore; DePuy Orthopaedics, Warsaw, IN). Mean patient age was 32 years. At last follow-up of 3–6 years, 75 % of patients remained satisfied, and five had proceeded to surface replacement arthroplasty. All patients made statistically significant improvements in pain scores, range of motion (ROM), American Shoulder and Elbow Surgeons (ASES) score, UCLA shoulder rating, Rowe, Constant-Murley, and SF-12 scores.

A second cohort of patients treated with an all-arthroscopic biologic glenoid resurfacing was reported by de Beer et al. [3] in 2010. Thirty-two consecutive patients underwent biologic glenoid resurfacing with an acellular human dermal scaffold (Graftjacket; Wright Medical Technology, Inc., Memphis, TN). The Constant and Murley score increased significantly from a median of

40 points preoperatively to 64.5 points at final assessment. The results were categorized as excellent in 28 %, satisfactory in 44 %, and unsatisfactory in 28 %. Overall, the procedure was considered successful in 72 %. Five patients had a complication, including one reaction to the graft material and one case of synovitis and five patients were converted to prosthetic arthroplasty.

Namdari et al. [9] performed a systematic review of published studies for biologic glenoid resurfacing for glenohumeral osteoarthritis. Seven studies met inclusion criteria; all were case series with level IV evidence published between 2007 and 2010. Weighted mean age of all 180 patients was 46.4 years, with 73.2 % males, and the most common operative indication was primary osteoarthritis in 59.4 % of cases. Half of the patients (50.6 %) had undergone previous surgery on the operative shoulder. Patients were followed at a weighted mean of 46.6 months. Visual analog scale (VAS) scores for pain improved from 7.5 preoperatively to 2.5 postoperatively. Range of motion improved in active forward elevation (82–136°) and active external rotation (12–44°). Multiple outcome measures were reported, and all improved from preoperative to postoperative, including ASES scores (32.7–76.7), Constant scores (23.5–68.8), simple shoulder test (SST) scores (3.2–7.6), UCLA scores (15–29), and Rowe scores (55–81). Two studies utilized Neer's criteria for outcome assessment and reported a total of 27 excellent, 27 satisfactory, and 14 unsatisfactory results. Overall, 81 % of patients were satisfied with their outcome. There was no difference in functional outcomes between the cohort of patients treated arthroscopically (two studies) and those treated with an open approach (five studies).

Namdari [9] found the overall complication rate for the procedure was 13.3 %. Complications across all studies included infection (8, 4.6 %), stiffness (6, 3.5 %), instability (3, 1.7 %), brachial neuritis (3, 1.7 %), graft reaction/synovitis (2, 1.2 %), and deep vein thrombosis (1, 0.6 %). None of the patients treated arthroscopically (52 patients) developed a postoperative infection compared with 6.6 % (8/121 patients) of those treated open. However, two of the patients treated arthroscopically with a commercially available graft had evidence of a graft-related reaction or synovitis. The overall rate of reoperation was 26.0 % with 12.7 % converting to TSA. In the two series of arthroscopic cases without humeral-sided resurfacing, 19 % of patients underwent a repeat surgical procedure to resurface the humerus or convert to a prosthetic arthroplasty. The authors conclude that biologic glenoid resurfacing demonstrates the potential for successful short-term outcomes but that patients and surgeons must be willing to accept a significant complication rate and likelihood for reoperation.

Recent studies show inconsistent results. Lee and colleagues [17] reported on 19 shoulders treated with meniscal allograft glenoid resurfacing and shoulder hemiarthroplasty followed for a minimum of 2 years and mean of 4.25 years. The authors report inconsistent results with a high complication rate of 32 %, all requiring additional surgery. Three patients underwent TSA and one patient underwent revision hemiarthroplasty, and the authors urge strong consideration should be given to performing TSA in all patients in whom conservative treatment options have failed.

Strauss and colleagues [12] reported disappointing results for biologic resurfacing in 2014. These authors reviewed 31 patients who were resurfaced with lateral meniscus allograft and 10 patients resurfaced with human acellular dermal tissue matrix. The mean age was 42.2 years, and all patients had either a hemiarthroplasty or humeral head prosthetic resurfacing. They reported an overall failure rate of 51.2 % at a mean of 2.8 years. The lateral meniscal allograft cohort had a failure rate of 45.2 % with a mean time to failure of 3.2 years. The human acellular dermal tissue matrix group had a failure rate of 70 % with a mean time to failure of 2.2 years. Significant improvements were seen compared to baseline in pain scores, ROM, ASES score, and SST score. However, high clinical failure rates were observed at intermediate time frames.

Muh et al. [8] also found disappointing results with biologic resurfacing at intermediate follow-up. These authors reviewed 16 patients who had undergone open humeral head arthroplasty with soft tissue interposition grafting of the glenoid. The soft tissue interposition graft was human acellular dermal matrix in seven patients and Achilles tendon allograft in nine patients. At a mean follow-up of 60 months with minimum 24-month follow-up, modest improvements were made in pain, ROM, and ASES scores. Conversion to a total shoulder arthroplasty was performed in seven patients (44 %) at a mean of 36 months. The authors conclude that because of these results, biologic resurfacing of the glenoid with humeral head resurfacing is no longer their primary treatment option for young patients with arthritis, and it should be used with caution.

It has long been our policy in these young patients not to combine the glenoid resurfacing and the humeral head surgery. The initial reconstructive surgery is usually arthroscopic glenoid resurfacing, followed several years later by humeral resurfacing and then eventually TSA. In some cases, humeral resurfacing may be performed as the initial reconstructive option if primary wear is confined to the humerus and followed later by either biologic resurfacing or TSA. Millet et al. [7, 18] have shown promising results with arthroscopic treatment of the arthritic shoulder by extensive debridement, removal of humeral spurs, and an axillary nerve neurolysis. This procedure is similar to the one presented in this chapter, with the exception of step biologic resurfacing of the glenoid.

Summary

Glenohumeral arthritis in the young patient or active patient is a difficult problem to treat. It can cause significant pain, stiffness, and functional limitations. When conservative measures fail to provide relief, and arthroscopic debridement does not adequately alleviate pain, shoulder arthroplasty may be the only surgical option. Total shoulder arthroplasty is a reliable option in older patients with low functional demand. In contrast, younger patients with longer life expectancy and energetic patients with increased activity levels create a dilemma for prosthetic replacement of the glenoid. These patients are at increased risk of complications including polyethylene wear, osteolysis, glenoid loosening, or progressive glenoid wear [1, 2]. In these active patients, biologic glenoid resurfacing is an attractive option.

Outcome studies reveal that biologic resurfacing of the glenoid has mixed results. While early reports demonstrated good clinical outcomes [10, 11], more recent studies reveal a failure rate of 50 % at 3 years [8, 12]. Biologic glenoid resurfacing remains a viable treatment option for a difficult patient population that has exhausted conservative means, especially when significant humeral head flattening is absent. It can offer pain relief and improved function for an intermediate time period and may serve as a bridge before prosthetic arthroplasty becomes necessary.

References

1. Sperling JW, Cofield RH, Rowland CM. Neer hemiarthroplasty and Neer total shoulder arthroplasty in patients fifty years old or less. J Bone Joint Surg Am. 1998;80:464–73.
2. Sperling JW, Cofield RH, Rowland CM. Minimum fifteen-year follow-up of Neer hemiarthroplasty and total shoulder arthroplasty in patients aged fifty years or younger. J Shoulder Elbow Surg. 2004;13:604–13.
3. De Beer JF, Bhatia DN, van Rooyen KS, Du Toit DF. Arthroscopic debridement and biological resurfacing of the glenoid in glenohumeral arthritis. Knee Surg Sports Traumatol Arthrosc. 2010;18:1767–73.
4. Savoie III FH, Brislin KY, Argo D. Arthroscopic glenoid resurfacing as a surgical treatment for glenohumeral arthritis in the young patient: midterm results. Arthroscopy. 2009;25:864–71.
5. Elhassan B, Ozbaydar M, Diller D, Higgins LD, Warner JJ. Soft-tissue resurfacing of the glenoid in the treatment of glenohumeral arthritis in active patients less than fifty years old. J Bone Joint Surg Am. 2009;91:419–24.
6. Gartsman GM, Roddey TS, Hammerman SM. Shoulder arthroplasty with or without resurfacing of the glenoid in patients who have osteoarthritis. J Bone Joint Surg Am. 2000;82:26–34.
7. Millett PJ, Gaskill TR. Arthroscopic management of glenohumeral arthrosis: humeral osteoplasty, capsular release, and arthroscopic axillary nerve release as a joint-preserving approach. Arthroscopy. 2011;27(9):1296–303.
8. Muh SJ, Streit JJ, Shishani Y, Dubrow S, Nowinski RJ, Gobezie R. Biologic resurfacing of the glenoid

with humeral head resurfacing for glenohumeral arthritis in the young patient. J Shoulder Elbow Surg. 2014;23(8):e185–90. doi:10.1016/j.jse.2013.11.016.
9. Namdari S, Alosh H, Baldwin K, Glaser D, Kelly JD. Biologic glenoid resurfacing for glenohumeral osteoarthritis: a systematic review. J Shoulder Elbow Surg. 2011;20:1184–90.
10. Burkhead Jr WZ, Hutton KS. Biologic resurfacing of the glenoid with hemiarthroplasty of the shoulder. J Shoulder Elbow Surg. 1995;4:263–70.
11. Krishnan SG, Nowinski RJ, Harrison D, Burkhead WZ. Humeral hemiarthroplasty with biologic resurfacing of the glenoid for glenohumeral arthritis. Two to fifteen year outcomes. J Bone Joint Surg Am. 2007;89:727–34.
12. Strauss EJ, Verma NN, Salata MJ, McGill KC, Klifto C, Nicholson GP, Cole BJ, Romeo AA. The high failure rate of biologic resurfacing of the glenoid in young patients with glenohumeral arthritis. J Shoulder Elbow Surg. 2014;23(3):409–19.
13. Lee KT, Bell S, Salmon J. Cementless surface replacement arthroplasty of the shoulder with biologic resurfacing of the glenoid. J Shoulder Elbow Surg. 2009;18:915–9.
14. Nicholson GP, Goldstein JL, Romeo AA, Cole BJ, Hayden JK, Twigg SL. Lateral meniscus allograft biologic glenoid arthroplasty in total shoulder arthroplasty for young shoulders with degenerative joint disease. J Shoulder Elbow Surg. 2007;16:S261–6.
15. Wirth MA. Humeral head arthroplasty and meniscal allograft resurfacing of the glenoid. J Bone Joint Surg Am. 2009;91:1109–19.
16. Wong I, Burns J, Snyder S. Arthroscopic Graftjacket repair of rotator cuff tears. J Shoulder Elbow Surg. 2010;19:104–9.
17. Lee BK, Vaishnav S, Hatch III GFR, Itamura JM. Biologic resurfacing of the glenoid with meniscal allograft: long-term results with minimum 2-year follow-up. J Shoulder Elbow Surg. 2013;22:253–60.
18. Millett PJ, Horan MP, Pennock AT, Rios D. Comprehensive Arthroscopic Management (CAM) procedure: clinical results of a joint-preserving arthroscopic treatment for young, active patients with advanced shoulder osteoarthritis. Arthroscopy. 2013;29(3):440–8.

Adhesive Capsulitis: Diagnosis, Etiology, and Treatment Strategies

14

Joshua Asher Gordon, Eric Breitbart, Daniel C. Austin, Christos D. Photopoulos, and John D. Kelly IV

Adhesive capsulitis (AC), often referred to as frozen shoulder (FS), is a common condition affecting approximately 2–3 % of the general population and up to 5 % in some specific populations [1–5]. The condition was originally described by Duplay in 1837 and further defined in Codman's classic text on the shoulder published in 1934. While the definition of FS has been a point of contention, it is widely accepted that hallmarks of this condition include gradual onset of pain near the deltoid insertion, sleep disturbance, and painful limitation of active and passive forward elevation and external rotation in the context of normal radiographs [3, 6–9]. A great deal has been written on the topic, and, since its earliest descriptions by Duplay, Codman, and Neviaser, we have learned much about the natural history, contributing risk factors, macro- and microscopic appearance of disease, biologic changes associated with the condition, and efficacy of various treatment methods; however, a complete understanding of disease pathogenesis and the development of rapidly effective treatment modalities have eluded the medical community [6, 7, 10].

J.A. Gordon, MD (✉) • C.D. Photopoulos, MD
Department of Orthopaedic Surgery, Hospital of the University of Pennsylvania, Philadelphia, PA, USA
e-mail: joshua.gordon@uphs.upenn.edu

E. Breitbart, MD
Department of Orthopaedic Surgery, University of Pennsylvania Health Systems, Philadelphia, PA, USA

D.C. Austin, MD
Department of Orthopaedic Surgery, Dartmouth Hitchcock Medical Center, Labanon, NH, USA

J.D. Kelly IV, MD
Department of Orthopedics, University of Pennsylvania, Philadelphia, PA, USA

Diagnosis, Classification, and Diagnostic Tests

The diagnosis of this condition is largely clinical and can often be made based on patient history and physical exam alone. Most frequently, the disease occurs in female patients between 40 and 60 years of age [4, 11–13]. The development of FS is often associated with injuries in or about the shoulder as well as specific systemic illnesses, most notably diabetes and thyroid dysfunction [5, 11, 12, 14–23]. In 20–30 % of patients, the condition will also develop in the contralateral shoulder [24]. The history may reveal a trivial traumatic injury or the gradual development of substantial pain with shoulder movement in the absence of injury; in either case, limitation of motion, particularly active and passive external rotation, develops and can be measured and compared with the opposite side. Few conditions lead to such a specific loss of external rotation; the list is predominantly limited to posterior dislocations, osteoarthritis, and FS. The other notable

J.D. Kelly IV (ed.), *Elite Techniques in Shoulder Arthroscopy*,
DOI 10.1007/978-3-319-25103-5_14

finding on physical examination is painful restriction of forward elevation. The diagnosis is further supported by a history of sleep disturbance and normal radiographs. Despite these classic hallmarks, significant confusion remains regarding the nomenclature and classification of the disease.

FS is described in stages which functionally describe the natural history arc of progression, from the pre-adhesive stage to the freezing, frozen, and thawing phases [25]. Alternatively, these stages can be referred to by symptoms or numerically as follows:

Stage 1: (pre-adhesive) pain, particularly at night
Stage 2: (freezing) limitation of motion with pain
Stage 3: (frozen) limitation of motion with pain occurring only at the end range of motion
Stage 4: (thawing) a gradual return to normal movement

The classic teaching is that the disease is self-limited with patients routinely progressing to complete resolution. Codman has frequently been quoted as stating that "even the most protracted cases recover with or without treatment in about two years" [3, 6, 26]. However this has not been unanimously accepted, and the literature does not confirm such universal recovery [3, 6, 19, 26]. More contemporary researchers paint a more complex picture, with variable patterns of recovery and even long-term disability [19, 26–29].

The confusion regarding FS and its diagnosis has been fueled by ambiguous and variable nomenclature and imprecise definitions. Even one of the most commonly used names for this condition, adhesive capsulitis, is misleading; adhesions in the shoulder have never been documented as being a cause or component of the disease [26, 30]. Similarly the name frozen shoulder, first used by Codman, has been criticized as an imprecise "wastebasket" term for the stiff shoulder that does not adequately specify the involved pathology [1, 25]. Perhaps the confusion regarding nomenclature for this diagnosis is best illustrated by the sheer number of names by which the condition has been known: adhesive capsulitis, frozen shoulder, pericapsulitis, Duplay disease, and, in its earliest incarnation as described by Duplay, humeral scapular periarthritis [7–10, 31]. Recent efforts have been made to improve the specificity of the current nomenclature [8, 9, 31, 32]. In a recent review of the literature exploring optimized treatment modalities, the lack of agreement about the definition of FS was cited as one of the most substantial obstacles to successful identification of best practices [32].

Sourcing expert opinions, Zuckerman and colleagues have worked to better define the condition and develop consensus. In their survey-based study, "frozen shoulder" was defined as a condition "characterized by functional restrictions of both active and passive motion for which radiographs of the glenohumeral joint are essentially unremarkable except for the possible presence of osteopenia or calcific tendonitis" [9]. This classification was further subdivided into primary FS arising without other underlying etiology and secondary FS, which was divided into intrinsic, extrinsic, and systemically derived disease. Intrinsic FS arises from pathology limited to shoulder structural failure and originates from rotator cuff dysfunction and other pathologies of the shoulder proper. Extrinsic FS refers to etiologies residing outside the shoulder such as neurological deficits after a cerebrovascular accident (CVA) or restricted motion due to injuries of adjacent structures. Systemic illness, such as diabetes or thyroid disorders, is the root cause for the third category of secondary disease [9]. These definitions were confirmed by survey; most shoulder and elbow surgeons queried felt these definitions appropriately defined the condition. Responses were largely affirmative but were not unanimous, highlighting the difficulty in defining the disease and the need for continued discussion. While this definition and categorization can be found through long-standing writings on the topic, it is notable that this classification makes progress toward standardizing these definitions [1, 6, 9, 19, 33]. Importantly, although these definitions are helpful for clarity of discussion and, particularly, literature review, they do not classify the disorder in such a way that has prognostic or therapeutic value.

Diagnosis

In making the diagnosis of FS, imaging can be helpful, primarily in a confirmatory capacity. As noted, conventional X-rays are negative, apart from osteopenia which may occur in the proximal humerus [34]. Magnetic resonance imaging (MRI) can be helpful [35]; MRI findings correspond well with the gross pathological process and include a reduced axillary recess volume, thickening of the axillary pouch, rotator interval thickening, narrowing of the interval between subscapularis and supraspinatus, rotator interval gadolinium enhancement, obliteration of the fat triangle under the coracoid process, coracohumeral ligament thickening, enhancement in the superior subscapular recess, and biceps tendon sheath effusion [34, 36–40]. The thickness of the axillary recess has been measured and found to be a specific marker of disease; a capsule and synovial thickness of greater than 4 mm was found to be 95 % sensitive and 70 % specific for FS [34, 41]. Post-gadolinium rotator interval enhancement has also been documented as a reliable marker of the disease; in one small study, Carrillon and colleagues were able to demonstrate this enhancement in 22/25 patients with FS, while only 1/15 of patients with a rotator cuff tear demonstrated this finding [38]. MR arthrograms have also been investigated and may improve diagnostic accuracy; however, in the context of a thorough history, physical examination, and, in some cases, less complex imaging studies, it is unlikely to be required for confirmation of the diagnosis and as such would not be recommended in routine workup. Findings of FS using this technique include an increased thickness of the coracohumeral ligament, increased rotator interval thickness, and decreased volume in both the glenohumeral joint as a whole and, more specifically, the axillary recess [34, 42, 43]. Mengiardi and colleagues found that thickening of the rotator cuff interval to 7 mm or more was 86 % specific and 64 % sensitive for the condition [42]. MR arthrography might be most useful when additional pathology is suspected [44].

Ultrasound evaluation performed with Doppler flow measurement can identify several key findings associated with FS including increased thickness of the rotator interval structures, peritendinous effusion about the long head of the biceps tendon, increased vascular flow, and abnormal contour of the supraspinatus beneath the acromion [34, 45]. This technique is also valuable in that it can be applied dynamically and symptoms can be evaluated at the time of the study.

Although these imaging techniques have been proven to be valuable in their confirmatory capacity, the diagnosis remains clinical and is chiefly based on the history and physical exam alone. In those cases that require confirmation, we recommend the use of ultrasound due to the reduced comparative cost and the ability to evaluate structures dynamically. If there is a strong suspicion of underlying pathology, an MRI may be warranted. Further, we find the term frozen shoulder and the definitions as set out by Zuckerman and colleagues to be the most current and appropriate.

Pathophysiology

In 1945, Neviaser reported on the microscopic appearance of tissues affected by FS. He initiated what would be a long-running investigation into the underlying pathophysiology and coined the term adhesive capsulitis in reference to what he observed as a chronic inflammatory fibrosis existing in the capsule, bursa, or both [10]. Since then, histologic studies have emphasized a fibrotic as opposed to direct inflammatory histologic appearance [46]. Neviaser, among others, described the histologic appearance of the diseased tissue and included hypervascularized synovium, tightening of the axillary recess, thickening of the shoulder capsule, scarring of the rotator interval, and decreased joint space; all associated with fibrosis and infiltration of fibroblasts seen on microscopy [10, 33, 47, 48]. These findings are congruous with those observed using modern imaging modalities.

In one of the most complete histologic evaluations to date, Rodeo and colleagues described the gross pathology and histology along with immunohistochemical characteristics of the disease. They identified synovial cells and fibroblasts as the dominant cell populations occurring in the presence of abundant type I and type III collagen, indicating new collagen deposition [49]. Additionally, they identified increased staining for platelet-derived growth factor (PDGF) and its receptor, transforming growth factor-β (TGF-β) and its receptor, interleukin 1-β (IL1-β), tumor necrosis factor-α (TNF-α), and hepatocyte growth factor in adhesive capsulitis tissues. Many of these same signaling proteins were upregulated, albeit in a distinct pattern, in samples diagnosed with nonspecific synovitis. These changes were not observed in normal tissues. Bunker concisely described previous histological studies, validated earlier findings, and clarified the histology of FS when he described it as a predominantly fibroproliferative condition associated with hypervascularity and characterized by abundant myofibroblasts, similar to Dupuytren's disease of the hand [1, 47, 50, 51]. Others have noted an increased expression of neuronal elements in adhesive capsulitis tissue [52]. Taken together, this information demonstrates the complex nature of this disorder with multiple responsive molecular signaling pathways leading to the biological changes that manifest in frozen shoulder. Although the resultant pathology is predominantly fibroproliferative, there has been some historical debate regarding a fibrotic versus an inflammatory etiology [49]. With the complex course and the time-dependent nature of this process, it is difficult to discern the specific roles of inflammation versus fibroproliferation through the course of the disease. Seemingly, the resultant pathology does appear to be dominated by fibrotic as opposed to inflammatory changes; however, this remains controversial [1, 3, 46]. Perhaps even further complicating this picture, Hagiwara and colleagues reported an additional increase in chondrogenic phenotype of tissues affected by FS [53]. It remains difficult to discern whether a mechanical change precipitates altered mechanotransductive signaling or altered signaling leads to changes in the mechanical tissue properties. Little work has been done to explore this balance. Elucidating a specific inciting factor for the disease remains an area of active investigation.

Efforts have been made in recent years to try to better understand the biology of the disease. Kim and colleagues were able to demonstrate that intercellular adhesion molecule-1 (ICAM-1) was increased in the affected capsule as well as the synovial fluid and serum of patients with adhesive capsulitis. Further, they demonstrated that the treatment of synovial cells with ICAM-1 in culture increased expression of inflammatory and fibroproliferative mediators [54]. Interestingly, efforts more generally exploring the reaction of fibroblasts to joint aspirates from patients with adhesive capsulitis indicated the presence of growth factors that stimulated fibroblastic proliferation [55]. Consistent with these findings, PCR analysis of tissue from patients with frozen shoulder has indicated an increased expression of cytokines associated with inflammation as well as fibrosis [56, 57]. In a different model system, upregulated TGF-β signaling demonstrated an increase in fibroproliferation as well as chondrogenic phenotype in the rat knee [58]. These findings are particularly interesting in that Hagiwara had previously demonstrated that TGF-β expression in synovium of the rat knee is increased during periods of immobilization, a factor known to be associated with frozen shoulder as well [59]. Investigation of Dupuytren's disease has generated further implication of TGF-β signaling in the activation of the P-38 MAPK pathway contributing to fibrosis. Further, the IGF-2 and β-catenin signaling pathways, both implicated in Dupuytren's disease, have been found to be upregulated in FS [60]. It appears that a complex set of regulatory mechanisms are shared by the two diseases, and epidemiology, histology, and basic science support this association. What has been learned regarding Dupuytren's disease will potentially provide clues to the biology of FS, although neither complex disease is fully understood. Genome-wide microarray expression confirms a complex dynamic pathologic process that involves multiple signaling pathways which lead to frozen shoulder. In a recent microarray analysis of FS capsule specimens, over 30 genes were found to be significantly upregulated and more than 10 significantly downregulated; upregulated genes were most associated with fibrogenic, chondrogenic, angiogenic, and to a lesser extent, neurogenic changes [53].

Although there are numerous disease processes that have been epidemiologically linked to FS (Table 14.1), the specific means by which they increase such risk has not been described. Models of these diseases have been increasingly investigated and may lead to an understanding of the

Table 14.1 Epidemiology and associated diseases of frozen shoulder

Associations with frozen shoulder (FS)		
Associated condition	Author/year	Results/conclusions
Gender		
Female	Austin et al. (2014) [11]	In a series of patients with FS, 59 % were women and 41 % were men
Female	White et al. (2011) [4]	Women had an observed rate of FS of 3.38 per 1000 person-years in comparison with 2.36 in men
Age		
Increasing age	White et al. (2011) [4]	In women, every 10-year incremental increase in age resulted in an 8 % greater FS rate
Increasing age	Balci et al. (1999) [13]	Average patient age of 59.2 with FS vs. 53.6 without disease in type II diabetes mellitus (DM)
Increasing age	Arkkila et al. (1996) [12]	Average patient age of 46.7 with FS vs. 31.7 without disease in type I diabetes and 65.3 with FS vs. 59.9 without disease in type II DM
Trauma		
Minor trauma	Austin et al. (2014) [11]	In 38 % of patients with FS a history of minor trauma was reported
Minor trauma	Hand et al. (2008) [19]	In 22 % of patients a history of minor trauma was reported
Minor trauma	Bulgen et al. (1984) [18]	In 34 % of patients a history of minor trauma was reported
Postsurgical		
Post-shoulder or upper limb surgery	Austin et al. (2014) [11]	In 21 % of patients a history of previous upper limb surgery was reported
Post-cardiac surgery	Tuten et al. (2000) [61]	Noted a 3.3 % incidence of postoperative development of FS in male cardiac surgery patients
Post-acute cerebral aneurysm surgery	Tanishima and Yoshimasu (1997) [62]	Up to 41 % of patients develop FS following acute aneurysm surgery possibly due to immobilization
Post-catheterization of brachial artery	Pineda et al. (1994) [63]	Case series of seven patients who developed FS post-cardiac catheterization of the brachial artery
Post-radical neck dissection	Patten and Hillel (1993) [64]	Reported that 70 % of patients undergoing a radical neck dissection developed shoulder disability consistent with FS
Post-neurosurgical	Bruckner and Nye (1981) [65]	23 % of patients developed FS after neurosurgical procedures. Within this group, there was an association with hemiparesis
Cardiovascular disease		
Hypertension	Austin et al. (2014) [11]	A 50 % increase in the prevalence of anti-hypertension medications observed within FS patients
Myocardial infarction/ coronary heart disease	Arkkila et al. (1996) [12]	Reported an odds ratio for myocardial infarction of 13.7 (95 % CI 1.3–139.5) in type I DM patients with FS. Higher prevalence of FS in type I DM with coronary artery disease
Ischemic heart disease	Bridgeman (1972) [17]	It was observed that 8 of 14 nondiabetic patients with FS also had ischemic heart disease
Peripheral vascular disease (PVD)	Arkkila et al. (1996) [12]	Prevalence of FS of 28.9 % in type I diabetics with PVD while only 7.4 % in those without PVD
Hypertension	Arkkila et al. (1996) [12]	Prevalence of FS of 21.7 % in type I DM with HTN while only 6.3 % in those without HTN
Diabetes mellitus (DM)		
Diabetes	Lo et al. (2014) [5]	Incidence of FS was three times greater in patients with DM in comparison with controls
Diabetes	Huang et al. (2013) [23]	After onset of DM, patients had a hazard ratio of 1.32 (95 % CI 1.22–1.42) for developing FS in comparison with controls

(continued)

Table 14.1 (continued)

Associations with frozen shoulder (FS)		
Associated condition	Author/year	Results/conclusions
Diabetes	Austin et al. (2014) [11]	Prevalence of diabetic medications in FS patients was over two times that observed in the general population
Diabetes Severity of diabetes	Ramchurn et al. (2009) [22]	In diabetics, 25 % had FS or shoulder tendonitis compared to 2 % of control group. Poor glycemic control associated with increased risk of upper limb disability
Diabetes or prediabetes	Tighe and Oakley (2008) [16]	When testing patients diagnosed with FS, 38.6 % had diabetes and 33.0 % had prediabetes. In this series, 2 % were newly diagnosed with diabetes and 28.4 % with prediabetes
Diabetes Duration of diabetes	Thomas et al. (2007) [21]	In diabetics, 4.3 % had FS in comparison with 0.5 % of control group. Observed a positive association with duration of diabetes
Diabetes Duration of diabetes Diabetes complications	Balci et al. (1999) [13]	It was reported that 29 % of diabetics have FS. Patients with FS had diabetes for 7.5 years on average vs. 6.0 years without FS. Significant association observed between FS and retinopathy in diabetics
Diabetes Duration of diabetes Diabetes complications	Arkkila et al. (1996) [12]	FS observed in 10.3 % of type I and 22.4 % of type II DM. Associated with duration of type I DM. Significantly increased odds ratio for autonomic neuropathy in diabetics with FS
Diabetes Severity of diabetes	Bridgeman (1972) [17]	In diabetics, 10.8 % have FS compared to 2.3 % of nondiabetics. Insulin-dependent diabetics have higher rates of FS than non-insulin-dependent
Metabolic disorders		
Hyperlipidemia	Lo et al. (2014) [5]	Hyperlipidemia independently increased risk of FS with a hazard ratio of 1.29 (95 % CI 1.11–1.49)
Hypercholesterolemia Hypertriglyceridemia	Bunker and Esler (1995) [66]	Patients with FS had significantly higher serum cholesterol and serum triglyceride concentrations
Hormonal disorders		
Hyperthyroidism	Huang et al. (2014) [20]	Patients with hyperthyroidism had an adjusted hazard ratio of 1.22 for developing FS
Hypothyroidism Hyperthyroidism	Cakir et al. (2003) [15]	Overall, 10.3 % of patients with thyroid dysfunction have FS. Observed in 17.4 % of those with subclinical thyrotoxicosis and 13 % in hypothyroidism
ACTH deficiency	Choy et al. (1991) [67]	Case report of bilateral FS in an ACTH-deficient patient
Hypothyroidism	Bowman et al. (1988) [14]	Case report of bilateral FS, oligoarthropathy, and myopathy in hypothyroidism
Hyperthyroidism	Wohlgethan (1987) [68]	Case report of bilateral FS in a patient with hyperthyroidism
Musculoskeletal		
Limited joint mobility	Balci et al. (1999) [13]	Reported an odds ratio of 2.1 (95 % CI 1.2–3.7) of limited joint mobility in diabetic patients with FS
Limited joint mobility	Arkkila et al. (1996) [12]	Prevalence of FS of 28.4 % in type II DM with limited joint mobility but only 13.2 % in those without
Dupuytren's disease	Smith et al. (2001) [50]	In patients with FS, 52 % have evidence of Dupuytren's disease, which is 8.27 (95 % CI 6.25–11.2) greater than the general population
Dupuytren's disease	Balci et al. (1999) [13]	Anodds ratio of 2.4 (95 % CI 1.3–4.4) of Dupuytren's disease in diabetic patients with FS was reported
Dupuytren's disease	Arkkila et al. (1996) [12]	Prevalence of FS of 25.0 % in type I DM with Dupuytren's disease while only 7.6 % in those without
Tennis elbow (lateral epicondylitis)	Hakim et al. (2003) [69]	FS and tennis elbow are observed together in individuals 2–3 times more often than expected. Although investigated in a twin study, the association was not thought to be genetic

(continued)

Table 14.1 (continued)

Associations with frozen shoulder (FS)		
Associated condition	Author/year	Results/conclusions
Neurologic conditions		
Stroke	Kang et al. (2010) [70]	After developing FS, patients had an adjusted hazard ratio of stroke of 1.22 (95 % CI 1.06–1.40)
Stroke	Lo et al. (2003) [43]	FS is responsible for 50 % of cases of shoulder pain following stroke, making it a common post-stroke morbidity
Parkinson's disease	Riley et al. (1989) [71]	In patients with Parkinson's disease, 12.7 % had FS in comparison with 1.7 % of control group. FS may be a presenting symptom of the disease
Hemiparesis Impaired consciousness	Bruckner and Nye (1981) [65]	Hemiparesis and impairment of consciousness were associated with FS in post-neurosurgical patients
Psychological		
Depressed personality	Bruckner and Nye (1981) [65]	Depressive personality was associated with the development of FS in post-neurosurgical patients. More recent studies have suggested personality traits may not be associated with adhesive capsulitis [72]
Drug induced		
Vaccinations (influenza and pneumococcal)	Bodor and Montalvo (2007) [73]	A case series of two patients who developed FS and additional shoulder pathology following injection. Likely injected into the sub-acromial bursa
Highly active antiretroviral therapy (HIV medications)	De Ponti et al. (2006) [74]	A case series of six patients who developed FS while on HIV therapy
Fluoroquinones (antibiotic)	Freiss et al. (2000) [75]	A case series of two patients who developed FS following antibiotic therapy
Protease inhibitors: indinavir (HIV medications)	Grasland et al. (2000) [76]	A series of eight patients is presented who developed FS (four bilaterally) while taking the medication
Matrix metalloproteinase inhibitor (chemotherapy)	Hutchinson et al. (1998) [77]	In a case series of patients treated with this drug, 6 out of 12 developed FS
Triple antiretroviral therapy (HIV)	Zabraniecki et al. (1998) [78]	A series of three patients who developed arthrography confirmed FS without other causes
Flunarizine (calcium channel blockers)	Franck and Beurrier (1996) [79]	A case report of a patient who developed severe bilateral FS that resolved after discontinuation of the medication
Others		
Malignancy	Gheita et al. (2010) [80]	In patients with known malignancies, 15 % of them have FS
Osteopenia	Okamura and Ozaki (1999) [81]	In women with FS, there was a significant decrease in bone mineral density in the proximal humerus

precise relationship to FS. Models of frozen shoulder resulting from secondary disease present an excellent opportunity to explore specific mechanisms of FS pathogenesis. Diabetes is potentially the most strongly linked disease to FS prevalence. Thomas and colleagues explored the specific effects of streptozocin-induced hyperglycemia on the rat shoulder and identified both a diminution of external rotation and an increase in inflammatory markers including advanced glycation end products (AGE) and IL-1β in the rotator interval region. They further observed increased TNF-α in the superior capsule. This finding may provide clues into some early biologic events leading to FS pathogenesis. Animal models exploring arthrofibrosis and Dupuytren's disease have similarly helped to discern some specific mechanisms that may lead to downstream fibrosis. Finally, a potential link of FS and general autoimmune disorders has been posited. This stands to reason given the shared inflammatory elements of both FS and autoimmune disorder.

These and other studies merely confirm that the pathophysiology of FS is complex and there are seemingly multiple pathways contributing to disease initiation and progression. It is the senior author's (JDK) contention that the term "idiopathic" FS will be ultimately abandoned as a causal link with some proinflammatory state will eventually be demonstrated in most cases.

Although the outcomes and treatment modalities in patients with different risk factors for FS may differ, we still know little about how each specific risk factor precisely contributes to pathologic changes.

Treatment and Outcomes

Historically, conservative management has been the treatment of choice for FS. Surgical measures have been reserved for patients failing nonoperative treatment for more than 6 months [25]. However, the time course for improvement and recovery in patients varies. With such uncertainty, some patients may prefer options with potential to expedite recovery. Additionally some data supports the use of earlier arthroscopic intervention. Baums and colleagues showed that after only 6 months of failed conservative management, arthroscopic release was an effective treatment. Further, their group noted significant difficulty experienced by patients waiting for resolution of a painful frozen shoulder [82]. In a small case series, Sabat and colleagues demonstrated that arthroscopic release was an effective treatment as early as 3 months and after only 6 weeks of failed conservative management. In that series, all patients returned to work in 3–5 months [83]. Despite results such as these, conservative management continues to be the gold standard for the initial treatment of FS [1, 6, 25, 34]. There are many forms of noninvasive treatment including physical therapy, anti-inflammatory medications, corticosteroid injections (CSI), sodium hyaluronate injections, acupuncture, and extracorporeal shockwave therapy. There remains a frustrating lack of consensus regarding which therapies, individual or combined, lead to the best outcomes (see Table 14.2).

Table 14.2 Conservative treatment options

Conservative treatments for FS				
Study/year	Study group	Interventions	Follow-up	Results/conclusions
Corticosteroids				
Yoon et al. (2013) [84]	Randomized controlled trial of 53 patients with primary FS in the freezing stage with symptoms for at least 1 month. Cases of secondary FS including diabetics were excluded	1. High-dose intra-articular corticosteroid injection (40 mg triamcinolone) 2. Low dose intra-articular corticosteroid injection (20 mg triamcinolone) 3. Placebo injection	12 weeks	Both cortisone injection treatment groups showed significant improvements in shoulder disability, pain, and range of motion in comparison with placebo. There was not a significant difference between the two doses administered. All treatment groups showed significant improvement with time
Roh et al. (2012) [85]	Randomized controlled trial of 45 diabetic patients with FS who had failed conservative therapy (stretching and NSAIDs) for at least 3 months. Patients were excluded if they had other shoulder pathology or systemic causes of disease	1. Intra-articular corticosteroid injection (40 mg triamcinolone) and home exercise with NSAIDs 2. Home exercise with NSAIDs	24 weeks	At the 4-week follow-up, the steroid injection group had significantly less pain than the home exercise group. At the 12-week follow-up, the steroid injection group has significantly greater range of motion. There were no significant differences in range of motion or pain scores between groups at the 24-week follow-up

(continued)

Table 14.2 (continued)

Conservative treatments for FS				
Study/year	Study group	Interventions	Follow-up	Results/conclusions
Bal et al. (2008) [86]	Randomized controlled trial of 80 patients with FS who had been symptomatic for 6 weeks to 6 months. Patients with previous surgery or diabetes were excluded	1. Intra-articular corticosteroid injection (40 mg methylprednisolone with 12 weeks of home exercise) 2. Intra-articular injection of saline with 12 weeks of home exercise	12 weeks	At week 2, shoulder pain and disability scores were significantly reduced in the corticosteroid group in comparison with the placebo. At the week 12 visit, there were no significant differences in pain or disability scores between the groups
Buchbinder et al. (2006) [87]	Cochrane review of oral steroids for FS	1. Oral corticosteroids 2. Other interventions including placebo	Various	Concluded that oral steroids provide significant short-term benefits in pain and disability but that these benefits may not last beyond 6 weeks. However, there were not enough studies to complete a meta-analysis
Buchbinder et al. (2004) [88]	Randomized controlled trial of 46 patients with FS for more than 3 weeks. Patients were excluded if they had other shoulder pathology or systemic causes of disease	1. Oral corticosteroid (30 mg prednisolone) 2. Placebo	12 weeks	The oral corticosteroid group showed significant improvement in pain, disability, and range of motion at 3 weeks. At 6 weeks and 12 weeks, there were no significant differences in any measures between the groups
Widiastuti-Samekto and Sianturi (2004) [89]	Randomized prospective trial of 26 patients in the frozen or thawing stage of FS. Patients were excluded if they had other shoulder pathology or systemic causes of disease	1. Triamcinolone intra-articular injection (40 mg) 2. Oral triamcinolone	3 weeks	Significantly more patients were considered cured at week 1 in the intra-articular injection group. There were no significant differences in cure rates at week 2 or week 3
Buchbinder et al. (2003) [90]	Cochrane review of intra-articular corticosteroid injections for shoulder pain	1. Intra-articular corticosteroids 2. Other interventions including placebo	Various	Concluded that intra-articular corticosteroid injections may be of limited short-term benefit in FS; however, there were not enough high-quality studies to complete a meta-analysis
Corticosteroids vs. physiotherapy				
Ryans et al. (2005) [91]	Randomized controlled trial of 80 patients with FS symptoms from 1 to 6 months' duration. Patients were excluded if they had other shoulder pathology or systemic causes of disease	1. Corticosteroid injection (20 mg triamcinolone) and eight sessions of physical therapy 2. Corticosteroid injection 3. Placebo injection and physical therapy 4. Placebo injection	16 weeks	At 6 weeks, corticosteroid injections were associated with significantly less patient-reported shoulder disability, while physical therapy was associated with an increased range of motion. At 16 weeks, there were no significant differences between any of the groups

Table 14.2 (continued)

Conservative treatments for FS				
Study/year	Study group	Interventions	Follow-up	Results/conclusions
Carette et al. 2003 [92]	Randomized controlled trial of 93 individuals. Only patients with idiopathic FS were included although the study did not exclude diabetic patients	1. Corticosteroid injection (40 mg triamcinolone) 2. Corticosteroid injection with physical therapy 3. Saline injection with physical therapy 4. Saline injection	12 months	Cortisone injection alone provided significantly more improvement than other groups. At 12 months, all interventions were equal for all outcome measures. Concluded that a single steroid injection with simple home exercises is best and that physical therapy alone has limited utility
Arslan and Celiker (2001) [93]	Randomized trial of 20 individuals with FS in the setting of no other shoulder abnormalities	1. Intra-articular corticosteroid injection (40 mg methylprednisolone) 2. Physiotherapy consisting of hot pack application, ultrasound, passive stretching, pendulum exercises, and NSAIDs	12 weeks	Both groups demonstrated significant improvements in range of motion with no significant differences between the groups. Both interventions resulted in significantly improved pain scores
Physiotherapy				
Russell et al. (2014) [94]	Randomized controlled trial of 75 patients with primary idiopathic FS and at least 3 months of symptoms. Patients were excluded if they had other shoulder pathology or systemic causes of disease	1. Group exercise classes twice per week with a physical therapist 2. Individual sessions twice per week with a physical therapist 3. Home exercises and an informational booklet	12 months	Patients in the group exercise class had significantly less symptoms at 1 year than those in the individual or home-based therapy groups. Both individual and group therapy had significantly greater range of motion than home-based patients. Significant improvements were seen in all three interventions
Dundar et al. (2009) [95]	Randomized prospective trial of 57 patients with primary FS in the painful or stiff phases. Patients with additional shoulder pathology were excluded	1. Continuous passive motion for 1 h/day for 20 days 2. Daily physical therapy with active stretching and pendulum exercises for 20 days	12 weeks	Patients in the CPM group showed significantly greater reductions in pain than those in the physical therapy group. All patients showed significant decreases in pain and increases in range of motion regardless of treatment protocol
Diercks and Stevens (2004) [96]	Cohort study of 77 patients with idiopathic FS. Patients were excluded if they had other shoulder pathology or systemic causes of disease	1. Intensive physical therapy including passive stretching and manual mobilization 2. Supportive therapy with home exercises within pain limits (supervised neglect)	24 months	Significantly more improved shoulder function in supervised neglect group at all points between 3 and 24 months follow-up. At the end of 24-month follow-up, 89 % of supervised neglect patients had normal or near-normal function vs. 63 % in the intensive physical therapy group
Green et al. (2003) [97]	Cochrane review of physical therapy interventions for shoulder pain.	1. Physical therapy 2. Other modalities	Various	Concluded that there is no evidence physical therapy alone is beneficial for FS. Also concluded that there is no evidence that ultrasound is of benefit in FS; however, there is evidence that laser therapy is superior to placebo

(continued)

Table 14.2 (continued)

Conservative treatments for FS				
Study/year	Study group	Interventions	Follow-up	Results/conclusions
Acupuncture				
Green et al. (2005) [98]	Cochrane review of acupuncture for shoulder pain	1. Acupuncture 2. Other modalities	Various	Due to lack of quality studies, there was not enough evidence to support or refute acupuncture as an effective intervention for FS
Sun et al. (2001) [99]	Randomized trial of 35 patients with FS for 1–12 months' duration. Patients were excluded if they had other shoulder pathology or systemic causes of disease	1. Acupuncture and exercise 2. Exercise alone	20 weeks	At the 20-week follow-up, patients in the acupuncture group had significantly higher shoulder scores in comparison with the control group. Both groups showed significant improvements in comparison with their baseline
Other interventions				
Dehghan et al. (2013) [100]	Randomized trial of 57 diabetics with FS of less than 6 months' duration. Patients were excluded if they had other shoulder pathology or additional systemic causes of disease	1. NSAIDs (500 mg naproxen twice daily) and home exercises 2. Intra-articular corticosteroid injection (40 mg triamcinolone) and home exercises	23 weeks	Both groups showed significant improvements in pain and shoulder range of motion during the time period of the study. No significant differences were observed between the treatment modalities
Leung and Cheing (2008) [101]	A randomized trial of 30 patients with primary FS and symptoms for at least 8 weeks. Patients were excluded if they had a history of other shoulder pathology or trauma	1. Shortwave diathermy (deep heating) and stretching 2. Heating pack (superficial heating) and stretching 3. Stretching alone	8 weeks	Shoulder score improvements were significantly better within the deep heating group in comparison with the superficial heating and placebo groups. All three groups showed significant improvements in pain and function during the study
Stergioulas (2008) [102]	A randomized trial of 63 patients with FS. Patients were excluded if they had received alternative treatments within 6 months and had underlying systemic diseases or additional shoulder pathology	1. Laser therapy applied to eight points on shoulder for 12 sessions (3B Laser M 1000) 2. Placebo laser treatments	16 weeks	There were significantly greater decreases in shoulder pain and disability observed in the laser therapy group at 4 weeks, 8 weeks, and at 16 weeks after the start of treatments. There were no significant differences observed in range of motion between groups
Calis et al. (2006) [103]	A randomized trial of 95 patients with FS with symptoms of at least 1 month duration. Patients were excluded if they had other shoulder pathology or systemic causes of disease	1. Sodium hyaluronate (Orthovisc 30 mg) 2. Intra-articular corticosteroid (40 mg triamcinolone) 3. Physical therapy 4. Home exercises	3 months	At 3 months, all interventions showed significantly more improved shoulder scores than the control group. The physical therapy group displayed the most clinical improvement. Authors concluded that sodium hyaluronate may be an alternative to steroid injections

(continued)

Table 14.2 (continued)

Conservative treatments for FS				
Study/year	Study group	Interventions	Follow-up	Results/conclusions
Page et al. (2014) [104]	Cochrane review of electrotherapy modalities applied for the treatment of FS	Review of all electrotherapy modalities in randomized controlled trials or quasi-randomized trials. Evaluating low-level laser therapy (LLLT) and pulsed electromagnetic field therapy (PEMFT)	1 month	Of electrotherapy modalities, only LLLT and PEMFT were compared to placebo. Although the quality of studies was not high, there was some evidence that LLLT and LLLT with exercise were effective in improving pain at 4 weeks and function up to 4 months. It remained unclear if PEMFT was more effective than placebo. Taken together, there was inadequate evidence to support or refute the use of electrotherapy modalities and additional trials would be needed
Dahan et al. (2000) [104]	Randomized trial of 34 patients with an average duration of shoulder pain of 1 year	1. Three indirect suprascapular nerve blocks with bupivacaine (10 cc) 7 days apart 2. Placebo injections with saline	1 month	At 2 weeks following the final injections, the bupivacaine group reported significantly lower pain scores in comparison with the placebo group; however there was not a significant difference in shoulder function or range of motion

Physical Therapy

Due to a lack of high-quality randomized studies, a Cochrane review of physical therapy (PT) failed to demonstrate that PT alone is beneficial for FS; nevertheless, it continues to be the foundation of FS treatment [97]. Only one paper concluded a negative effect of early aggressive PT as compared with home exercises alone [96]. This article, based on a study performed by Diercks and Stevens in 2004, reported that supervised neglect and home range of motion exercises within pain limits outperformed formal PT in terms of restoring function. Although described as a randomized cohort study consisting of 77 patients, the authors failed to describe how their randomization process was performed, assessors were not blinded, and the patient distribution between men and women was unequal. In view of these factors, this study is clearly associated with a high risk of bias. The authors concluded that all follow-up points between 3 and 24 months had significant improvements in shoulder function with supervised neglect when compared with formal PT. At the end of a 2-year period, they found that 89 % of the supervised neglect group had near normal or normal function versus 63 % in the PT group [96]. Other subsequent studies have reported results in favor of formal PT programs. Jewell and colleagues, using a database of 2370 patients diagnosed with FS, concluded in 2009 that joint mobilization and exercises were associated with improved outcomes as compared to controls [105]. In 2014, Russell and colleagues conducted a randomized controlled trial of 75 patients and showed that after 1 year of treatment, patients who received formal PT, either individually or in groups, outperformed patients with a home exercise program only [94].

Corticosteroid Injections

A Cochrane review performed by Buchbinder and colleagues in 2003 concluded that while intra-articular corticosteroid injections may have the limited benefit of providing short-term relief from symptoms of FS, long-term benefits could not be proven due to the paucity of high-quality studies [90]. In a more recent study, Roh and colleagues conducted a randomized controlled trial of 45 diabetic patients. Subjects injected with 40 mg of triamcinolone showed improved pain at 4 weeks and improved motion at 12 weeks, with no difference observed at 24 weeks' follow-up [85]. Similarly, Bal and colleagues randomized 80 patients into two groups: the first group received an injection of 40 mg of methylprednisolone plus 12 weeks of home exercises, and the second group received a placebo injection with 12 weeks of home exercise [86]. While at 2 weeks post-injection, pain and disability scores were improved in the CSI group, no differences were seen at week 12. In contrast, the most recent randomized controlled trial in the literature, by Yoon and colleagues, showed a significant improvement in shoulder dysfunction, pain, and range of motion 12 weeks following intra-articular CSI as compared with findings in patients who received placebo treatment [84].

Manipulation Under Anesthesia

Manipulation under anesthesia (MUA), while essentially a nonoperative approach, carries the risk of humeral fracture. There is limited evidence supporting this means of treatment. The only randomized controlled trial in the literature that investigates MUA was conducted by Kivimaki and colleagues in 2007 [106]. This study included 127 patients and failed to report any difference in function as a result of MUA compared with home exercises during the 1-year trial period. Other iatrogenic damage to the shoulder, such as labral tears and rotator cuff injuries, may occur during MUA, adding increased risk to the procedure [107]. Similarly hydrodilatation, or forcibly distending the joint capsule with fluid, is a theoretical means of disrupting the restrictive and fibrotic capsule. This technique has not been strongly supported by evidence, although some suggest it may be superior to MUA [108, 109].

Operative Management

Indications for operative management of FS remain controversial. There are no randomized controlled trials in the literature comparing the efficacy of conservative and surgical management. A review was undertaken by Rookmoneea and colleagues. They could not draw any firm conclusions regarding the effectiveness of nonsurgical versus surgical modalities of treatment [32]. The greatest stumbling block to forming firm conclusions was the lack of high-quality or randomized controlled studies [32]. Another recent review by Grant and colleagues analyzed 22 studies that included a total of 989 patients. This review failed to find differences in range of motion or Constant scores between patients who underwent MUA compared with those who were treated with a capsular release [110]. The highest quality case series reporting the effects of arthroscopic capsular release had an average length of follow-up of 10 months with a range of 3–29 months. This study showed a significant improvement in function, disability, and range of motion after capsular release. Unfortunately, this study lacked a control group that received conservative management. Another case series followed 43 patients who had arthroscopic capsular release with a mean follow-up of 7 years, with a range of 5–13 years [111]. This study showed improved shoulder function with ultimate range of motion comparable to that of the contralateral side and significant reduction in frequency and severity of pain.

Current thoughts on when to proceed from conservative to surgical management with the treatment of FS are patient-centric. Although the majority of cases of FS are expected to resolve over the course of 1–2 years with conservative management, many patients with a high level of activity prefer surgical capsular release with manipulation under anesthesia as a means to potentially expedite recovery. Certain patients have long-term dysfunction without surgery and up to 50 % continue to have symptoms after 4–7 years. Thus, there appear to be subsets of patients who would substantially benefit from early surgical intervention [19, 26, 112]. This is especially true in view of studies showing recovery of pain-free motion averaging less than 3 months following arthroscopic release [113, 114]. This additional information could convince the active patient to consider surgical intervention. Some patients may adjust to their minor disability rather than fully recovering; this phenomenon has been noted since early descriptions of the disease. Codman acknowledged that complete recovery was not routine but that patients were often able to return to good function, and he is quoted as saying "it is pretty hard even for the patient to say when they are well [3, 6]."

Our recommendation for proceeding to arthroscopic capsular release with manipulation is the failure to see improvement of symptoms after at least 3 months of conservative management consisting of a CSI and physical therapy. Even modest gains in motion or pain would preclude surgical intervention, providing the patient is reasonably comfortable. The inability to sleep and the presence of inordinate pain also influence the recommendation for arthroscopic intervention. The typical arthroscopic findings in FS are a contracted rotator interval and an inflamed, contracted capsule (Fig 14.1a). An associated biceps synovitis may also be encountered (Fig. 14.1b). Our preferred approach is to first measure passive ROM once the patient is placed supine and under anesthesia. Scalene block anesthetic is preferred. A gentle manipulation is performed using the following order: forward flexion, abduction external rotation, abduction and adduction, and finally abduction/internal rotation. If at least 90 % of motion is not attained, or a solid "end feel" of the capsule is encountered, the patient is positioned in the lateral decubitus position for arthroscopic release. Anterior superior and anterior portals are made in addition to the standard posterior portal. The tightened structures are released first through

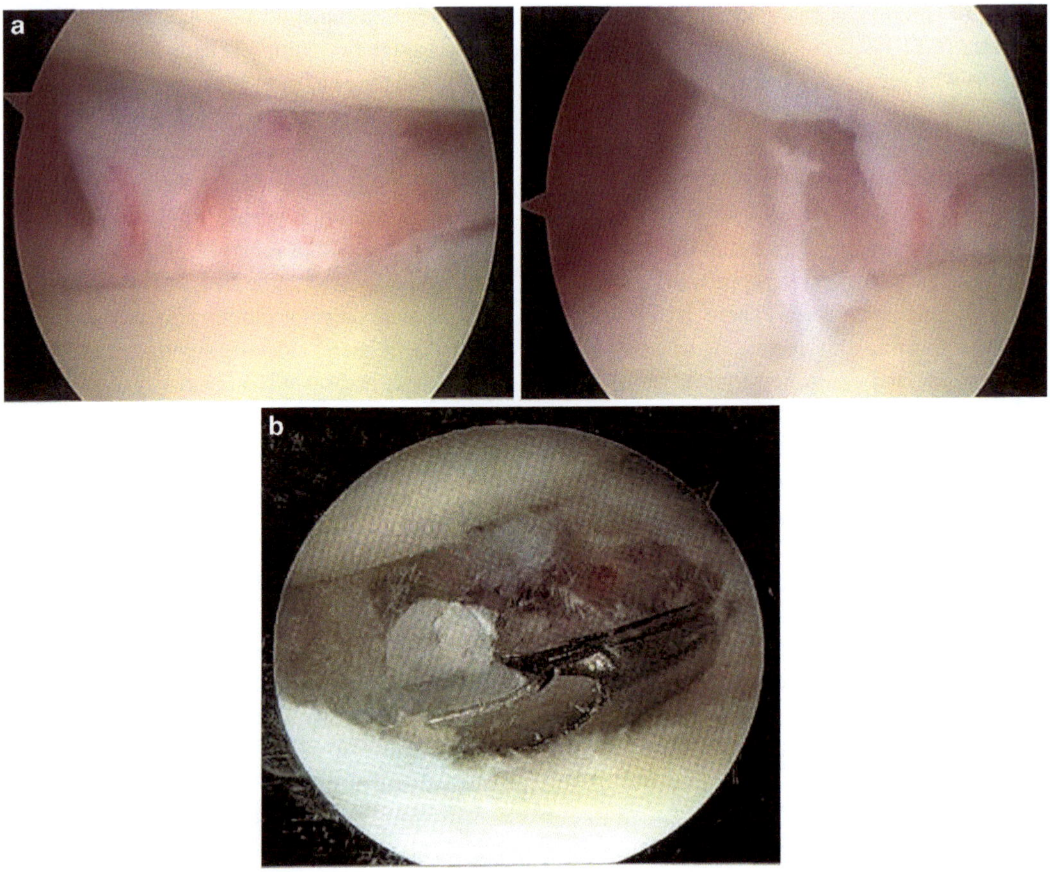

Fig. 14.1 (**a**) Arthroscopic image of tightened and irritated capsular structures prior to release. (**b**) Inflamed superior capsule and rotator interval

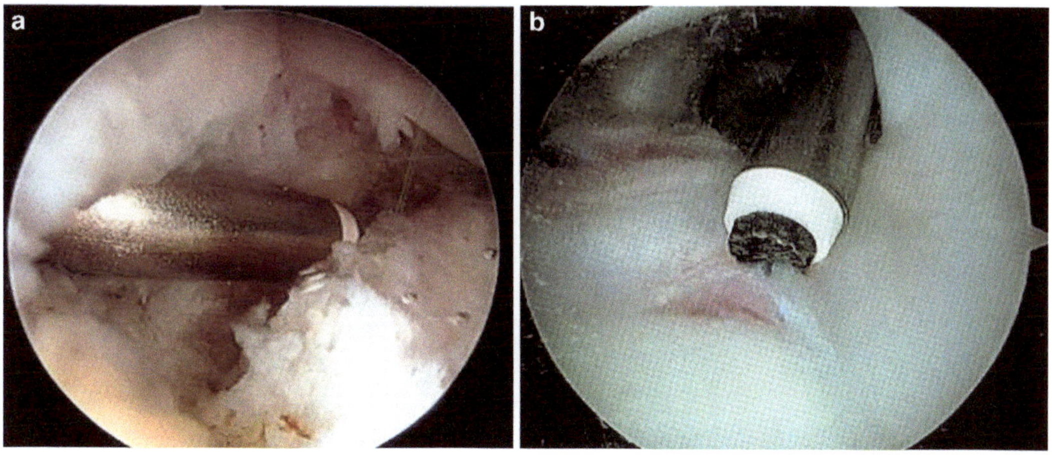

Fig. 14.2 (**a**) Arthroscopic release of capsule using electrocautery. (**b**) Thermal instrument in the interval after release

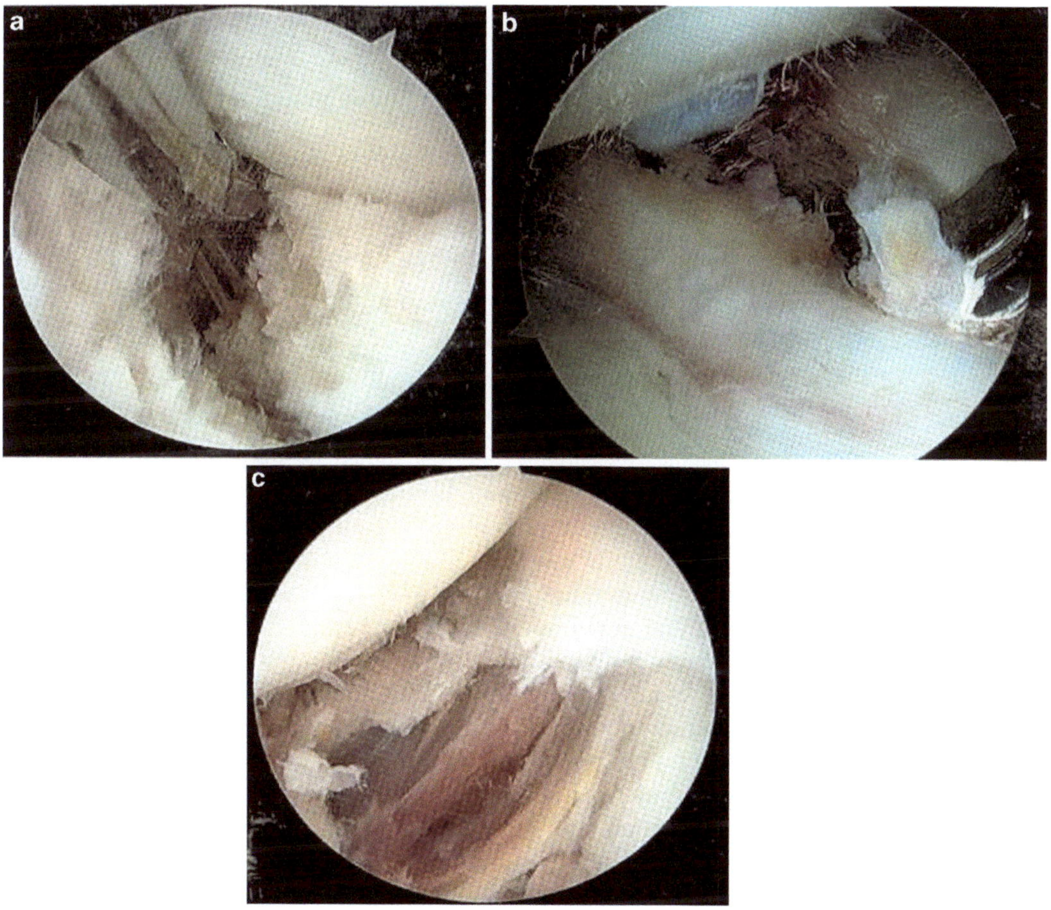

Fig. 14.3 (**a**) Anterior inferior capsular release. (**b**) Anterior capsular release. (**c**) Posterior capsular release

a posterior arthroscopic portal, using a capsular punch or electrothermal device, followed by an arthroscopic shaver to ***excise*** the contracted capsule. The rotator interval is fully released with a thermal device (Fig. 14.2), and the coracoid process is skeletonized to ensure complete release of the coracohumeral ligament. While viewing anterior superiorly (Fig. 14.3a), the anterior inferior

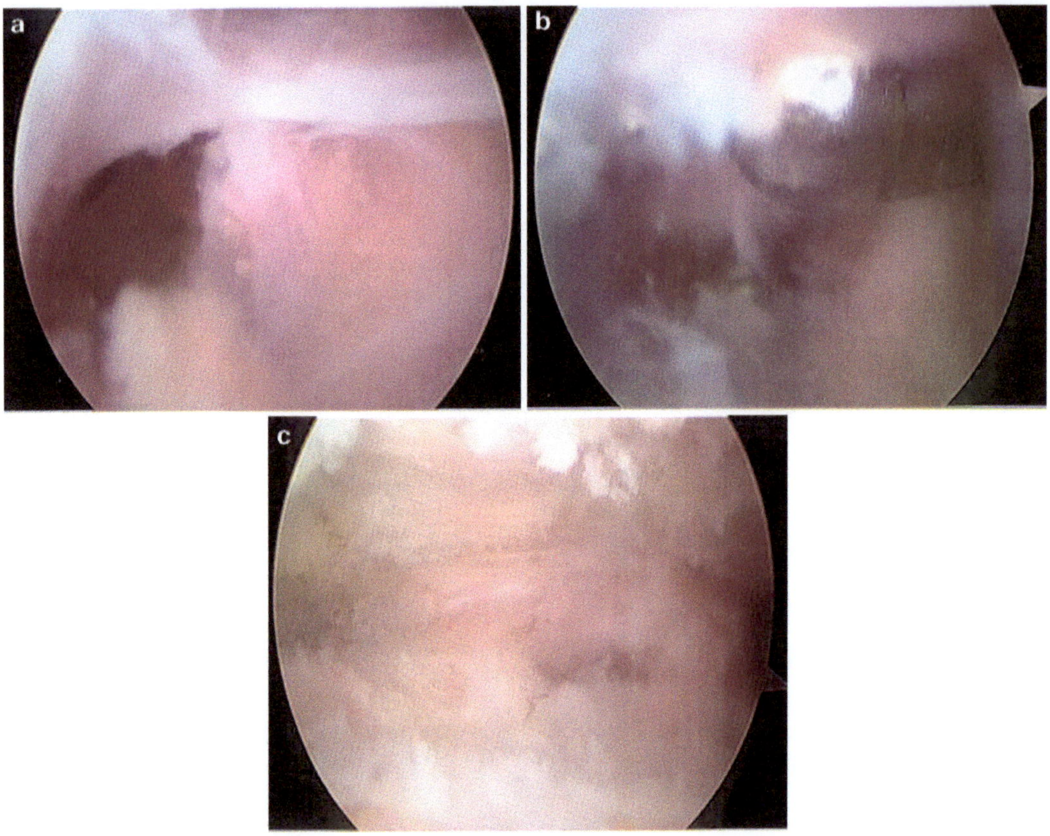

Fig. 14.4 Subacromial fibrosis (**a**) pre-release, (**b**) during release, and (**c**) post-release

capsule is released (Fig. 14.3b) hugging the glenoid in order to avert axillary nerve injury. Finally a 70 degree scope may be helpful to view from the front and visualize the inferior pouch, which may be approached via anterior, posterior, or modified "7 o'clock" inferior lateral portal. A posterior capsular release can best be achieved with fine tip electrocautery or with capsular punch instruments with care to "hug" the glenoid to avoid axillary nerve injury (Fig. 14.3c). Finally, the subacromial space is explored arthroscopically through the posterior portal, and adhesions present are visualized and released through a lateral portal (Fig. 14.4a–c). Once satisfied with the releases, the patient's arm is manipulated through a full range of motion in order to confirm adequate release. Physical therapy is started postoperatively the following day with passive range of motion started immediately and active isotonic exercises started by the second or third week. Full, unrestricted use of the shoulder should be achieved in most patients by 3–4 months.

Conclusion

Although often considered to have an excellent prognosis, full recovery is variable and there is substantial and often enduring morbidity associated with frozen shoulder. Improvements in the treatment of frozen shoulder from both a medical and a surgical standpoint are being made and will translate to preserving shoulder function. Basic science studies have yielded elements of both a fibroproliferative and an inflammatory process at work in the genesis of FS.

Some have challenged the long-held belief in conservative treatment for this disorder and have suggested early arthroscopic intervention. Although the senior author (JDK) supports a considerable trial of conservative management before entertaining surgery, some data supports relatively early arthroscopic release. Recent work has improved our definitions of disease, but prognostic grading systems continue to elude us. There is a continued need for deeper insight into the disease pathogenesis with the hopes that safe and effective means of prevention and treatment will become manifest. Perhaps by understanding the contribution of and controlling individual risk factors for FS, overall disease burden will be lessened.

Much has been learned about the pathogenesis of frozen shoulder, with many great clinicians and scientists having contributed substantially to progress in understanding this disease. However, the topic remains an area of exciting investigation and provides future researchers with a tremendous opportunity to help those impacted by this vexing condition.

References

1. Hsu JE, Anakwenze OA, Warrender WJ, Abboud JA. Current review of adhesive capsulitis. J Shoulder Elbow Surg. 2011;20:502–14.
2. Pomeranz SJ, Modi N. Adhesive capsulitis. J Surg Orthop Adv. 2014;23:119–21.
3. Bunker TD. Frozen shoulder: unravelling the enigma. Ann R Coll Surg Engl. 1997;79:210–3.
4. White D, Choi H, Peloquin C, Zhu Y, Zhang Y. Secular trend of adhesive capsulitis. Arthritis Care Res. 2011;63:1571–5.
5. Lo S-F, et al. Diabetes mellitus and accompanying hyperlipidemia are independent risk factors for adhesive capsulitis: a nationwide population-based cohort study (version 2). Rheumatol Int. 2014;34:67–74.
6. Codman EA. The shoulder: rupture of the supraspinatus tendon and other lesions in or about the subacromial bursa. Boston, MA: Thomas Todd Company; 1934.
7. Duplay S. De la péri-arthrite scapulo-humérale et des raideurs de l'epaule qui en sont la consequénce. Arch Gen Méd. 1872;20:513–42.
8. Robinson CM, Seah KTM, Chee YH, Hindle P, Murray IR. Frozen shoulder. J Bone Joint Surg Br. 2012;94-B:1–9.
9. Zuckerman JD, Rokito A. Frozen shoulder: a consensus definition. J Shoulder Elbow Surg Am Shoulder Elbow Surg Al. 2011;20:322–5.
10. Neviaser JS. Adhesive capsulitis of the shoulder. J Bone Joint Surg. 1945;27:211–22.
11. Austin DC, Gans I, Park MJ, Carey JL, Kelly JD. The association of metabolic syndrome markers with adhesive capsulitis. J Shoulder Elbow Surg Am Shoulder Elbow Surg Al. 2014;23:1043–51.
12. Arkkila PE, Kantola IM, Viikari JS, Rönnemaa T. Shoulder capsulitis in type I and II diabetic patients: association with diabetic complications and related diseases. Ann Rheum Dis. 1996;55:907–14.
13. Balci N, Balci MK, Tüzüner S. Shoulder adhesive capsulitis and shoulder range of motion in type II diabetes mellitus: association with diabetic complications. J Diabetes Complications. 1999;13:135–40.
14. Bowman CA, Jeffcoate WJ, Pattrick M, Doherty M. Bilateral adhesive capsulitis, oligoarthritis and proximal myopathy as presentation of hypothyroidism. Br J Rheumatol. 1988;27:62–4.
15. Cakir M, Samanci N, Balci N, Balci MK. Musculoskeletal manifestations in patients with thyroid disease. Clin Endocrinol (Oxf). 2003;59:162–7.
16. Tighe CB, Oakley WS. The prevalence of a diabetic condition and adhesive capsulitis of the shoulder. South Med J. 2008;101:591–5.
17. Bridgman JF. Periarthritis of the shoulder and diabetes mellitus. Ann Rheum Dis. 1972;31:69–71.
18. Bulgen DY, Binder AI, Hazleman BL, Dutton J, Roberts S. Frozen shoulder: prospective clinical study with an evaluation of three treatment regimens. Ann Rheum Dis. 1984;43:353–60.
19. Hand C, Clipsham K, Rees JL, Carr AJ. Long-term outcome of frozen shoulder. J Shoulder Elbow Surg. 2008;17:231–6.
20. Huang S-W, et al. Hyperthyroidism is a risk factor for developing adhesive capsulitis of the shoulder: a nationwide longitudinal population-based study. Sci Rep. 2014;4:4183.
21. Thomas SJ, et al. Prevalence of symptoms and signs of shoulder problems in people with diabetes mellitus. J Shoulder Elbow Surg Am Shoulder Elbow Surg Al. 2007;16:748–51.
22. Ramchurn N, et al. Upper limb musculoskeletal abnormalities and poor metabolic control in diabetes. Eur J Intern Med. 2009;20:718–21.
23. Huang Y-P, et al. Association of diabetes mellitus with the risk of developing adhesive capsulitis of the shoulder: a longitudinal population-based followup study. Arthritis Care Res. 2013;65:1197–202.
24. Sheridan MA, Hannafin JA. Upper extremity: emphasis on frozen shoulder. Orthop Clin North Am. 2006;37:531–9.
25. Neviaser AS, Neviaser RJ. Adhesive capsulitis of the shoulder. J Am Acad Orthop Surg. 2011;19:536–42.
26. Shaffer B, Tibone JE, Kerlan RK. Frozen shoulder. A long-term follow-up. J Bone Joint Surg Am. 1992;74:738–46.
27. Griggs SM, Ahn A, Green A. Idiopathic adhesive capsulitis. A prospective functional outcome study

of nonoperative treatment. J Bone Joint Surg Am. 2000;82-A:1398–407.
28. Binder AI, Bulgen DY, Hazleman BL, Roberts S. Frozen shoulder: a long-term prospective study. Ann Rheum Dis. 1984;43:361–4.
29. Reeves B. The natural history of the frozen shoulder syndrome. Scand J Rheumatol. 1975;4:193–6.
30. Lewis J. Frozen shoulder contracture syndrome – aetiology, diagnosis and management. Man Ther. 2014. doi:10.1016/j.math.2014.07.006.
31. Bunker T. Time for a new name for frozen shoulder—contracture of the shoulder. Shoulder Elbow. 2009;1:4–9.
32. Rookmoneea M, et al. The effectiveness of interventions in the management of patients with primary frozen shoulder. J Bone Joint Surg Br. 2010;92:1267–72.
33. Lundberg J. The frozen shoulder. Clinical and radiographical observations. The effect of manipulation under general anesthesia. Structure and glycosaminoglycan content of the joint capsule. Local bone metabolism. Acta Orthop Scand. 1969;119(Suppl):1–59.
34. Harris G, Bou-Haidar P, Harris C. Adhesive capsulitis: review of imaging and treatment. J Med Imaging Radiat Oncol. 2013;57:633–43.
35. Binder AI, Bulgen DY, Hazleman BL, Tudor J, Wraight P. Frozen shoulder: an arthrographic and radionuclear scan assessment. Ann Rheum Dis. 1984;43:365–9.
36. Zhao W, et al. An MRI study of symptomatic adhesive capsulitis. PLoS One. 2012;7, e47277.
37. Carbone S, Napoli A, Gumina S. MRI of adhesive capsulitis of the shoulder: distension of the bursa in the superior subscapularis recess is a suggestive sign of the pathology. Eur J Radiol. 2014;83:345–8.
38. Carrillon Y, Noel E, Fantino O, Perrin-Fayolle O, Tran-Minh VA. Magnetic resonance imaging findings in idiopathic adhesive capsulitis of the shoulder. Rev Rhum Engl Ed. 1999;66:201–6.
39. Sharma P, Morrison WB, Cohen S. Imaging of the shoulder with arthroscopic correlation. Clin Sports Med. 2013;32:339–59.
40. Beltran LS, Beltran J. Biceps and rotator interval: imaging update. Semin Musculoskelet Radiol. 2014;18:425–35.
41. Emig EW, Schweitzer ME, Karasick D, Lubowitz J. Adhesive capsulitis of the shoulder: MR diagnosis. AJR Am J Roentgenol. 1995;164:1457–9.
42. Mengiardi B, Pfirrmann CWA, Gerber C, Hodler J, Zanetti M. Frozen shoulder: MR arthrographic findings. Radiology. 2004;233:486–92.
43. Lo S-F, et al. Arthrographic and clinical findings in patients with hemiplegic shoulder pain. Arch Phys Med Rehabil. 2003;84:1786–91.
44. Yoo JC, Ahn JH, Lee YS, Koh KH. Magnetic resonance arthrographic findings of presumed stage-2 adhesive capsulitis: focus on combined rotator cuff pathology. Orthopedics. 2009;32:22.
45. Lee JC, Sykes C, Saifuddin A, Connell D. Adhesive capsulitis: sonographic changes in the rotator cuff interval with arthroscopic correlation. Skeletal Radiol. 2005;34:522–7.
46. Bunker TD, Anthony PP. The pathology of frozen shoulder. A Dupuytren-like disease. J Bone Joint Surg Br. 1995;77-B:677–83.
47. Wiley AM. Arthroscopic appearance of frozen shoulder. Arthroscopy. 1991;7:138–43.
48. Uitvlugt G, Detrisac DA, Johnson LL, Austin MD, Johnson C. Arthroscopic observations before and after manipulation of frozen shoulder. Arthroscopy. 1993;9:181–5.
49. Rodeo SA, Hannafin JA, Tom J, Warren RF, Wickiewicz TL. Immunolocalization of cytokines and their receptors in adhesive capsulitis of the shoulder. J Orthop Res. 1997;15:427–36.
50. Smith SP, Devaraj VS, Bunker TD. The association between frozen shoulder and Dupuytren's disease. J Shoulder Elbow Surg Am Shoulder Elbow Surg Al. 2001;10:149–51.
51. Hand GCR, Athanasou NA, Matthews T, Carr AJ. The pathology of frozen shoulder. J Bone Joint Surg Br. 2007;89:928–32.
52. Xu Y, Bonar F, Murrell GAC. Enhanced expression of neuronal proteins in idiopathic frozen shoulder. J Shoulder Elbow Surg Am Shoulder Elbow Surg Al. 2012;21:1391–7.
53. Hagiwara Y, et al. Coexistence of fibrotic and chondrogenic process in the capsule of idiopathic frozen shoulders. Osteoarthr Cartil OARS Osteoarthr Res Soc. 2012;20:241–9.
54. Kim Y-S, et al. Intercellular adhesion molecule-1 (ICAM-1, CD54) is increased in adhesive capsulitis. J Bone Joint Surg Am. 2013;95:e181–8.
55. Mullett H, Byrne D, Colville J. Adhesive capsulitis: human fibroblast response to shoulder joint aspirate from patients with stage II disease. J Shoulder Elbow Surg Am Shoulder Elbow Surg Al. 2007;16:290–4.
56. Kabbabe B, Ramkumar S, Richardson M. Cytogenetic analysis of the pathology of frozen shoulder. Int J Shoulder Surg. 2010;4:75–8.
57. Bunker TD, Reilly J, Baird KS, Hamblen DL. Expression of growth factors, cytokines and matrix metalloproteinases in frozen shoulder. J Bone Joint Surg Br. 2000;82:768–73.
58. Watson RS, et al. Gene delivery of TGF-β1 induces arthrofibrosis and chondrometaplasia of synovium in vivo. Lab Invest. 2010;90:1615–27.
59. Hagiwara Y, et al. Expression of transforming growth factor-beta1 and connective tissue growth factor in the capsule in a rat immobilized knee model. Ups J Med Sci. 2008;113:221–34.
60. Raykha CN, et al. IGF2 expression and β-catenin levels are increased in Frozen Shoulder Syndrome. Clin Investig Med Médecine Clin Exp. 2014;37, E262.
61. Tuten HR, et al. Adhesive capsulitis of the shoulder in male cardiac surgery patients. Orthopedics. 2000;23:693–6.

62. Tanishima T, Yoshimasu N. Development and prevention of frozen shoulder after acute aneurysm surgery. Surg Neurol. 1997;48:19–22.
63. Pineda C, Arana B, Martínez-Lavín M, Dábague J. Frozen shoulder triggered by cardiac catheterization via the brachial artery. Am J Med. 1994;96:90–1.
64. Patten C, Hillel AD. The 11th nerve syndrome. Accessory nerve palsy or adhesive capsulitis? Arch Otolaryngol Head Neck Surg. 1993;119:215–20.
65. Bruckner FE, Nye CJ. A prospective study of adhesive capsulitis of the shoulder ("frozen shoulder") in a high risk population. Q J Med. 1981;50:191–204.
66. Bunker TD, Esler CN. Frozen shoulder and lipids. J Bone Joint Surg Br. 1995;77:684–6.
67. Choy EH, Corkill MM, Gibson T, Hicks BH. Isolated ACTH deficiency presenting with bilateral frozen shoulder. Br J Rheumatol. 1991;30:226–7.
68. Wohlgethan JR. Frozen shoulder in hyperthyroidism. Arthritis Rheum. 1987;30:936–9.
69. Hakim AJ, Cherkas LF, Spector TD, MacGregor AJ. Genetic associations between frozen shoulder and tennis elbow: a female twin study. Rheumatology. 2003;42:739–42.
70. Kang J-H, Sheu J-J, Lin H-C. Increased risk of stroke after adhesive capsulitis: a population-based study. Stroke J Cereb Circ. 2010;41:1044–7.
71. Riley D, Lang AE, Blair RD, Birnbaum A, Reid B. Frozen shoulder and other shoulder disturbances in Parkinson's disease. J Neurol Neurosurg Psychiatry. 1989;52:63–6.
72. Debeer P, Franssens F, Roosen I, Dankaerts W, Claes L. Frozen shoulder and the Big Five personality traits. J Shoulder Elbow Surg Am Shoulder Elbow Surg Al. 2014;23:221–6.
73. Bodor M, Montalvo E. Vaccination-related shoulder dysfunction. Vaccine. 2007;25:585–7.
74. De Ponti A, Viganò MG, Taverna E, Sansone V. Adhesive capsulitis of the shoulder in human immunodeficiency virus-positive patients during highly active antiretroviral therapy. J Shoulder Elbow Surg Am Shoulder Elbow Surg Al. 2006;15:188–90.
75. Freiss S, Lecocq J, Isner ME, Vautravers P. Frozen shoulder and fluoroquinones. Two case reports. Joint Bone Spine Rev Rhum. 2000;67:245–9.
76. Grasland A, Ziza JM, Raguin G, Pouchot J, Vinceneux P. Adhesive capsulitis of shoulder and treatment with protease inhibitors in patients with human immunodeficiency virus infection: report of 8 cases. J Rheumatol. 2000;27:2642–6.
77. Hutchinson JW, Tierney GM, Parsons SL, Davis TR. Dupuytren's disease and frozen shoulder induced by treatment with a matrix metalloproteinase inhibitor. J Bone Joint Surg Br. 1998;80:907–8.
78. Zabraniecki L, et al. Frozen shoulder: a new delayed complication of protease inhibitor therapy? Rev Rhum Engl Ed. 1998;65:72–4.
79. Franck JL, Beurrier P. Can flunarizine induce frozen shoulder? Rev Rhum Engl Ed. 1996;63:457.
80. Gheita TA, Ezzat Y, Sayed S, El-Mardenly G, Hammam W. Musculoskeletal manifestations in patients with malignant disease. Clin Rheumatol. 2010;29:181–8.
81. Okamura K, Ozaki J. Bone mineral density of the shoulder joint in frozen shoulder. Arch Orthop Trauma Surg. 1999;119:363–7.
82. Baums MH, et al. Functional outcome and general health status in patients after arthroscopic release in adhesive capsulitis. Knee Surg Sports Traumatol Arthrosc. 2007;15:638–44.
83. Sabat D, Kumar V. Early arthroscopic release in stiff shoulder. Int J Shoulder Surg. 2008;2:36–40.
84. Yoon S-H, Lee HY, Lee HJ, Kwack K-S. Optimal dose of intra-articular corticosteroids for adhesive capsulitis: a randomized, triple-blind, placebo-controlled trial. Am J Sports Med. 2013;41:1133–9.
85. Roh YH, et al. Intra-articular corticosteroid injection in diabetic patients with adhesive capsulitis: a randomized controlled trial. Knee Surg Sports Traumatol Arthrosc. 2012;20:1947–52.
86. Bal A, et al. Effectiveness of corticosteroid injection in adhesive capsulitis. Clin Rehabil. 2008;22:503–12.
87. Buchbinder R, Green S, Youd JM, Johnston RV. Oral steroids for adhesive capsulitis. Cochrane Database Syst Rev. 2006;CD006189. doi:10.1002/14651858.CD006189.
88. Buchbinder R, et al. Short course prednisolone for adhesive capsulitis (frozen shoulder or stiff painful shoulder): a randomised, double blind, placebo controlled trial. Ann Rheum Dis. 2004;63:1460–9.
89. Widiastuti-Samekto M, Sianturi GP. Frozen shoulder syndrome: comparison of oral route corticosteroid and intra-articular corticosteroid injection. Med J Malaysia. 2004;59:312–6.
90. Buchbinder R, Green S, Youd JM. Corticosteroid injections for shoulder pain. Cochrane Database Syst Rev. 2003;CD004016. doi:10.1002/14651858.CD004016.
91. Ryans I, Montgomery A, Galway R, Kernohan WG, McKane R. A randomized controlled trial of intra-articular triamcinolone and/or physiotherapy in shoulder capsulitis. Rheumatol Oxf Engl. 2005;44:529–35.
92. Carette S, et al. Intraarticular corticosteroids, supervised physiotherapy, or a combination of the two in the treatment of adhesive capsulitis of the shoulder: a placebo-controlled trial. Arthritis Rheum. 2003;48:829–38.
93. Arslan S, Celiker R. Comparison of the efficacy of local corticosteroid injection and physical therapy for the treatment of adhesive capsulitis. Rheumatol Int. 2001;21:20–3.
94. Russell S, et al. A blinded, randomized, controlled trial assessing conservative management strategies for frozen shoulder. J Shoulder Elbow Surg Am Shoulder Elbow Surg Al. 2014;23:500–7.

95. Dundar U, Toktas H, Cakir T, Evcik D, Kavuncu V. Continuous passive motion provides good pain control in patients with adhesive capsulitis. Int J Rehabil Res Int Z Für Rehabil Rev Int Rech Réadapt. 2009;32:193–8.
96. Diercks RL, Stevens M. Gentle thawing of the frozen shoulder: a prospective study of supervised neglect versus intensive physical therapy in seventy-seven patients with frozen shoulder syndrome followed up for two years. J Shoulder Elbow Surg Am Shoulder Elbow Surg Al. 2004;13:499–502.
97. Green S, Buchbinder R, Hetrick S. Physiotherapy interventions for shoulder pain. Cochrane Database Syst Rev. 2003;CD004258. doi:10.1002/14651858.CD004258.
98. Green S, Buchbinder R, Hetrick S. Acupuncture for shoulder pain. Cochrane Database Syst Rev. 2005;CD005319. doi:10.1002/14651858.CD005319.
99. Sun KO, Chan KC, Lo SL, Fong DY. Acupuncture for frozen shoulder. Hong Kong Med J Xianggang Yi Xue Za Zhi Hong Kong Acad Med. 2001;7:381–91.
100. Dehghan A, et al. Comparison between NSAID and intra-articular corticosteroid injection in frozen shoulder of diabetic patients; a randomized clinical trial. Exp Clin Endocrinol Diabetes. 2013;121:75–9.
101. Leung MSF, Cheing GLY. Effects of deep and superficial heating in the management of frozen shoulder. J Rehabil Med. 2008;40:145–50.
102. Stergioulas A. Low-power laser treatment in patients with frozen shoulder: preliminary results. Photomed Laser Surg. 2008;26:99–105.
103. Calis M, et al. Is intraarticular sodium hyaluronate injection an alternative treatment in patients with adhesive capsulitis? Rheumatol Int. 2006;26:536–40.
104. Page MJ, et al. Electrotherapy modalities for adhesive capsulitis (frozen shoulder). Cochrane Database Syst Rev. 2014;10, CD011324.
105. Jewell DV, Riddle DL, Thacker LR. Interventions associated with an increased or decreased likelihood of pain reduction and improved function in patients with adhesive capsulitis: a retrospective cohort study. Phys Ther. 2009;89:419–29.
106. Kivimäki J, et al. Manipulation under anesthesia with home exercises versus home exercises alone in the treatment of frozen shoulder: a randomized, controlled trial with 125 patients. J Shoulder Elbow Surg Am Shoulder Elbow Surg Al. 2007;16:722–6.
107. Loew M, Heichel TO, Lehner B. Intraarticular lesions in primary frozen shoulder after manipulation under general anesthesia. J Shoulder Elbow Surg Am Shoulder Elbow Surg Al. 2005;14:16–21.
108. Tveitå EK, Tariq R, Sesseng S, Juel NG, Bautz-Holter E. Hydrodilatation, corticosteroids and adhesive capsulitis: a randomized controlled trial. BMC Musculoskelet Disord. 2008;9:53.
109. Quraishi NA, Johnston P, Bayer J, Crowe M, Chakrabarti AJ. Thawing the frozen shoulder. A randomised trial comparing manipulation under anaesthesia with hydrodilatation. J Bone Joint Surg Br. 2007;89:1197–200.
110. Dahan TH, et al. Double blind randomized clinical trial examining the efficacy of bupivacaine suprascapular nerve blocks in frozen shoulder. J Rheumatol. 2000;27:1464–9.
111. Grant JA, Schroeder N, Miller BS, Carpenter JE. Comparison of manipulation and arthroscopic capsular release for adhesive capsulitis: a systematic review. J Shoulder Elbow Surg Am Shoulder Elbow Surg Al. 2013;22:1135–45.
112. Le Lievre HMJ, Murrell GAC. Long-term outcomes after arthroscopic capsular release for idiopathic adhesive capsulitis. J Bone Joint Surg Am. 2012;94:1208–16.
113. Mehta SS, Singh HP, Pandey R. Comparative outcome of arthroscopic release for frozen shoulder in patients with and without diabetes. Bone Joint J. 2014;96-B:1355–8.
114. Warner JJ, Allen A, Marks PH, Wong P. Arthroscopic release for chronic, refractory adhesive capsulitis of the shoulder. J Bone Joint Surg Am. 1996;78:1808–16.

Part IV

Rotator Cuff

15 Ultrasound in Rotator Cuff Evaluation

Christos D. Photopoulos, Ann Marie Kelly, and Viviane Khoury

Abbreviations

US Ultrasound/ultrasonography
MRI Magnetic resonance imaging

Introduction

Rotator cuff disease is a very common cause of shoulder pain in the adult. The use of US in the evaluation of the shoulder was first described by Seltzer et al. in 1979 when it was used to detect intra-articular effusions in a study of rhesus monkeys [1]. Subsequently, studies investigating the role of sonography in diagnosis of rotator cuff tears began to surface in the 1980s [2]. Although initially fraught by poor resolution and lack of inter-examiner reliability, technical advancements as well as standardized protocols have significantly improved sonographic results and reliability [3]. Today, the diagnostic accuracy of US in the evaluation of the rotator cuff is equivalent to that of MRI and has gained wide acceptance as a useful and versatile modality to evaluate soft tissue about the shoulder [4–7]. Several components of the shoulder can be evaluated in both healthy and pathologic states. The goal of this chapter is to provide a comprehensive overview of US in rotator cuff evaluation.

Shoulder Imaging

In the evaluation of the painful shoulder, several noninvasive imaging modalities exist to help guide diagnosis and treatment. These include radiography, ultrasonography, magnetic resonance imaging, magnetic resonance arthrography, computed tomography, and computed tomographic arthrography [8].

Radiography is routinely used as a first-line imaging tool to rule out osseous abnormalities, including fractures and dislocations, glenohumeral and acromioclavicular arthropathy, and osseous neoplastic lesions. Radiographs may also show signs that are suggestive of chronic rotator cuff disease. Cortical irregularities at the greater tuberosity have been shown to be predictive of supraspinatus tendon tears (with 90 % sensitivity,

C.D. Photopoulos, MD (✉)
Department of Orthopaedic Surgery, Hospital of the University of Pennsylvania, Philadelphia, PA, USA
e-mail: christos.photopoulos@uphs.upenn.edu

A.M. Kelly, BA
Department of Orthopedics, University of Pennsylvania, Philadelphia, PA, USA

V. Khoury, BSc, MD
Division of Musculoskeletal Imaging, University of Pennsylvania Health System, Philadelphia, PA, USA

J.D. Kelly IV (ed.), *Elite Techniques in Shoulder Arthroscopy*,
DOI 10.1007/978-3-319-25103-5_15

96 % negative predictive value), subacromial enthesophytes are frequently associated with subacromial impingement, and periarticular calcifications may be associated with calcific tendonitis and/or bursitis [8].

MRI is an effective way to evaluate the soft tissue structures of the shoulder and historically has served as the gold standard imaging modality for rotator cuff evaluation. Specifically, MRI is useful in diagnosing full-thickness rotator cuff tears (92.1 % sensitivity, 92.9 % specificity) and partial-thickness tears (63.6 % sensitivity, 91.7 % specificity) [8] and is an effective tool in evaluating surrounding soft tissue structures. These include the long head of the biceps tendon, the glenoid labrum, the hyaline cartilage of the glenohumeral joint, and the osseous/bone marrow abnormalities. Drawbacks to the use of MRI do however exist, including high cost, length of study, patient tolerance (claustrophobia, inability to lie supine or still), and contraindications (morbid obesity, metallic implants such as pacemakers).

As an imaging modality, US provides the distinct advantages of being inexpensive and accessible, having no contraindications, and using no ionizing radiation. An especially unique advantage of US use in the musculoskeletal system is the capacity to perform dynamic maneuvers, including motion of an extremity, probe compression, and position change of the patient. As such, US can diagnose conditions that are better or only visible dynamically [5, 9–11].

In experienced hands, diagnostic accuracy of US for rotator cuff pathology is comparable to that of MRI. Recent studies have shown that US provides 92.3 % sensitivity with 94.4 % specificity in diagnosing full-thickness rotator cuff tears and 66.7 % sensitivity with 93.5 % specificity in diagnosing partial-thickness rotator cuff tears [8, 9]. In addition, US can effectively diagnose rotator cuff muscle atrophy and fatty infiltration of the supraspinatus, infraspinatus, and teres minor.

The major drawback of US as an imaging modality for the shoulder is its limited ability to evaluate intra-articular structures (glenoid labrum and cartilage) and osseous structures (bone lesions, marrow abnormalities). Additionally, given the intervening coracoid process, evaluation for subscapularis muscle atrophy and fatty infiltration is not feasible.

Ultrasound Technique

Ultrasound as an imaging tool relies on the emission of high-frequency sound waves from a transducer that is held against the body. The reflection of these sound waves off structures of interest and their subsequent reception by the emitting transducer ultimately helps to format a sonographic image. A structure's echogenicity refers to its ability to reflect these ultrasound waves, and the juxtaposition of structures of variable echogenicity helps generate the ultrasound-created image [12]. Dense and robust structures, such as a healthy long head of the biceps tendon, reflect sound waves well and will appear hyperechoic (or white/bright). Tendons, ligaments, fluid, and articular cartilage appear hypoechoic (or dark/black). Osseous structures appear as a hyperechoic line representing the cortex, beyond which the bone cannot be visualized, as the sound waves cannot be transmitted through the bone (which therefore appears dark) [9].

Evaluation of the structure of interest depends on the orientation of the US transducer relative to that structure. When the long axis of the transducer is held longitudinally to the orientation of a desired tendon, parallel echogenic lines are visualized. This orientation is referred to as "longitudinal," "long axis," or "parallel." When evaluating rotator cuff tendons, these echogenic lines represent the fascicles of the tendon, and the apparent fibrillar appearance results from the tightly packed collagen fibers [4, 10] (Fig. 15.1a). When the transducer is rotated so its long axis is perpendicular to the tendon fibers, fascicles appear as points or lines [10] (Fig. 15.1b). This orientation is otherwise referred to as "short axis" or "transverse."

During an US examination, the transducer must be moved slowly and meticulously, so as not to miss any abnormalities. It is likewise

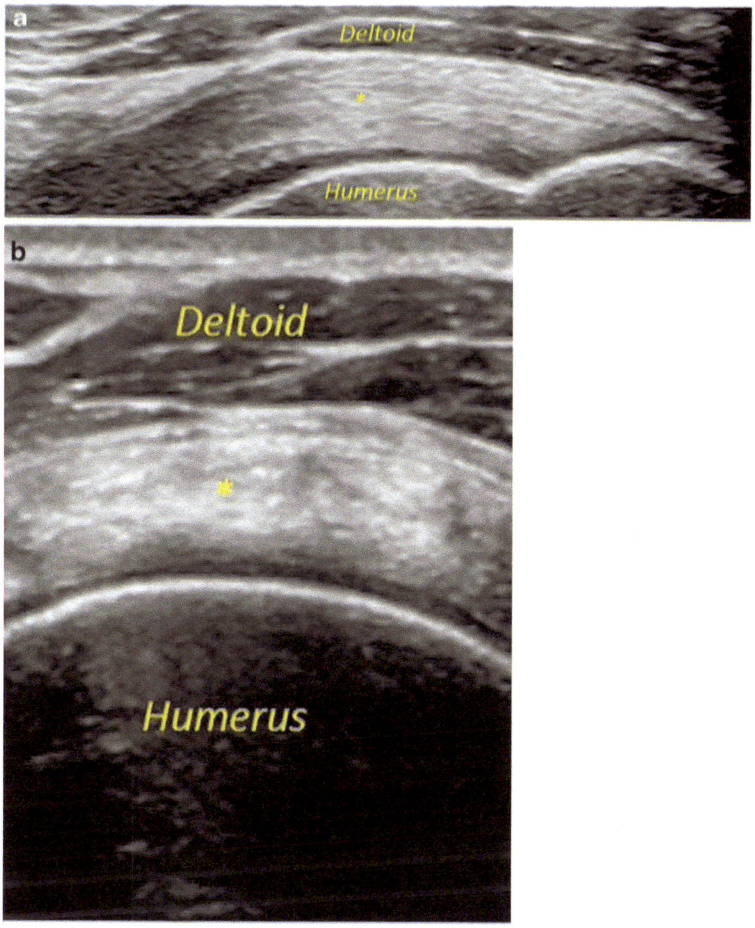

Fig. 15.1 (**a**) Supraspinatus tendon, long axis (*asterisk*). Note the fibrillar appearance of tightly packed collagen fibers. (**b**) Supraspinatus tendon, short axis (*asterisk*). Note that in this cross-sectional axis, fascicles have a round or dot-like appearance

paramount that the transducer body is always kept at 90° to the structure of interest, as any variation in this angle may alter the echogenicity of the structures of interest and result in false positives or false negatives due to an artifact named "anisotropy" [13]. Stability of the examiner's hand is also important, and it is often found helpful if the examiner rests their fifth finger or lateral aspect of their palm on the patient's skin during examination [3].

Sequence

For optimal positioning, the patient is asked to sit upright on a revolving chair, thus allowing for 360° access to the shoulder. The examiner stands at an angled position relative to the patient, thus allowing visualization of both the patient's shoulder and the ultrasound monitor. In order to perform a complete assessment of the shoulder and visualize all pathology, a standardized sequence must be followed. Although this varies by examiner, a typical shoulder sequence includes the following: (1) evaluation of the long head of the biceps tendon; (2) evaluation of the subscapularis tendon with dynamic evaluation for subluxation/subluxation of the long head of the biceps tendon; (3) evaluation of the supraspinatus tendon, rotator interval, and subacromial-subdeltoid bursa; (4) evaluation of the infraspinatus and teres minor tendons; (5) evaluation of the posterior glenohumeral joint recess; (6) evaluation of the supraspinatus, infraspinatus, and teres minor muscles; and (7) dynamic maneuvers to evaluate for subacromial impingement.

Evaluation: Long Head of the Biceps Tendon

The long head of the biceps tendon, comprised of both intra-articular and extra-articular components, is, as stated, typically the first structure that is evaluated. The intra-articular component originates from the supraglenoid tubercle and the glenoid labrum and traverses extrasynovially through the rotator interval. Upon exiting this interval, the tendon becomes extra-articular and resides within the bicipital groove between the greater and lesser tuberosities. The long head of the biceps is frequently affected in pathologic states of the rotator cuff. To evaluate this tendon, the seated patient is asked to keep their elbow flexed to 90°, with their hand fully supinated in order to achieve external rotation of the glenohumeral joint, thereby allowing the patient to present their bicipital groove anteriorly [9] (Fig. 15.2a).

On US evaluation, the extra-articular component of the tendon is usually easily visualized, whereas its intra-articular segment is not. When the transducer is held perpendicularly to the orientation of the biceps (short axis), the tendon is seen as a hyperechoic, round structure between the supraspinatus and the subscapularis (Fig. 15.2b). Rotating the transducer so that it is parallel to the orientation of the tendon (long axis), the biceps takes on a narrow and striated appearance (Fig. 15.2c). This normal striation pattern can be often compromised, especially in setting of partial or complete tears, whereupon the longitudinal anechoic fissures can become apparent. A small amount of fluid surrounding the biceps is usually a normal finding; however, larger

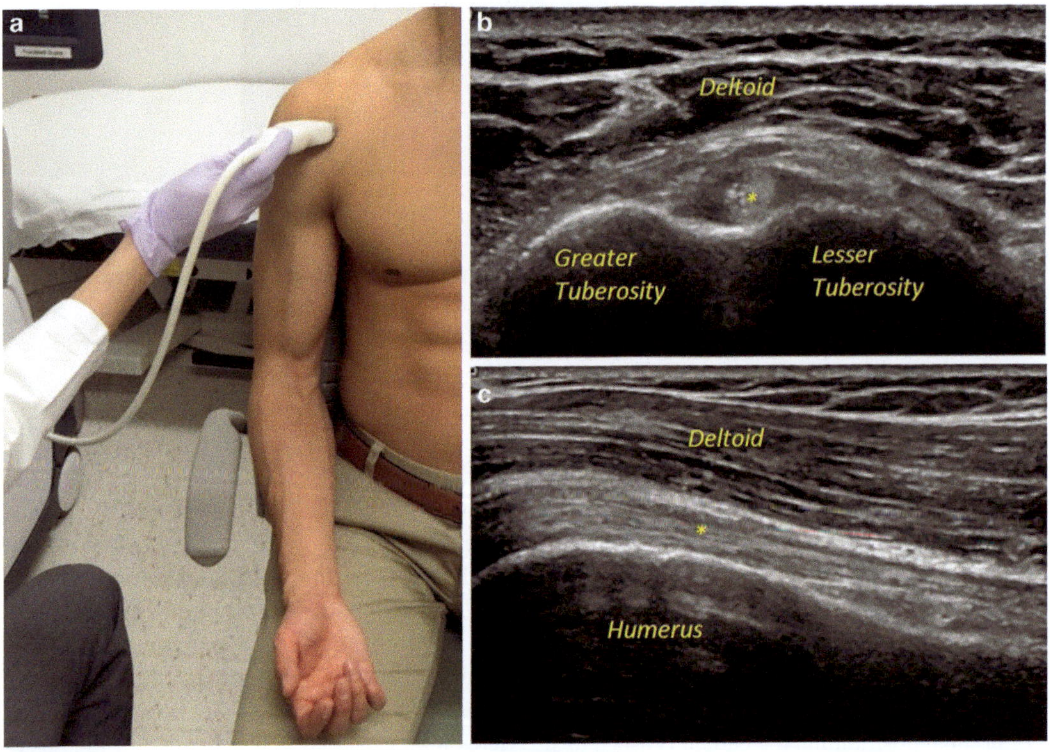

Fig. 15.2 (**a**) Patient positioning during examination of long head of the biceps tendon. Note that the elbow remains flexed, with the forearm supinated. (**b**) Normal long head of the biceps tendon, short axis (*asterisk*). (**c**) Normal long head of the biceps tendon, long axis (*asterisk*)

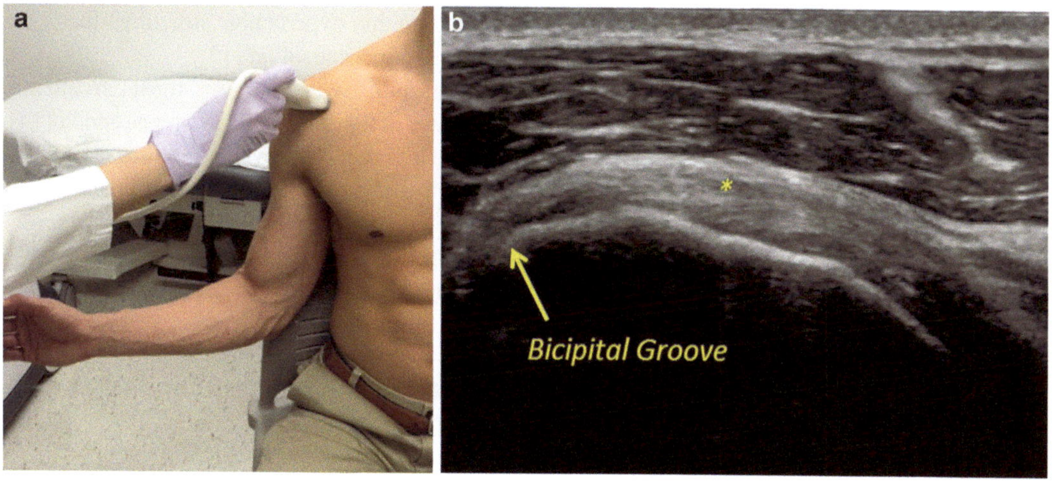

Fig. 15.3 (**a**) Patient positioning during examination of subscapularis tendon. Note that the elbow is flexed and the shoulder is externally rotated. (**b**) Normal subscapularis tendon, long axis (*asterisk*)

bicipital tendon sheath effusions signal either a glenohumeral joint effusion or bicipital tenosynovitis. Dynamic conditions, such as biceps instability, can likewise be evaluated by asking the patient to externally and internally rotate their shoulder while the transducer is held in place [11, 14].

Evaluation: Subscapularis Tendon

Following evaluation of the long head of the biceps tendon, the adjacent subscapularis tendon can be readily identified. This anterior and largest rotator cuff muscle originates within the subscapular fossa, courses anteriorly over the humeral head, and inserts on the lesser tuberosity. Innervated by the upper and lower subscapular nerves, the subscapularis facilitates internal rotation and adduction of the arm.

For ease of evaluation, the patient is asked to keep their elbow flexed at 90°. The shoulder is then externally rotated, allowing for visualization of the entire tendon, seen as a hyperechoic fibrillar structure inserting on the lesser tuberosity [6] (Fig. 15.3a, b).

It is important to note that the tendon typically courses superiorly and laterally. As such, for optimal visualization, a cranial tilt of the transducer is required [3]. Although pathology can occur at any point within the tendon, most subscapularis tendon tears originate at the superior portion of the tendon, and careful attention must be paid to this area when moving cranially to caudally during evaluation [9]. Dynamic evaluation can likewise help better delineate any tendinous retraction. With the transducer held in the short axis, gentle internal and external rotation of the arm allows for full evaluation of the tendon thickness as it courses toward the lesser tuberosity.

Evaluation: Supraspinatus Tendon

Evaluation of the supraspinatus tendon is of particular interest, as it is the rotator cuff tendon most frequently associated with tendinopathy or tears [4]. Originating from the supraspinous fossa on the superior aspect of the scapula and inserting onto the superior facet of the greater tuberosity of the humerus, the supraspinatus is innervated by the suprascapular nerve and functions to assist the deltoid in arm abduction.

Sonographic visualization is best completed with the patient's arm in internal rotation and extension, thus presenting the supraspinatus anteriorly relative to the otherwise anechoic acromion. This is typically achieved with the patient's arm placed in the Crass position (elbow flexed to 90°, forearm internally rotated to behind patient's back). However, in patients with rotator cuff pathology, this degree of internal rotation may be difficult, and the modified Crass (patient's palm placed over the ipsilateral buttock with the elbow flexed and directed medially) can be utilized [14] (Fig. 15.4a).

As with identification of the subscapularis tendon, the long head of the biceps tendon can be used for orienting the examiner to the location of the supraspinatus, as both structures run adjacently and parallel to each other. When visualized longitudinally (long axis), the tendon should appear uniformly echogenic and it should taper as it approaches its insertion onto the greater tuberosity (Fig. 15.4b). Visualized transversely (short axis), the biceps tendon should be visualized just anterior to the supraspinatus tendon, within the rotator interval [3] (Fig. 15.4c). The subacromial–subdeltoid bursa, which resides just superficial to the supraspinatus tendon, is normally a thin hyperechoic structure, due to the presence of peribursal fat [13].

Supraspinatus pathology most frequently originates at the anterior edge of the tendon [14]. Thus, the sequence of evaluating the supraspinatus typically begins with a longitudinal view of the tendon, starting anteriorly and moving posteriorly, followed by evaluation in the transverse axis, moving in the medial–lateral plane.

Evaluation: Infraspinatus and Teres Minor Tendons

The infraspinatus and teres minor make up the posterior rotator cuff complex. The infraspinatus muscle originates in the infraspinous fossa of the scapula and is innervated by the suprascapular nerve. The teres minor originates at the dorsolateral border of the scapula and is innervated by the axillary nerve. Infraspinatus and teres minor

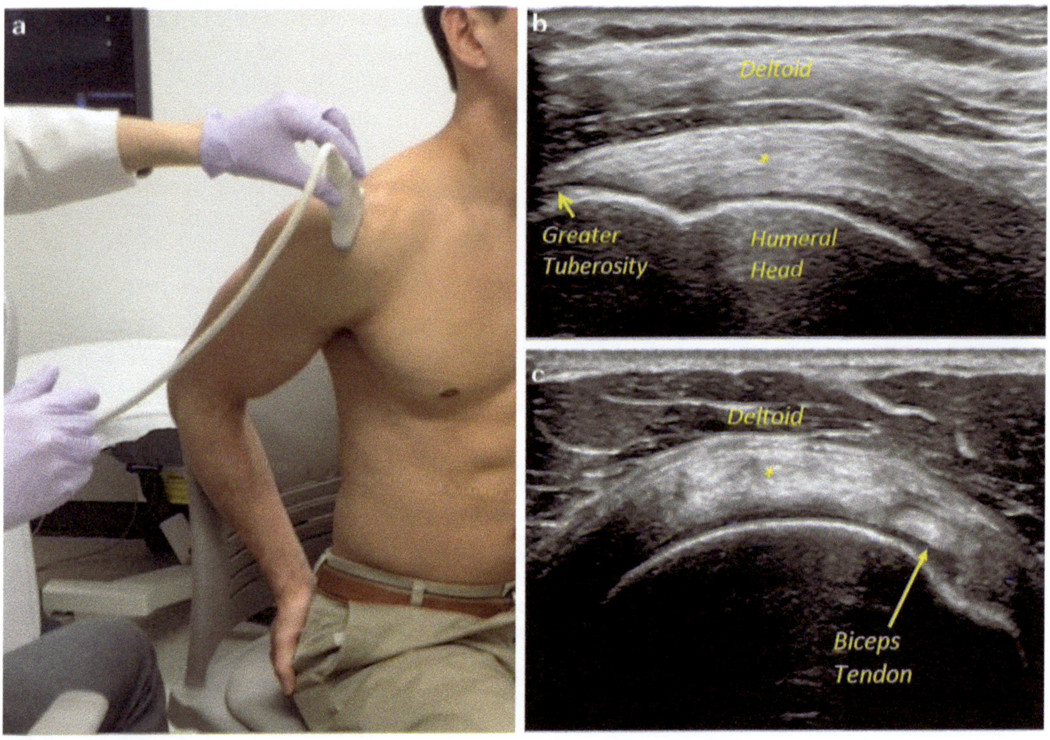

Fig. 15.4 (**a**) Patient positioning during examination of supraspinatus (modified Crass position). Note that the arm is extended and internally rotated. (**b**) Normal supraspinatus tendon, long axis (*asterisk*). Note the hyperechoic subacromial–subdeltoid bursa above supraspinatus tendon. (**c**) Normal supraspinatus tendon, short axis (*asterisk*)

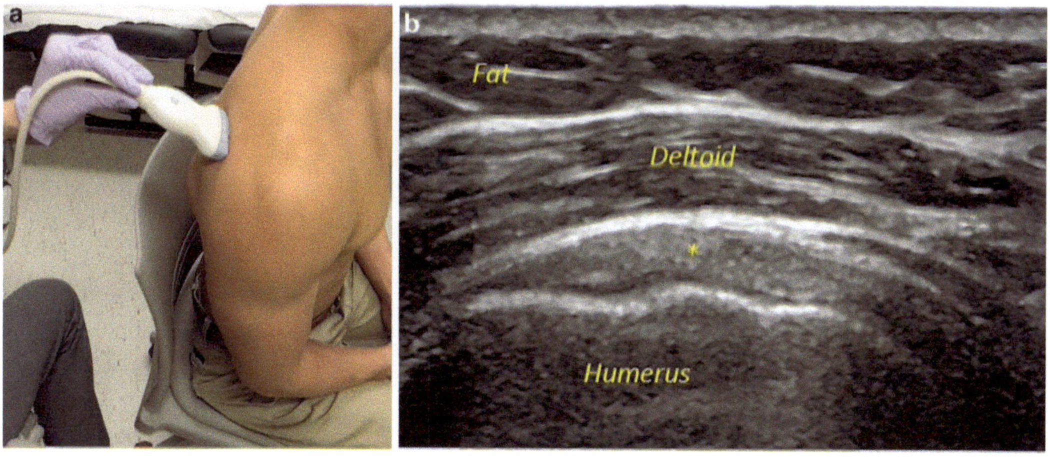

Fig. 15.5 (**a**) Patient positioning during examination of the infraspinatus and teres minor. (**b**) Normal infraspinatus muscle tendon, long axis (*asterisk*)

tendons insert on the posterior aspect of the superior facet and the inferior facet of the greater tuberosity, respectively, and facilitate external rotation of the shoulder.

To best visualize these external rotators, the probe is placed on the posterior aspect of the shoulder with the arm placed in the resting position (Fig. 15.5a). Additionally, the palm of the patient's hand can be placed atop their contralateral shoulder. This, in effect, abducts and internally rotates the arm, thus putting these two external rotators under tension and allowing for ease of visualization.

Due to their common insertion as well as their shared border, sonographic differentiation between these two tendons can be difficult [14] (Fig. 15.5b). To better delineate any pathology, it is often helpful to ask patients to isometrically externally rotate their arms against resistance. Doing this, any tears or retracted components of the tendons frequently become more apparent [14].

Evaluation: Rotator Cuff Muscles

Three of the four rotator cuff muscles can be evaluated by US; there is a very limited visualization of the subscapularis muscle since it is obscured by the overlying coracoid process of the scapula. With the shoulder in neutral position, the supraspinatus muscle can be localized by locating the suprascapular notch in the coronal oblique plane (in the plane of the scapula). The transducer can then be moved to the posterior aspect of the shoulder to evaluate the infraspinatus muscle superiorly and the teres minor muscle inferiorly. The rotator cuff muscles appear as a relatively hypoechoic structures with a muscle belly tapering to a tendon distally (Fig. 15.6a). Atrophy manifests as loss of muscle bulk, and fatty infiltration appears as hyperechogenicity of the muscle [15] (Fig. 15.6b).

Evaluation: Subacromial Impingement (Dynamic)

Dynamic sonography can be used to diagnose external shoulder impingement by directly visualizing the subacromial space during active arm elevation [11, 16]. For dynamic sonography, the patient is seated on a rotating stool, and two impingement-evoking maneuvers may be utilized. In the first maneuver, "the empty can test," the transducer is placed in the coronal oblique plane with its medial margin at the anterolateral edge of the acromion. The shoulder is abducted anterolaterally (flexion and abduction) while in internal rotation (thumb down). In the second maneuver, the "Neer sign," the transducer is

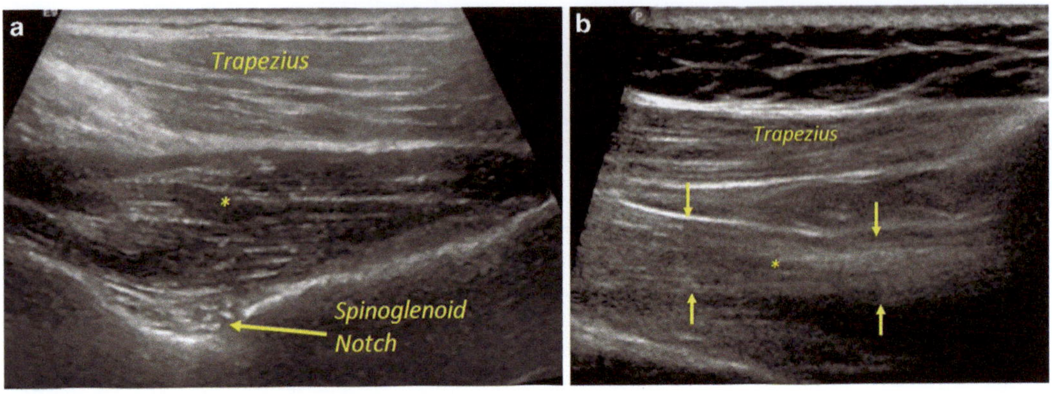

Fig. 15.6 (**a**) Normal supraspinatus muscle, long axis (*asterisk*). (**b**) Supraspinatus muscle atrophy with fatty infiltration, long axis (*asterisk* between *arrows*)

Fig. 15.7 Long-axis image showing bunching up of subacromial–subdeltoid fluid (*asterisk*) lateral to the acromion during shoulder abduction

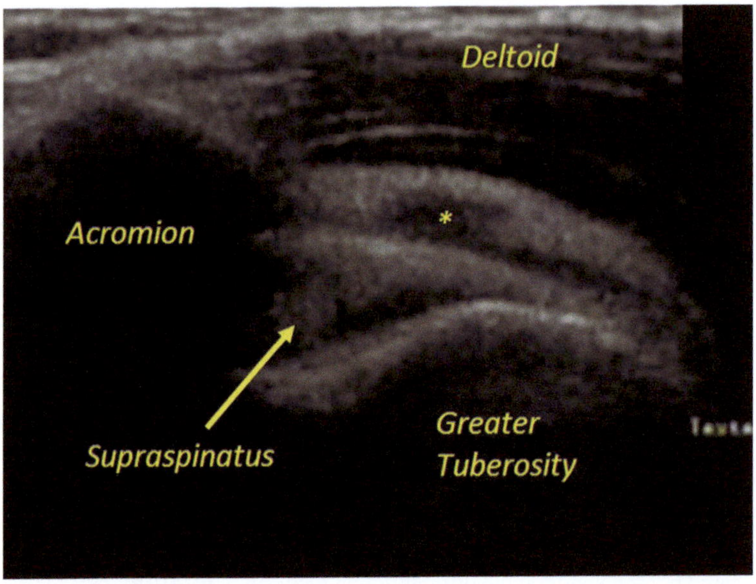

placed in a similar fashion; the shoulder is abducted while in the neutral position and the elbow is flexed for ease.

With impingement, there is accumulation of subacromial–subdeltoid bursal synovium or fluid lateral to the acromion (Fig. 15.7). With progressive impingement, the supraspinatus tendon may catch on the acromion (ratchet motion.) With severe impingement, there is superior migration of the humeral head and the tendon bunches up or bulges laterally, and the greater tuberosity does not glide under the acromial acoustic shadow.

Rotator Cuff Tears

Rotator cuff tears can have several different sonographic appearances. The US appearance depends on tear size, tear retraction, and the concomitant presence of any fluid or focalized synovitis [2]. Long-axis views delineate partial and full-thickness tears most clearly, with small motions of the arm to help better resolve the images [14]. Full-thickness tears extend from the articular surface to the bursal side of the tendon

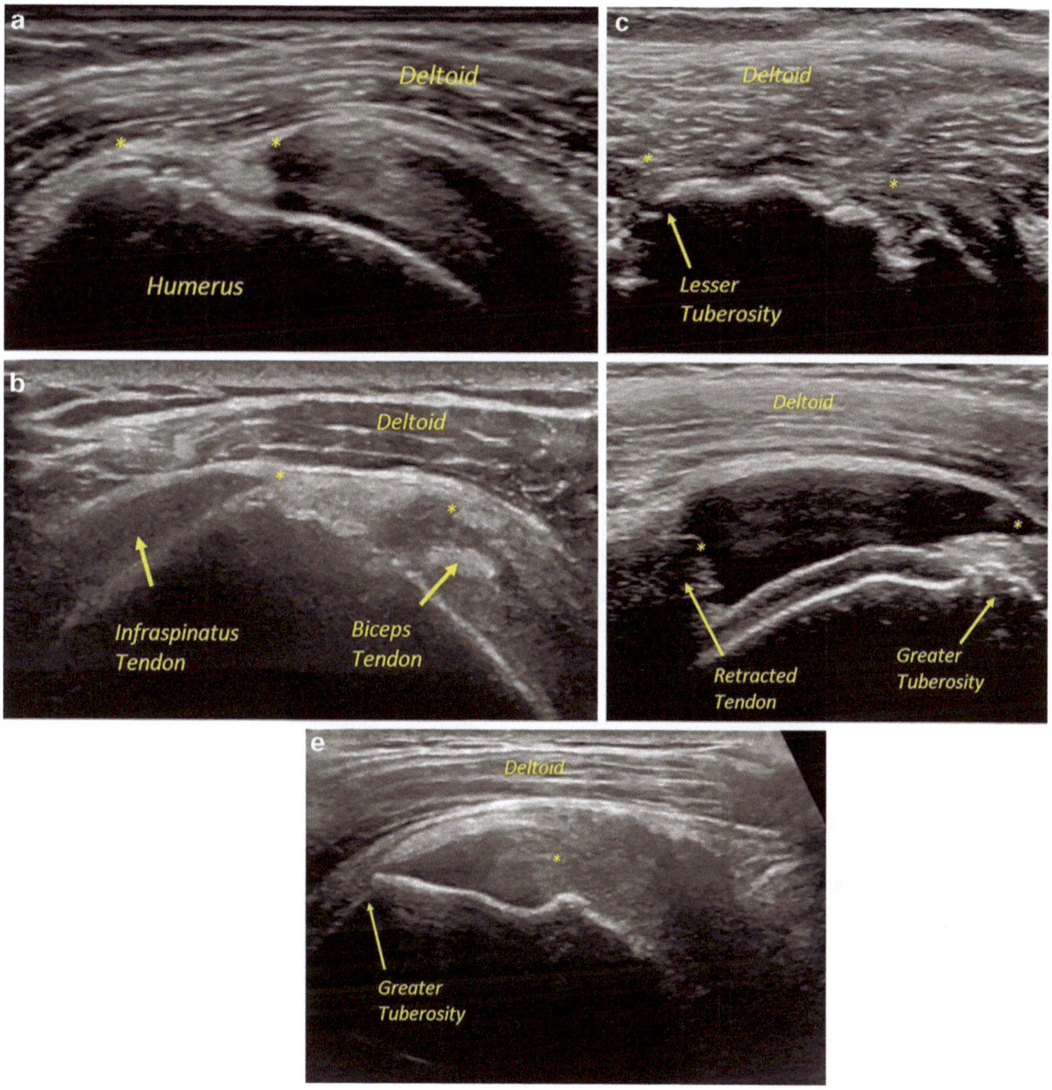

Fig. 15.8 (**a**) Small full-thickness tear of supraspinatus tendon in long axis (tear is between *asterisks*). Note the adjacent cortical irregularity of greater tuberosity. (**b**) Full-thickness tear of the supraspinatus tendon in short axis (tear is between *asterisks*). (**c**) Full-thickness retracted tear of the subscapularis tendon in long axis (tear is between *asterisks*). (**d**) Large retracted full-thickness tear of the supraspinatus tendon in long axis (tear with large fluid-filled defect is between *asterisks*). (**e**) Severe supraspinatus tendinosis, long axis (*asterisk*). Note hypoechogenicity, loss of fibrillar pattern, and thickening of the tendon

and must be visualized on both short- and long-axis scanning (Fig. 15.8a–c). In the acute setting, exposure of the articular surface with the presence of anechoic fluid can usually be identified at the site injury (Fig. 15.8d). In the more chronic setting, full-thickness tears can become more difficult to identify, as echogenic debris or scarring often replace fluid at the site of injury [2, 13].

Partial-thickness tears typically take on one of three forms. These include articular-sided tears, bursal-sided tears, and intrasubstance (interstitial) tears. Articular-sided partial-thickness tears reveal intact rotator cuff tendon fibers on the bursal side with concomitant hybrid hypoechoic and hyperechoic signal on the articular side. Bursal-sided partial-thickness tears are usually denoted by a loss of tendon convexity, often with bursal tissue or deltoid muscle occupying the space of the lesion. Intrasubstance tears may be difficult to visualize, as neither the bursal nor articular-sided surfaces are compromised. They are frequently characterized as focal hypoechoic or anechoic defects within the tendon substance.

Rotator cuff tendinosis is characterized by an inflammatory response to a tendon followed by a degenerative process. Sonographically, tendinosis typically manifests as tendon thickening with hypoechogenicity and loss of the fibrillar pattern (Fig. 15.8e). Contralateral extremity sonographic evaluations may be helpful in equivocal cases to help discern pathology from normal anatomy [4].

Conclusion

The utility of US in rotator cuff evaluation has evolved considerably over the last three decades. With the emergence of more refined techniques as well as standardized protocols, US has gained widespread acceptance and has paved its way into the current-day practices of radiology and orthopedic surgery. As an imaging modality used in rotator cuff evaluation, US allows for safe, cost-effective, and accessible examinations with diagnostic accuracy comparable to that of MRI. As such, it may be considered as a first-line imaging modality for the evaluation of shoulder pain in the adult patient. It can accurately diagnose rotator cuff disease, long head of biceps tendon disease, and rotator cuff muscle atrophy and fatty infiltration. As imaging technologies continue to evolve, ultrasonography will undoubtedly remain a valuable tool in diagnosis, preoperative planning, and treatment of rotator cuff disorders.

References

1. Seltzer SE, et al. Arthrosonography: gray-scale ultrasound evaluation of the shoulder. Radiology. 1979;132(2):467–8.
2. Middleton WD. Ultrasonography of rotator cuff pathology. Top Magn Reson Imaging. 1994;6(2):133–8.
3. Rutten MJ, et al. Ultrasound of the rotator cuff with MRI and anatomic correlation. Eur J Radiol. 2007;62(3):427–36.
4. Yablon CM, et al. Ultrasonography of the shoulder with arthroscopic correlation. Clin Sports Med. 2013;32(3):391–408.
5. Fotiadou AN, et al. Ultrasonography of symptomatic rotator cuff tears compared with MR imaging and surgery. Eur J Radiol. 2008;68(1):174–9.
6. Bretzke CA, et al. Ultrasonography of the rotator cuff. Normal and pathologic anatomy. Invest Radiol. 1985;20(3):311–5.
7. Kelly AM, Fessell D. Ultrasound compared with magnetic resonance imaging for the diagnosis of rotator cuff tears: a critically appraised topic. Semin Roentgenol. 2009;44(3):196–200.
8. Nazarian LN, et al. Imaging algorithms for evaluating suspected rotator cuff disease: Society of Radiologists in Ultrasound consensus conference statement. Radiology. 2013;267(2):589–95.
9. Corazza A, et al. Dynamic high-resolution ultrasound of the shoulder: How we do it. Eur J Radiol. 2015;84(2): 266–77.
10. Weinreb JH, et al. Tendon structure, disease, and imaging. Muscles Ligaments Tendons J. 2014;4(1): 66–73.
11. Khoury V, Cardinal E, Bureau NJ. Musculoskeletal sonography: a dynamic tool for usual and unusual disorders. AJR Am J Roentgenol. 2007;188(1): W63–73.
12. Ihnatsenka B, Boezaart AP. Ultrasound: basic understanding and learning the language. Int J Shoulder Surg. 2010;4(3):55–62.
13. Beggs I. Shoulder ultrasound. Semin Ultrasound CT MR. 2011;32(2):101–13.
14. Churchill RS, et al. Rotator cuff ultrasonography: diagnostic capabilities. J Am Acad Orthop Surg. 2004;12(1):6–11.
15. Khoury V, Cardinal E, Brassard P. Atrophy and fatty infiltration of the supraspinatus muscle: sonography versus MRI. AJR Am J Roentgenol. 2008;190(4): 1105–11.
16. Farin PU, et al. Shoulder impingement syndrome: sonographic evaluation. Radiology. 1990;176(3): 845–9.

16 Indications for Repair: Who Really Needs Surgery?

Robert W. Westermann and Brian R. Wolf

Incidence

The incidence and prevalence of rotator cuff disease is important information for patients and providers when considering treatment options in symptomatic patients. Rotator cuff tears are a common cause of morbidity, resulting in shoulder pain, arm dysfunction, and sleep disturbances; the prevalence of tears increases with age [1–3]. The three most traditional means to assess incidence of rotator cuff tears are (1) cadaveric studies, (2) ultrasound (US), and (3) magnetic resonance imaging (MRI). Overall, the incidence of *any* rotator cuff tear (partial or full thickness) in cadaveric studies approaches 30 % [4]. Cadaveric studies are highly variable. Neer reported 25 full-thickness rotator cuff tears in 500 cadaveric shoulders (5 %) in 1983 [5]. Petersson [6] reported 32 rotator cuff tears in 99 cadaveric shoulders (32.3 %) (14 full thickness, 18 partial thickness). Ozaki et al. [7] reported 96 rotator cuff tears (48 %) (27 full thickness, 69 partial thickness) in 200 cadaveric shoulders. Reilley et al. [4] reviewed and combined nine studies that evaluated tears in 2553 cadaveric shoulders with complete data; it was determined that the overall prevalence of any tear was 30 % (12 % full thickness, 18 % partial thickness) in cadavers with a mean age of 70 years.

The incidence of rotator cuff tear diagnosed by ultrasound is also variable and has been strongly correlated with age [2, 3] and presence of shoulder pain. In a review of 100 clinically symptomatic patients, Teefey et al. [8] reported an incidence of 80 % (65 full thickness, 15 partial thickness). Milgrom et al. [2] evaluated 180 asymptomatic patients by ultrasound and discovered 31 partial-thickness tears (17.2 %) and 32 full-thickness tears (17.7 %, 35 % overall). Reilley et al. [4] reviewed the incidence of rotator cuff tears by ultrasound in 11 papers (1449 subjects) and determined the overall prevalence to be 40.7 %.

MRI is a common modality used to diagnose rotator cuff tears in current practice. The incidence of rotator cuff tears diagnosed by MRI is also variable. Sher et al. [9] reported 14 full-thickness and 22 partial-thickness rotator cuff tears in 96 asymptomatic subjects for a total incidence of 34.3 %. The mean age of patients in Sher's study was 54 years. Torstensen and Hollinshead [10] evaluated 57 symptomatic patients (average age 41) and discovered 40 (70.2 %) full-thickness rotator cuff tears by MRI. Reilley et al. [4] reviewed the incidence of rotator cuff tears diagnosed by MRI in 13 papers (761 subjects) and determined the overall prevalence to be 41.1 %. Rotator cuff tears are likely present in between 30 and 40 % of the population.

R.W. Westermann, MD • B.R. Wolf, MD, MS (✉)
Department of Orthopaedics and Rehabilitation,
University of Iowa Hospitals and Clinics,
Iowa City, IA, USA
e-mail: brian-wolf@uiowa.edu

J.D. Kelly IV (ed.), *Elite Techniques in Shoulder Arthroscopy*,
DOI 10.1007/978-3-319-25103-5_16

Tears are more common in symptomatic patients [4, 8, 10], and the prevalence of tears increases with age [2, 3].

Natural History

The natural history of rotator cuff pathology also impacts decision making for patients with rotator cuff problems. Neer conceptualized rotator cuff pathology as a spectrum of diseases [5] beginning with edema and hemorrhage of the tendon bursa early and progressing to fibrosis, tendonitis, and, in later stages, partial and complete tendon tearing. Debate regarding the etiology of these changes continues inclusive of intrinsic tendon degeneration and extrinsic mechanical factors. The fate of partial-thickness tears has been described by Yamanaka et al. [11] who performed repeat arthrography on 40 conservatively treated partial-thickness rotator cuff tears at a mean interval of 412 days; during this interval, 10 % of tears healed, 10 % decreased in size, 53 % increased in size, and 28 % progressed to full-thickness tears. Increased incidence of tears has also been associated with increasing age [2, 3]. There is therefore strong evidence that tear size and incidence increase with time.

Population studies suggest rotator cuff tears are prevalent in asymptomatic shoulders. Patients in their 50s have a 13 % rate of asymptomatic tears, compared to 20 % of patients in their 60s, 31 % of patients in their 70s, and between 50 and 80 % of patients greater than 80 [2, 3]. Longitudinal studies suggest subsequent development of pain in previously asymptomatic shoulders over time. Moosmayer et al. evaluated initially asymptomatic rotator cuff tears at 3-year follow-up and determined 18 of 50 (36 %) became symptomatic [12]. Similarly, Yamaguchi et al. [13] observed 23 of 45 (51 %) initially asymptomatic patients go on to become symptomatic over a mean of 2.8 years. Mall et al. [14] observed development of symptoms in 34 of 69 (49 %) previously asymptomatic tears over a 1.9 year period. Patients who are initially identified as "asymptomatic" are at risk for both symptom development and tear progression over time.

Demographic Variables

Patient demographics are usually among the first variables considered when deciding to recommend rotator cuff repair to patients.

Age

Older chronological age should not preclude appropriate and symptomatic patients from operative interventions. Although increased age is classically thought to correlate with poorly repairable tissue and worse outcomes [15, 16], postoperative pain relief and improved function have proven reliable in older patients. Cofield et al. report outcomes 13 years after rotator cuff repair and determined that advanced age was associated with worse results in terms of motion and strength but not satisfaction, pain relief, or reoperation [15]. Rhee et al. [17] evaluated outcomes of rotator cuff tears in patients in their 60s versus their 70s; they determined that there was no difference with respect to age, and outcomes were more closely related to the size of tear. Pai and Lawson [18] report good to excellent results in 78 % of patients undergoing rotator cuff repair over the age of 70. Hattrup reported a comparison of outcomes between patients under and over the age of 65. The under 65-year-old cohort demonstrated excellent results in 88.6 % of cases, compared to 77.2 % of cases over the age of 65 [19]. Good and excellent results are achievable when performing rotator cuff repairs in elderly patients. No strict age cutoff for surgical indication is appropriate as there is significant interpersonal variability in activity level, and good outcomes are achievable.

Younger chronological age and physiologically young patients with full-thickness rotator cuff tears are often indicated for surgical intervention sooner than chronologically or physiologically older patients. Younger patients tend to be more active and are more likely to be working in occupations that require a strong arm. One of the predictors of failure of nonoperative treatment for rotator cuff tears has been shown to be activity level, which tends to be higher in chronologically and physiologically younger patients (MOON data—unpublished—Warren Dunn correspondence). Younger patients also have higher life expectancies and, given that rotator cuff tears rarely heal on their own but rather tend to progress, repair may be more desirable in this population. There is no agreed upon age where early repair should be performed, but younger than 50–55 years of age is a frequently used cutoff by many surgeons.

Gender

While there is some inconsistency in the literature [17, 19], female gender has been correlated with inferior results after rotator cuff surgery [15, 16]. Cofield et al. [15] evaluated 105 patients who underwent repair of chronic rotator cuff tears at a mean follow-up of 13 years. Female gender was associated with worse outcomes in terms of pain relief and active motion at final follow-up, but gender did not predict patient satisfaction or reoperation. Romeo et al. [16] evaluated 72 patients (44 men and 28 women) at an average follow-up of 4.5 years. Worse outcomes were seen in women over the age of 65 with regard to the simple shoulder test and Constant-Murley scores, while no such correlations were present in men [16]. Rhee et al. [17] performed a retrospective review of 238 patients ages 60–79 who underwent rotator cuff repair. They created a sex- and tear size-matched model and determined there was no difference in outcomes with respect to gender. Good outcomes have been demonstrated in males and females and gender should not factor into surgical indications. However, outcomes after surgery may differ based on gender.

Workers' Compensation

Pending workers' compensation claims are associated with poor satisfaction with nonoperative treatment of rotator cuff tears [20]. In addition, McKee and Yoo [21] determined that patients who had filed a workers' compensation claim and who underwent surgical repair had lower shoulder pain and disability index scores as well as SF-36 scores both preoperatively and postoperatively compared to those who had not filed claims. In a retrospective review, Misamore et al. [22] reported outcomes of rotator cuff repairs in 103 consecutive patients; of these, 54 % of patients with open workers' compensation claims were rated good or excellent at 45 months compared to 92 % good and excellent results in those without claims. Workers' compensation was also associated with lower satisfaction and worse ASES scores in patients with recurrent rotator cuff tears [23]. In conclusion, workers' compensation is associated with poor tolerance for physical therapy, inferior preoperative status, and worse postoperative outcomes.

Patient History and Physical Exam

Duration of Symptoms

Not all patients with rotator cuff tears are symptomatic [2, 9]; however, progression of initially asymptomatic tears often occurs [12–14]. Pain is typically over the lateral shoulder or deltoid, and it often occurs at night and with overhead activities [24]. There remains significant controversy in the literature regarding duration of clinical symptoms as an indication for rotator cuff repair. Prior studies suggest nonoperative treatment initiated early is associated with improved outcomes, while late initiation of nonoperative treatment (>1 year) is associated with less favorable results [25]. Bokor et al. [26] evaluated 53 patients at an average of 7.6 years after arthroscopically diagnosed full-thickness rotator cuff tears treated nonoperatively. They noted 86 % of patients that initiated nonoperative management within 3 months of symptoms had satisfactory results, compared to 56 % of patients who had shoulder pain for >6 months prior to presentation. Bartolozzi et al. [25] reported a series of 136 patients treated nonoperatively for rotator cuff disease. They concluded that a greater than 1-year history of pretreatment clinical symptoms correlated with unfavorable clinical outcomes with nonoperative treatment.

More recent studies suggest the duration of symptoms has no effect on outcomes. The MOON Shoulder group, a multicenter cohort, evaluated 450 patients stratified by the duration of symptoms at the time of presentation [27]. They determined that there was no correlation of prolonged pretreatment symptoms with rotator cuff disease severity or patient outcomes. This study, however, did not exclude patients who had already begun nonoperative treatment modalities.

Increased symptom duration does not necessarily translate to inferior surgical results. Bjorkenheim et al. [28] evaluated 78 rotator cuff repairs at 5–10 year follow-up and concluded preoperative symptom duration did not correlate with outcome of surgery.

Acute versus Chronic Tears: Surgical Timing

Determining chronicity of rotator cuff tears is often difficult. In some circumstances, patients may suffer complete traumatic full-thickness tears after a fall or shoulder dislocation [29]. Acute rotator cuff tears are thought to account for less than 10 % of patients presenting with symptomatic rotator cuff disease [16, 29, 30]. Bassett and Cofield performed a retrospective review of 37 patients who had surgical repair within 3 months of an acute rotator cuff tear. The average follow-up was 7 years, and the authors determined that early surgical repair (defined as <3 weeks) was associated with the better shoulder function at follow-up [29]. Hantes et al. [31] evaluated 35 patients with traumatic rotator cuff tears; 15 patients had early repair (<3 weeks) while 20 patients had delayed repairs (>3 weeks). Average follow-up for the two groups was 34 and 38 months, respectively. Postoperatively, the early repair group demonstrated significantly better UCLA scores, Constant scores, and range of motion. However, there is some evidence that delayed rotator cuff repair for acute tears has no effect on outcome [16, 32, 33]. The matter of surgical timing was summarized in a recent systematic review by Mukovozov et al. [34] who identified 15 studies reporting the interval to surgical management of acute rotator cuff tears. The acute surgery group, defined as <3 months between injury and surgery, was inclusive of 7 studies and 209 patients. Eight studies including 162 patients comprised the surgical delay group of acute rotator cuff tears. This systematic review determined that early repair (<3 months) was associated with significantly improved Constant scores, UCLA shoulder scores, and better abduction and elevation [34].

Range of Motion

Active and passive ranges of motion are important concerns in the indication for surgical repair of rotator cuff tears. Poor preoperative range of motion has been correlated with inferior results after rotator cuff repair. Patients who are unable to achieve 100° of active abduction preoperatively commonly have compromised postoperative results [35, 36]. Feng et al. [36] followed a cohort of 1067 patients for an average of 7.9 years and determined those who had greater than 90° of active abduction preoperatively had improved postoperative outcomes. Pai and Lawson [18] corroborated these findings when they observed good and excellent results more frequently in patients with preoperative abduction greater than 90°. While improved preoperative active range of motion is associated with superior outcomes, close evaluation of passive ROM is crucial to rule out concomitant adhesive capsulitis or "frozen shoulder." Rotator cuff tears may be observed concurrently with adhesive capsulitis. In general, adhesive capsulitis should be successfully addressed before rotator cuff pathology is surgically managed [37]. Tauro [38] determined that patients with a total range of motion deficit of 70° or more (a combination of loss of abduction, forward flexion, and internal and external rotation) were more likely to have lasting postoperative adhesive capsulitis and poor results of rotator cuff repairs [38].

It is critically important to evaluate both active and passive range of motion prior to recommending rotator cuff repair to patients. Good preoperative active range of motion clearly correlates with improved outcomes. Furthermore, it is crucial to diagnose and treat adhesive capsulitis prior to addressing rotator cuff pathology. It is much preferable to get passive range of motion restored prior to performing surgery of a rotator cuff tear, given that a period of immobilization typically occurs postoperatively.

Strength

The loss of strength and function in rotator cuff disease is often used as an indication for repair [39, 40]. Patients with objective weakness on physical exam often fail physical therapy or other conservative modalities [25]. In a study performed by Bartolozzi et al. [25], patients without weakness at the time of presentation obtained good and excellent results with physical therapy 74 % of the time. Patients presenting with moderate and severe weakness (grade 3 or less out of 5) experienced good and excellent outcomes only between 13 and 33 % of the time with conservative management. The mean follow-up in their study was 20 months. Furthermore, Bartolozzi found that functional impairment at the time of presentation was associated with poor outcomes with conservative management. This finding has been disputed by recent MOON cohort data as preoperative weakness was not associated with failure of physical therapy programs [41]. Surgery should be considered when weakness is present in young and active patients who wish to regain strength; in elderly patients, a full course of structured physical therapy is prudent as improvements in strength are often observed [40].

Preoperative weakness has been associated with worse outcomes after rotator cuff repair [25, 35, 36]. Ellman et al. [35] evaluated 50 patients at an average of 3.5 years after rotator cuff repair; he determined patients with preoperative external rotation strength grade less than 3 had significantly worse outcomes than those with preoperative strength 4 or 5. In conclusion, indications for rotator cuff repair based on strength should include both those with good strength who fail conservative treatments and young active patients with weakness who need or want return of strength.

Physical Exam

Impingement signs described by Hawkins [42, 43] and Neer [44, 45] are positive in most patients presenting with rotator cuff disease. MacDonald et al. [46] prospectively evaluated the diagnostic accuracy of these impingement signs in 85 consecutive patients undergoing shoulder arthroscopy. The sensitivity of the Neer and Hawkins signs for detecting rotator cuff tears is 85 % and 88 %, respectively [46]. Leroux et al. [47] demonstrated similar sensitivities (89 % and 87 %) of Neer and Hawkins signs. Some propose a further exam with an impingement tests [5] (i.e., subacromial injection with local anesthetic after a positive impingement sign and repeating exam to assess for improvement). While the impingement test has proven reliable in detecting rotator cuff disease, correlations with patient outcomes have proven inconsistent [48, 49].

Imaging

Plain films are often obtained in the initial workup of patients with shoulder pain. The acromiohumeral distance measured from the superior aspect of the humerus to the inferior boarder of the acromion on anteroposterior or true AP shoulder plain films has been associated with chronicity of rotator cuff tears. Distances 7 mm or less have been shown to correlate with larger tears and decreased strength, motion, and satisfaction after surgical repair [35, 50]. Plain shoulder radiographs are often used to evaluate acromial shape preoperatively. Bigliani characterized acromion morphology as flat, curved, or hooked [51]. Acromion morphology has not been demonstrated to correlate with outcomes following repair [36, 52]. Classically, type 2 or 3 (curved or hooked) acromions were thought to contribute to external subacromial impingement [44]. A prospective, randomized controlled trial has shown no differences in patient outcomes between rotator cuff tears treated with repair and acromioplasty and those treated with repair alone [52]. MacDonald et al. [52], however, did report higher reoperation in patients treated with repair alone at 2-year follow-up. As part of the AAOS clinical practice guidelines for rotator cuff problems, the academy suggests routine acromioplasty is not required at the time of rotator cuff repair [53, 54].

MRI

Advanced imaging allows clinicians to accurately evaluate rotator cuff tear characteristics when deciding to indicate patients for repair. While multiple modalities have proven reliable, MRI and US are the techniques most commonly used [55–57]. It is important to evaluate tear size, tendon retraction, muscle atrophy, and fatty infiltration as these factors are associated with reparability.

Tear Size and Retraction

It should be recognized that tear size is a dynamic variable as small tears have been shown to increase in size over time [13, 58]. Also, in general, the size of tears generally increases with patient age [15]. Surgeons can reliably differentiate partial from full-thickness tears on advanced imaging but cannot reliably measure the size of full-thickness tears in millimeters. A study by Kuhn et al. [59] demonstrated that agreement among surgeons is poor when trying to measure full-thickness rotator cuff tear size on MRI. They suggest cuff tear size is best assessed by the anatomic level of retraction (i.e., adjacent to the footprint, at the level of the humeral head, and at the level of the glenoid) as described by Patte [60].

Maman et al. [58] performed an MRI follow-up study on patients treated conservatively for rotator cuff disease. He noted progression of tears was associated with advanced age, full-thickness tears, and fatty infiltration of rotator cuff musculature. Large tears have classically been demonstrated to be a negative predictor of outcome in patients treated without surgery [61]. This finding was contradicted by data from the MOON cohort [41] who showed increased tear size and retraction were not associated with failure of a physical therapy program.

The size of the rotator cuff tear has been demonstrated to correlate strongly with patient outcome after surgical repair [15, 16, 19, 36, 62]. Cofield et al. [15] evaluated 105 patients at a mean of 13.4 years after rotator cuff repair. They determined increased size of the tear at the time of treatment was associated with worse postoperative motion, strength, and patient satisfaction score. Reoperations were also higher in patients with larger tears during the follow-up period. Massive tears with significant retraction may be more challenging to repair, and some may be deemed irreparable. However, with contemporary arthroscopic techniques, all but the most retracted and atrophic tears can at least be repaired partially.

Muscle Atrophy and Fatty Infiltration

Muscle bodies of the rotator cuff commonly degenerate after their associated tendons tear and detach. This muscle degeneration is characterized by decrease in volume (atrophy) and fatty infiltration [35, 50, 63]. Coleman et al. [64] observed a 12-fold increase in intramuscular fat content after simulated full-thickness rotator cuff injury in a sheep model. Atrophy of the rotator cuff musculature at the time of presentation has been associated with worse pretreatment pain and function measured by the Western Ontario Rotator Cuff (WORC) Index and the American Shoulder and Elbow Surgeons (ASES) scores [65]. These MRI findings, however, do not seem to predict failure of conservative management [41]. The presence of fatty infiltration has been associated with decreased rates of tendon healing after surgery; however, they are not associated with worse postoperative subjective outcomes [66–68].

Nonoperative Treatment

The primary indication for operative management of rotator cuff tears is failure of nonoperative management. Physical therapy has been demonstrated to be effective in 67–83 % of patients with atraumatic symptomatic rotator cuff pathology [40, 69, 70]. Data from the MOON cohort [40] suggests physical therapy is effective in managing up to 75 % of full-thickness atraumatic rotator cuff tears. They also demonstrated patients who failed nonoperative management tended to do so in the first 12 weeks of their physical therapy program. In a retrospective review of 616 patients, Morrison et al. [69] found that 67 % of partial-thickness tears were treated successfully with physical therapy.

In contrast, Moosmayer et al. [70] performed a controlled trial of 103 patients randomized to either physical therapy (PT) of rotator cuff repair. They determined that operative repair resulted in superior constant scores, ASES scores, improved pain-free abduction, and overall reduction in pain as compared to treatment with PT. Interestingly, only 9 of the 51 (17 %) patients randomized to physical therapy in their study failed nonoperative treatment and elected to undergo surgical repair [70] (Figs. 16.1 and 16.2).

Data from the MOON cohort [41] suggests patient expectations regarding physical therapy are the strongest predictor of nonoperative management failure. In other words if the patient

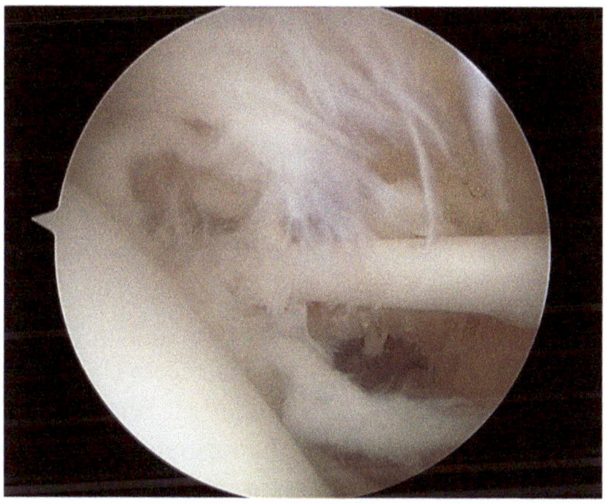

Fig. 16.1 Intra-articular view of a partial-thickness rotator cuff tear with significant intra-articular fraying

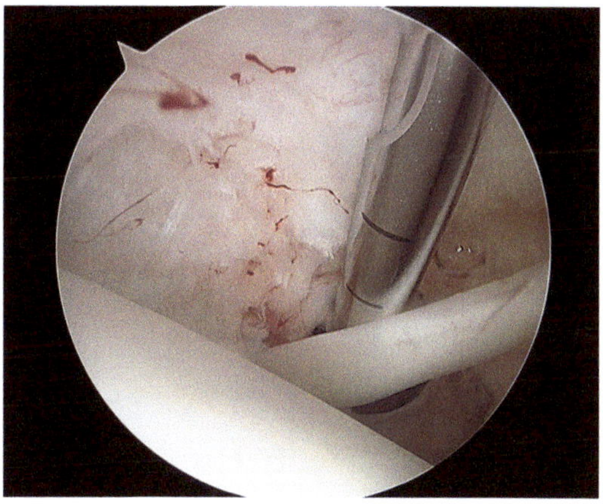

Fig. 16.2 Intra-articular view of a partial-thickness rotator cuff tear after debridement

believes therapy will work for them, then it probably will. If the patient does not think therapy will help them then it likely will not. Furthermore, they identified younger age, higher activity level, and abstinence from smoking as independent factors that predict failure of physical therapy programs for treatment of symptomatic full-thickness rotator cuff tears. Nonetheless, 6–12 weeks of a structured physical therapy program should be generally prescribed prior to offering surgery for patients with atraumatic, symptomatic, full-thickness rotator cuff tears.

It should be recognized that the MOON cohort [40, 41] excluded acute and traumatic rotator cuff tears. Conservative management likely has a limited role in these patients. As mentioned, there is evidence that patients surgically treated within 3 months of an acute injury [34] have improved outcomes; some even advocate repair within 3 weeks of injury [29, 31]. Physical therapy, therefore, should have a limited role in the preoperative treatment of acute rotator cuff tears from traumatic events. A proposed treatment algorithm for management is displayed in Fig. 16.3.

Partial-Thickness Tears

Operative management of partial-thickness rotator cuff tears is controversial. Management options for partial-thickness tears that fail physical

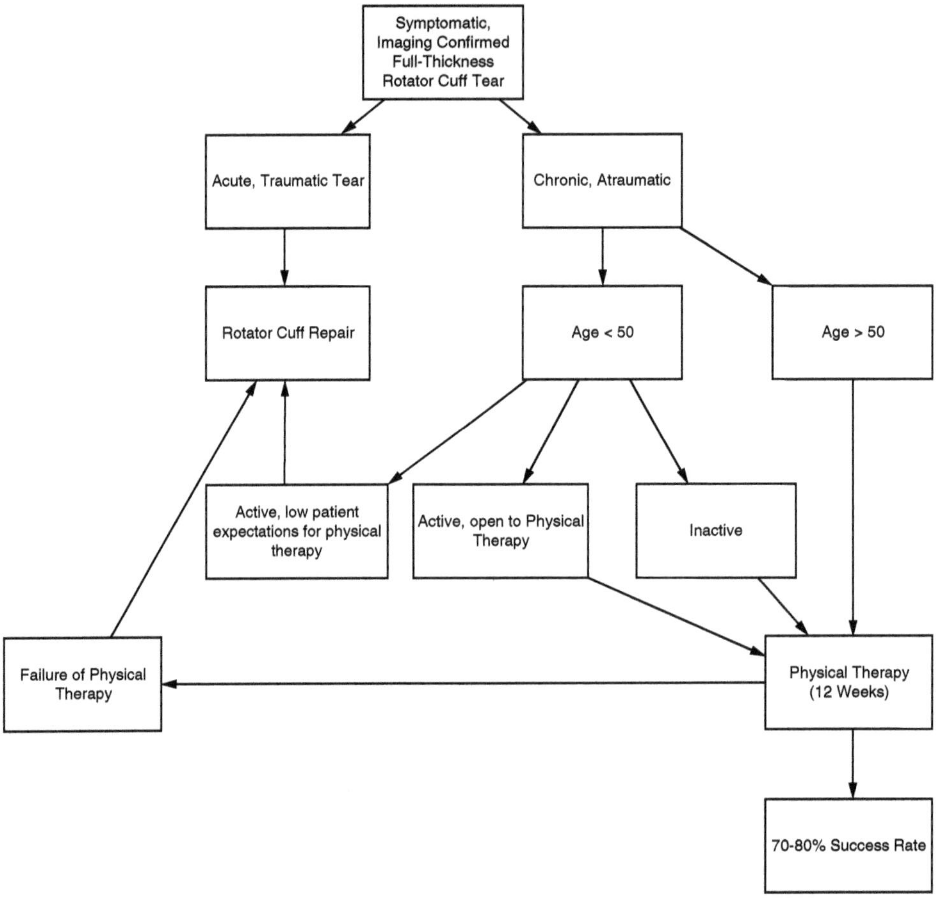

Fig. 16.3 A proposed treatment algorithm for patients with imaging-confirmed, full-thickness rotator cuff tears

therapy include tendon debridement, acromioplasty, and excision with repair. In general, symptomatic partial-thickness tears in patients that fail conservative management may be offered surgical intervention which can include debridement or repair depending on tear depth.

Partial-thickness rotator cuff tears involving more than 50 % of the affected tendon are often offered tear completion and subsequent repair. Dugas et al. [71] studied the insertional anatomy of the rotator cuff in 20 cadaveric shoulders. They determined that the mean medial-lateral diameter of the supraspinatus insertion is 14.7 mm. Symptomatic high-grade partial-thickness rotator cuff tears (defects >5–7 mm) who fail conservative treatment may be offered tear completion and repair with good expected results. There is evidence that symptomatic partial-thickness tears involving >50 % of the tendons are best treated with conversion to a full-thickness tear and repair [72, 73]. Webber et al. [72] compared 32 patients with partial-thickness RTC tears treated with debridement compared to 33 patients treated with conversion to full-thickness tears followed by repair. All tears in their series involved >50 % of the affected tendon defined by a >6 mm RTC defect; they found reoperation to be significantly higher in patients who underwent debridement alone. They also reported higher UCLA scores in patients treated with repair of partial rotator cuff tears compared to those treated with debridement. Bursal-sided tears may be resistant to nonoperative care and subacromial decompression alone [74]. Kim et al. [75] reported similar outcomes in patients undergoing repair of bursal- and articular-sided

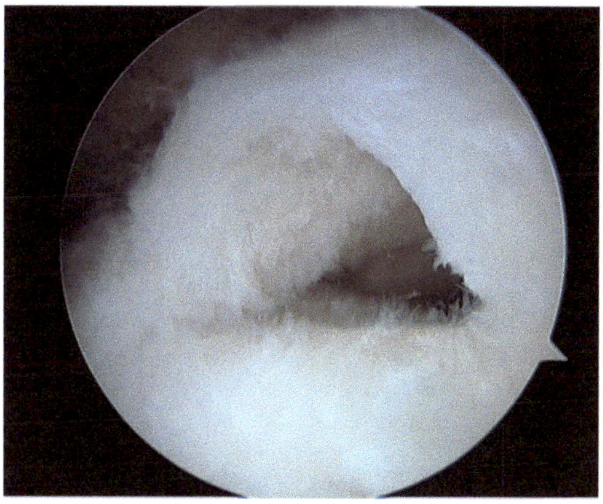

Fig. 16.4 Full-thickness rotator cuff tear

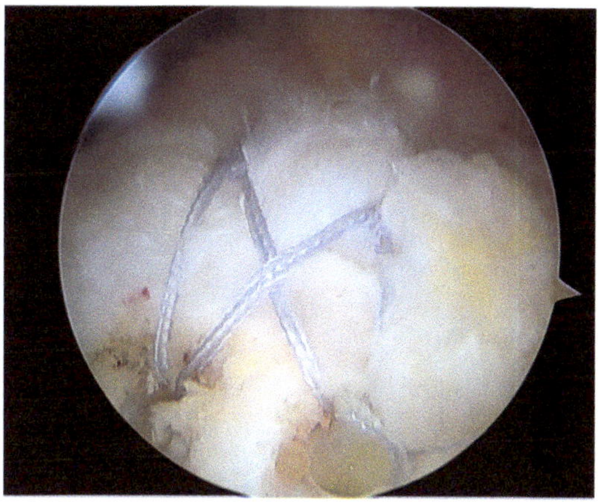

Fig. 16.5 Full-thickness rotator cuff tear status postrepair

partial-thickness tears at a mean follow-up of 36 months. Other techniques have also been described for repair of partial-thickness tears. These include transtendinous PASTA (partial articular-sided tendon avulsion) repair [76] and the all-inside articular-sided rotator cuff repair as described by Spencer [77]. The indications for repair using these other techniques are the same as described above for completion and repair of the tear, and no real data exists demonstrating superiority of one technique over another.

Partial rotator cuff tears that effect <50 % of the tendon may be offered debridement if conservative management fails [78, 79]. Partial-thickness tears result in significant intra-articular fraying that can irritate the glenoid labrum or the long head of biceps tendon with shoulder motion. This is not an uncommon scenario in young active/athletic patients with partial rotator cuff injuries (Figs. 16.4 and 16.5). Debridement of partial-thickness rotator cuff tears in elite throwers has been demonstrated to have good results in 75 % of patients including returning to competitive pitching [80]. Repair of partial-thickness rotator cuff tears in the throwing athlete is rarely indicated as shoulder stiffness may ensue [79]. Patients with partial-thickness rotator cuff tears involving <5–7 mm of the tendon footprint who fail physical therapy may be offered debridement; careful inspection and possible repair of other intra-articular structures in the throwing athlete may also be indicated.

Summary

The indications for rotator cuff repair are still evolving. The prevalence of cuff pathology in asymptomatic patients suggests that many patients can do well without surgery. In addition, the body of evidence is improving regarding indications for surgery. Factors such as patient activity level and patient expectations have been proven to be important considerations for recommending treatment. The rimportance of structural factors such as size of tear and characteristics on MRI remains controversial and requires more investigation.

References

1. Kannus P, Jozsa L. Histopathological changes preceding spontaneous rupture of a tendon. A controlled study of 891 patients. J Bone Joint Surg Am. 1991;73(10):1507–25.
2. Milgrom C, et al. Rotator-cuff changes in asymptomatic adults. The effect of age, hand dominance and gender. J Bone Joint Surg Br. 1995;77(2):296–8.
3. Tempelhof S, Rupp S, Seil R. Age-related prevalence of rotator cuff tears in asymptomatic shoulders. J Shoulder Elbow Surg. 1999;8(4):296–9.
4. Reilly P, et al. Dead men and radiologists don't lie: a review of cadaveric and radiological studies of rotator cuff tear prevalence. Ann R Coll Surg Engl. 2006;88(2):116–21.
5. Neer II CS. Impingement lesions. Clin Orthop Relat Res. 1983;173:70–7.

6. Petersson CJ. Ruptures of the supraspinatus tendon: cadaver dissection. Acta Orthop. 1984;55(1):52–6.
7. Ozaki J, et al. Tears of the rotator cuff of the shoulder associated with pathological changes in the acromion. A study in cadavera. J Bone Joint Surg. 1988;70(8):1224–30.
8. Teefey SA, et al. Ultrasonography of the rotator cuff a comparison of ultrasonographic and arthroscopic findings in one hundred consecutive cases. J Bone Joint Surg. 2000;82(4):498.
9. Sher JS, et al. Abnormal findings on magnetic resonance images of asymptomatic shoulders. J Bone Joint Surg. 1995;77(1):10–5.
10. Torstensen ET, Hollinshead RM. Comparison of magnetic resonance imaging and arthroscopy in the evaluation of shoulder pathology. J Shoulder Elbow Surg. 1999;8(1):42–5.
11. Yamanaka K, Matsumoto T. The joint side tear of the rotator cuff. A followup study by arthrography. Clin Orthop Relat Res. 1994;304:68–73.
12. Moosmayer S, et al. The natural history of asymptomatic rotator cuff tears: a three-year follow-up of fifty cases. J Bone Joint Surg Am. 2013;95(14):1249–55.
13. Yamaguchi K, et al. Natural history of asymptomatic rotator cuff tears: a longitudinal analysis of asymptomatic tears detected sonographically. J Shoulder Elbow Surg. 2001;10(3):199–203.
14. Mall NA, et al. Symptomatic progression of asymptomatic rotator cuff tears: a prospective study of clinical and sonographic variables. J Bone Joint Surg Am. 2010;92(16):2623–33.
15. Cofield RH, et al. Surgical repair of chronic rotator cuff tears. A prospective long-term study. J Bone Joint Surg Am. 2001;83-A(1):71–7.
16. Romeo AA, et al. Repair of full thickness rotator cuff tears. Gender, age, and other factors affecting outcome. Clin Orthop Relat Res. 1999;367:243–55.
17. Rhee YG, Cho NS, Yoo JH. Clinical outcome and repair integrity after rotator cuff repair in patients older than 70 years versus patients younger than 70 years. Arthroscopy. 2014;30(5):546–54.
18. Pai VS, Lawson DA. Rotator cuff repair in a district hospital setting: outcomes and analysis of prognostic factors. J Shoulder Elbow Surg. 2001;10(3):236–41.
19. Hattrup SJ. Rotator cuff repair: relevance of patient age. J Shoulder Elbow Surg. 1995;4(2):95–100.
20. Hawkins RH, Dunlop R. Nonoperative treatment of rotator cuff tears. Clin Orthop Relat Res. 1995;321:178–88.
21. McKee MD, Yoo DJ. The effect of surgery for rotator cuff disease on general health status. Results of a prospective trial. J Bone Joint Surg Am. 2000;82-A(7):970–9.
22. Misamore GW, Ziegler DW, Rushton II JL. Repair of the rotator cuff. A comparison of results in two populations of patients. J Bone Joint Surg Am. 1995;77(9):1335–9.
23. Kim HM, et al. Factors affecting satisfaction and shoulder function in patients with a recurrent rotator cuff tear. J Bone Joint Surg Am. 2014;96(2):106–12.
24. Duckworth DG, et al. Self-assessment questionnaires document substantial variability in the clinical expression of rotator cuff tears. J Shoulder Elbow Surg. 1999;8(4):330–3.
25. Bartolozzi A, Andreychik D, Ahmad S. Determinants of outcome in the treatment of rotator cuff disease. Clin Orthop Relat Res. 1994;308:90–7.
26. Bokor DJ, et al. Results of nonoperative management of full-thickness tears of the rotator cuff. Clin Orthop Relat Res. 1993;294:103–10.
27. M.S.G., et al. The duration of symptoms does not correlate with rotator cuff tear severity or other patient-related features: a cross-sectional study of patients with atraumatic, full-thickness rotator cuff tears. J Shoulder Elbow Surg. 2014;23(7):1052–8.
28. Bjorkenheim JM, et al. Surgical repair of the rotator cuff and surrounding tissues. Factors influencing the results. Clin Orthop Relat Res. 1988;236:148–53.
29. Bassett RW, Cofield RH. Acute tears of the rotator cuff: the timing of surgical repair. Clin Orthop Relat Res. 1983;175:18–24.
30. Cofield RH. Rotator cuff disease of the shoulder. J Bone Joint Surg Am. 1985;67(6):974–9.
31. Hantes ME, et al. A comparison of early versus delayed repair of traumatic rotator cuff tears. Knee Surg Sports Traumatol Arthrosc. 2011;19(10):1766–70.
32. Bjornsson HC, et al. The influence of age, delay of repair, and tendon involvement in acute rotator cuff tears: structural and clinical outcomes after repair of 42 shoulders. Acta Orthop. 2011;82(2):187–92.
33. Wolfgang GL. Surgical repair of tears of the rotator cuff of the shoulder. Factors influencing the result. J Bone Joint Surg Am. 1974;56(1):14–26.
34. Mukovozov I, et al. Time to surgery in acute rotator cuff tear. A systematic review. Bone Joint Res. 2013;2(7):122–8.
35. Ellman H, Hanker G, Bayer M. Repair of the rotator cuff. End-result study of factors influencing reconstruction. J Bone Joint Surg. 1986;68(8):1136–44.
36. Feng S, et al. Prognostic indicators for outcome following rotator cuff tear repair. J Orthop Surg. 2003;11(2):110–6.
37. Hannafin JA, Chiaia TA. Adhesive capsulitis. A treatment approach. Clin Orthop Relat Res. 2000;372:95–109.
38. Tauro JC. Stiffness and rotator cuff tears: incidence, arthroscopic findings, and treatment results. Arthroscopy. 2006;22(6):581–6.
39. Wolf BR, Dunn WR, Wright RW. Indications for repair of full-thickness rotator cuff tears. Am J Sports Med. 2007;35(6):1007–16.
40. Kuhn JE, et al. Effectiveness of physical therapy in treating atraumatic full-thickness rotator cuff tears: a multicenter prospective cohort study. J Shoulder Elbow Surg. 2013;22(10):1371–9.
41. Dunn WR, et al. Predictors of success of nonoperative treatment for full-thickness rotator cuff tears: a multicenter cohort study. Arthroscopy. 2013;29(10):e125–6.

42. Hawkins RJ, Abrams JS. Impingement syndrome in the absence of rotator cuff tear (stages 1 and 2). Orthop Clin North Am. 1987;18(3):373–82.
43. Hawkins RJ, Kennedy JC. Impingement syndrome in athletes. Am J Sports Med. 1980;8(3):151–8.
44. Neer II CS. Anterior acromioplasty for the chronic impingement syndrome in the shoulder: a preliminary report. J Bone Joint Surg Am. 1972;54(1):41–50.
45. Neer II CS, Welsh RP. The shoulder in sports. Orthop Clin North Am. 1977;8(3):583–91.
46. MacDonald PB, Clark P, Sutherland K. An analysis of the diagnostic accuracy of the Hawkins and Neer subacromial impingement signs. J Shoulder Elbow Surg. 2000;9(4):299–301.
47. Leroux JL, et al. Diagnostic value of clinical tests for shoulder impingement syndrome. Rev Rhum Engl Ed. 1995;62(6):423–8.
48. Kirkley A, et al. The use of the impingement test as a predictor of outcome following subacromial decompression for rotator cuff tendinosis. Arthroscopy. 2002;18(1):8–15.
49. Oh JH, et al. Modified impingement test can predict the level of pain reduction after rotator cuff repair. Am J Sports Med. 2010;38(7):1383–8.
50. Gerber C, Fuchs B, Hodler J. The results of repair of massive tears of the rotator cuff. J Bone Joint Surg Am. 2000;82(4):505–15.
51. Bigliani L. The morphology of the acromion and its relationship to rotator cuff tears. Orthop Trans. 1986;10:228.
52. MacDonald P, et al. Arthroscopic rotator cuff repair with and without acromioplasty in the treatment of full-thickness rotator cuff tears. A multicenter, randomized controlled trial. J Bone Joint Surg. 2011;93(21):1953–60.
53. Tashjian RZ. AAOS clinical practice guideline: optimizing the management of rotator cuff problems. J Am Acad Orthop Surg. 2011;19(6):380–3.
54. Pedowitz RA, et al. Optimizing the management of rotator cuff problems. J Am Acad Orthop Surg. 2011;19(6):368–79.
55. Farin PU, et al. Site and size of rotator-cuff tear: findings at ultrasound, double-contrast arthrography, and computed tomography arthrography with surgical correlation. Invest Radiol. 1996;31(7):387–94.
56. Iannotti JP, et al. Accuracy of office-based ultrasonography of the shoulder for the diagnosis of rotator cuff tears. J Bone Joint Surg. 2005;87(6):1305–11.
57. Teefey SA, et al. Detection and quantification of rotator cuff tears. Comparison of ultrasonographic, magnetic resonance imaging, and arthroscopic findings in seventy-one consecutive cases. J Bone Joint Surg. 2004;86(4):708–16.
58. Maman E, et al. Outcome of nonoperative treatment of symptomatic rotator cuff tears monitored by magnetic resonance imaging. J Bone Joint Surg Am. 2009;91(8):1898–906.
59. Kuhn JE, et al. Interobserver agreement in the classification of rotator cuff tears. Am J Sports Med. 2007;35(3):437–41.
60. Patte D. Classification of rotator cuff lesions. Clin Orthop Relat Res. 1990;254:81–6.
61. Itoi E, Tabata S. Conservative treatment of rotator cuff tears. Clin Orthop Relat Res. 1992;275:165–73.
62. Motycka T, Kriegleder B, Landsiedl F. Results of open repair of the rotator cuff–a long-term review of 79 shoulders. Arch Orthop Trauma Surg. 2001;121(3):148–51.
63. Goutallier D, et al. Fatty muscle degeneration in cuff ruptures: pre-and postoperative evaluation by CT scan. Clin Orthop Relat Res. 1994;304:78–83.
64. Coleman SH, et al. Chronic rotator cuff injury and repair model in sheep. J Bone Joint Surg. 2003;85(12):2391–402.
65. Harris JD, Pedroza A, Jones GL. Predictors of pain and function in patients with symptomatic, atraumatic full-thickness rotator cuff tears: a time-zero analysis of a prospective patient cohort enrolled in a structured physical therapy program. Am J Sports Med. 2012;40(2):359–66.
66. Cho NS, Rhee YG. The factors affecting the clinical outcome and integrity of arthroscopically repaired rotator cuff tears of the shoulder. Clin Orthop Surg. 2009;1(2):96–104.
67. Chung SW, et al. Arthroscopic repair of massive rotator cuff tears: outcome and analysis of factors associated with healing failure or poor postoperative function. Am J Sports Med. 2013;41(7):1674–83.
68. Vastamaki M, Lohman M, Borgmastars N. Rotator cuff integrity correlates with clinical and functional results at a minimum 16 years after open repair. Clin Orthop Relat Res. 2013;471(2):554–61.
69. Morrison DS, Frogameni AD, Woodworth P. Non-operative treatment of subacromial impingement syndrome. J Bone Joint Surg Am. 1997;79(5):732–7.
70. Moosmayer S, et al. Comparison between surgery and physiotherapy in the treatment of small and medium-sized tears of the rotator cuff: a randomised controlled study of 103 patients with one-year follow-up. J Bone Joint Surg Br. 2010;92(1):83–91.
71. Dugas JR, et al. Anatomy and dimensions of rotator cuff insertions. J Shoulder Elbow Surg. 2002;11(5):498–503.
72. Weber SC. Arthroscopic debridement and acromioplasty versus mini-open repair in the treatment of significant partial-thickness rotator cuff tears. Arthroscopy. 1999;15(2):126–31.
73. McConville OR, Iannotti JP. Partial-thickness tears of the rotator cuff: evaluation and management. J Am Acad Orthop Surg. 1999;7(1):32–43.
74. Cordasco FA, et al. The partial-thickness rotator cuff tear: is acromioplasty without repair sufficient? Am J Sports Med. 2002;30(2):257–60.
75. Kim KC, et al. Repair integrity and functional outcome after arthroscopic conversion to a full-thickness rotator cuff tear: articular- versus bursal-side partial tears. Am J Sports Med. 2014;42(2):451–6.
76. Abrams J. Partial articular-sided tendon avulsion transtendon rotator cuff repair. In: Abrams J, Bell R, editors. Arthroscopic rotator cuff surgery. New York, NY: Springer; 2008. p. 143–58.

77. Spencer Jr EE. Partial-thickness articular surface rotator cuff tears: an all-inside repair technique. Clin Orthop Relat Res. 2010;468(6):1514–20.
78. Park JY, Yoo MJ, Kim MH. Comparison of surgical outcome between bursal and articular partial thickness rotator cuff tears. Orthopedics. 2003;26(4):387–90. discussion 390.
79. Wolff AB, et al. Partial-thickness rotator cuff tears. J Am Acad Orthop Surg. 2006;14(13):715–25.
80. Reynolds SB, et al. Debridement of small partial-thickness rotator cuff tears in elite overhead throwers. Clin Orthop Relat Res. 2008;466(3):614–21.
81. Dunn WR, et al. Variation in orthopaedic surgeons' perceptions about the indications for rotator cuff surgery. J Bone Joint Surg Am. 2005;87(9):1978–84.
82. Oh LS, et al. Indications for rotator cuff repair: a systematic review. Clin Orthop Relat Res. 2007;455:52–63.

Biologic Augmentation of Rotator Cuff Repair

17

Jon-Michael E. Caldwell, Xinzhi Zhang, Helen H. Lu, and William N. Levine

Introduction

More than 75,000 rotator cuff repairs are conducted annually in the United States with an average total cost of over $10,000 per surgery [1]. The prevailing wisdom in the orthopedic community declares that these patients generally do well and have a high degree of satisfaction with the surgical outcomes. This belief is bolstered by prospective cost-effectiveness studies that demonstrate that while expensive, these procedures provide a significant benefit to a patient's quality of life. However, the literature also demonstrates that rotator cuff tears repaired using the current best practices have a high rate of failure and re-tear, widely reported to be from 20 % to over 90 % [2, 3]. The incongruity between the surgical community's perceptions of high patient satisfaction in the face of high failure rates was recently reexamined. Patients with a failure of their rotator cuff repair are not, in fact, as satisfied with their shoulder function as are patients with intact repairs [4]. This high rate of repair failure in spite of the best techniques available has stimulated the development of biological augmentation devices to improve the long-term durability of rotator cuff repairs.

Many hypotheses exist as to why rotator cuff repairs fail so frequently. From a mechanical point of view, inadequate fixation can lead to failure in achieving a lasting anatomic repair. Studies to optimize mechanical fixation have examined various suture patterns including single- vs. double-row techniques, suture bridges, as well as bone anchoring options ranging from implantable suture anchors to transosseous tunneling [5–7]. Mechanical failure can also result from excessive tension at the repair site. Following injury, the rotator cuff muscles retract to varying degrees, presenting challenges to the surgeon to perform an anatomic repair without undue tension. Inadequate postoperative immobilization can also result in gradual failure of the healing site. Biological factors may prove equally important in determining the success or failure of a rotator cuff repair. The tissue at the repair site is often of poor quality. Injured rotator cuff muscles often undergo rapid fatty atrophy following injury, which greatly compromises tissue quality (Fig. 17.1). Meanwhile, inflammatory cascades are triggered by the surgical procedure, leading to the release of pro-inflammatory cytokines and cellular migration. When healing does occur, these injured tendon stumps form disorganized fibrotic scar tissue that is mechanically inferior to

J.-M.E. Caldwell, MD • W.N. Levine, MD (✉)
Department of Orthopaedic Surgery, New York Presbyterian—Columbia University Medical Center, New York, NY, USA
e-mail: wnl1@columbia.edu

X. Zhang, PhD • H.H. Lu, PhD
Department of Biomedical Engineering, Columbia University, New York, NY, USA

J.D. Kelly IV (ed.), *Elite Techniques in Shoulder Arthroscopy*,
DOI 10.1007/978-3-319-25103-5_17

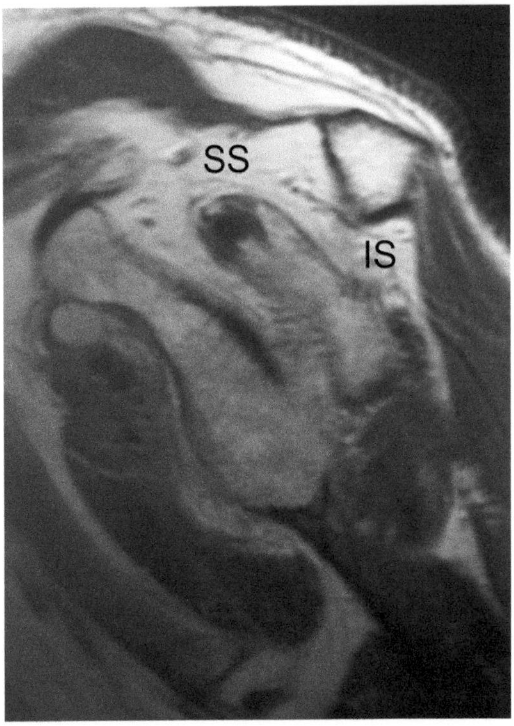

Fig. 17.1 Advanced fatty infiltration of the rotator cuff muscle bellies following rotator cuff tear. *SS* supraspinatus, *IS* infraspinatus (Figure courtesy of Columbia University Center for Shoulder, Elbow and Sports Medicine)

native tissue and fails to anatomically recreate the graduated tendon-bone insertion.

In an effort to address the myriad physical and biologic challenges in performing a durable rotator cuff repair, the orthopedic research community has pursued biologic augmentation strategies. Biological augmentation describes any tissue-based or organic-synthetic device or technique which improves, supports, or directs the native healing response. Different methods of biological augmentation have been proposed ranging from novel arthroscopic techniques and instrumentation to tissue-engineered synthetic and biologic scaffolds, to systemic and local therapy, growth factors, and stem cells. This chapter will examine the principles and evidence supporting the various products that are currently available to the practicing surgeon. Emerging and promising technologies on the immediate horizon will also be discussed.

Regulatory Standards

When evaluating any bioengineered products and techniques, the clinician must be aware of the regulatory standards under which the product is marketed. Most biologic augmentation strategies for the rotator cuff can be divided broadly into cellular-/tissue-based products (e.g., stem cell injections) or synthetic medical devices (e.g., poly(lactic-co-glycolic acid) (PLGA) scaffold). The Food and Drug Administration (FDA) regulates human cell- and tissue-based products (HCT/Ps) under 21 CFR Part 1271 using a tiered risk stratified approach [8, 9]. New products meeting the regulatory definition of "articles containing or consisting of human cells or tissues that are intended for implantation, transplantation, infusion, or transfer into a human recipient" are regulated under FDA Part 361 of the Public Health Service Act (PHSA) if they are determined to be low risk or FDA Part 351 if they are considered high risk. Notably, this regulation applies only to cadaveric or living human donor-derived tissue; it does not extend to xenografts (animal based) or extracted products (e.g., growth factors). To be considered a low-risk biological product, the following four conditions must be met: (1) minimal manipulation during manufacturing, (2) homologous use: the product carries out the same biologic function it normally would, (3) noncombination product: it cannot be combined with any other substance except for simple electrolyte or preservative solutions, and (4) nonsystemic effect or autologous origin: the product must be derived from the intended recipient or a close relative to minimize the risk of an immune reaction [8, 9]. Products meeting these conditions are only required to be manufactured using Current Good Tissue Practice (CGTP) and do not require any formal pre-market review for efficacy or safety. HCT/Ps not meeting the guidelines for Part 361 approval are regulated under the more stringent Part 351. This regulatory pathway encompasses the complex pre-market approval process which requires multiple preclinical studies to establish safety and proof of concept, Investigational New Drug approval leading to regulated clinical trials, and final FDA review of safety and efficacy prior to marketing [8]. Biological augmentations such as platelet-rich plasma (PRP) and human-derived growth factors often fall under the more lenient Part 361. Stem cell therapies including autologous peripherally derived stem cells have recently fallen under increased scrutiny [8, 10]. In a February 2014 decision, the US Court of Appeals in *United States v. Regenerative Sciences, LLC* upheld an earlier district court ruling that autologous stem cells cultured ex vivo and later reintroduced to patients did not meet the Part 361 standard and were subject to full FDA regulation [11].

Similarly to HCT/Ps, devices such as synthetic scaffolds are regulated by the FDA under the Medical Device Amendments of 1976 to the Federal Food, Drug, and Cosmetic Act: 21 CFR 807(E). Devices are classified as Class I, II, or III in a stratified system based on risk potential with a respectively increasing level of regulatory scrutiny. Low-risk devices (Classes I and II), including most rotator cuff repair augmentation devices, are often introduced through the 510(k) process based on the concept of "substantial equivalence" to a "predicate" device already on the market. A device is considered substantially equivalent to an existing product if (1) it has the same intended use and (2) it has the same technological characteristics as the predicate device OR; if it has different technical characteristics, they do not raise new questions of safety and effectiveness and demonstrate equivalence to the predicate [12]. This 510(k) approval process does not require any preclinical proof of efficacy or controlled trials prior to marketing [13, 14]. Class III devices, those with the highest risk or that do not demonstrate substantial equivalence to an existing device, require a full pre-market approval process including preclinical trials, establishment of safety and effectiveness, and controlled human trials prior to FDA approval. Under the current FDA guidelines, most biologic and synthetic augmentations for rotator cuff repair enter the market under the less stringent regulatory bar set forth in Part 361 and 510(k) without a requirement for formal preclinical evaluation establishing safety and efficacy.

Preclinical Evaluation of Biologic Augmentations

The preclinical evaluation of rotator cuff repair augmentations relies on animal models. However, the currently available models of rotator cuff injury all have significant limitations. Ideally, an animal model should (1) mimic the biomechanics of a human shoulder while sharing functional and structural similarities, (2) be large enough to allow appropriate and reproducible surgical techniques, and (3) contain muscles, tendons, and other tissues that exhibit a similar biological response to injury as that seen in the human shoulder (e.g., fatty atrophy of chronically torn cuff muscles) [15]. The general limitations of animal models include different soft tissue and bony anatomy, biomechanics, and injury response in the forelimbs. In many animals, the acromion, clavicle, and coracoid are generally vestigial or nonexistent and do not cover the rotator cuff. Biomechanically, animals are quadrupeds and rely on the rotator cuff to both accelerate a pendular extremity and actively stabilize a weight-bearing shoulder joint. The rotator cuff tendons themselves exhibit a parallel fiber orientation (with the exception of high primates), unlike the interdigitated patterns found in humans [15]. This can lead to decreased suture purchase and compromised pullout strength. In many animals the rotator cuff tendons are extra-articular and are not exposed to the unique milieu of proteins, nutrients, and growth factors that are present in the synovial fluid and can influence healing. Finally, animals form interposed scar following cuff tearing, unlike the persistent gap and fatty atrophy of muscle found in humans with chronic tears.

The rat is one of the most frequently used models in the literature. Unlike other animals, the rat has an overriding coracoacromial arch, a well-documented genome, and readily available reagents for immunohistochemistry. Furthermore, rats tolerate bilateral procedures well and use the forelimb for limited overhead reaching [15]. However, the rat shoulder is small and unsuitable for many clinically relevant repair techniques.

Rats also heal with a robust interposed scar tissue mass bridging the tear to the tuberosity and do not undergo fatty degeneration. Rabbits are less frequently used, and the majority of studies involving them are limited to histological and mechanical studies following supraspinatus detachment. However, recent studies have shown that the torn rabbit subscapularis muscle undergoes fatty infiltration and atrophy while exhibiting some biomechanical resemblance to the torn human supraspinatus complex [16]. Canines have larger shoulders allowing more accurate evaluation of clinically relevant repair techniques. In addition, these animals can tolerate casting, slinging, treadmills, and swimming and have well-established orthopedic rehabilitation protocols in the veterinary literature. However, their status as a companion animal presents ethical and social challenges to research use [17]. Sheep represent the most common large-animal model used in rotator cuff studies. The sheep infraspinatus tendon is similar in size and shape to the human supraspinatus and is readily accessible through a simple surgical approach [18]. This allows accurate reproduction of clinical techniques, the use of standard instrumentation and implants, and evaluation with accepted imaging modalities. However, unlike the human shoulder, the sheep infraspinatus tendon is completely extracapsular, necessitating a capsulotomy if exposure to synovial fluid is desired. Sheep do not have a coracoacromial arch overriding the tendon and are notoriously resistant to postoperative immobilization or reduced weight bearing, leading to almost universal rotator cuff repair failure [19]. Additionally sheep have extremely dense bone and, like other animals, form a fibrous scar in the tendon-bone gap; therefore, this model has many limitations as well [18]. Higher primates (such as the baboon and chimpanzee) have a nearly identical bony and muscular anatomy to humans; however, lower primates (including monkeys) lack the interdigitation of the rotator cuff tendons proximal to their humeral insertion [20]. These animals are immunologically similar to humans and exhibit an analogous healing response [21]. However, high cost and significant ethical considerations limit their use in orthopedic research. Cadaveric human shoulders offer the most accurate physical model, but are obviously limited to time-zero studies.

In conclusion, preclinical models are chiefly used for histological analysis of repair microstructure and biomechanical analysis of the repair construct. Unfortunately, very few studies are able to show consistent results in either realm. The quality of biomechanical testing is technique dependent and varies highly between investigators. Further, the reported metrics are inconsistent in the literature and often of limited clinical relevance. Each preclinical model used to evaluate rotator cuff augmentation devices presents unique strengths and weaknesses; unfortunately, none are ideal.

Biological Augmentation with Scaffolds and Grafts

Scaffolds and grafts have been used to augment rotator cuff repair procedures that involve large defects. These devices seek to improve the physiologic healing response, improve the physical strength of the repair by mechanical reinforcement, or both [13]. To accomplish these goals, rotator cuff scaffolds must have several characteristics: (1) Biocompatibility: the implant must not encourage an inflammatory response over its lifespan and if degradable and must not produce toxic metabolites. A favorable host response in terms of tendon regeneration, recreation of the tendon-bone interface, and formation of a functional muscle-tendon-bone unit should be achieved. (2) Mechanically robust construction: a successful scaffold must be able to both hold sutures securely and endure or transmit any applied forces. This is particularly important for augmentation-style implants which are designed to "off-load" tensile forces from the injured tendon-bone interface. (3) Surgical compatibility: the device should be implantable with reproducible surgical techniques in either an open or arthroscopic approach. The implantation technique should not be overly complex or present additional operative risk to the patient.

Based on the materials used, these grafts can be considered as biologic, synthetic, or a hybrid of both. Most biologic tendon grafts are based on decellularized allogeneic or xenogenic extracellular matrix (ECM) [22–25]. Synthetic grafts are usually made of biocompatible and biodegradable polymers that erode or break down into non-toxic metabolites in the body. Compared to ACL grafts, of which there are currently no FDA-approved commercial products, there are several rotator cuff tendon grafts available on the market. In addition, numerous efforts have been devoted to developing new tendon grafts that aim to improve tendon-bone healing. In the subsequent section, currently commercially available rotator cuff grafts and those promising technologies nearing clinical trials will be reviewed.

Commercially Available Rotator Cuff Grafts

Table 17.1 summarizes commonly used commercialized rotator cuff patches. Most of them are based on biological materials derived from ECM, such as small intestinal submucosa (SIS) and dermis. These patches provide a chemical and 3D structural framework, native matrix composition, and residual remodeling biomolecules that direct repair and remodeling of the rotator cuff tendons by the host cells [13]. However, their clinical use, especially that of SIS, has been in question due to suboptimal outcomes observed in human trials [26, 27]. Several reported adverse outcomes have been attributed to a mismatch in mechanical properties and rapid matrix remodeling inherent in the graft within the demanding and often poor host environment of the shoulder joint. A systematic comparison of four commercially available ECM patches (Restore® of porcine SIS, CuffPatch® of porcine SIS, GraftJacket® of human dermis, and TissueMend® of bovine dermis) was conducted using a canine model [28]. All four patches were inferior mechanically to the native tendon and underwent premature graft resorption. To improve the mechanical properties of rotator cuff patches, synthetic materials have been developed with the goal of providing initial mechanical reinforcement as well as lasting reinforcement over time [13]. One concern with

Table 17.1 Commercially available rotator cuff augmentation grafts

Product	Material	Company
Extracellular matrix grafts		
Restore	SIS (porcine)	Depuy Orthopaedics
CuffPatch	SIS (porcine cross-linked)	Organogenesis
GraftJacket	Dermis (human)	Wright Medical
ArthroFlex	Dermis (human)	Arthrex
Conexa	Dermis (porcine a-Gal-reduced)	Tornier
TissueMend	Dermis (fetal bovine)	Stryker Orthopaedics
Zimmer Collagen Repair	Dermis (porcine cross-linked)	Zimmer
Bio-Blanket	Dermis (bovine cross-linked)	Kensey Nash
OrthADAPT Bioimplant	Pericardium (equine cross-linked)	Pegasus Biologics
Synthetic grafts		
SportMesh Soft Tissue Reinforcement	Poly(urethaneurea)	Biomet Sports Medicine
X-Repair	Poly-L-lactide	Synthasome
Biomerix RCR Patch	Polycarbonate poly(urethaneurea)	Biomerix
Hybrid grafts		
OrthoADAPT PR Bioimplant	Cross-linked equine pericardium with woven polymer	Pegasus Biologics

Reproduced from E. T. Ricchetti, A. Aurora, J. P. Iannotti, and K. A. Derwin, 'Scaffold Devices for Rotator Cuff Repair', *J Shoulder Elbow Surg*, 21 (2012), 251–65, with permission from Elsevier using all-synthetic materials is the risk of an undesirable host response. Two studies have been performed to test such response of synthetic patches in canine and rat models [29, 30]. Results showed that both patches (X-Repair®, made of poly-L-lactide, and Biomerix RCR Patch®, made of polycarbonate polyurethane) showed a biocompatible host cell response with tissue infiltration and minimal inflammation response, indicating the feasibility of using this synthetic material. Hybrid rotator cuff patches are designed with the aim of combining the benefits of both poly-L-lactide and polyurethane. However, very limited data is available for the performance of these scaffolds. Currently, Tornier BioFiber-CM®, a patch made by adding bovine collagen I to poly-4-hydroxybutyrate, is in clinical trials for full-thickness rotator cuff tear repair. Trial completion is expected by June 2015.

Although rotator cuff patches are frequently used in surgery, systematic follow-up studies that evaluate performance of such scaffolds are sparse. Results from the limited number of follow-up studies available demonstrated a mixed performance of commercially available patches. Specifically, for a SIS-based scaffold (Restore®), an early study reported that when compared to preoperative levels, shoulders repaired with the Restore® patch improved in strength, motion, and function with no increased risk in infection at 24 months [31]. However, subsequent studies failed to confirm these findings. In one study, no difference between preoperative and postoperative shoulder scores was observed with use of this product [27]. Another study showed no improvement in the rate of tendon healing or clinical outcome scores compared to repair without the Restore® patch [26]. Walton et al. showed several persisting deficits with no recognizable benefit compared to controls in addition to a severe inflammatory reaction in 20% of the patients [32]. As a result, the authors concluded that SIS-based scaffolds are not recommended for rotator cuff repair [32]. The Zimmer Collagen Repair Patch® also similarly showed inconsistent performance. In one study, four patients underwent rotator cuff repair surgery augmented with this patch. Despite a promising early postoperative period, all grafts failed within 3–6 months after surgery [33]. However; in another study, repairs augmented with this product showed improved pain scores and shoulder movement compared to the preoperative shoulder and an acceptable re-tear rate [34]. Compared to the SIS-based scaffold and Zimmer Collagen Repair Patch®, published results evaluating GraftJacket® (Fig. 17.2) have demonstrated more consistent results. In a prospective, randomized study, patients with a massive rotator cuff tear repaired with GraftJacket® showed improved pain scores and a higher ratio of intact tendon at the 24-month follow-up compared to the patients with shoulders repaired without the graft [35]. In other studies, results demonstrated that augmentation with GraftJacket® led to a lower re-tear rate, improved pain score, and increased shoulder functionality compared to the preoperative condition with no inflammatory response [36–38]. Currently, only one study is available reporting the performance of the synthetic Biomerix RCR Patch®. In this study, patients showed improved pain scores, satisfactory range of shoulder movement at 6 and 12 months, a low re-tear rate (10 %), and no adverse reactions [39].

Even with the limited number of follow-up studies performed, it is clear that despite a wide selection of commercial patches, very limited success has been found in early clinical trials. Surgical outcomes are also associated with other non-patch factors such as age of the patient, size and severity of the tear, and surgical techniques used. Surgeons should keep these factors in mind when evaluating the literature and be cautious when selecting an augmentation graft.

Tendon-Bone Insertion Scaffolds

In the rotator cuff, tendon naturally inserts to the bone through a complex fibrocartilaginous tissue. This insertion can be divided into four zones: tendon, noncalcified and calcified fibrocartilage, and bone. Each zone has distinct cell populations, matrix composition, and mechanical properties. As a result of this controlled heterogeneity, the insertion serves to minimize stress concentration, mediates load transfer, and supports communication of multiple cell types at the tendon-bone interface [40–43]. Therefore, regeneration of this multifaceted structure is an essential quality of a durable tendon graft. However, despite a variety of selections, none of the currently commercially available rotator cuff tendon products are designed for tendon-bone insertion regeneration. Rather, they focus solely on potentiating tendon repair. An augmentation that recaptures the organization of the interface, with region-dependent change in mineral content, will be highly advantageous for tendon-bone repair [44]. One way to control scaffold mineral distribution is to create a gradient of mineral in the patch. In one design, using a novel extrusion system, calcium phosphate nanoparticles were incorporated into polycaprolactone (PCL) nanofibers to create a gradient of mineral distribution across the depth of the PCL scaffold. In vitro analysis showed that when MC3T3 cells were cultured on the scaffold, a gradient of calcified matrix was formed on it within 4 weeks [45]. In another study, using a simulated body fluid immersion method, a calcium phosphate coating was deposited on a layer of gelatin-coated PCL nanofibers in a graded manner. This gradient led to controlled modulation of stiffness across the scaffold, which corresponded to varying mouse MC3T3 cell attachment on the scaffold [46]. However, these scaffold designs are still at a very early stage of development. On the other hand, Moffat et al. designed a composite nanofiber system of a poly(lactic-co-glycolic acid) (PLGA) layer and a PLGA layer

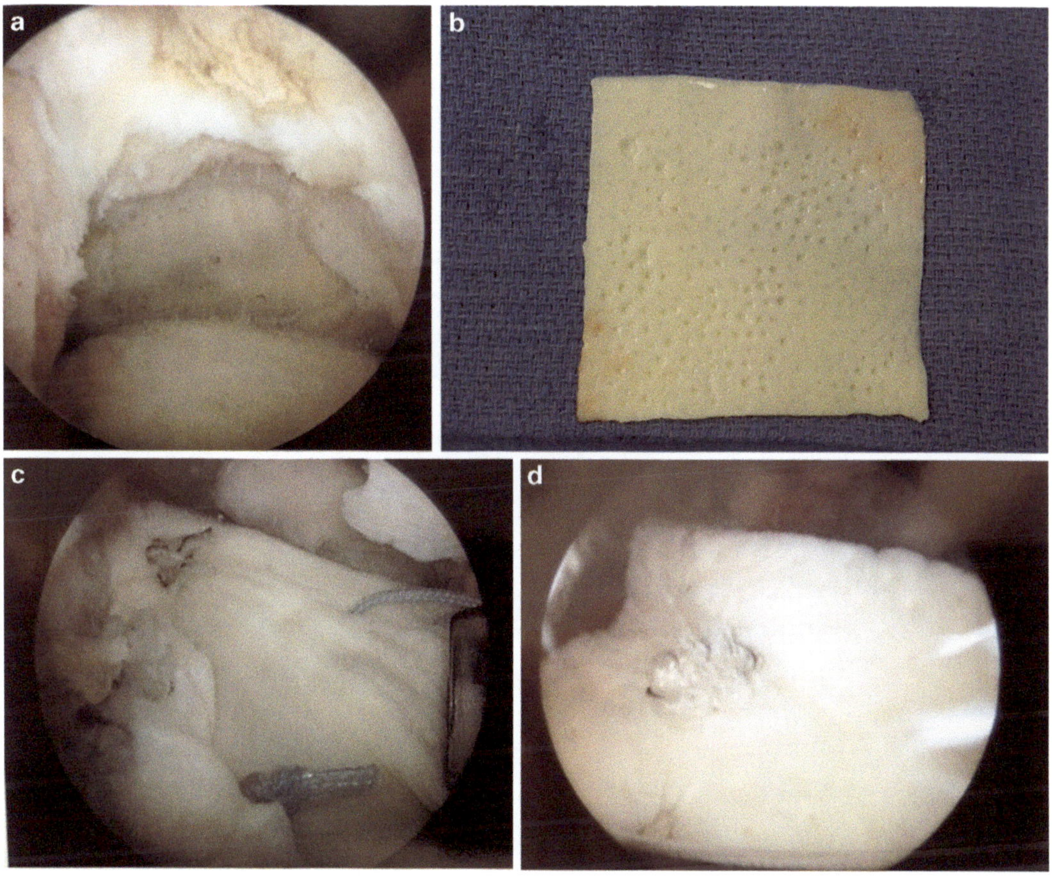

Fig. 17.2 (**a**) Large supraspinatus tear prior to repair. (**b**) GraftJacket (Wright Medical) prior to implantation. (**c**) GraftJacket in situ over defect. (**d**) Completed GraftJacket augmentation [Figure courtesy of Columbia University Center for Shoulder, Elbow, and Sports Medicine (**b**), Dr. John Kelly (**a**, **c**, **d**)]

loaded with hydroxyapatite (HA) nanoparticles aimed at regenerating both the noncalcified and calcified regions of the native insertion [47–49]. When seeded with bovine chondrocytes and cultured in vitro, a continuous layer of noncalcified and calcified fibrocartilaginous tissue was formed on the biphasic scaffold. Following this, a series of in vivo studies were performed to evaluate the function of the biphasic scaffold. First, biocompatibility of the scaffold and osteointegration between PLGA-HA phase and bone was confirmed. Then, the biphasic scaffold was used to repair acute, full-thickness rotator cuff tears in a rat model with results demonstrating that an insertion-like, fibrocartilaginous tissue was indeed formed only in the shoulders using the biphasic scaffold. Lastly, the efficacy of the biphasic scaffold to repair acute, full-thickness rotator cuff tears was confirmed in a sheep model. Collectively, these results demonstrate the potential of the biomimetic, biphasic scaffold for integrative, tendon-bone repair.

In summary, grafts are being clinically used and researched to augment rotator cuff repair. Currently, there are numerous commercially available products. However, caution must be taken when using these scaffolds since their performance may be inconsistent. In addition, none of them are designed specifically to fully reproduce regeneration of the tendon-bone junction, a prerequisite for integrative and truly functional rotator cuff repair. To achieve this, several research groups have been focusing on developing a scaffold that recapitulates the controlled

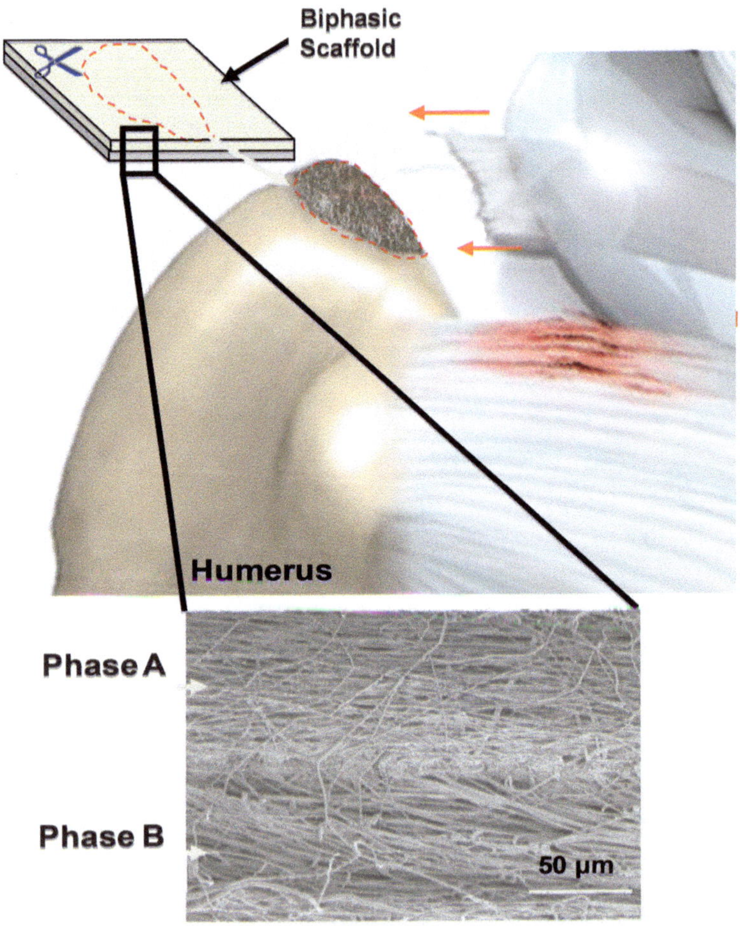

Fig. 17.3 Schematic demonstration a biologic scaffold uses as an inlay between the torn rotator cuff and the greater tuberosity footprint (Figure courtesy of Dr. Helen Lu)

heterogeneity of the tendon-bone insertion, specifically mineral distribution across the scaffold. Currently, a bilayered scaffold that consists of a PLGA layer and a PLGA-HA layer demonstrates a great potential for integrative and functional rotator cuff repair (Fig. 17.3).

Non-scaffold Biologic Augmentations

In addition to grafts, augmentation of rotator cuff repair can be achieved through biological and systemic enhancement. The three main categories of adjunctive therapy are growth factors, stem cells, and systematic interventions. In this section, current approaches in each category will be reviewed, followed by discussion of future directions and promising approaches.

Growth Factors and Cytokines

Tendon healing is a complicated and well-orchestrated process that involves several biological elements, including growth factors. Specifically, at the initial healing phase, transforming growth factor (TGF)-β is upregulated and stimulates cell migration and proliferation within the repair zone [50, 51]. Platelet-derived growth factors (PDGFs) promote expression of other excreted factors such as insulin-like growth factor (IGF)-1, which in turn further enhances the migration and proliferation of cells to the wound site [52, 53]. Basic fibroblast growth factor (bFGF) is also associated with cell proliferation and migration and is expressed by fibroblasts and inflammatory cells [54, 55]. Studies have shown that administration of such growth factors improves healing of tendon lacerations at different stages of tendon healing [56–58]. Up-regulation of the listed growth factors as well as others has been well documented in rotator cuff tendon healing studies performed in different animal models [59, 60]. Human growth hormone (HGH) has also been examined for rotator cuff repair, though the results are inconsistent. Intra-articular injection of GH improved histologic and gross appearance of focal articular cartilage injuries [61, 62]. However, when examined in a rotator cuff model, it did not improve any biomechanical parameter with daily injection and actually had a detrimental effect when dosed twice daily [63].

Augmentation of rotator cuff repair with local or systemic administration of these growth factors is being tested in vivo in a variety of studies, as listed in Table 17.2. In spite of recent advances, rotator cuff repair supplementation with growth factors remains a complicated and controversial process. First of all, in order to improve the retention rate of the growth factor at repair site, a carrier needs to be used. Therefore, in all studies, growth factors are either loaded in sutures or on a biological based matrix that act as a reservoir for sustained growth factor release. Second, the dose of growth factor is critical for the healing process. Local concentrations of the growth factor should be high enough for it to be effective, but if the concentration is too high, it could be detrimental to healing [75, 76]. In addition, healing is achieved through organized expression of a series of sequentially released growth factors, not the isolated action of any single one. Therefore, despite positive results reported in animal models thus far, single growth factor augmented repair has not gain popularity in clinical practice.

Platelet-Rich Plasma

Currently, one of the most common clinically used biologic augmentations is the application of autologous platelet-rich plasma (PRP) or platelet-rich fibrin matrix (PRFM) prepared from the patient's blood. PRP is rich in a mixture of growth factors including the ones mentioned above that are important for tendon healing [51]. PRP is harvested by centrifuging blood at a defined speed to separate it to three layers: the top layer which is platelet-poor plasma, the middle layer which is platelet-rich plasma, and the bottom layer which consists of mostly red blood cells. Currently, there are several commercially available systems for on-site PRP harvesting for use in a variety of

Table 17.2 Animal studies evaluating growth factor augmented rotator cuff repairs

Author	Growth factor	Animal model	Carrier type	Time point	Results
Chen et al. (2011) [64]	BMP-2	Rabbit	Poly(ethylene glycol) diacrylate gel(PEGDA) with BMP-2 tethered PEG gel, mixed with periosteal progenitor cells	4 and 8 weeks	Fibrocartilage formation and higher maximum pullout in BMP-2-loaded group
Seeherman et al. (2008) [65]	BMP-12	Sheep	Collagen and hyaluronic sponges	8 weeks	Accelerated healing with BMP-12
Murray et al. (2007) [66]	BMP-13	Rat	Collagen sponge	2, 3, 4, and 6 weeks	More organized healing and higher mechanical properties at weeks 4 and 6 in BMP-13 loaded group
Gulotta et al. (2010) [67]	BMP-13 transduced mesenchymal stem cells	Rat	Repair with 106 BMP-13 transduced MSCs	2 and 4 weeks	No difference in cartilage formation, collagen fiber orientation and peak stress at failure, stiffness compared to non-transduced MSCs
Dines et al. (2007) [68]	rhBMP-14	Rat	Suture	3 and 6 weeks	Accelerated healing at 3 weeks in rhBMP-14 loaded group
Uggen et al. (2010) [69]	rhPDGF-BB	Sheep, repair at 2 weeks after detachment	Suture	6 weeks	Increase in histology score but not in mechanical properties compared to without rhPDGF-BB
Hee et al. (2011) [70]	rhPDGF-BB	Sheep	Collagen sponge loaded with rhPDGF-BB at 75, 150 and 500 μg	12 weeks	75 and 150 μg showed significant increase in ultimate load and tendon-bone interdigitation compared to control and 500 μg
Ide et al. (2009) [71]	FGF-2	Rat	Acellular dermal matrix	2, 6, and 12 weeks	Accelerated healing with FGF-2
Ide et al. (2009) [72]	FGF-2	Rat	Fibrin sealant with	2, 4, and 6 weeks	Accelerated healing with FGF-2
Manning et al. (2011) [73]	TGF-β3	Rat	Heparin/fibrin	2, 4, and 6 weeks	Increased healing at early time points, increased mechanical properties at 4 and 6 weeks
Kovacevic et al. [74]	TGF-β3	Rat	Ca-P matrix	2 and 4 weeks	Increased tendon strength at week 4, lead to a more physiological COL I/COL III expression ratio

orthopedic applications including rotator cuff repair (Fig. 17.4). Despite the popular use of PRP, to date, results from numerous clinical studies (summarized in Table 17.3) do not provide solid evidence that supports its use. Although animal studies and early clinical studies suggested that PRP improved shoulder performance relative to preinjection levels, more contemporary and well-controlled studies, in which the outcome of repair is compared between shoulders with or without PRP augmentation, showed that PRP did not significantly improve shoulder function or repair integrity. The inconsistency in PRP performance is likely due to several factors. First, the quality of PRP cannot be uniformly ensured. Multiple vendors offer varied systems and protocols for plasma preparation. The potency of the administered PRP depends on the platelet concentration of the sample, which can vary widely among healthy individuals and within a single donor [88, 89]. Thus, the attempt to procure the optimal dose is fraught with difficulty. Second, there is no standardized technique to apply PRP. Suggested protocols have varied between advocating a single percutaneous injection of PRP into a torn tendon, a series of injections around the site of an injury, or as an incorporated component of an augmentation graft. These varied dosing strategies can contribute to substantial differences in performance and make comparing outcomes across studies difficult. Finally, the severity and chronicity of rotator cuff tears vary widely with the ideal candidate for PRP therapy yet to be defined.

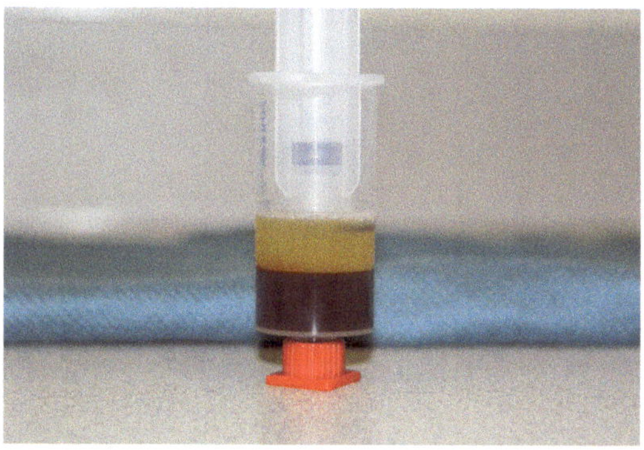

Fig. 17.4 Double-syringe system demonstrating post-centrifuge separation of red blood cells (*bottom layer*) and autologous conditioned plasma (ACP) (*top layer*) (Figure courtesy of Columbia University Center for Shoulder, Elbow and Sports Medicine)

Although both single growth factor-based approaches and PRP show potential for clinical applications in rotator cuff repair, to date, neither strategy has been proven to be effective in well-controlled prospective clinical trials. Surgeons must weigh this paucity of data when considering the use of growth factor augmentation in their clinical practice.

Autologous Mesenchymal Stem Cells

Mesenchymal stem cells have also been investigated as a means to augment tendon healing. The rotator cuff healing process is mediated by cells at the injury site, which include fibroblasts in tendon, fibrochondrocytes at the tendon-bone insertion region, and osteoblasts in the bone region. However, these differentiated cells have limited regenerative capability in adults. To overcome this hurdle, a stem cell-based approach is considered since these cells have unlimited self-renewal and differentiation potentials. Specifically for rotator cuff repair, bone marrow and adipose tissue-derived mesenchymal stem cell (MSCs) are being considered. It has been shown that during arthroscopic rotator cuff repair, bone marrow can be harvested through the anchor tunnel of the humeral head, and MSCs can be isolated from the bone marrow [90]. Furthermore, the ability of MSCs to differentiate into fibroblastic, chondrocytic, and osteocytic lineages has been demonstrated [90–92]. Given this, several animal studies have been performed to test the feasibility of augmenting rotator cuff repair with MSCs in animal models.

Gulotta et al. performed a series of studies using MSCs to repair rotator cuff in a rat model [93–95]. In the first study [93], MSCs were seeded on a fibrin carrier and used for repair. Despite being metabolically active, the addition of MSCs did not improve the structure, composition, or strength of the healing tendon at weeks 2 and 4 post-surgery. This apparent failure was thought to be due to lack of guided differentiation

Table 17.3 Clinical studies evaluating PRP for rotator cuff tears

Author	Method	Follow-up time	Compared to	Results
Maniscalco et al. (2008) [77]	One patient, PRP membrane sutured to close side to side 10 mm tear	6 months	Preoperative shoulder	MRI showed complete integrity of cuff under the membrane
Randelli et al. (2008) [78]	Rotator cuff tear repaired with PRP intraoperatively and with autologous thrombin component	6, 12, and 24 months	Preoperative shoulder	Significant decrease in pain and increase in function scores at all time points No adverse events
Jo et al. (2011) [79]	Rotator cuff tear repaired with PRP applied to a suture during surgery	3, 6, 9, and 12 months	Repair without PRP	A trend of lower re-tear rate (not significantly different) in PRP group
Ruiz-Moneo et al. (2013) [80]	PRP injection and spread over suture at end of surgery	1 year	Repair without PRP	No difference in functional outcome scores, healing rat and patient satisfaction
Castricini et al. (2011) [81]	Small and medium rotator cuff tears. Repaired with PRFM	16 months	Repair without PRFM	No difference in functional outcome score and integrity
Rodeo et al. (2012) [82]	Rotator cuff tear repaired with PRFM during surgery	6 and 12 weeks	Repair without PRFM	No difference in functional outcomes and strength Platelet count has no effects on healing Regression analysis suggests PRFM may have a negative impact
Bergeson et al. (2012) [83]	Rotator cuff tears at risk of re-tear repaired with PRFM	1 year	Repair without PRFM	No difference in functional outcome scores Significant higher re-tear rate in PRFM group Two infections in the PRFM group
Weber et al. (2013) [84]	Rotator cuff repaired with PRFM	1 year	Repair without PRFM	No significant outcome difference
Antuña et al. (2013) [85]	PRF to repair site after surgery	2 years	Repair without PRF	No difference in clinical outcome and healing rate
Rha et al. (2013) [86]	Partial tendon tear, PRP injection at 4-week intervals	6 months after initial injection	Dry needle injection	Increased functional outcome scores in PRP group No severe side effects from PRP
Kesikburun et al. (2013) [87]	Chronic rotator cuff tear, injected with PRP	1 year	Saline injection	No difference in outcome measurement

of the MSCs or retention of cells at injury site. Therefore, in the following two studies, MSCs modified with membrane type 1 matrix metalloproteinase (MT1-MMP), which is upregulated during development of tendon-bone insertion in embryo [94], and MSCs modified with scleraxis (Scx) [95], a gene that is related to tendon development in embryo, were used to augment rotator cuff repairs respectively. Results show that both MT1-MMP- and Scx-transduced MSCs lead to more fibrocartilage production at the tendon-bone insertion and higher mechanical properties at week 4. This finding has also been reported in rabbit models. A recent study showed that addition of MSCs to a polyglycolic acid (PGA) graft enhanced regeneration of both tendon and tendon-bone insertion in terms of more fibrocartilage formation at week 8 and higher mechanical properties at week 16 post surgery compared to the PGA only repair [96]. To date, one clinical study was reported regarding the use of autologous MSCs in rotator cuff repair [97]. In this study, 14 patients with full-thickness rotator cuff tears were repaired with a mini-open procedure, and autologous MSCs were subsequently injected to the surgical site. 1-year follow-up results showed that the procedure was safe and there was an increase in shoulder functional scores compared to preoperative shoulders. Although these initial results look promising, no control groups such as a repair without MSCs were included in the study.

In summary, although MSC-based therapy shows potential to enhance rotator cuff healing, there is presently only limited support in the literature due to the general lack of testing in large-animal models, as well as prospective, comprehensive clinical studies. As a result, considerable research efforts are needed before this technology becomes commonplace in the clinic.

Systemic Treatments

In addition to locally delivered growth factors and stem cells, a variety of systemic agents have been investigated to augment rotator cuff healing. This approach attempts to modulate the physiologic injury response or correct underlying biologic factors that could cause suboptimal healing. Oral doxycycline administration following rotator cuff repair has been shown to decrease matrix metalloproteinase activity in the acute postoperative period leading to enhanced enthesis regeneration while also protecting against *P. acnes* infection—another inhibitor of healing. However, this effect was not sustained past 4 weeks [62, 98, 99]. Preliminary data suggests that systemic administration of atorvastatin inhibits a COX-2-mediated inflammatory mechanism after rotator cuff injury which improves the biomechanical outcomes of repair [100]. Systemic TNF-α inhibition has also been investigated to decrease acute inflammation after cuff injury. This therapy demonstrated mixed success in improving repair load to failure and some histological parameters, but did not sustain these benefits at 8 weeks [101]. Likewise, vitamin D deficiency has been associated with poor collagen fiber organization and decreased bone formation at injury sites in an animal model, though no biomechanical difference was found with controls between 2 and 4 weeks [102].

Biologically Active Repair and Postoperative Care

The surgical technique and instrumentation used to repair a rotator cuff injury can positively influence the biological healing response. Some groups hypothesize that hematogenous or marrow-derived factors improve tendon-bone healing. To this end, techniques employed for increasing exposure of the repair site to these factors have been attempted in the shoulder. Microfracture is a surgical technique commonly used for treating articular cartilage damage in the knee [103]. In one investigation, microfracture of the greater tuberosity performed during the repair of full-thickness rotator cuff tears yielded no significant change on MRI regarding the structural integrity of the repair, but a subgroup analysis demonstrated that patients with large tears involving both the supraspinatus and infraspinatus experienced significantly improved healing with this treatment [104]. Vented suture anchors contain lateral windows in communication with a central cannula to permit blood and marrow contents to communicate with the repair site. Although intriguing, evidence supporting this feature is sparse. Preoperative temporary paralysis of the injured rotator cuff muscles using botulinum toxin has also been proposed to off-load the damaged tendon during recovery. While animal studies have demonstrated improvements in tendon organization and collagen content using botulinum toxin, they have not established biomechanical superiority [105].

Summary and Future Directions

The quest to improve the long-term success rate of rotator cuff repairs has spurred the development of a wide range of biologic augmentation strategies. Scaffolds and grafts have been developed to improve the mechanical integrity of repairs and stimulate healing through a variety of mechanisms. Systemic and locally delivered growth factors, stem cell therapies, and medications have been described to decrease inflammation and encourage regeneration, while surgical techniques have been optimized to maximize the integrity of the repaired tendon. However, the evidence supporting the clinical use of many such products and strategies is limited. The reasons for this paucity of convincing evidence are many. The regulatory standards applied to many of these devices require minimal clinical evidence establishing efficacy. Additionally, the preclinical models for the rotator cuff are imperfect, making accurate and reproducible studies difficult to conduct. As seen in some of the preclinical studies cited in this chapter, improvements in histology do not always correlate with biomechanical improvement. This disparity is due, in part, to the reliance on mechanical testing protocols and instruments which are not designed to evaluate the complexities of biological structures or assess long-term function. It is also due to the high and frequently unpredictable variation between subjects, be they animal or human. In addition, the structure of the tendon-bone insertion is a critical determinant of the biomechanical strength of the rotator cuff. This tendon-bone insertion has limited regenerative capacity, leading to diminished mechanical integrity after injury, even after repair with the current best practices. Although grafts are designed to augment rotator cuff repair, none of the commercially available devices have demonstrated the ability to produce a biomechanically superior, anatomic regeneration of this junction. The facilitation of an integrative rotator cuff repair with biological regeneration of the native enthesis remains the goal pursued by a number of research groups. To date, the most commonly pursued approach is to design a patch that recapitulates the compositional and structural heterogeneities of the native insertion site, which will guide the regeneration of this critical region. In vitro and in vivo studies evaluating these next-generation scaffolds in large-animal models have shown great promise.

Biological augmentation remains one of the most active areas in biomedical and orthopedic research. The current generation of commercially available technologies and those still in development represent exciting potential to solve one of the most frustrating clinical problems in shoulder surgery.

References

1. Vitale MA, Vitale MG, Zivin JG, Braman JP, Bigliani LU, Flatow EL. Rotator cuff repair: an analysis of utility scores and cost-effectiveness. J Shoulder Elbow Surg/Am Shoulder Elbow Surg. 2007;16:181–7.
2. Galatz LM, Ball CM, Teefey SA, Middleton WD, Yamaguchi K. The outcome and repair integrity of completely arthroscopically repaired large and massive rotator cuff tears. J Bone Joint Surg Am. 2004;86-A:219–24.
3. Gazielly DF, Gleyze P, Montagnon C. Functional and anatomical results after rotator cuff repair. Clin Orthop Relat Res. 1994;304:43–53.
4. Kim HM, Caldwell JM, Buza JA, et al. Factors affecting satisfaction and shoulder function in patients with a recurrent rotator cuff tear. J Bone Joint Surg Am. 2014;96:106–12.
5. Quigley RJ, Gupta A, Oh JH, et al. Biomechanical comparison of single-row, double-row, and transosseous-equivalent repair techniques after healing in an animal rotator cuff tear model. J Orthop Res. 2013;31:1254–60.

6. Mall NA, Lee AS, Chahal J, et al. Transosseous-equivalent rotator cuff repair: a systematic review on the biomechanical importance of tying the medial row. Arthrosc Journal Arthrosc Rel Surg. 2013;29:377–86.
7. Salata MJ, Sherman SL, Lin EC, et al. Biomechanical evaluation of transosseous rotator cuff repair: do anchors really matter? Am J Sports Med. 2013;41:283–90.
8. Anz AW, Hackel JG, Nilssen EC, Andrews JR. Application of biologics in the treatment of the rotator cuff, meniscus, cartilage, and osteoarthritis. J Am Acad Orthop Surg. 2014;22:68–79.
9. "361" Human Cells, Tissues, and Cellular and Tissue-Based Products (HCT/Ps). Office of Cellular, Tissue, and Gene Therapies, United States Food and Drug Administration. http://www.fda.gov/downloads/biologicsbloodvaccines/newsevents/UCM251330.ppt. Accessed 25 Mar 2014.
10. Malarkey, MA. Warning Letter to IntelliCell Biosciences, Inc. Letter to Dr. Steven Victor. 13 Mar 2012. Inspections, Compliance, Enforcement, and Criminal Investigations. U.S. Food and Drug Administration, 26 Mar 2012. Web. 27 Oct 2015.
11. United States of America, Appellee v. Regenerative Science, LLC, A Corporation, et al. Appellants No. 12–5254. Appeal from the United States District Court for the District of Columbia. 4 Feb 2014. USCourts.gov, n.d. Web. 27 Oct. 2015.
12. 510(k) Overview. United States Food and Drug Administration; 2011. http://www.fda.gov/downloads/MedicalDevices/ResourcesforYou/Industry/ucm126293.pdf. Accessed 25 Mar 2014.
13. Ricchetti ET, Aurora A, Iannotti JP, Derwin KA. Scaffold devices for rotator cuff repair. J Shoulder Elbow Surg/Am Shoulder Elbow Surg. 2012;21:251–65.
14. De Deyne PG, Dauria RE, Bruder SP. The introduction of an extracellular matrix-based scaffold to the marketplace. J Shoulder Elbow Surg/Am Shoulder Elbow Surg. 2007;16:S164–70.
15. Soslowsky LJ, Carpenter JE, DeBano CM, Banerji I, Moalli MR. Development and use of an animal model for investigations on rotator cuff disease. J Shoulder Elbow Surg/Am Shoulder Elbow Surg. 1996;5:383–92.
16. Gupta R, Lee TQ. Contributions of the different rabbit models to our understanding of rotator cuff pathology. J Shoulder Elbow Surg/Am Shoulder Elbow Surg. 2007;16:S149–57.
17. Derwin KA, Baker AR, Iannotti JP, McCarron JA. Preclinical models for translating regenerative medicine therapies for rotator cuff repair. Tissue Eng Part B Rev. 2010;16:21–30.
18. Turner AS. Experiences with sheep as an animal model for shoulder surgery: strengths and shortcomings. J Shoulder Elbow Surg/Am Shoulder Elbow Surg. 2007;16:S158–63.
19. Lewis CW, Schlegel TF, Hawkins RJ, James SP, Turner AS. The effect of immobilization on rotator cuff healing using modified Mason-Allen stitches: a biomechanical study in sheep. Biomed Sci Instrum. 2001;37:263–8.
20. Sonnabend DH, Young AA. Comparative anatomy of the rotator cuff. J Bone Joint Surg. 2009;91:1632–7.
21. Sonnabend DH, Howlett CR, Young AA. Histological evaluation of repair of the rotator cuff in a primate model. J Bone Joint Surg. 2010;92:586–94.
22. Schlegel TF, Hawkins RJ, Lewis CW, Motta T, Turner AS. The effects of augmentation with Swine small intestine submucosa on tendon healing under tension: histologic and mechanical evaluations in sheep. Am J Sports Med. 2006;34:275–80.
23. Badylak SF. The extracellular matrix as a scaffold for tissue reconstruction. Semin Cell Dev Biol. 2002;13:377–83.
24. Coons DA, Alan Barber F. Tendon graft substitutes-rotator cuff patches. Sports Med Arthrosc Rev. 2006;14:185–90.
25. Dejardin LM, Arnoczky SP, Ewers BJ, Haut RC, Clarke RB. Tissue-engineered rotator cuff tendon using porcine small intestine submucosa. Histologic and mechanical evaluation in dogs. Am J Sports Med. 2001;29:175–84.
26. Iannotti JP, Codsi MJ, Kwon YW, Derwin K, Ciccone J, Brems JJ. Porcine small intestine submucosa augmentation of surgical repair of chronic two-tendon rotator cuff tears. A randomized, controlled trial. J Bone Joint Surg Am. 2006;88:1238–44.
27. Sclamberg SG, Tibone JE, Itamura JM, Kasraeian S. Six-month magnetic resonance imaging follow-up of large and massive rotator cuff repairs reinforced with porcine small intestinal submucosa. J Shoulder Elbow Surg/Am Shoulder Elbow Surg. 2004;13:538–41.
28. Derwin KA, Baker AR, Spragg RK, Leigh DR, Iannotti JP. Commercial extracellular matrix scaffolds for rotator cuff tendon repair. Biomechanical, biochemical, and cellular properties. J Bone Joint Surg Am. 2006;88:2665–72.
29. Derwin KA, Codsi MJ, Milks RA, Baker AR, McCarron JA, Iannotti JP. Rotator cuff repair augmentation in a canine model with use of a woven poly-L-lactide device. J Bone Joint Surg Am. 2009;91:1159–71.
30. Cole BJ, Gomoll AH, Yanke A, et al. Biocompatibility of a polymer patch for rotator cuff repair. Knee Surg Sports Traumatol Arthrosc. 2007;15:632–7.
31. Metcalf MH, Savoie Iii FH, Kellum B. Surgical technique for xenograft (SIS) augmentation of rotator-cuff repairs. Oper Techniques Orthop. 2002;12:204–8.
32. Walton JR, Bowman NK, Khatib Y, Linklater J, Murrell GA. Restore orthobiologic implant: not recommended for augmentation of rotator cuff repairs. J Bone Joint Surg Am. 2007;89:786–91.
33. Soler JA, Gidwani S, Curtis MJ. Early complications from the use of porcine dermal collagen implants (Permacol) as bridging constructs in the repair of

massive rotator cuff tears. A report of 4 cases. Acta Orthop Belg. 2007;73:432–6.
34. Badhe SP, Lawrence TM, Smith FD, Lunn PG. An assessment of porcine dermal xenograft as an augmentation graft in the treatment of extensive rotator cuff tears. J Shoulder Elbow Surg/Am Shoulder Elbow Surg. 2008;17:35S–9.
35. Barber FA, Burns JP, Deutsch A, Labbe MR, Litchfield RB. A prospective, randomized evaluation of acellular human dermal matrix augmentation for arthroscopic rotator cuff repair. Arthrosc J Arthrosc Rel Surg. 2012;28:8–15.
36. Bond JL, Dopirak RM, Higgins J, Burns J, Snyder SJ. Arthroscopic replacement of massive, irreparable rotator cuff tears using a GraftJacket allograft: technique and preliminary results. Arthrosc J Arthrosc Rel Surg. 2008;24:403–9. e1.
37. Wong I, Burns J, Snyder S. Arthroscopic Graft Jacket repair of rotator cuff tears. J Shoulder Elbow Surg/Am Shoulder Elbow Surg. 2010;19:104–9.
38. Burkhead Jr WZ, Schiffern SC, Krishnan SG. Use of Graft Jacket as an augmentation for massive rotator cuff tears. Semin Arthroplasty. 2007;18:11–8.
39. Encalada-Diaz I, Cole BJ, Macgillivray JD, et al. Rotator cuff repair augmentation using a novel polycarbonate polyurethane patch: preliminary results at 12 months' follow-up. J Shoulder Elbow Surg/Am Shoulder Elbow Surg. 2011;20:788–94.
40. Benjamin M, Evans EJ, Copp L. The histology of tendon attachments to bone in man. J Anat. 1986;149:89–100.
41. Cooper RR, Misol S. Tendon and ligament insertion. A light and electron microscopic study. J Bone Joint Surg Am. 1970;52:1–20.
42. Thomopoulos S, Williams GR, Gimbel JA, Favata M, Soslowsky LJ. Variation of biomechanical, structural, and compositional properties along the tendon to bone insertion site. J Orthop Res. 2003;21:413–9.
43. Woo SL, Buckwalter JA. AAOS/NIH/ORS workshop. Injury and repair of the musculoskeletal soft tissues. Savannah, Georgia, June 18–20, 1987. J Orthop Res. 1988;6:907–31.
44. Zhang X, Bogdanowicz D, Erisken C, Lee NM, Lu HH. Biomimetic scaffold design for functional and integrative tendon repair. J Shoulder Elbow Surg/Am Shoulder Elbow Surg. 2012;21:266–77.
45. Erisken C, Kalyon DM, Wang H. Functionally graded electrospun polycaprolactone and beta-tricalcium phosphate nanocomposites for tissue engineering applications. Biomaterials. 2008;29:4065–73.
46. Li X, Xie J, Lipner J, Yuan X, Thomopoulos S, Xia Y. Nanofiber scaffolds with gradations in mineral content for mimicking the tendon-to-bone insertion site. Nano Lett. 2009;9:2763–8.
47. Moffat KL, Cassilly R, Subramony SD, et al. In vivo evaluation of a bi-phasic nanofiber-based scaffold for integrative rotator cuff repair. Proceeding of 56th Annual Meeting of the Orthopaedic Research Society; 2010 Mar 6–9; New Orleans, LA. Accessed 27 Oct 2015.
48. Moffat KL, Zhang X, Greco S, et al. In vitro and in vivo evaluation of a bi-phasic nanofiber scaffold for integrative rotator cuff repair. Proceeding of 57th Annual Meeting of the Orthopaedic Research Society; 2011 Jan 13–16; Long Beach, CA. Accessed 27 Oct 2015.
49. Zhang X, Caldwell J, Easley J, et al. In vivo evaluation of a biomimetic biphasic scaffold in sheep. Proceeding of 60th Annual Meeting of the Orthopaedic Research Society; 2014 Mar 15–18; New Orleans, LA. Accessed 27 Oct 2015.
50. Kashiwagi K, Mochizuki Y, Yasunaga Y, Ishida O, Deie M, Ochi M. Effects of transforming growth factor-beta 1 on the early stages of healing of the Achilles tendon in a rat model. Scand J Plast Reconstr Surg Hand Surg/Nordisk plastikkirurgisk forening [and] Nordisk klubb for handkirurgi. 2004;38:193–7.
51. James R, Kesturu G, Balian G, Chhabra AB. Tendon: biology, biomechanics, repair, growth factors, and evolving treatment options. J Hand Surg. 2008;33:102–12.
52. Kurtz CA, Loebig TG, Anderson DD, DeMeo PJ, Campbell PG. Insulin-like growth factor I accelerates functional recovery from Achilles tendon injury in a rat model. Am J Sports Med. 1999;27:363–9.
53. Tsuzaki M, Brigman BE, Yamamoto J, et al. Insulin-like growth factor-I is expressed by avian flexor tendon cells. J Orthop Res. 2000;18:546–56.
54. Chang J, Most D, Thunder R, Mehrara B, Longaker MT, Lineaweaver WC. Molecular studies in flexor tendon wound healing: the role of basic fibroblast growth factor gene expression. J Hand Surg. 1998;23:1052–8.
55. Khan U, Edwards JC, McGrouther DA. Patterns of cellular activation after tendon injury. J Hand Surg. 1996;21:813–20.
56. Lou J, Tu Y, Burns M, Silva MJ, Manske P. BMP-12 gene transfer augmentation of lacerated tendon repair. J Orthop Res. 2001;19:1199–202.
57. Bolt P, Clerk AN, Luu HH, et al. BMP-14 gene therapy increases tendon tensile strength in a rat model of Achilles tendon injury. J Bone Joint Surg Am. 2007;89:1315–20.
58. Aspenberg P, Forslund C. Enhanced tendon healing with GDF 5 and 6. Acta Orthop Scand. 1999;70:51–4.
59. Wurgler-Hauri CC, Dourte LM, Baradet TC, Williams GR, Soslowsky LJ. Temporal expression of 8 growth factors in tendon-to-bone healing in a rat supraspinatus model. J Shoulder Elbow Surg/Am Shoulder Elbow Surg. 2007;16:S198–203.
60. Kobayashi M, Itoi E, Minagawa H, et al. Expression of growth factors in the early phase of supraspinatus tendon healing in rabbits. J Shoulder Elbow Surg/Am Shoulder Elbow Surg. 2006;15:371–7.

61. Strauss E, Joshi BB, Daher RJ, Dunn AR, Jazrawi LM. Can intraarticular growth hormone improve repair tissue quality after marrow stimulation techniques? AAOS Annual Meeting Proceedings. CD-ROM. Paper No. 183. Rosemont, IL: American Academy of Orthopaedic Surgeons; 2013. p. 933.
62. O'Brien MJ. Update on biologics in the treatment of rotator cuff disease. J Am Acad Orthop Surg. 2013;21:642–3.
63. Baumgarten KM, Oliver HA, Foley J, et al. Human growth hormone may be detrimental when used to accelerate recovery from acute tendon-bone interface injuries. J Bone Joint Surg Am. 2013;95:783–9.
64. Chen C-H, Chang C-H, Wang K-C, et al. Enhancement of rotator cuff tendon–bone healing with injectable periosteum progenitor cells-BMP-2 hydrogel in vivo. Knee Surg Sports Traumatol Arthrosc. 2011;19:1597–607.
65. Seeherman HJ. rhBMP-12 accelerates healing of rotator cuff repairs in a sheep model. J Bone Joint Surg (Am). 2008;90:2206.
66. Murray DH, Kubiak EN, Jazrawi LM, et al. The effect of cartilage-derived morphogenetic protein 2 on initial healing of a rotator cuff defect in a rat model. J Shoulder Elbow Surg. 2007;16:251–4.
67. Gulotta LV, Kovacevic D, Packer JD, Ehteshami JR, Rodeo SA. Adenoviral-mediated gene transfer of human bone morphogenetic protein-13 does not improve rotator cuff healing in a rat model. Am J Sports Med. 2010;39:180–7.
68. Dines JS, Weber L, Razzano P, et al. The effect of growth differentiation factor-5-coated sutures on tendon repair in a rat model. J Shoulder Elbow Surg. 2007;16:S215–21.
69. Uggen C, Dines J, McGarry M, Grande D, Lee T, Limpisvasti O. The effect of recombinant human platelet-derived growth factor BB–coated sutures on rotator cuff healing in a sheep model. Arthrosc J Arthrosc Rel Surg. 2010;26:1456–62.
70. Hee CK, Dines JS, Dines DM, et al. Augmentation of a rotator cuff suture repair using rhPDGF-BB and a type I bovine collagen matrix in an ovine model. Am J Sports Med. 2011;39:1630–9.
71. Ide J, Kikukawa K, Hirose J, Iyama K-I, Sakamoto H, Mizuta H. The effects of fibroblast growth factor-2 on rotator cuff reconstruction with acellular dermal matrix grafts. Arthrosc J Arthrosc Rel Surg. 2009;25:608–16.
72. Ide J, Kikukawa K, Hirose J, et al. The effect of a local application of fibroblast growth factor-2 on tendon-to-bone remodeling in rats with acute injury and repair of the supraspinatus tendon. J Shoulder Elbow Surg. 2009;18:391–8.
73. Manning CN, Kim HM, Sakiyama-Elbert S, Galatz LM, Havlioglu N, Thomopoulos S. Sustained delivery of transforming growth factor beta three enhances tendon-to-bone healing in a rat model. J Orthop Res. 2011;29:1099–105.
74. Kovacevic D, Fox AJ, Bedi A, et al. Calcium-phosphate matrix with or without TGF- 3 improves tendon-bone healing after rotator cuff repair. Am J Sports Med. 2011;39:811–9.
75. Liu X, Kang H, Shahnazari M, et al. A novel mouse model of trauma induced heterotopic ossification. J Orthop Res. 2014;32:183–8.
76. Sand JP, Kokorina NA, Zakharkin SO, Lewis Jr JS, Nussenbaum B. BMP-2 expression correlates with local failure in head and neck squamous cell carcinoma. Otolaryngol Head Neck Surg. 2014;150:245–50.
77. Pietro Maniscalco DG, Lunati A, et al. The "Cascade" membrane: a new PRP device for tendon ruptures. Description and case report on rotator cuff tendon. Acta Biomed. 2008;79:223–6.
78. Randelli PS, Arrigoni P, Cabitza P, Volpi P, Maffulli N. Autologous platelet rich plasma for arthroscopic rotator cuff repair. A pilot study. Disabil Rehabil. 2008;30:1584–9.
79. Jo CH, Kim JE, Yoon KS, et al. Does platelet-rich plasma accelerate recovery after rotator cuff repair? A prospective cohort study. Am J Sports Med. 2011;39:2082–90.
80. Ruiz-Moneo P, Molano-Muñoz J, Prieto E, Algorta J. Plasma rich in growth factors in arthroscopic rotator cuff repair: a randomized, double-blind, controlled clinical trial. Arthrosc J Arthrosc Rel Surg. 2013;29:2–9.
81. Castricini R, Longo UG, De Benedetto M, et al. Platelet-rich plasma augmentation for arthroscopic rotator cuff repair: a randomized controlled trial. Am J Sports Med. 2010;39:258–65.
82. Rodeo SA, Delos D, Williams RJ, Adler RS, Pearle A, Warren RF. The effect of platelet-rich fibrin matrix on rotator cuff tendon healing: a prospective, randomized clinical study. Am J Sports Med. 2012;40:1234–41.
83. Bergeson AG, Tashjian RZ, Greis PE, Crim J, Stoddard GJ, Burks RT. Effects of platelet-rich fibrin matrix on repair integrity of at-risk rotator cuff tears. Am J Sports Med. 2011;40:286–93.
84. Weber SC, Kauffman JI, Parise C, Weber SJ, Katz SD. Platelet-rich fibrin matrix in the management of arthroscopic repair of the rotator cuff: a prospective, randomized, double-blinded study. Am J Sports Med. 2012;41:263–70.
85. Samuel Antuña RB, Martínez Díez JM, et al. Platelet-rich fibrin in arthroscopic repair of massive rotator cuff tears: a prospective randomized pilot clinical trial. Acta Orthop Belg. 2013;79:25–30.
86. Rha DW, Park GY, Kim YK, Kim MT, Lee SC. Comparison of the therapeutic effects of ultrasound-guided platelet-rich plasma injection and dry needling in rotator cuff disease: a randomized controlled trial. Clin Rehabil. 2012;27:113–22.
87. Kesikburun S, Tan AK, Yilmaz B, Yasar E, Yazicioglu K. Platelet-rich plasma injections in the treatment of chronic rotator cuff tendinopathy: a

randomized controlled trial with 1-year follow-up. Am J Sports Med. 2013;41:2609–16.
88. Russell RP, Apostolakos J, Hirose T, Cote MP, Mazzocca AD. Variability of platelet-rich plasma preparations. Sports Med Arthrosc Rev. 2013;21:186–90.
89. Miller CH, Rice AS, Garrett K, Stein SF. Gender, race and diet affect platelet function tests in normal subjects, contributing to a high rate of abnormal results. Br J Haematol. 2014;165:842–53.
90. Mazzocca AD, McCarthy MB, Chowaniec DM, Cote MP, Arciero RA, Drissi H. Rapid isolation of human stem cells (connective tissue progenitor cells) from the proximal humerus during arthroscopic rotator cuff surgery. Am J Sports Med. 2010;38:1438–47.
91. Pittenger MF, Mackay AM, Beck SC, et al. Multilineage potential of adult human mesenchymal stem cells. Science. 1999;284:143–7.
92. Altman GH, Horan RL, Martin I, et al. Cell differentiation by mechanical stress. FASEB J. 2002;16:270–2.
93. Gulotta LV, Kovacevic D, Ehteshami JR, Dagher E, Packer JD, Rodeo SA. Application of bone marrow-derived mesenchymal stem cells in a rotator cuff repair model. Am J Sports Med. 2009;37:2126–33.
94. Gulotta LV, Kovacevic D, Montgomery S, Ehteshami JR, Packer JD, Rodeo SA. Stem cells genetically modified with the developmental gene MT1-MMP improve regeneration of the supraspinatus tendon-to-bone insertion site. Am J Sports Med. 2010;38:1429–37.
95. Gulotta LV, Kovacevic D, Packer JD, Deng XH, Rodeo SA. Bone marrow-derived mesenchymal stem cells transduced with scleraxis improve rotator cuff healing in a rat model. Am J Sports Med. 2011;39:1282–9.
96. Yokoya S, Mochizuki Y, Natsu K, Omae H, Nagata Y, Ochi M. Rotator cuff regeneration using a bioabsorbable material with bone marrow-derived mesenchymal stem cells in a rabbit model. Am J Sports Med. 2012;40:1259–68.
97. Ellera Gomes JL, da Silva RC, Silla LM, Abreu MR, Pellanda R. Conventional rotator cuff repair complemented by the aid of mononuclear autologous stem cells. Knee Surg Sports Traumatol Arthrosc. 2012;20:373–7.
98. Bedi A, Fox AJ, Kovacevic D, Deng XH, Warren RF, Rodeo SA. Doxycycline-mediated inhibition of matrix metalloproteinases improves healing after rotator cuff repair. Am J Sports Med. 2010;38:308–17.
99. Bedi A, Kovacevic D, Hettrich C, et al. The effect of matrix metalloproteinase inhibition on tendon-to-bone healing in a rotator cuff repair model. J Shoulder Elbow Surg/Am Shoulder Elbow Surg. 2010;19:384–91.
100. Chechik O, Dolkart O, Alhajajra FY, Gigi R, Mozes G, Maman E. Atorvastatin increases the biomechanical strength of the repaired rotator cuff by the cyclo-oxygenase-2 mechanism. AAOS Annual Meeting Proceedings. CD-ROM. Paper No. 310. Rosemont, IL: American Academy of Orthopaedic Surgeons; 2013. p. 774–775.
101. Gulotta LV, Kovacevic D, Cordasco F, Rodeo SA. Evaluation of tumor necrosis factor alpha blockade on early tendon-to-bone healing in a rat rotator cuff repair model. Arthrosc J Arthrosc Rel Surg. 2011;27:1351–7.
102. Angeline ME, Ma R, Pascual-Garrido C, et al. Effect of diet-induced vitamin D deficiency on rotator cuff healing in a rat model. Am J Sports Med. 2014;42:27–34.
103. Redler LH, Caldwell JM, Schulz BM, Levine WN. Management of articular cartilage defects of the knee. Phys Sportsmed. 2012;40:20–35.
104. Milano G, Saccomanno MF, Careri S, Taccardo G, De Vitis R, Fabbriciani C. Efficacy of marrow-stimulating technique in arthroscopic rotator cuff repair: a prospective randomized study. Arthrosc J Arthrosc Rel Surg. 2013;29:802–10.
105. Ficklscherer A, Hartl TK, Scharf M, et al. Effects of selective paralysis of the supraspinatus muscle using botulinum neurotoxin a in rotator cuff healing in rats. J Orthop Res. 2013;31:716–23.

18 Indications and Techniques for Double-Row Fixation

Lauren Wessel, Joshua Sykes, Jason B. Anari, and David Glaser

Introduction

Rotator cuff tears are among the most common problems treated in the medical profession. Each year, approximately 200,000 Americans require shoulder surgery related to repair of the rotator cuff, and an additional 400,000 Americans have surgery for related rotator cuff tendonitis or for partial tears [1]. The annual volume of procedures is increasing rapidly with the aging of the population, as rotator cuff tears are reported to have a prevalence of 22 % in those aged 65 years or over [2]. The vast majority of these tears are chronic in nature due to degenerative changes. Thus, with increasing longevity and larger proportions of an aged populace, tear incidence is expected to markedly increase. Improvements in surgical technique and instrumentation have made arthroscopic repair commonplace, largely eliminating open and mini-open approaches to the rotator cuff [3–5]. Arthroscopic repair provides a minimally invasive means of addressing pain, motion limitations, and quality of life. However, retear rates are still substantial, being reported within a broad range, but in a published recent meta-analysis average 21.7 % [6].

Anatomy and Biomechanics of the Rotator Cuff

The rotator cuff footprint is comprised of the insertions of the supraspinatus, infraspinatus, teres minor, and subscapularis tendons on the greater and lesser tuberosities. Multiple anatomic studies have been performed in efforts to define the dimensions of these insertions and variations in dimensions are largely attributable to patient size and body habitus. Knowledge of insertion dimensions is critical in order to achieve anatomic rotator cuff repairs. Curtis et al. measured and found average maximum insertion lengths and widths in 20 cadaver specimens finding that the subscapularis insertion measured 40 mm × 20 mm, supraspinatus 23 mm × 16 mm, infraspinatus 29 mm × 19 mm, and teres minor 29 mm × 21 mm [7]. Similarly, Mochizuki et al. studied the insertion dimensions of the rotator cuff in study included 113 shoulders from 64 cadavers and found that the supraspinatus insertion was much smaller than previously believed and that much of the area of insertion on the greater tuberosity is in fact occupied by the insertion of the infraspinatus tendon [8] (Table 18.1).

L. Wessel, BS
Department of Orthopaedic Surgery, Washington University in St. Louis, Houston, TX, USA

J. Sykes, MD (✉) • J.B. Anari, MD • D. Glaser, MD
Department of Orthopaedic Surgery, University of Pennsylvania, Philadelphia, PA, USA
e-mail: sykes.josh@gmail.com

J.D. Kelly IV (ed.), *Elite Techniques in Shoulder Arthroscopy*, DOI 10.1007/978-3-319-25103-5_18

Table 18.1 Rotator cuff tendon anatomy [8]

Tendon	Anatomic landmark	Dimensions (mm)
Supraspinatus	Maximum medial-to-lateral length	6.9±1.4
	Anteroposterior width of medial margin	12.6±2.0
	Anteroposterior width of lateral margin	1.3±1.4
Infraspinatus	Maximum medial-to-lateral length	10.2±1.6
	Anteroposterior width of medial margin	20.2±6.2
	Anteroposterior width of lateral margin	32.7±3.4
Articular capsule	Medial-to-lateral length at posterior edge of the supraspinatus footprint	4.5±0.5

The rotator cuff serves as a dynamic stabilizer for the glenohumeral joint and dynamically compresses the head of the humerus into the glenoid socket. Study of individual tendon origins and insertions highlights rotator cuff vectors of force and predicts individual tendon function. The subscapularis internally rotates the humeral head in relation to the scapula. The infraspinatus and teres minor externally rotate the humerus. The primary function of the supraspinatus is to initiate the first 30° of forward elevation and assist the deltoid in the first 90° of abduction. In addition, it serves as a humeral head compressor. The supraspinatus also plays a role in rotation. From a neutral or externally rotated starting position, the supraspinatus externally rotates the humerus, and when starting from a position of internal rotation, the supraspinatus internally rotates the humeral head [9, 10]. It has been hypothesized that interaction between cuff regions may explain why some patients retain strength after partial rotator cuff tears [10]. Restoration of the anterior and posterior force couple may adequately restore the centering force of the rotator cuff and provide a stable fulcrum for glenohumeral motion. Some studies have demonstrated that partial repair of the posterior portion of an irreparable two-tendon tear may restore function to a cuff-deficient shoulder [11]. Rotator cuff repair surgery aims to alleviate symptoms and reestablish rotator cuff function.

The enthesal sites of insertion are composed of specialized fibrocartilaginous tissue, which serve to minimize stress concentrations at the tendon-bone interface [12]. The enthesis is composed of well-organized zones of tissue, including the tendon proper, fibrocartilage, mineralized fibrocartilage, and bone [13]. Interruption of the enthesis does not spontaneously heal after initial injury, and these zones of interface are not histologically preserved after rotator cuff repair. Thus, structural integrity is compromised, and healing proceeds with disorganization and decreased strength as compared to the native rotator cuff construct [13]. Several studies have documented a correlation between symptomatic and functional results of rotator cuff repair and quality of healing [14–23]. As such, a robust repair that allows for anatomic healing is the primary goal of rotator cuff repair, and techniques to maximize tendon healing are of great interest for their potential to improve clinical outcomes.

History of Rotator Cuff Repair

Traditionally, both open and arthroscopic rotator cuff repairs were performed using a single row of suture anchors. The suture anchors are traditionally placed linearly along the anterior to posterior aspect of the greater tuberosity. Investigators have attempted to correlate the integrity of these repairs with postoperative function with varying results [24–27]. Outcomes after repair have been hypothesized to be related to biomechanical strength, contact area, implant failure, and suturing pattern. Concerns over the adequacy of the strength of single-row techniques have motivated the development of new repair approaches. One such development has been double-row fixation, which better restores the anatomic footprint of the rotator cuff and provides a biomechanically stronger construct compared to single-row repair [28]. This represents a major advancement in arthroscopic technique, incorporating a linear row of anchors placed medially at the articular margin and a second row along the lateral aspect of the rotator cuff footprint on the tuberosity [29–31].

Repair Failures

Individual rotator cuff tears vary greatly in their configuration and prognosis. Clinical outcomes are reported as good to excellent in only about 85 % of repairs [24, 32–35] and are worse with increasing preoperative tear size and poorer tissue quality [22, 23, 25, 28, 36–38]. Gerber et al. hypothesized that initial fixation strength and minimal gap formation upon stress would improve rates of healing for rotator cuff repair [39]. Tendon-bone healing has been a much-debated topic of recent research investigations. Studies have demonstrated that the degree of rotator cuff atrophy and fatty infiltration, quality of repair, and postoperative restoration of shoulder flexibility and strength have all proven to be important determinants of the ultimate success of rotator cuff repair [25–27, 40, 41]. Reasons for failure can be roughly grouped into four categories: technical, biologic, mechanical, and anatomic.

Increased surgeon comfort with arthroscopy and improvements in suture material, anchor, and arthroscopic technology have reduced concern for technical causes of rotator cuff repair failure such as suture anchor failure [42]. Additionally, recent studies have demonstrated that functional results after arthroscopic repair versus those after open or mini-open repair are equivalent, and patients report less postoperative pain and increased satisfaction with this method [5, 35, 43–49]. In addition, technical advances have fostered improvement in fixation via suture anchor design. As stronger suture materials have been introduced, constructs have greatly surpassed previously achieved biomechanical strength parameters and have shown impressive healing rates after arthroscopic rotator cuff repair [50].

Biologic failures are those related to tendon-bone healing. These failure modalities are often highly dependent on the individual patient and can be attributable to factors such as age, smoking status, history of corticosteroid injection, diabetes, vascular disease, or tear chronicity, resulting in fatty atrophy of muscle [51]. Of these factors, age appears to be the leading biological determinant regarding success or failure of rotator cuff repair. Tashjian et al. reported that of 49 repairs, only 51 % were healed by examination on ultrasound 6 months postoperatively, with age at surgery and longer duration of follow-up being significantly associated with lower healing rates after rotator cuff repair [52]. Intrinsic patient factors such as tobacco use have been less well established by the literature, with conflicting findings reported in various publications. For example, animal studies have demonstrated nicotine's effect in delay of tendon-to-bone healing; however, these effects have not been consistently confirmed clinically [53–56].

Mechanical failures are related to the inability of the repair to overcome the exertional force placed upon the repaired tendon. The rotator cuff endures significant mechanical forces with shoulder motion and loading. Forces on the cuff muscles differ according to position during loading. The durability of cuff repair is dependent on repaired tendons to maintain integrity in the setting of forces applied across the glenohumeral joint. Specifically, most tears originate at the junction between the supraspinatus and infraspinatus tendons, roughly 13–17 mm posterior to the biceps tendon [57], and force vectors applied across these tendons will cause differential relative stress across the tendons. The supraspinatus experiences maximal loading in a position of internal rotation and abduction [58]. Conversely, the infraspinatus experiences maximum force in a position of external rotation and adduction [58]. Finally, anterior cuff tears are less common and result in tears to the subscapularis tendon, which endures relatively high forces in both internal rotation with abduction and adduction [58]. Given differential tendon loading, some surgeons advise tailored postoperative rehabilitation protocols based on tear size and location, though there is no definitive study on the effectiveness of this strategy and more research is required to advise these strategies. In general, however, it is known that early motion and loading may compromise tendon-bone healing. A study by Lee et al. demonstrated that aggressive early passive rehabilitation was associated with retear rate more than twice that of limited passive rehabilitation [59].

Anatomical failures are related to inability to restore the native insertional footprint of the rotator cuff or failure to restore resting tension of the tendons. Apreleva et al. introduced the concept of the anatomical footprint of the rotator cuff [60], and, since, multiple studies have sought to develop techniques to improve upon the restoration of repair site insertion. It is hypothesized that superior restoration of the native footprint of the rotator cuff fosters improved healing of the tendinous insertion, as the footprint is thought of as the maximum two-dimensional healing zone [61]. Repairs that do not restore the cuff footprint endure greater force across the repaired site and suture anchors and may predispose these repairs to higher failure rates [31].

Double-row repair, while mechanically advantageous, may present unique problems. Unlike the typical modes of leading edge failure related to rotator cuff repair in general, double-row cuff repairs appear to present a previously unreported mode of failure. Trantalis et al. reported this unique failure pattern in patients who underwent double-row rotator cuff repair in a subset of five patients. In these patients footprint repair appeared to be well fixed to the greater tuberosity with normal thickness. However, on arthroscopic examination, each of these patients incurred a full-thickness tendon tear medial to the intact footprint [62]. Such failures have been hypothesized to be related to tension overload of the suture-tendon interface at the medial repair site. This mechanism of loading has been supported by Mazzocca et al., who demonstrated that cyclic loading of a double-row repair first resulted in failure of the medial site by mattress sutures pulling through the tendon medial to the repair site [63]. Similar findings were reported in a case report by Yamakado et al. in which the authors found tendon avulsion at the medial row with concomitant exposure of knots on the bony surface of the rotator cuff footprint [64]. The authors hypothesize that the requirement of pulling the tendon more laterally for double-row repair results in a relatively high tensile stress compare to single-row repair [65]. In spite of these reports, double-row rotator cuff repair appears to be successful and further studies are required to evaluate the long-term impact of medial row stress on repair as well as the incidence of failures.

Rationale for Double-Row Rotator Cuff Repair

Double-row rotator cuff repair has been hypothesized to result in superior fixation for a number of reasons including increased restoration of the rotator cuff footprint, increased mechanical strength and contact pressure, as well as decreased gap formation across the repair.

Restoration of Rotator Cuff Footprint

Success of rotator cuff repair is dependent on tendon-to-bone healing. Tendon healing is initiated by the development of fibrovascular tissue interface [66]. Woven bone formation begins at the bone-tendon interface, eventually resulting in collagen fiber continuity between tendon and bone [67]. Aoki et al. demonstrated that an increase in available healing surface at the bone-tendon junction increased the potential for bone-to-tendon healing and formation of such a collagenous interface. Thus, repairs with greater coverage of the native footprint of the rotator cuff theoretically offer greater healing potential than those that do not provide as much interface, with the footprint being described as the maximum two-dimensional healing zone.

Meier et al. utilized three-dimensional mapping to determine the area of the footprint recreated with transosseous simple suture technique, fixation with a single row of suture anchors, and double-row suture anchor technique fixation. This study demonstrated that double-row suture anchor fixation consistently reproduced 100 % of the original supraspinatus footprint. In contrast, single-row suture anchor fixation and transosseous simple suture techniques reproduced only 46 % and 71 % of the insertion site, respectively [68]. Brady et al. demonstrated similar results, finding that after an isolated lateral-row repair, 52.7 ± 9.2 % of the rotator cuff footprint remains uncovered, and, on average, the double-row repair offered over twice the footprint coverage yielded by a single-row repair [69]. Thus, double-row fixation may provide a tendon-bone interface better suited for biologic healing and restoration of normal anatomy.

Mechanical Strength

In biomechanical studies of the initial mechanical strength of rotator cuff repair, double-row repair has proven to have superior strength as compared to single-row repair. In a study by Meier and Meier, the authors studied repair strength in 30 fresh-frozen cadaveric shoulders with full-thickness supraspinatus tears; the authors found that the fixation strength of the double-row repair suture anchor technique proved to be significantly greater than that of single-row suture anchor repair or transosseous technique. Samples were subjected to cyclic load testing from 5 N to 180 N at a rate of 33 mm/s until complete failure or a total of 5000 cycles. The transosseous repair group failed at an average of 75.3 ± 22.49 cycles, single-row repairs failed at an average of 798.3 ± 73.28 cycles, and the double-row suture anchor repair group had no failures because all samples were stopped when 5000 cycles had been completed [68]. Thus, both the increased footprint apposition and increased strength afforded by double-row constructs minimize gap formation during cyclic loading.

Contact Area and Pressure

In addition to the establishment of the native footprint of the rotator cuff, contact pressure is an important factor in the establishment of native cuff dynamics. Tuoheti et al. studied full-thickness cuff tears treated with transosseous, single-row, and double-row repairs in ten cadaveric specimens and determined that contact area of the double-row technique was 42 % greater than that of the transosseous technique and 60 % greater than that of the single-row technique. Moreover, the average pressures of the single-row and double-row techniques were 18 % and 16 % greater, respectively, than that of the transosseous technique. There was no demonstrated significant difference between contact pressure in the single-row and double-row techniques [70]. In the study of time zero contact pressure over the rotator cuff footprint in an established sheep model, Baums et al. investigated contact pressure across rotator cuff repair sites in 40 fresh-frozen shoulders, demonstrating that contact pressure was lowest for single-row repair and for simple stitch configurations. Double-row repair and arthroscopic Mason-Allen/horizontal mattress stitches significantly increased repair contact pressure [71]. Park et al. demonstrated that a transosseous-equivalent (TOE) rotator cuff repair via tendon suture bridges improves pressurized contact between the tendon and tuberosity when compared with a double-row technique [72]. These results support the use of double-row repair, more complex arthroscopic Mason-Allen stitches, and suture bridging techniques in the setting of a complex tear requiring additional aid in healing. Such techniques may improve the environment for healing of the repaired rotator cuff tendons and should be weighed against the risk of potential increased tension, tissue strangulation, and devascularization that TOE configurations may confer.

Gap Formation

As alluded to above, the minimization of gap formation is another key factor in the restoration of the anatomical configuration and mechanical performance of tendon-bone insertion to sufficiently sustain loading associated with functional activity. In a study by Smith et al., the investigators found that gap formation during *static* loading was significantly greater in the single-row group than in the double-row group [73]. Under *cyclic* loading gap formation was not found to be significantly different between groups; however, double-row repairs endured significantly greater loading forces prior to failure [73]. Thus, double-row repair reconstruction may provide a more reliable construct with superior resistance to gap formation and greater loading prior to failure. The early postoperative period is a critical phase prior to healing, during which time the load transfer from tendon to bone is entirely carried through the means of the repair construct. Thus, it is reasonable to presume that if a repair is predisposed to increased gap formation, this would be detrimental for appropriate healing as tendon-bone contact would be reduced. This is of particular concern in the setting of constant postoperative static loading with the patient's arm held in a sling.

Repair Techniques

A number of techniques are available to the shoulder surgeon in order to execute the repair appropriate for any given patient. Among these, the workhorse repairs include simple single- and double-row repairs and can be additionally augmented by suture linking techniques as well as TOE repair.

Single-Row Repair

The single-row technique involves repair of a rotator cuff tear with a single row of medial anchors. Different types of anchors are available with variation in size, screw thread pattern, material, number of preloaded sutures, and type of fixation. These properties all result in variation in strength of fixation. Vented anchors are now available, which are hypothesized to cause migration of bone marrow elements to the repair site through the holes of the anchor (Fig. 18.1).

Double-Row Repair

The double-row technique implies two rows of anchors: a medial row and a lateral row. Similar to single-row repair, this technique may include the use of suture anchor with a broad variation in properties. Additionally, these repairs vary in configuration of suture anchor placement (Fig. 18.2).

Linked Double-Row Repair

Linked double-row repair represent a variation in double-row repair. This technique links the medial and lateral rows by passing limbs of suture from medial to lateral row, thus creating a crisscross suture configuration, ensuring large contact area and contact pressure at the bone-tendon interface (Fig. 18.3).

Anchorless and Transosseous-Equivalent Double-Row Repair

Anchorless repairs have been introduced in order to improve upon current cuff repair options. This technique involves the creation of two converging bone tunnels: one where medial anchors are generally placed and one where lateral anchors are placed in parallel line. With this system, it is possible to perform a transosseous technique in a reproducible fashion. This novel technique combines the clinical advantages of minimally invasive arthroscopic surgery and the biomechanical advantages of open transosseous procedures [74]. The TOE repair involves the creation of a medial row of suture anchors that utilize mattress repairs and lateral fixation points, roughly 1-cm distal-lateral to the lateral edge of the tuberosity footprint insertion. After the medial row is repaired, the suture limbs are then used to create suture bridges over the tendon [72].

TOE anchorless repair has controversial supporting data. The repair was developed in order to maximize the utility of a single-row repair technique by preserving the suture limbs of the medial single-row and bridging these sutures over the footprint insertion with distal-lateral interference screw suture fixation [72]. The geometry of the construct is thought to compress the tendon, optimizing tendon-to-tuberosity contact dimensions while additionally providing appropriate repair strength to withstand forces placed on the rotator cuff. In a study by Park et al., transosseous rotator cuff repair technique was shown to restore greater anatomic footprint contact and provide greater ultimate strength, compared with a double-row repair technique [75, 76]. A follow-up study by Salata et al. compared TOE repair to a curved bone tunnel and with a repair technique utilizing a simple or *X-box* suture configuration. TOE resulted in superior contact area, pressure, and failure rates compared to non-bridging double-row repair [72, 77].

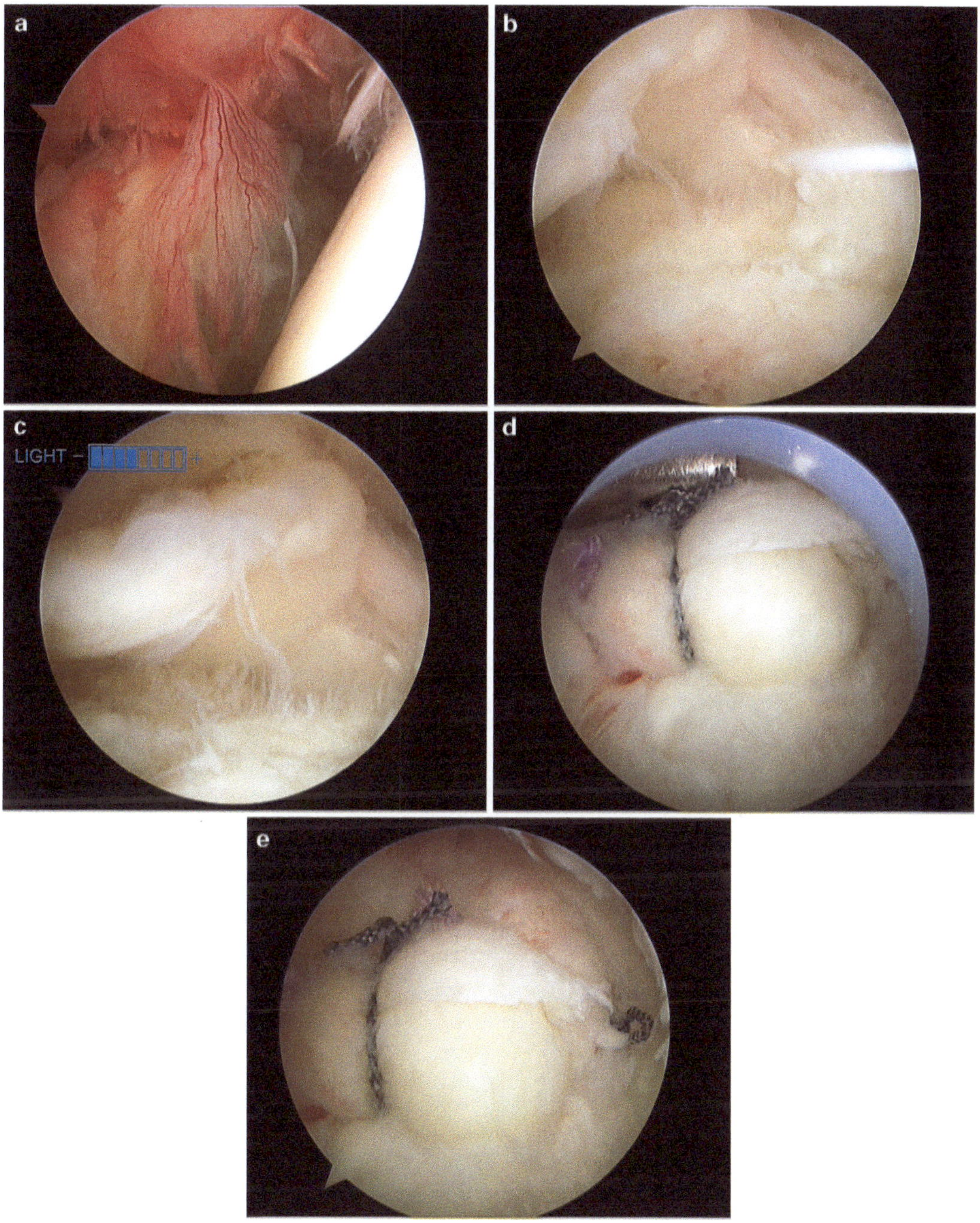

Fig. 18.1 Single-row rotator cuff repair, performed in this case secondary to significant synovitis and concern for postoperative stiffness. (**a**) Beach chair position, right arm, viewing from posterior portal demonstrating extensive synovitis. (**b** and **c**) Beach chair position, subacromial space of right shoulder demonstrating rotator cuff tear. (**d** and **e**) Viewing from lateral portal, repaired rotator cuff with single row

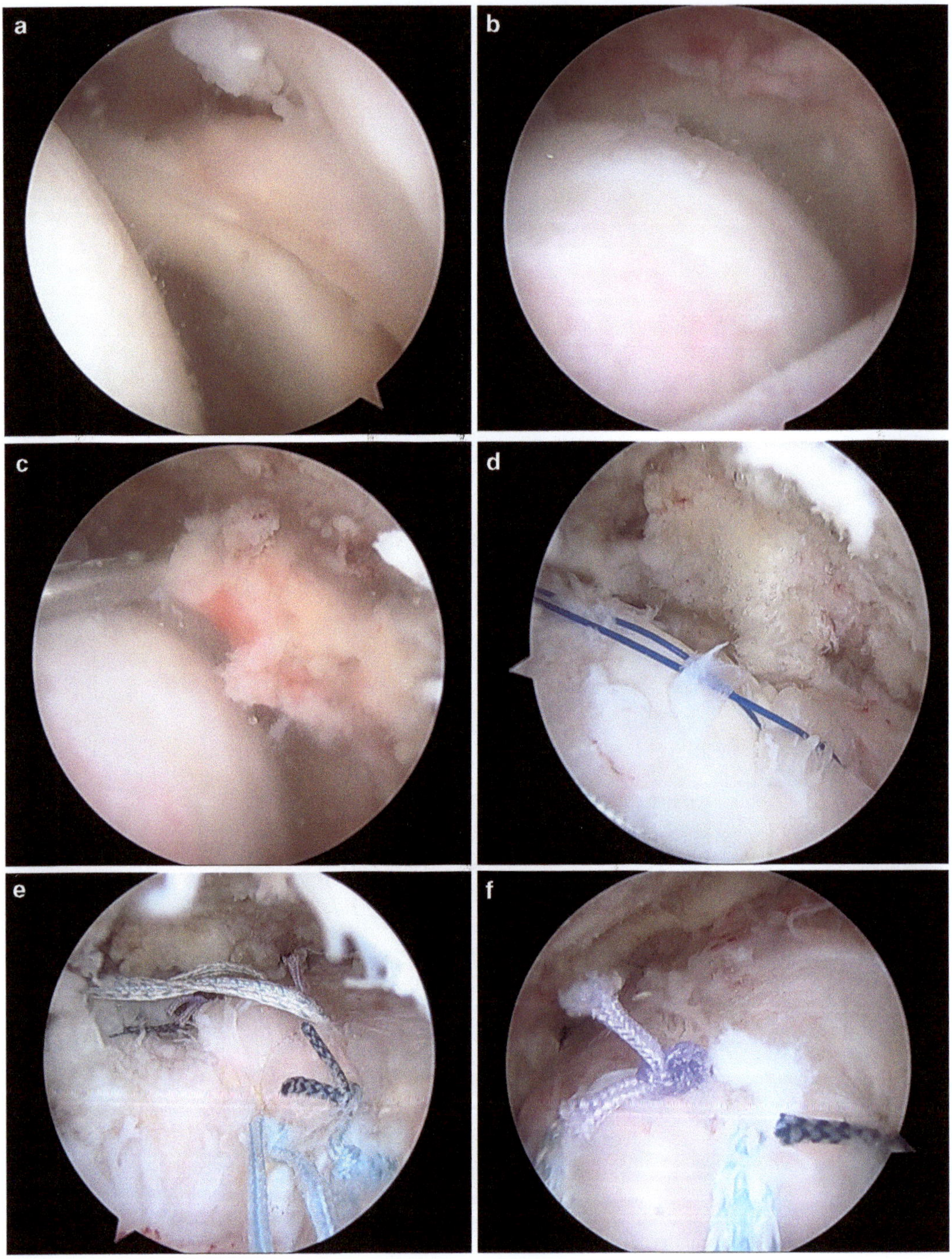

Fig. 18.2 Single-row rotator cuff repair with a tension relaxing stitch to a lateral-row anchor performed because the repair was felt to be under high tension after a single-row repair. (**a** and **b**) Beach chair position viewing from posterior, left shoulder, showing retraction of rotator cuff to glenoid. (**c** and **d**) Viewing from posterior demonstrating difficulty to mobilize cuff to footprint using arthroscopic grasper and a traction suture. (**e–h**) Repair completed with single-row technique in "**e**" and then additional sutures that were passed through the rotator cuff in a horizontal mattress fashion were taken to lateral-row anchors to take tension off of the medial row repair

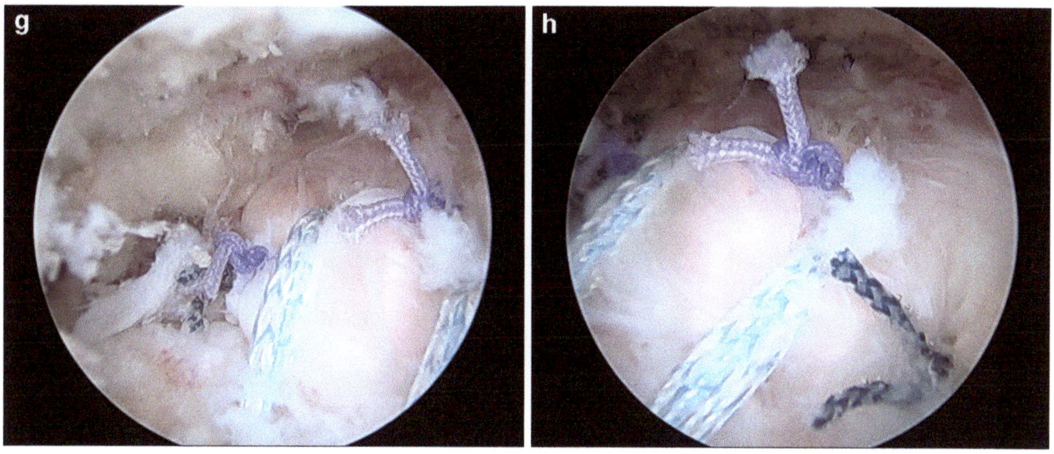

Fig. 18.2 (continued)

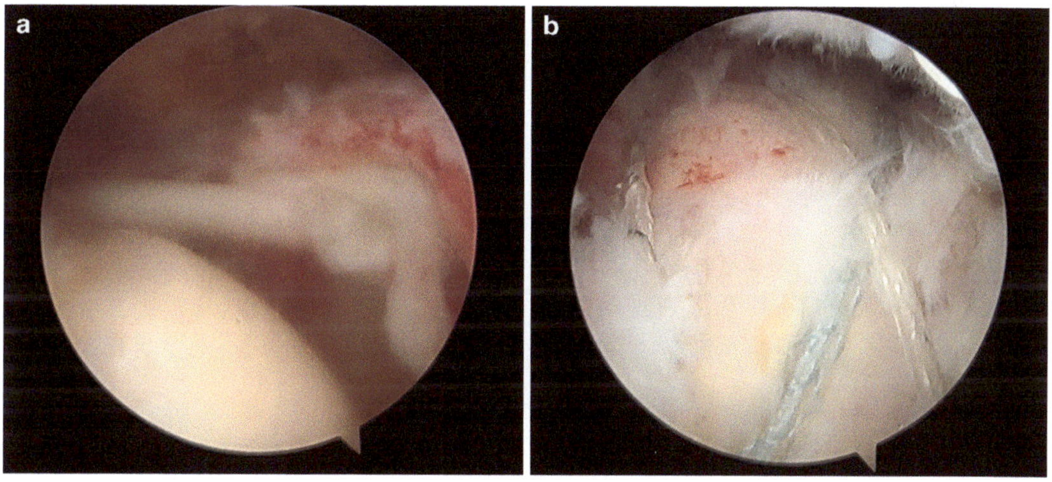

Fig. 18.3 Double-row rotator cuff repair performed in this case as the tendon was easily mobilized to the footprint, and there was no sign of synovitis or arthritis on diagnostic arthroscopy of the glenohumeral joint. (**a**) Beach chair position, left shoulder, viewing from posterior demonstrating a rotator cuff tear retracted almost to the level of the glenoid, which mobilized easily to the footprint when traction was applied. (**b**) Completed double-row repair viewing from a lateral portal

Clinical Outcomes

Clinical outcomes of single- and double-row rotator cuff repair have borne out to be roughly equivalent. Multiple studies have investigated the effects of double-row repair with various outcomes scores and have failed to delineate differences in clinical outcomes based on the repair technique; however, in a study by Parks et al., the authors delineated groups based on preoperative tear size and found an improved functional outcomes scores with double-row fixation for large or massive tears (>3 cm), suggesting that double-row repair configurations may have a clinically relevant role in the treatment of large to massive cuff tears [78]. A meta-analysis by Millet et al. also suggested that stratification of tear size suggests superiority of double-row repair in treatment of large rotator cuff tears [79]. This investigation additionally suggested that longer-term

Table 18.2 Single versus double-row outcomes [80]

Study	Intervention	*N*	Population difference	Tear length (sagittal plane)	Mean follow-up (months)	Outcomes	Relevant findings
Gartsman et al. (2013)	SR versus DR retear rate	83 (40 SR, 43 DR)	Included any repairable full-thickness tear; excluded smokers, steroid users, bilateral cuff repairs, suprascapular nerve decompressions	SR: <2.5 cm DR: <2.5 cm	SR: N/R DR: N/R Mean: 10 (6–12)	*Subjective*: N/R *Objective*: N/R *Imaging*: US	DR had significantly decreased retear rate (7 %) compared with SR (25 %) (P=0.024)
Carbonel et al. (2012)	SR versus DR; clinical outcome and retear rate	160 (80 SR, 80 DR)	Excluded OA, tears >5 cm, Fuchs >4, steroid users	SR 1–3 cm: 51 SR 3–5 cm: 29 DR 1–3 cm: 53 DR 3–5 cm: 27	SR: 24 DR: 24 MRI SR: 24 MRI DR: 24	*Subjective*: ASES, UCLA, constant *Objective*: physical examination, SSI, ROM in degrees *Imaging*: MRI	DR significantly improved over SR in 1- to 3-cm tears with respect to degrees of flexion and abduction, internal rotation SSI, and external rotation SSI; DR significantly improved over SR with respect to all measured variables in 3- to 5-cm tears except for Constant score, abduction SSI, and external rotation SSI
Lapner et al. (2012)	SR versus DR; clinical outcome and retear rate	80 (40 SR, 40 DR)	Included any full-thickness tear; excluded SSx <6 months, GFDI >3, ACH distance <7 mm	SR: mean 1.89 cm DR: mean 2.38 cm	SR: 24 DR: 24 MRI SR: 24 MRI DR: 24	*Subjective*: ASES, WORC, constant *Objective*: strength (kg) *Imaging*: MRI/US	DR had significantly decreased retear rate; smaller coronal tear sizes resulted in improved healing rate; patients with retears had larger initial tear sizes; those with retears had significantly decreased strength
Koh et al. (2011)	SR versus DR; clinical outcome and retear rate	71 (37 SR, 34 DR)	Included OA, smokers; excluded those without complete footprint coverage on postoperative MRI	SR: mean 1.72 cm DR: mean 1.75 cm (all tears 2–4 cm in sagittal oblique or coronal oblique plane)	SR: 31.0 DR: 32.8 MRI SR: 27.4 MRI DR: 27.6	*Subjective*: ASES, UCLA, VAS *Objective*: ROM (FF, IR, ER) in degrees *Imaging*: MRI	DR showed improvement over SR with respect to internal rotation capacity (approaches statistical significance; P=0.53); no other clinical or radiographic differences between DR and SR groups reported
Burks et al. (2009)	SR versus DR; clinical outcome and retear rate	40 (20 SR, 20 DR)	Excluded smokers, steroid users, U tears, and workers' compensation; included OA	SR 1–3 cm: 18 SR >3 cm: 2 DR 1–3 cm: 15 DR >3 cm: 5	SR: 12 DR: 12	*Subjective*: ASES, UCLA, constant, SANE, WORC *Objective*: ROM, strength (IR/ER in N-m) *Imaging*: MRI	No differences in clinical or radiographic outcomes between SR and DR

Grasso et al. (2009)	SR versus DR; clinical outcome	80 (40 SR, 40 DR)	Excluded OA, AC arthritis, workers' compensation, very small or very large tears	SR: mean 1.56 cm DR: mean 1.61 cm	SR: N/R DR: N/R Mean: 24.8	*Subjective*: DASH, WorkDASH, constant *Objective*: strength (lbs) *Imaging*: N/R	No difference in clinical outcomes between SR and DR
Franceschi et al. (2007)	SR versus DR; clinical outcome and retear rate	60 (30 SR, 30 DR)	Included SSx 3 months, OA; excluded tendon retraction, SSx instability	SR 3–5 cm: 18 SR >5 cm: 8 DR 3–5 cm: 21 DR >5 cm: 5	SR: N/R DR: N/R Mean: 22.5 MRA: N/R	*Subjective*: UCLA *Objective*: FF, ER, IR (in degrees) *Imaging*: MRA	No differences in clinical or radiographic outcomes between SR and DR

studies might be necessary to delineate clinical effects of repair method as the progression to full-thickness retear may be more commonly seen in single-row repairs and be correlated with poorer clinical outcomes [79] (Table 18.2). Given these results, it is reasonable to consider tear size and patient age in consideration of approach to rotator cuff repair, though larger-sized and longer-term clinical trials are required to better understand the implications of repair in these patients.

Pearls and Pitfalls for Double-Row Rotator Cuff Repair

Rotator cuff repair is a relatively successful operation commonly performed by shoulder surgeons. Successful repair results in decreased pain and improved shoulder function for the patient. Success of repair is dependent on a number of factors including patient age, tissue quality, repair technique and integrity, as well as postoperative therapy. The choice of surgical technique is nuanced and patient and tear factors should be carefully considered in operative planning. To this end, a general set of guidelines is useful for consideration.

Tear Size

As stated, tear size is an important factor related to prognosis of rotator cuff repair and utility of repair method. Rate of rotator cuff tear recurrence have been associated with increasing tear size [22, 81, 82]. A 2012 level I study by Carbonel et al. demonstrated that patients with tears measuring between 3 and 5 cm had improved subjective and objective results following double-row repair as compared to single-row repair after 2-year follow-up [83]. Park et al. also found clinically superior results in repairs of larger tears with double-row repair, though no significant difference was noted when all tears were included in analysis [78]. In a prospective randomized level II study, Ma et al. demonstrated that tears with >3 cm in sagittal length had increased strength when repaired with double-row repair as compared to single-row repair [84]. Similarly, Lorbach et al. found that increased initial tear size was an independent predictor of inferior mechanical properties after repair of rotator cuff repair [85]. These results suggest that the generalized finding of equivalent clinical outcomes between double- and single-row repairs may be related to the inability to detect clinical difference in groups with mixed tear sizes and that subgroup analysis should be studied further. With these findings in mind, we suggest that acute tears >3 cm should be repaired with double-row repair technique.

Tendon Retraction

Mobility of tendon ends of the rotator cuff prerepair contributes to the likelihood of failure of repair due to overtensioning of the repair site and failure at the muscle-tendon junction, which can be catastrophic. Overtensioning raises concern for medial row failure. Hersche and Gerber demonstrated that active force generation by the supraspinatus muscle will be compromised after surgery and that the high strain after repair may expose the musculotendinous unit to further damage [86]. Such phenomena have borne out clinically as reported in case series of medial row failures in double-row repair, which primarily occurs at the musculotendinous junction. Furthermore, the remnant tendon needs to be of sufficient length to allow for a double-row repair. In a recent study by Kim et al., the single-row repair technique was demonstrated to provide superior rotator cuff integrity with remnant tendons <10 mm in length [87]. Thus, it is of the authors' opinion that in the setting of a chronic tear with preoperative tendon retraction >3 cm or remnant tendon length <10 mm, a double-row cuff will have an increased likelihood of failure due to greater likelihood of medial row failure. This is general guideline to guide treatment, however, and each tear should be treated with consideration of the intraoperative ease of cuff mobilization to cover the footprint—if the surgeon is unable to easily mobilize the cuff and perform margin convergence, then a single-row repair will likely be the better option.

Preoperative Arthritis

Glenohumeral osteoarthritis decreases the likelihood of cuff tear given decreased motion at the glenohumeral joint; however, the two pathologies are not mutually exclusive. At primary arthroscopic examination, Gartsman et al. reported minor glenohumeral cartilage abnormality in 8.5 % and major abnormality in 4.5 % of patients with partial thickness cuff tears [88]. It has been suggested that patients with evidence of arthritis and other intra-articular pathology might have an increased rate of stiffness or failure after rotator cuff repair. Kukkonen et al. demonstrated that patients with glenohumeral osteoarthritis treated with rotator cuff repairs have lower pre- and postoperative functional scores as compared to those without glenohumeral osteoarthritis [89]. Though there is limited data investigating a cohort of patients with glenohumeral osteoarthritis in addition to rotator cuff pathology, there is a notably increased incidence of glenohumeral osteoarthritis in patients undergoing revision rotator cuff repair. In a study of revision rotator cuff surgeries, Piasecki et al. reported glenohumeral arthritis visible on radiograph in 18.5 % of patients [90]. This finding supports the prevailing belief that rotator cuff repair in such patients more frequently leads to further surgeries such as revision rotator cuff repair or reverse total shoulder arthroplasty. As such, it is of the authors' opinion that these patients may not benefit from a double-row rotator cuff repair and that, should these patients be treated with primary cuff repair, it should be a single-row repair as this preserves options for revision surgery and is less likely to introduce additional shoulder stiffness.

Conclusion

Rotator cuff repair is a relatively successful operation regardless of repair technique. Double-row rotator cuff repair has shown to have greater biomechanical integrity with regard to restoration of anatomic footprint, mechanical strength, contact area, and pressure as well as gap formation. However, clinical studies have not yet demonstrated a conclusive benefit from double-row repair. Current studies have not adequately delineated preoperative tear size with regard to effect on outcome of rotator cuff repair, which may be of greater importance with larger-sized lesions. Additionally, lack of evidence regarding techniques is due to relative novelty of these approaches. Further research will be required to clearly delineate indications and contraindications for double-row rotator cuff repair.

Given the current evidence, the surgeon must look at the overall patient picture in order to make an effective evaluation regarding the most appropriate repair type. For example, factors that have controversial evidence such as preoperative tear size, osteoarthritis, and tendon retraction should cause the shoulder surgeon to critically think through the costs and benefits of double-row repair. Increased time and cost of performing double-row repair should be carefully considered in such cases in order to ensure appropriate intervention.

References

1. Yamaguchi K. New guideline on rotator cuff problems; 2011. http://www.aaos.org/news/aaosnow/jan11/cover1.asp
2. Fehringer EV, Sun J, VanOeveren LS, Keller BK, Matsen FA. Full-thickness rotator cuff tear prevalence and correlation with function and co-morbidities in patients sixty-five years and older. J Shoulder Elbow Surg. 2008;17(6):881–5.
3. Kim S-H, Ha K-I, Park J-H, Kang J-S, Oh S-K, Oh I. Arthroscopic versus mini-open salvage repair of the rotator cuff tear: outcome analysis at 2 to 6 years' follow-up. Arthroscopy. 2003;19(7):746–54.
4. Severud EL, Ruotolo C, Abbott DD, Nottage WM. All-arthroscopic versus mini-open rotator cuff repair: a long-term retrospective outcome comparison. Arthroscopy. 2003;19(3):234–8.
5. Wilson F, Hinov V, Adams G. Arthroscopic repair of full-thickness tears of the rotator cuff. Arthroscopy. 2002;18(2):136–44.
6. Russell RD, Knight JR, Mulligan E, Khazzam MS. Structural integrity after rotator cuff repair does not correlate with patient function and pain: a meta-analysis. J Bone Joint Surg Am. 2014;96-A(4):265–71.
7. Curtis AS, Burbank KM, Tierney JJ, Scheller AD, Curran AR. The insertional footprint of the rotator cuff: an anatomic study. Arthroscopy. 2006;22(6):603–9.
8. Mochizuki T, Sugaya H, Uomizu M, et al. Humeral insertion of the supraspinatus and infraspinatus. New anatomical findings regarding the footprint of the rotator cuff. J Bone Joint Surg Am. 2008;90(5):962–9.

9. Ihashi K, Matsushita N, Yagi R, Handa Y. Rotational action of the supraspinatus muscle on the shoulder joint. J Electromyogr Kinesiol. 1998;8(5):337–46.
10. Langenderfer JE, Patthanacharoenphon C, Carpenter JE, Hughes RE. Variation in external rotation moment arms among subregions of supraspinatus, infraspinatus, and teres minor muscles. J Orthop Res. 2006; 24(8):1737–44.
11. Hsu J, Reuther K, Sarver J, et al. Restoration of anterior-posterior rotator cuff force balance improves shoulder function in a rat model of chronic massive tears. J Orthop Res. 2011;29(7):1028–33.
12. Thomopoulos S, Williams GR, Gimbel JA, Favata M, Soslowsky LJ. Variation of biomechanical, structural, and compositional properties along the tendon to bone insertion site. J Orthop Res. 2003;21(3):413–9.
13. Benjamin M, Kumai T, Boszczyk A, Ralphs J. The skeletal attachment of tendons—tendon "entheses.". Comp Biochem Physiol A Mol Integr Physiol. 2002; 133(4):931–45.
14. Anderson K, Boothby M, Aschenbrener D, van Holsbeeck M. Outcome and structural integrity after arthroscopic rotator cuff repair using 2 rows of fixation: minimum 2-year follow-up. Am J Sports Med. 2006;34(12):1899–905.
15. Cole BJ, McCarty LP, Kang RW, Alford W, Lewis PB, Hayden JK. Arthroscopic rotator cuff repair: prospective functional outcome and repair integrity at minimum 2-year follow-up. J Shoulder Elbow Surg. 2007; 16(5):579–85.
16. Flurin P-H, Landreau P, Gregory T, et al. Cuff integrity after arthroscopic rotator cuff repair: correlation with clinical results in 576 cases. Arthroscopy. 2007;23(4):340–6.
17. Huijsmans PE, Pritchard MP, Berghs BM, van Rooyen KS, Wallace AL, de Beer JF. Arthroscopic rotator cuff repair with double-row fixation. J Bone Joint Surg Am. 2007;89(6):1248–57.
18. Lafosse L, Brzoska R, Toussaint B, Gobezie R. The outcome and structural integrity of arthroscopic rotator cuff repair with use of the double-row suture anchor technique. J Bone Joint Surg Am. 2008;90(Supp 2, Part 2):275–86.
19. Lichtenberg S, Liem D, Magosch P, Habermeyer P. Influence of tendon healing after arthroscopic rotator cuff repair on clinical outcome using single-row Mason-Allen suture technique: a prospective, MRI controlled study. Knee Surg Sports Traumatol Arthrosc. 2006;14(11):1200–6.
20. Liem D, Bartl C, Lichtenberg S, Magosch P, Habermeyer P. Clinical outcome and tendon integrity of arthroscopic versus mini-open supraspinatus tendon repair: a magnetic resonance imaging–controlled matched-pair analysis. Arthroscopy. 2007;23(5):514–21.
21. Liem D, Lichtenberg S, Magosch P, Habermeyer P. Magnetic resonance imaging of arthroscopic supraspinatus tendon repair. J Bone Joint Surg Am. 2007;89(8):1770–6.
22. Sugaya H, Maeda K, Matsuki K, Moriishi J. Repair integrity and functional outcome after arthroscopic double-row rotator cuff repair. J Bone Joint Surg Am. 2007;89(5):953–60.
23. Thomazeau H, Boukobza E, Morcet N, Chaperon J, Frantz L. Prediction of rotator cuff repair results by magnetic resonance imaging. Clin Orthop Relat Res. 1997;344:275–83.
24. Baker CL, Liu SH. Comparison of open and arthroscopically assisted rotator cuff repairs. Am J Sports Med. 1995;23(1):99–104.
25. Galatz LM, Ball CB, Teefey SA, Middleton WD, Yamaguchi K. The outcome and repair integrity of completely arthroscopically repaired large and massive rotator cuff tears. J Bone Joint Surg Am. 2004;86(2):219–24.
26. Liu SH, Baker CL. Arthroscopically assisted rotator cuff repair: correlation of functional results with integrity of the cuff. Arthroscopy. 1994;10(1):54–60.
27. Harryman DT, Mack LA, Wang KY, Jackins SE, Richardson ML, Matsen FA. Repairs of the rotator cuff: correlation of functional results with integrity of the cuff. J Bone Joint Surg Am. 1991;73(7):982–9.
28. Sugaya H, Maeda K, Matsuki K, Moriishi J. Functional and structural outcome after arthroscopic full-thickness rotator cuff repair: single-row versus dual-row fixation. Arthroscopy. 2005;21(11):1307–16.
29. Fealy S, Kingham TP, Altchek DW. Mini-open rotator cuff repair using a two-row fixation technique. Arthroscopy. 2002;18(6):665–70.
30. Waltrip R, Zheng N, Dugas J, Andrews J. Rotator cuff repair. A biomechanical comparison of three techniques. Am J Sports Med. 2003;31(4):493–7.
31. Lo IK, Burkhart SS. Double-row arthroscopic rotator cuff repair: re-establishing the footprint of the rotator cuff. Arthroscopy. 2003;19(9):1035–42.
32. Blevins F, Hayes W, Warren R. Rotator cuff injury in contact athletes. Am J Sports Med. 1996;24(3):263–7.
33. Paulos L, Kody M. Arthroscopically enhanced "miniapproach" to rotator cuff repair. Am J Sports Med. 1994;22(1):19–25.
34. Posada A, Uribe JW, Hechtman KS, Tjin-A-Tsoi EW, Zvijac JE. Mini-deltoid splitting rotator cuff repair: do results deteriorate with time? Arthroscopy. 2000; 16(2):137–41.
35. Tauro J. Arthroscopic rotator cuff repair: analysis of technique and results at 2- and 3-year follow-up. Arthroscopy. 1998;14(1):45–51.
36. Boileau P, Brassart N, Watkinson DJ, Carles M, Hatzidakis A, Krishnan SG. Arthroscopic repair of full-thickness tears of the supraspinatus: does the tendon really heal? J Bone Joint Surg Am. 2005;87(6): 1229–40.
37. Gazielly D, Gleyze P, Montagnon C. Functional and anatomical results after rotator cuff repair. Clin Orthop Relat Res. 1994;304:43–53.
38. Gerber C, Fuchs B, Hodler J. The results of repair of massive tears of the rotator cuff. J Bone Joint Surg Am. 2000;82(4):505–15.
39. Gerber C, Schneeberger AG, Beck M, Schlegel U. Mechanical strength of repairs of the rotator cuff. J Bone Joint Surg Br. 1994;76-B(3):371–80.

40. Gore D, Murray M, Sepic S, Gardner G. Shoulder-muscle strength and range of motion following surgical repair of full-thickness rotator-cuff tears. J Bone Joint Surg Am. 1986;68(2):266–72.
41. Mansat P, Cofield RH, Kersten TE, Rowland CM. Complications of rotator cuff repair. Orthop Clin North Am. 1997;28(2):205–13.
42. Ma R, Chow R, Choi L, Diduch D. Arthroscopic rotator cuff repair: suture anchor properties, modes of failure and technical considerations. Expert Rev Med Devices. 2011;8(3):377–87.
43. Gartsmann GM, Khan M, Hammerman SM. Arthroscopic repair of full-thickness tears of the rotator cuff. J Bone Joint Surg Am. 1998;80(6): 832–40.
44. Burkhart SS, Tehrany AM. Arthroscopic subscapularis tendon repair. Arthroscopy. 2002;18(5):454–63.
45. Murray TF, Lajtai G, Mileski RM, Snyder SJ. Arthroscopic repair of medium to large full-thickness rotator cuff tears: outcome at 2- to 6-year follow-up. J Shoulder Elbow Surg. 2002;11(1):19–24.
46. Bennett WF. Arthroscopic repair of massive rotator cuff tears: a prospective cohort with 2- to 4-year follow-up. Arthroscopy. 2003;19(4):380–90.
47. Bennett WF. Arthroscopic repair of full-thickness supraspinatus tears (small to-medium): a prospective study with 2- to 4-year follow-up. Arthroscopy. 2003; 19(3):249–56.
48. Jones CK, Savoie FH. Arthroscopic repair of large and massive rotator cuff tears. Arthroscopy. 2003;19(6):564–71.
49. Youm T, Murray DH, Kubiak EN, Rokito AS, Zuckerman JD. Arthroscopic versus mini-open rotator cuff repair: a comparison of clinical outcomes and patient satisfaction. J Shoulder Elbow Surg. 2005; 14(5):455–9.
50. Denard PD, Burkhart SS. The evolution of suture anchors in arthroscopic rotator cuff repair. Arthroscopy. 2013;29(9):1589–95.
51. Rudzki JR, Adler RS, Warren RF, et al. Contrast-enhanced ultrasound characterization of the vascularity of the rotator cuff tendon: age- and activity-related changes in the intact asymptomatic rotator cuff. J Shoulder Elbow Surg. 2008;17:96S–100.
52. Tashjian R, Hollins A, Kim H, et al. Factors affecting healing rates after arthroscopic double-row rotator cuff repair. Am J Sports Med. 2010;38(12):2435–42.
53. Baumgarten KM, Gerlach D, Galatz LM, et al. Cigarette smoking increases the risk for rotator cuff tears. Clin Orthop Relat Res. 2010;468(6):1534–41.
54. Nho SJ, Brown BS, Lyman S, Adler RS, Altchek DW, MacGillivary JD. Prospective analysis of arthroscopic rotator cuff repair: prognostic factors affecting clinical and ultrasound outcome. J Shoulder Elbow Surg. 2009;18(1):13–20.
55. Galatz L, Silva M, Rothermich M, Zaegel M, Havlioglu N, Thomopoulos S. Nicotine delays tendon-to-bone healing in a rat shoulder model. J Bone Joint Surg Am. 2006;88(9):2027–34.
56. Prasad N, Odumala A, Elias F, Jenkins T. Outcome of open rotator cuff repair. An analysis of risk factors. Acta Orthop Belg. 2005;71(6):662–6.
57. Kim HM, Nirvikar D, Teefey SA, et al. Location and initiation of degenerative rotator cuff tears: an analysis of three hundred and sixty shoulders. J Bone Joint Surg Am. 2010;92-A(5):1088–96.
58. Hughes RE, An K-N. Force analysis of rotator cuff muscles. Clin Orthop Relat Res. 1996;330:75–83.
59. Lee BG, Cho NS, Rhee YG. Effect of two rehabilitation protocols on range of motion and healing rates after arthroscopic rotator cuff repair: aggressive versus limited early passive exercises. Arthroscopy. 2012;28(1):34–42.
60. Apreleva M, Ozbaydar M, Fitzgibbons PG, Warner JJ. Rotator cuff tears: the effect of the reconstruction method on three-dimensional repair site area. Arthroscopy. 2002;18(5):519–26.
61. Cole BJ, El-Attrache NS, Anbari A. Arthroscopic rotator cuff repairs: an anatomic and biomechanical rationale for different suture-anchor repair configurations. Arthroscopy. 2007;23(6):662–9.
62. Trantalis JN, Boorman RS, Pletsch K, Lo IK. Medial rotator cuff failure after arthroscopic double-row rotator cuff repair. Arthroscopy. 2008;24(6):727–31.
63. Mazzocca AD, Millett PJ, Guanche CA, Santangelo SA, Arciero RA. Arthroscopic single-row versus double-row suture anchor rotator cuff repair. Am J Sports Med. 2005;33(12):1861–8.
64. Yamakado K, Katsuo S, Mizuno K, Arakawa H, Hayashi S. Medial-row failure after arthroscopic double-row rotator cuff repair. Arthroscopy. 2010;26(3):430–5.
65. Kim D, El-Attrache N, TIbone J, et al. Biomechanical comparison of a single-row versus double-row suture anchor technique for rotator cuff repair. Am J Sports Med. 2005;34(3):407–14.
66. Rodeo S, Arnoczky S, Torzilli P, Hidaka C, Warren R. Tendon-healing in a bone tunnel. A biomechanical and histological study in the dog. J Bone Joint Surg Am. 1993;75(12):1795–803.
67. Aoki M, Oguma H, Fukushima S, Ishii S, Ohtani S, Murakami G. Fibrous connection to bone after immediate repair of the canine infraspinatus: the most effective bony surface for tendon attachment. J Shoulder Elbow Surg. 2001;10(2):123–8.
68. Meier SW, Meier JD. Rotator cuff repair: the effect of double-row fixation on three-dimensional repair site. J Shoulder Elbow Surg. 2006;15(6):691–6.
69. Brady PC, Arrigoni P, Burkhart SS. Evaluation of residual rotator cuff defects after in vivo single- versus double-row rotator cuff repairs. Arthroscopy. 2006;22(10):1070–5.
70. Tuoheti Y, Itoi E, Yamamoto N, et al. Contact area, contact pressure, and pressure patterns of the tendon-bone interface after rotator cuff repair. Am J Sports Med. 2005;33(12):1869–74.
71. Baums MH, Spahn G, Fischer A, Schultz W, Klinger H. Comparative evaluation of the tendon-bone interface

contact pressure in different single- versus double-row suture anchor repair techniques. Knee Surg Sports Traumatol Arthrosc. 2009;17(12): 1466–72.
72. Park MC, El-Attrache NS, Tibone JE, Ahmad CS, Jun B-J, Lee TQ. Part I: Footprint contact characteristics for a transosseous-equivalent rotator cuff repair technique compared with a double-row repair technique. J Shoulder Elbow Surg. 2007;16(4):461–8.
73. Smith CD, Alexander S, Hill AM, et al. A biomechanical comparison of single and double-row fixation in arthroscopic rotator cuff repair. J Bone Joint Surg Am. 2006;88(11):2425–31.
74. Garofalo R, Castagna A, Borroni M, Krishnan SG. Arthroscopic transosseous (anchorless) rotator cuff repair. Knee Surg Sports Traumatol Arthrosc. 2012;20(6):1031–5.
75. Park MC, El-Attrache NS, Ahmad CS, Tibone JE. "Transosseous-equivalent" rotator cuff repair technique. Arthroscopy. 2006;22(12):1360.e1–5.
76. Park MC, Tibone JE, El-Attrache NS, Ahmad CS, Jun B-J, Lee TQ. Part II: Biomechanical assessment for a footprint-restoring transosseous-equivalent rotator cuff repair technique compared with a double-row repair technique. J Shoulder Elbow Surg. 2007;16(4):469–76.
77. Salata M, Sherman S, Lin E, et al. Biomechanical evaluation of transosseous rotator cuff repair: do anchors really matter? Am J Sports Med. 2013;41(2):282–90.
78. Park J-Y, Lhee S-H, Choi J-H, Park H-K, Yu J-W, Seo J-B. Comparison of the clinical outcomes of single- and double-row repairs in rotator cuff tears. Am J Sports Med. 2008;36(7):1310–6.
79. Millett PJ, Warth R. Posterosuperior rotator cuff tears: classification, pattern recognition, and treatment. J Am Acad Orthop Surg. 2014;22(8):521–34.
80. Millett PJ, Warth RJ, Dornan GJ, Lee JT, Spiegl UJ. Clinical and structural outcomes after arthroscopic single-row versus double-row rotator cuff repair: a systematic review and meta-analysis of level I randomized clinical trials. J Shoulder Elbow Surg. 2014;23(4):586–97.
81. Ide J, Maeda S, Takagi K. A comparison of arthroscopic and open rotator cuff repair. Arthroscopy. 2005;21(9):1090–8.
82. Verma NN, Dunn W, Adler RS, et al. All-arthroscopic versus mini-open rotator cuff repair: a retrospective review with minimum 2-year follow-up. Arthroscopy. 2006;22(6):587–94.
83. Carbonel I, Martinez AA, Calvo A, Ripalda J, Herrera A. Single-row versus double-row arthroscopic repair in the treatment of rotator cuff tears: a prospective randomized clinical study. Int Orthop. 2012;36(9):1877–83.
84. Ma H-L, Chiang E-R, Wu H-TH, et al. Clinical outcome and imaging of arthroscopic single-row and double-row rotator cuff repair: a prospective randomized trial. Arthroscopy. 2012;28(1):16–24.
85. Lorbach O, Pape D, Raber F, Busch L, Kohn D, Kieb M. Influence of the initial rupture size and tendon subregion on three-dimensional biomechanical properties of single-row and double-row rotator cuff reconstructions. Knee Surg Sports Traumatol Arthrosc. 2012;20(11):2139–47.
86. Hersche O, Gerber C. Passive tension in the supraspinatus musculotendinous unit after long-standing rupture of its tendon: a preliminary report. J Shoulder Elbow Surg. 1998;7(4):393–6.
87. Kim YK, Moon SH, Cho SH. Treatment outcomes of single- versus double-row repair for larger than medium-sized rotator cuff tears the effect of preoperative remnant tendon length. Am J Sports Med. 2013;41(10):2270–7.
88. Gartsmann GM, Taverna E. The incidence of glenohumeral joint abnormalities associated with full-thickness, reparable rotator cuff tears. Arthroscopy. 1997;13(4):450–5.
89. Kukkonen J, Joukainen A, Lehtinen J, Aarimaa V. The effect of glenohumeral osteoarthritis on the outcome of isolated operatively treated supraspinatus tears. J Orthop Sci. 2013;18(3):405–9.
90. Piasecki D, Verma N, Nho SJ, et al. Outcomes after arthroscopic revision rotator cuff repair. Am J Sports Med. 2010;38(1):40–6.

Retracted Subscapularis Tears 19

Patrick J. Denard and Stephen S. Burkhart

Introduction

Tears of the subscapularis were once thought to be uncommon but are now recognized to be present in nearly 30 % of all arthroscopic shoulder procedures and approximately 50 % of rotator cuff repairs [1–4]. Although the subscapularis has historically received less attention than posterosuperior rotator cuff tears, recognition and repair of a complete retracted subscapularis tendon is critically important to restoring anatomy and therefore achieving the best functional outcome possible. The subscapularis is the largest and most powerful of the rotator cuff muscles [5] and is more important for arm elevation than either the supraspinatus or infraspinatus [6]. Because it is the only anterior rotator cuff muscle, repair must be accomplished in order to balance the posterior forces of the rotator cuff [7, 8]. The upper portion of the subscapularis is particularly important since the insertion is broadest superiorly [9], and this site serves as the anterior attachment of the rotator cable [8]. The rotator cable attachments and the subscapularis tendon in particular are vital to maintaining overhead function. We examined rotator cuff tear patterns and found that pseudoparalysis requires disruption of at least of one of the rotator cable attachments [10]. Another study demonstrated that pseudoparalysis is most common when there is a 100 % tear of the subscapularis tendon [11]. Finally, for tears extending into the supraspinatus, repair of the upper subscapularis decreases the stress on the adjacent repair of the supraspinatus since the two tendons are connected by the comma tissue (Fig. 19.1) [12]. Given that the majority of the retracted subscapularis tendon tears are associated with tears extending into the posterosuperior cuff, repair of the subscapularis will facilitate repair of the remainder of the rotator cuff tear.

Repair of the subscapularis tendon begins with proper recognition. Once recognized, a systematic approach can be utilized to arthroscopically repair all subscapularis tendon tears regardless of the degree of retraction or fatty degeneration. This chapter describes our current approach to arthroscopic management of retracted subscapularis tendon tears.

Surgical Technique

We repair *all* subscapularis tears arthroscopically and have found that these tears are essentially always repairable with meticulous mobilization. Three unique aspects of the subscapularis make it

P.J. Denard, MD (✉)
Southern Oregon Orthopedics, Medford, OR, USA
e-mail: pjdenard@gmail.com

S.S. Burkhart, MD
The San Antonio Orthopaedic Group,
San Antonio, TX, USA

J.D. Kelly IV (ed.), *Elite Techniques in Shoulder Arthroscopy*,
DOI 10.1007/978-3-319-25103-5_19

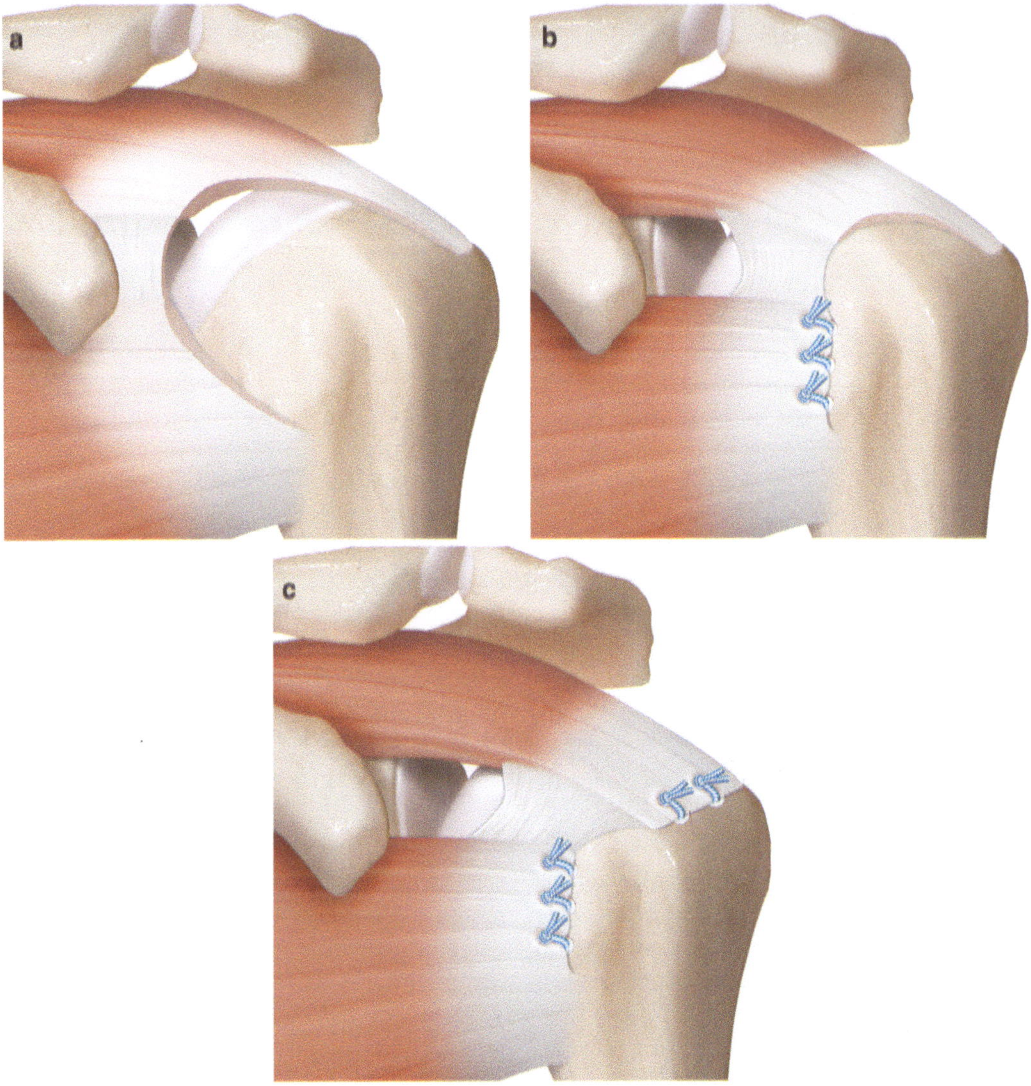

Fig. 19.1 Schematic of the relationship between subscapularis repair and the supraspinatus. (**a**) Massive retracted and contracted tear of the subscapularis and supraspinatus tendons. (**b**) Repair of the subscapularis partially reduces the supraspinatus retraction. (**c**) Repair of the supraspinatus can then be accomplished with minimal tension (Reproduced with permission from Burkhart SS, Lo IK, Brady PC, Denard PJ. *The Cowboy's Companion: A Trail Guide for the Arthroscopic Shoulder Surgeon*. Philadelphia: Lippincott, Williams, & Wilkins, 2012)

more challenging to repair than posterosuperior rotator cuff tears. First, the chronic subscapularis tear tends to retract much more than the remaining rotator cuff tendons, causing mobilization to be more difficult. Second, mobilization of the retracted subscapularis can be intimidating because it scars against the coracoid process, in close proximity to important neurovascular structures. Third, visualization, arthroscopic instrument manipulation, and knot tying in the limited subcoracoid space are more challenging compared to working in the subacromial space.

Order of Steps

Repair of the subscapularis requires working in the subcoracoid space. Since this space can become compromised rapidly by soft tissue swelling from fluid extravasation, it is critical to address the subscapularis prior to repairing the rest of the cuff. In general, when the subscapularis is torn, the order of steps is as follows:

1. Arthroscopic recognition
2. Biceps tenotomy and whipstitch in preparation for tenodesis
3. Creation of window in the rotator interval
4. If the subscapularis tendon is adhesed, skeletonization of the posterolateral coracoid, as well as a three-sided release
5. Coracoplasty if indicated (i.e., if subcoracoid coracohumeral distance is <7 mm)
6. Preparation of the lesser tuberosity bone bed
7. Repair of the subscapularis tendon
8. Completion of the biceps tenodesis
9. Repair of the remainder of the rotator cuff

Diagnostic Arthroscopy

The patient is placed in the lateral decubitus position and the arm is placed in balanced suspension or an articulating arm holder at 20–30° of abduction and 20° of forward flexion. The subscapularis is initially inspected with a 30° arthroscope viewing through a posterior portal. During subscapularis tendon repair, we view exclusively through a posterior portal and switch between 30° and 70° arthroscopes as needed.

Retracted tears are the most obvious and are located by a torn medial biceps sling which creates a "comma sign." [13] The medial sling, composed of the medial coracohumeral ligament and the superior glenohumeral ligament, normally inserts at the superior lesser tuberosity adjacent to the superolateral subscapularis footprint (Fig. 19.2). When the upper subscapularis tears away from its bone attachment, the medial sling also tears away from the bone and forms a distinctive comma-shaped arc of soft tissue (*comma sign*) at the superolateral corner of the subscapularis (Fig. 19.3). Identification of this structure therefore always leads to the superolateral subscapularis tendon, even when the tendon is severely retracted and adhesed medially. If the subscapularis tendon is not immediately visible at the front of the joint, it is probably retracted medially to the level of the glenoid margin. It can usually be located by placing the tip of a blunt instrument (e.g., a switching stickor shaver introduced

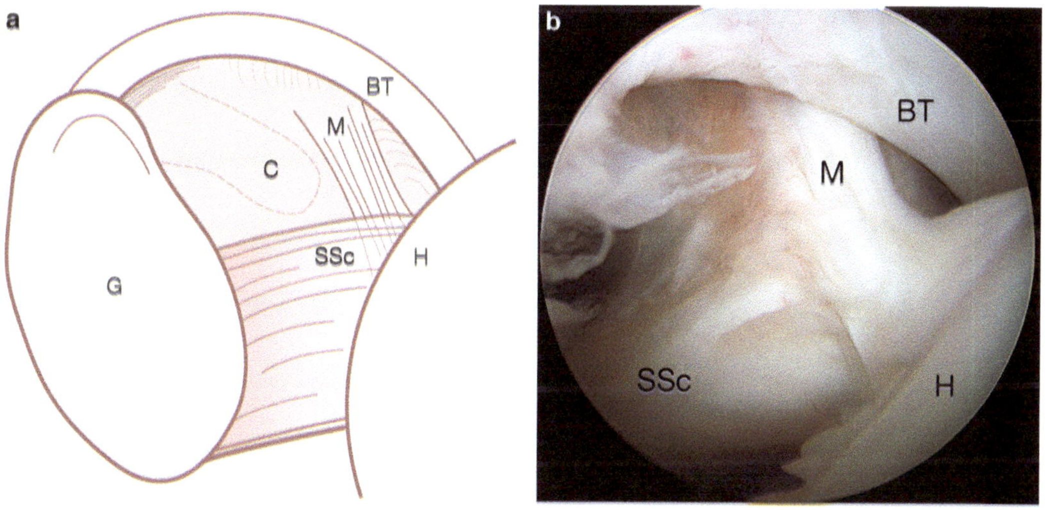

Fig. 19.2 This drawing (**a**) and corresponding arthroscopic photo (**b**) represent the view of the anterior structures from a posterior viewing portal of a right shoulder. The medial sling (M) of the biceps tendon (BT) inserts onto the lesser tuberosity of the humerus (H) along with the superolateral margin of the subscapularis (SSc). *C* coracoid, *G* glenoid (Reproduced with permission from Burkhart SS, Lo IK, Brady PC, Denard PJ. *The Cowboy's Companion: A Trail Guide for the Arthroscopic Shoulder Surgeon*. Philadelphia: Lippincott, Williams, & Wilkins, 2012)

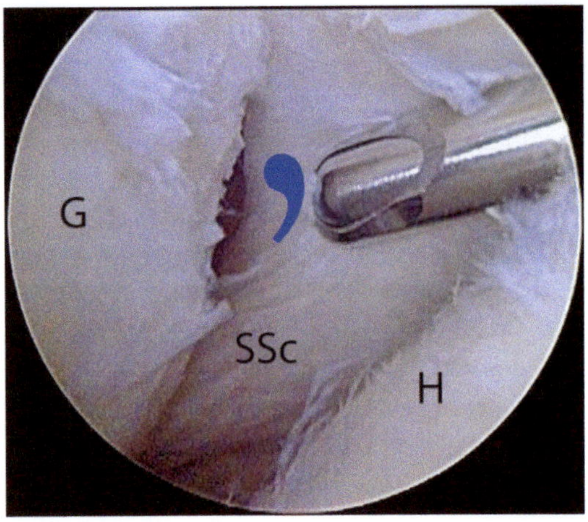

Fig. 19.3 Right shoulder, posterior viewing portal. In the setting of a retracted subscapularis tear, the medial sling tears away from the bone with the subscapularis tendon. The medial sling forms a distinctive comma-shaped arc of soft tissue (*blue comma* shape) at the superolateral corner of the subscapularis. As demonstrated in this photo, the comma sign serves as a landmark for locating a retracted subscapularis tendon. *G* glenoid, *H* humeral head, *SSc* subscapularis tendon (Reproduced with permission from Burkhart SS, Lo IK, Brady PC, Denard PJ. *The Cowboy's Companion: A Trail Guide for the Arthroscopic Shoulder Surgeon*. Philadelphia: Lippincott, Williams, & Wilkins, 2012)

through an anterosuperolateral portal) into the soft tissue adjacent to the glenoid rim at the level of the mid-glenoid notch. The mid-glenoid notch is the level at which the upper border of the subscapularis tendon usually crosses transversely. The tip of the switching stick is used to hook into the junction where the superolateral border of the subscapularis tendon joins the *comma tissue* at approximately a right angle.

With a posterior viewing portal, the subscapularis footprint can only be fully visualized by using a 70° arthroscope. Visualization can also be enhanced with a posterior lever push and internal rotation of the arm. In the case of retracted tears, the lesser tuberosity will be bare.

Biceps Tenodesis

With the exception of very young individuals and throwing athletes, we routinely perform a biceps tenodesis in conjunction with repair of a subscapularis tear. Tenotomy is reserved for patients over the age of 70 or with multiple comorbidities. Poorer results have been reported when the biceps is left in place in the setting of subscapularis repair [14]. After identifying a subscapularis tear, an anterosuperolateral (ASL) portal is established viewing with a 30° arthroscope, using an 18-gauge spinal needle as a guide. This portal is typically 1–2 cm lateral to the anterolateral acromion but can vary, and placement should be such that it provides a 5°–10° angle of approach to the lesser tuberosity and is parallel to the subscapularis tendon. An 8.25 mm threaded clear cannula is placed in this portal.

Our technique for arthroscopic biceps tenodesis is briefly summarized here but has been described in detail previously [15]. Through the ASL portal, 2 half-racking #2 FiberWire (Arthrex Inc., Naples, FL) sutures are placed as traction sutures in the biceps tendon and then a tenotomy is performed. The biceps is then exteriorized, secured with a whipstitch, sized, and left outside of the ASL portal for later tenodesis. Performing the biceps tenotomy first provides greater access to the subscapularis insertion.

Accessing the Subcoracoid Space

Accessing the subcoracoid space is an essential component of subscapularis repair. A 30° arthroscope is used to initially locate the coracoid tip. Using the 30° arthroscope helps to maintain proper orientation so as to avoid inadvertent dissection as all important neurovascular structures are greater than 2.5 cm from the tip of the coracoid [16]. In non-retracted tears, the coracoid tip is usually just anterior to the upper subscapularis tendon and can be palpated with an instrument inserted through the ASL portal. A shaver or electrocautery is used to make a window in the rotator interval just superior to the subscapularis tendon and medial to the comma tissue. We strongly believe it is important to preserve the comma tissue during this step because of the connection to the supraspinatus tendon and its ability to afford margin convergence suturing to the posterior cuff.

With retracted tears, the tendon is usually initially resting medial to the coracoid, and the coracoid tip is frequently hidden behind bursal leaders that extend from the lateral border of the subscapularis to the anterior internal deltoid fascia. These bursal leaders must be released to access the subcoracoid space. Once the comma sign is identified, an electrocautery can be used to free these adhesions by working parallel and slightly anterior to the comma tissue. Usually after just a few sweeps of the electrocautery, the conjoined tendon and coracoid tip will be visualized, providing access to the subcoracoid space. A 70° arthroscope is then inserted and attention is turned to the 3-sided release. The 70° arthroscope offers a much wider field of view medially for skeletonizing the coracoid neck and coracoid base.

Three-Sided Subscapularis Tendon Release

Retracted tears of the subscapularis require a three-sided release. A traction suture is placed in the superolateral tendon medial to the comma tissue using an antegrade suture passer (FastPass Scorpion; Arthrex, Inc., Naples, FL). In order to maintain freedom in the ASL working portal, it is helpful to briefly remove the cannula and replace it so that the traction suture remains in the ASL portal but outside of the cannula. A hemostat can be placed on the traction stitch to separate it from the biceps whipstitch sutures which exit the same portal. While pulling laterally on the traction suture, the coracoid is then identified and a window is created in the rotator interval as described previously (Fig. 19.4).

The posterolateral coracoid tip is skeletonized with an electrocautery and a shaver is used to remove the fibrofatty bursa between coracoid and the anterior aspect of the subscapularis tendon. This step constitutes the anterior release.

Next, a superior release is performed between the coracoid neck and the tendon with a 30° arthroscopic elevator. The elevator is inserted only to the base of its blade, which is enough to release the adhesions to the coracoid (Fig. 19.5). We performed a cadaveric study and found that the upper subscapular nerve innervates the muscle a mean of 3.2 cm medial to the base of the coracoid when the arm is in the neutral position and 2.4 cm medial with the arm in maximal external rotation [17]. The nerve was never closer than 11 mm. Since the blade of the arthroscopic elevator we use is 8 mm in length and the arm is typically internally rotated (which increases the distance between the nerve and coracoid), the method we describe is very safe. It is not necessary and potentially detrimental to neurovascular structures to dissect any farther medially than 8 mm. If there is an associated retracted tear of the posterosuperior cuff at this point, we also often use an electrocautery to release the CHL from the base of the coracoid (posteromedial to the subscapularis tendon). This step completes the anterior interval "slide in continuity" which is useful for mobilization of the posterosuperior cuff.

The posterior release of the subscapularis tendon is performed by introducing a 15° elevator between the posterior subscapularis tendon and the anterior glenoid neck (Fig. 19.6). This is a safe, relatively avascular plane in which the elevator can safely be manipulated blindly to do the posterior release. This completes the three-sided release (anterior, superior, posterior). We have not found it necessary to do an inferior release and such a release would risk axillary nerve injury. Following a three-sided release, we have found that we can always mobilize the subscapularis to the lesser tuberosity or at the very least to within 5 mm of its native insertion.

Coracoplasty

Prior to repair of the subscapularis, we always assess the coracohumeral interval. In the treatment of retracted tears, this is performed at the time of the anterior release of the subscapularis tendon. The width of the coracohumeral interval is estimated by comparing it to the known width of a 5-mm shaver. An interval of less than 7 mm is considered stenotic and is an indication for coracoplasty [18, 19]. If necessary, a high-speed

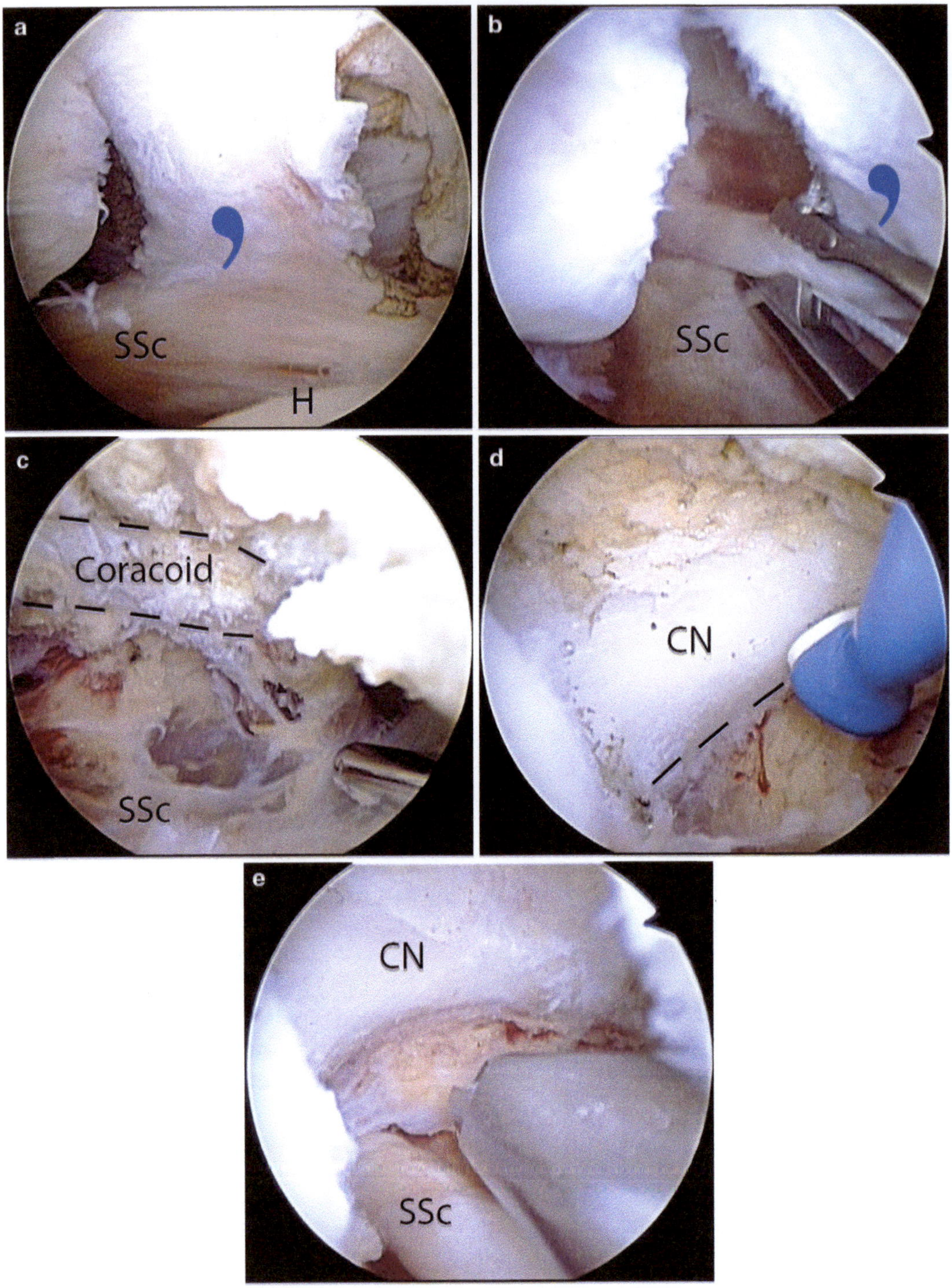

Fig. 19.4 Anterior release of a retracted adhesed subscapularis tendon tear in a right shoulder, viewed from a posterior glenohumeral portal. (**a**) While viewing with a 30° arthroscope the *comma sign* is identified. (**b**) A traction stitch is placed in the upper subscapularis tendon. (**c**) The arthroscope is placed through a window in the rotator interval to indentify the coracoid. (**d**) While viewing with a 70° arthroscope, the posterolateral coracoid is skeletonized to the level of the coracoid neck and coracoid base using an electrocautery. (**e**) After the anterior release is completed the coracoid neck and underlying subscapularis tendon are clearly visualized. *CN* coracoid neck, *H* humerus, *SSc* subscapularis tendon, *blue comma symbol*, *comma sign* (Reproduced with permission from Burkhart SS, Lo IK, Brady PC, Denard PJ. *The Cowboy's Companion: A Trail Guide for the Arthroscopic Shoulder Surgeon*. Philadelphia: Lippincott, Williams, & Wilkins, 2012)

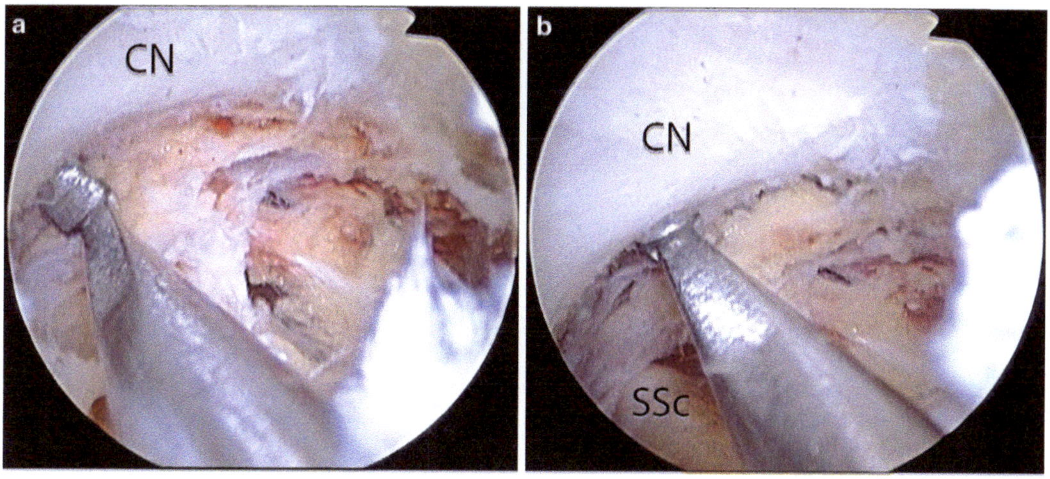

Fig. 19.5 Superior release of a retracted adhesed subscapularis tendon tear in a right shoulder viewed from a posterior portal with a 70° arthroscope. (**a**) A 30° elevator is introduced from an anterosuperolateral working portal. (**b**) Adhesions between the superior subscapularis and the coracoid neck are released. The elevator is inserted only to the base of its blade, which is enough to release the adhesions to the coracoid. *CN* coracoid neck, *SSc* subscapularis tendon (Reproduced with permission from Burkhart SS, Lo IK, Brady PC, Denard PJ. *The Cowboy's Companion: A Trail Guide for the Arthroscopic Shoulder Surgeon*. Philadelphia: Lippincott, Williams, & Wilkins, 2012)

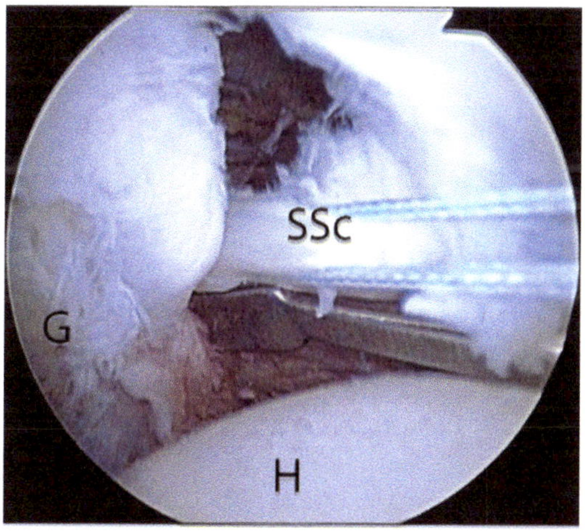

Fig. 19.6 Posterior release of a retracted adhesed subscapularis tendon tear in a right shoulder viewed from a posterior portal. A 15° elevator, introduced from an anterosuperolateral portal, frees the subscapularis from adhesions between its posterior border and the glenoid. *G* glenoid, *H* humerus, *SSc* subscapularis tendon (Reproduced with permission from Burkhart SS, Lo IK, Brady PC, Denard PJ. *The Cowboy's Companion: A Trail Guide for the Arthroscopic Shoulder Surgeon*. Philadelphia: Lippincott, Williams, & Wilkins, 2012)

burr is introduced through the anterosuperolateral portal and used to create a 7- to 10-mm space between the coracoid tip and the subscapularis.

Bone Bed Preparation

Next, the lesser tuberosity bone bed is prepared through the ASL portal with light use of a burr in order to create a bleeding base. Ring curettes are useful to create a sharp medial margin. For retracted tears, footprint restoration of the subscapularis tendon depends upon defining the medial and lateral margins of the lesser tuberosity. The normal medial margin is 2–3 mm lateral to the articular surface. The lateral margin can be less obvious to delineate but can be determined by identifying the bicipital groove which marks the lateral border of the lesser tuberosity. Even though there is usually a 2- to 3-mm gap between the articular cartilage and the anatomic footprint of the subscapularis, we prepare the lesser tuberosity footprint for repair all the way

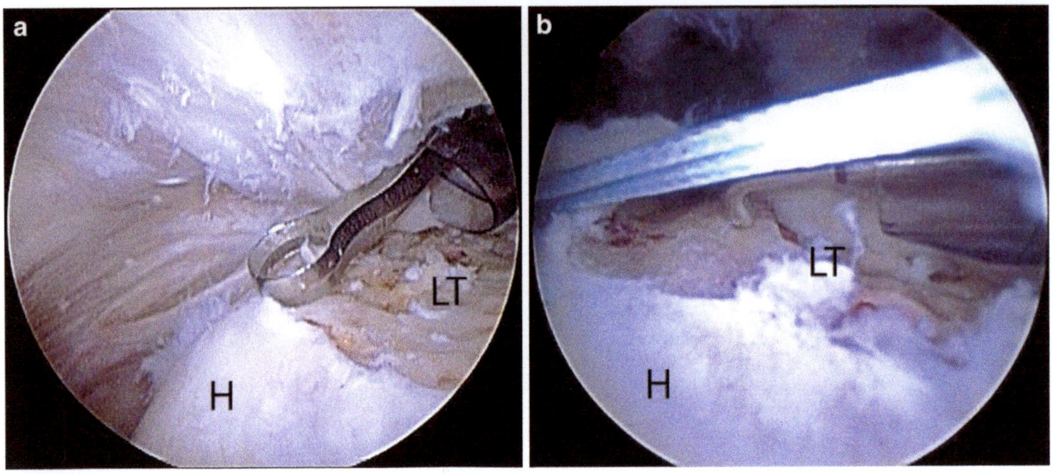

Fig. 19.7 Right shoulder, posterior glenohumeral viewing portal with a 70° arthroscope demonstrates medialization of the subscapularis footprint for repair of a subscapularis tendon tear with decreased lateral excursion after a three-sided release. (**a**) The medial margin of the subscapularis footprint is further medialized by using a ring curette. (**b**) The tip of a probe introduced from an anterosuperolateral portal demonstrates the native medial margin of the footprint. *H* humerus, *LT* lesser tuberosity (Reproduced with permission from Burkhart SS, Lo IK, Brady PC, Denard PJ. *The Cowboy's Companion: A Trail Guide for the Arthroscopic Shoulder Surgeon*. Philadelphia: Lippincott, Williams, & Wilkins, 2012)

to the articular margin. In cases where mobilization does not create enough lateral excursion for a true anatomic repair of the subscapularis, we medialize the footprint 5–7 mm and have observed no decrease in functional outcome with this medialized position (Fig. 19.7) [20].

Repair of the Subscapularis Tendon

Full-thickness tears can be repaired with a variety of techniques. If the subscapularis is minimally retracted, a double-row repair is sometimes possible, though we have found this to be possible in less than 25 % of cases.

The tendinous footprint of the subscapularis is roughly trapezoidal in shape, with its widest portion superior, and has a mean superior to inferior length of 2.5 cm [9]. We place one anchor for every superior to inferior cm of the subscapularis that is torn. Therefore, for full-thickness tears, a double-row repair requires two medial and two lateral anchors in order to adequate reestablish the footprint. We most commonly use a SutureBridge technique (Arthrex, Inc., Naples, FL). A double-loaded inferomedial anchor (5.5 mm BioComposite Corkscrew FT; Arthrex, Inc., Naples, FL) is first placed adjacent to the articular margin in a percutaneous fashion via an anterior portal. The anterior portal is established using an 18-gauge spinal needle with an outside-in technique. This is a percutaneous stab portal only which begins somewhat more medial than a standard anterior portal; in determining placement, the needle should pass just lateral to the coracoid tip and approach the lesser tuberosity at a 30–45° angle. The suture limbs are then passed as mattress stitches through the subscapularis tendon; most commonly an antegrade suture passer is utilized via the ASL portal, but a retrograde instrument may also be used via the anterior portal. The FastPass Scorpion is particularly useful for antegrade passage because its spring-loaded trapdoor in the upper jaw allows for "blind" capture of the suture, even with limited visualization in the subcoracoid space. These suture limbs are retrieved out the same portal used for anchor placement. The second medial anchor is then placed superomedially and these suture limbs are passed antegrade through the superolateral subscapularis tendon (medial to the comma tissue) as simple stitches. By placing the sutures there, the tendon edge inverts against the bone bed and the comma tissue acts as a rip-stop to suture cutout through soft tissue (since the fibers of the comma tissue are oriented at right angles to the fibers of the subscapularis tendon). The suture limbs are then tied sequentially from inferior to superior with a Surgeon's Sixth Finger Knot Pusher (Arthrex, Inc., Naples, FL). At least four suture limbs are preserved, crisscrossed, and secured laterally with two SwiveLock C anchors. Importantly, the superior suture limbs are passed anterior to the comma tissue when they are incorporated in the lateral row.

In the vast majority of chronic full-thickness subscapularis tears, however, footprint coverage is only adequate for a single-row repair. The steps are the same as just described, with the exception that the suture limbs are cut after being passed as simple sutures and no lateral row is performed (Fig. 19.8).

Biceps Tenodesis and Subsequent Rotator Cuff Repair

After the subscapularis has been repaired, the biceps tenodesis is performed at the top of the bicipital groove with a BioComposite Tenodesis screw. In the setting of a concomitant supraspinatus tendon repair, the placement of the anchor can be moved slightly posterior so that it will also serve as an anteromedial anchor for supraspinatus tendon repair. Then the scope is redirected to the subacromial space. The comma sign can be followed to the anterolateral border of the supraspinatus tendon, which can then be mobilized and repaired.

Postoperative Management

Postoperatively the patient is placed in a sling for 6 weeks. In the case of a complete tear, no external rotation is allowed past neutral during this period. No overhead motion is allowed for 6 weeks. Elbow flexion, wrist exercises, and hand exercises are encouraged. At 6 weeks the sling is discontinued and a stretching program of passive external rotation and forward flexion with a rope and pulley is begun. For isolated subscapularis tears, strengthening is initiated at 12 weeks, progressing from resistance bands to light weights. For massive rotator cuff tears or revision repairs, strengthening is delayed until 16 weeks. Unrestricted activity is allowed at 6–12 months, depending on the size of the tear.

Discussion

Arthroscopy has dramatically improved the ability to recognize and repair subscapularis tendon tears. In our opinion recognition and repair of these tears is critical to achieving the best outcome possible for both isolated subscapularis tears and combined rotator cuff tears involving the subscapularis. With the principles and techniques described in this article, repair of the subscapularis tendon has led to good or excellent functional outcomes at both short and long term in the vast majority of cases [21–23].

Burkhart and Tehrany first reported the preliminary results of arthroscopic subscapularis repair in 2002 [21]. Short-term outcomes (10.7 months) in 25 patients were encouraging with University of California Los Angeles (UCLA) scores improving from a 10.7 preoperatively to 30.5 postoperatively and forward flexion increasing from 96° to 146°. A subsequent report of 45 patients with median 5-year follow-up showed sustained results at the intermediate term [22]. Substantial improvements in functional outcome were observed in both American Shoulder and Elbow Surgeons (ASES) scores, which improved from 40.5 to 91.2, and in UCLA scores, which improved from 15.7 to 31.6. Overall, 80 % of patients had a good or excellent result and 83 % of patients returned to usual work or sport. More recently, we reviewed 79 patients at a minimum follow-up of 7 years and mean follow-up of 105 months [23]. Compared to preoperative values, UCLA mean scores improved from 16.5 to 30.1 and mean ASES scores improved from 40.8 to 88.5 ($p<0.001$). Results were rated as good or excellent in 83.3 % of cases, 92.4 % of patients returned to normal activities, and 92.4 % of patients were satisfied.

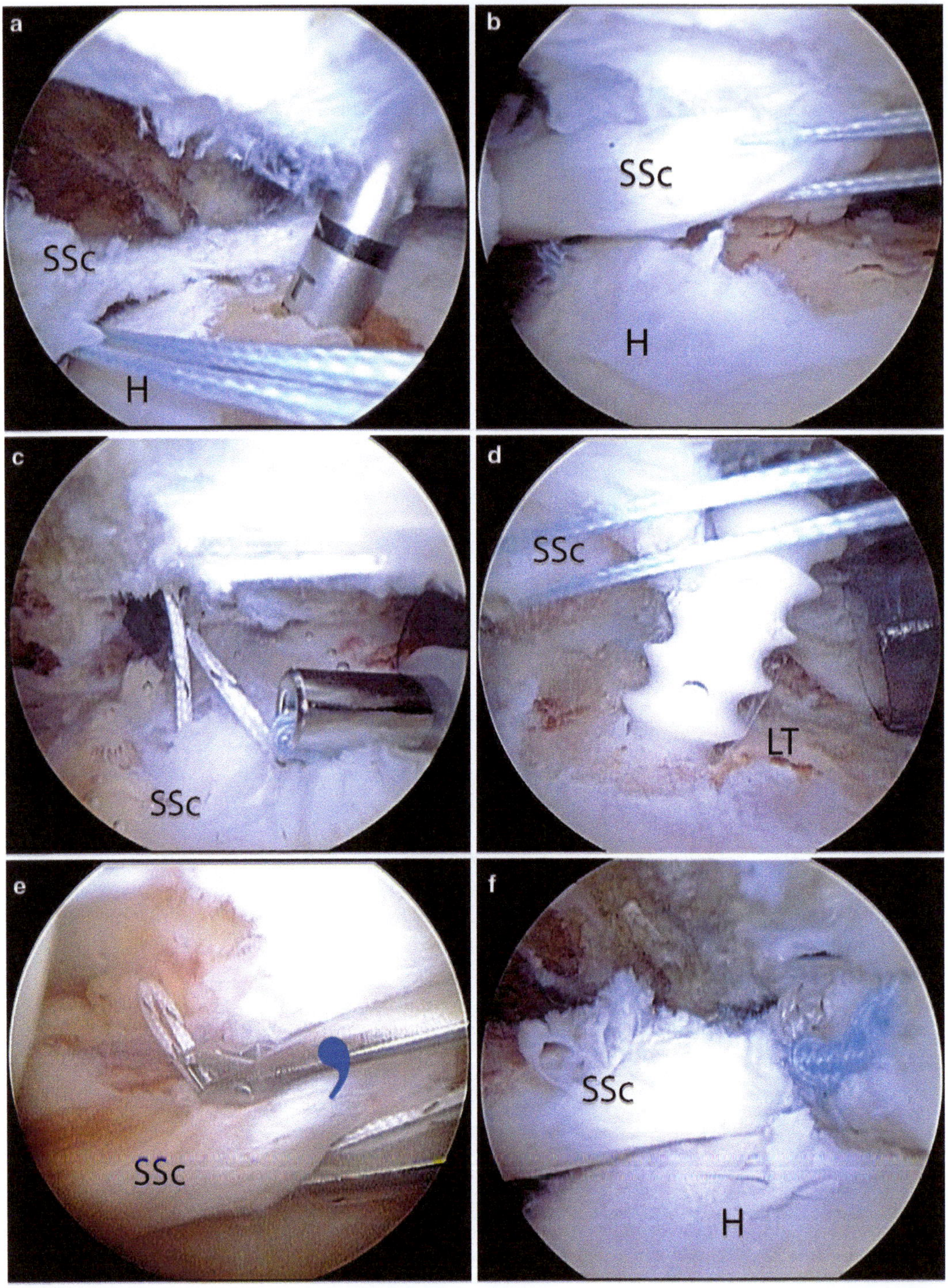

Fig. 19.8 Two-anchor repair of a retracted full-thickness subscapularis tendon tear in a right shoulder viewed form a posterior glenohumeral portal. (**a**) A bone socket is created in the inferior lesser tuberosity for placement of a BioComposite Corkscrew FT suture anchor (Arthrex, Inc., Naples, FL). (**b**) After suture passage, a provisional reduction is obtained with a traction stitch in the upper subscapularis tendon. (**c**) The arthroscope is placed through a window in the rotator interval and the sutures from the inferior anchor are tied while tension is maintained on the traction stitch. (**d**) A second anchor is then placed in the superior lesser tuberosity. (**e**) Sutures from the superior anchor are passed antegrade, medial to the comma tissue. (**f**) Completed repair, demonstrating restoration of the subscapularis footprint. H, humerus; LT, lesser tuberosity; SSc, subscapularis tendon; blue comma symbol, comma sign (Reproduced with permission from Burkhart SS, Lo IK, Brady PC, Denard PJ. *The Cowboy's Companion: A Trail Guide for the Arthroscopic Shoulder Surgeon*. Philadelphia: Lippincott, Williams, & Wilkins, 2012)

While the aforementioned reflect the combined results of different sizes of subscapularis tears, the results of arthroscopic repair of complete subscapularis tendon tears are also very good. We reviewed 23 patients at a mean of over 80 months after an arthroscopic repair of a 100 % subscapularis tendon tear [20]. Fourteen of the tears were anatomically repaired to the lesser tuberosity and 9 of the tears were repaired following 4–7 mm of footprint medialization. There was no difference in final functional outcome, patient satisfaction, or return to activity between the anatomic and medialized repair groups. Final forward flexion (158° and 164° respectively), UCLA scores (30.2 in both groups), and ASES scores (87.3 and 81.3 respectively) were comparable to the previously mentioned results.

References

1. Arai R, Sugaya H, Mochizuki T, Nimura A, Moriishi J, Akita K. Subscapularis tendon tear: an anatomic and clinical investigation. Arthroscopy. 2008;24: 997–1004.
2. Bennett WF. Subscapularis, medial, and lateral head coracohumeral ligament insertion anatomy. Arthroscopic appearance and incidence of “hidden” rotator interval lesions. Arthroscopy. 2001;17: 173–80.
3. Lafosse L, Jost B, Reiland Y, Audebert S, Toussaint B, Gobezie R. Structural integrity and clinical outcomes after arthroscopic repair of isolated subscapularis tears. J Bone Joint Surg Am. 2007;89:1184–93.
4. Barth JR, Burkhart SS, De Beer JF. The bear-hug test: a new and sensitive test for diagnosing a subscapularis tear. Arthroscopy. 2006;22:1076–84.
5. Keating JF, Waterworth P, Shaw-Dunn J, Crossan J. The relative strengths of the rotator cuff muscles. A cadaver study. J Bone Joint Surg (Br). 1993;75:137–40.
6. Kuechle DK, Newman SR, Itoi E, Morrey BF, An KN. Shoulder muscle moment arms during horizontal flexion and elevation. J Shoulder Elbow Surg. 1997;6:429–39.
7. Kelly BT, Williams RJ, Cordasco FA, et al. Differential patterns of muscle activation in patients with symptomatic and asymptomatic rotator cuff tears. J Shoulder Elbow Surg. 2005;14:165–71.
8. Burkhart SS, Esch JC, Jolson RS. The rotator crescent and rotator cable: an anatomic description of the shoulder's “suspension bridge”. Arthroscopy. 1993;9:611–6.
9. Richards DP, Burkhart SS, Tehrany AM, Wirth MA. The subscapularis footprint: an anatomic description of its insertion site. Arthroscopy. 2007;23: 251–4.
10. Denard PJ, Koo SS, Murena L, Burkhart SS. Pseudoparalysis: the importance of rotator cable integrity. Orthopedics. 2012;35:e1353–7.
11. Collin P, Matsumura N, Ladermann A, Denard PJ, Walch G. Relationship between massive chronic rotator cuff tear pattern and loss of active shoulder range of motion. J Shoulder Elbow Surg. 2014;23(8):1195–202.
12. Ticker JB, Burkhart SS. Why repair the subscapularis? A logical rationale. Arthroscopy. 2011;27:1123–8.
13. Lo IK, Burkhart SS. The comma sign: an arthroscopic guide to the torn subscapularis tendon. Arthroscopy. 2003;19:334–7.
14. Edwards TB, Walch G, Sirveaux F, et al. Repair of tears of the subscapularis. J Bone Joint Surg Am. 2005;87:725–30.
15. Lo IK, Burkhart SS. Arthroscopic biceps tenodesis using a bioabsorbable interference screw. Arthroscopy. 2004;20:85–95.
16. Lo IK, Burkhart SS, Parten PM. Surgery about the coracoid: neurovascular structures at risk. Arthroscopy. 2004;20:591–5.
17. Denard PJ, Duey RE, Dai X, Hanypsiak B, Burkhart SS. Relationship of the subscapular nerves to the base of the coracoid. Arthroscopy. 2013;29:986–9.
18. Lo IK, Burkhart SS. The etiology and assessment of subscapularis tendon tears: a case for subcoracoid impingement, the roller-wringer effect, and TUFF lesions of the subscapularis. Arthroscopy. 2003;19: 1142–50.
19. Richards DP, Burkhart SS, Campbell SE. Relation between narrowed coracohumeral distance and subscapularis tears. Arthroscopy. 2005;21:1223–8.
20. Denard PJ, Burkhart SS. Medialization of the subscapularis footprint does not affect functional outcome of arthroscopic repair. Arthroscopy. 2012;28:1608–14.
21. Burkhart SS, Tehrany AM. Arthroscopic subscapularis tendon repair: Technique and preliminary results. Arthroscopy. 2002;18:454–63.
22. Adams CR, Schoolfield JD, Burkhart SS. The results of arthroscopic subscapularis tendon repairs. Arthroscopy. 2008;24:1381–9.
23. Denard PJ, Jiwani AZ, Ladermann A, Burkhart SS. Long-term outcome of a consecutive series of subscapularis tendon tears repaired arthroscopically. Arthroscopy. 2012;28:1587–91.

Arthroscopic Repair of Massive Retracted Rotator Cuff Tears

20

Michael H. McGraw, Stuart D. Kinsella, Ann Marie Kelly, and John D. Kelly IV

Introduction

Rotator cuff tears are a common cause of pain and disability [1, 2]. With modern advances in arthroscopy and arthroscopic techniques, most rotator cuff tears can now be repaired arthroscopically, with several authors reporting successful results with even larger tears [3–7]. However, the optimal management of massive rotator cuff tears is controversial and is ever evolving [8].

In general, a massive rotator cuff tear is defined as a tear in which the major tear diameter is greater than 5 cm [9]. However, just as a fracture can be reduced, even the largest of tears can afford the arthroscopist at least a partial "reduction" of the tear. Since the rotator cuff tendons are each attached to their respective muscle bellies, the directional "pull" of the muscle-tendon unit determines the retraction pattern. Burkhart has classified massive cuff tears into one of three categories: crescent shaped, U shaped, and L shaped. Smaller crescent-shaped tears are mobile and reduce easily to the anatomic footprint without excess tension and are the result of direct medial retraction [10]. U-shaped tears extend medially with equal mobility of anterior and posterior limbs. L-shaped tears have a longitudinal component with one limb, anterior or posterior, demonstrating more mobility. Usually, the posterior limb (infraspinatus) demonstrates more mobility and can be "reduced" anteriorly and laterally. Thus, each massive tear holds a pattern for "reduction": once the arthroscopist masters tear recognition, even some of the most retracted tears may be repaired.

Open Repair

In the past, massive rotator cuff tears were managed with open repair with satisfactory outcomes. Good or excellent results were reported in 42 of 50 (84 %) of patients by Ellman et al. and 69 % of patients by Wolfgang [11, 12]. However, the open technique had several disadvantages. Despite the incision, visualization was still poor and allowed for poor access medially. The open technique also confers the morbidity of a larger incision including resulting inflammation and increased recovery times. In fact IL 6 levels have been shown to be significantly higher in open versus arthroscopic surgery [13]. As arthroscopic instrumentation and techniques evolved, there

M.H. McGraw, MD (✉)
Department of Orthopaedic Surgery, Hospital of the University of Pennsylvania, Philadelphia, PA, USA
e-mail: Michael.mcgraw@uphs.upenn.edu

S.D. Kinsella, MD, MTR
Department of Orthopaedic Surgery, Massachusetts General Hospital, Boston, MA, USA

A.M. Kelly, BA • J.D. Kelly IV, MD
Department of Orthopedics, University of Pennsylvania, Philadelphia, PA, USA

J.D. Kelly IV (ed.), *Elite Techniques in Shoulder Arthroscopy*,
DOI 10.1007/978-3-319-25103-5_20

has been a conversion from open to arthroscopic treatment of rotator cuff tears.

Arthroscopic Debridement

The majority of the early arthroscopic literature reported on arthroscopic debridement of massive rotator cuff tears. Early results of debridement were promising [8, 14–16]. The tears that were successfully treated with debridement were those where the force couple remained balanced in the coronal and transverse plane. As long as the force couple is maintained, the shoulder, although painful, remained functional regardless of the size of the tear. Pain relief from debridement was likely due to bursal removal, irrigation of inflammatory mediators, placebo, and "smoothing" out of acromial spurs on a prominent tuberosity (tuberoplasty). However, these results seemed to deteriorate with time [17, 18]. For example, in younger, more active patients, the results of rotator cuff debridement worsened with time [17, 18]. As repair techniques evolved, cuff debridement gradually fell out of favor for all tears except the small partial-thickness tears. The advancement of suture anchor techniques has brought us into the current era of arthroscopic repair of virtually all rotator cuff tears.

Reverse Total Shoulder Arthroplasty

There has been a recent broadening of the indications for reverse total shoulder arthroplasty (RTSA) for the treatment of non-arthritic patients with massive rotator cuff tears. The use of RTSA has now expanded to include shoulder pathology such as massive rotator cuff tears, failed shoulder arthroplasty, and fracture sequelae [19, 20]. The number of complications has increased, as well, with reported rates ranging from 19 to 68 % [21, 22]. Wierks et al. performed a retrospective review of 20 consecutive patients and observed a higher intraoperative and postoperative complication rate than previously reported [23]. Furthermore, there are few papers looking at the long-term results with RTSA. Therefore, the senior author cautions surgeons performing RTSA for massive rotator cuff tears, as the clinical outcome after arthroscopic repair is favorable with minimal risk, and RTSA has a high complication rate and uncertain long-term results [24, 25]. RTSA indications should be narrow. The performance of an arthroscopic cuff repair "burns no bridges" and, if skillfully performed, may obviate the need for eventual RTSA.

Arthroscopic Rotator Cuff Repair

The arthroscope provides several advantages to the shoulder surgeon. One of the greatest advantages of the arthroscope is that it frees the surgeon from spatial limitations. The surgeon can approach a pathologic area from anterior, posterior, medial, or lateral positions with equal facility. Likewise, arthroscopy allows less dissection and decreased postoperative inflammation and pain when compared to open or mini-open techniques. Unlike arthroscopic surgery, open surgery is restricted in its approach by the position of the incision. Therefore, if the surgeon makes an anterolateral incision for cuff repair, he or she must bring the torn edge of the cuff to the incision to facilitate repair.

Indications

Massive rotator cuff tears present in different clinical situations: acute traumatic, acute on chronic, and chronic atraumatic. Acute traumatic tears tend to occur in young active individuals while chronic atraumatic tears occur in elderly patients. Muscle atrophy typically is not seen in acute traumatic tears while atrophy is commonly present in patients with chronic atraumatic tears. Patients with acute or chronic tears either present with an acute exacerbation in pain in the presence of a chronic symptomatic tear or with the new onset of shoulder pain in the presence of a chronic asymptomatic tear.

Patients with history and physical examination findings of pain and/or weakness with the presence of a massive rotator cuff tear on MRI are excellent candidates for arthroscopic rotator cuff repair. Relative contraindications for arthroscopic repair include patients with Goutallier grade 4B fatty atrophy (greater than 75 % fat vs. muscle), patients with pseudoparalysis for more than 1 year, and failure of cuff repair by a skilled surgeon. In these patients other options such as tendon transfer or RTSA may be considered with the morbidity of RTSA mentioned above. Furthermore, the results of tendon transfer are less than reliable [26–28].

Burkhart and Denard reported good results with arthroscopic repair in patients with even up to Goutallier grade 4 fatty atrophy. They reported increases in UCLA and Constant scores in 22 patients who underwent arthroscopic repair with grade 3 and 4 fatty infiltration. They also reported clinical improvement in two out of five patients with advanced stage 4 degeneration [29]. Therefore, a detailed discussion should be undertaken with the patient regarding expectations and prognosis as clinical improvements can be achieved even in patients with significant fatty degeneration.

If a patient can abduct their shoulder to at least 90°, then at least some force couple remains, and it is the senior author's considered opinion that a properly executed arthroscopic cuff repair should be offered.

Margin Convergence

Prior orthopedic teaching encouraged a medial to lateral mobilization mindset when addressing retracted massive rotator cuff tears. This was likely due to the fact that most of these repairs were being performed via an open technique where the rotator cuff needed to be mobilized laterally into the field of view in order to facilitate repair. The pitfall of this mindset is that it ignored the actual morphology of the tear and resulted in massive mobilization and repairs under high tension which led to failure. These failures were secondary to tension overload at the apex of the tear repair.

Massive rotator cuff tears that initially seem retracted are often not retracted at all. They are merely exhibiting a resting position of an elastic, albeit detached, muscle-tendon unit. In fact, they have been described as L-shaped tear that has assumed a U shape by virtue of this elasticity of the muscle-tendon unit [10, 30]. In order to repair these tears with respect given to the tear configuration and minimize tension on the repair, authors have advocated a side-to-side repair followed by repair of the tendon to the humeral bone bed. Burkhart coined the phrase "margin convergence" to describe the mechanical advantage that ensues when the free margin of the tear converges toward the greater tuberosity as the side-to-side repair progresses (Fig. 20.1) [31]. As this margin converges, the strain at the free edge of the cuff is reduced dramatically, leaving a virtually tension-free converged cuff margin overlying the humeral bone bed for repair. This reduction in strain protects the repair which lowers the likelihood of failure of the fixation to the bone. Tension is to be abhorred as it interferes with biology. The senior author believes that most "double-row" hysteria ignores tear reduction and uses "more suture and more anchors" to effect an imperfect reduction.

Force Couple: Value of Subscapularis and Infraspinatus, True Humeral Head Depressors

The "force couple" is an important principal of rotator cuff repair and is essential to understand when treating massive cuff tears. The muscles of the rotator cuff and shoulder girdle are positioned to create moments about the shoulder that will produce stable rotational motion (Fig. 20.2). The shoulder can only maintain a stable fulcrum of motion when it maintains this balanced relationship in both the coronal and sagittal plane [14, 32]. With massive rotator cuff tears, these synergistic forces are disrupted and the shoulder can no longer maintain a stable fulcrum, resulting in decreased range of motion and sometimes pseudoparalysis. The superior pull of the deltoid overcomes the absent "concavity compression," usually afforded by the humeral head depressors. If repair of a massive rotator cuff tear is performed

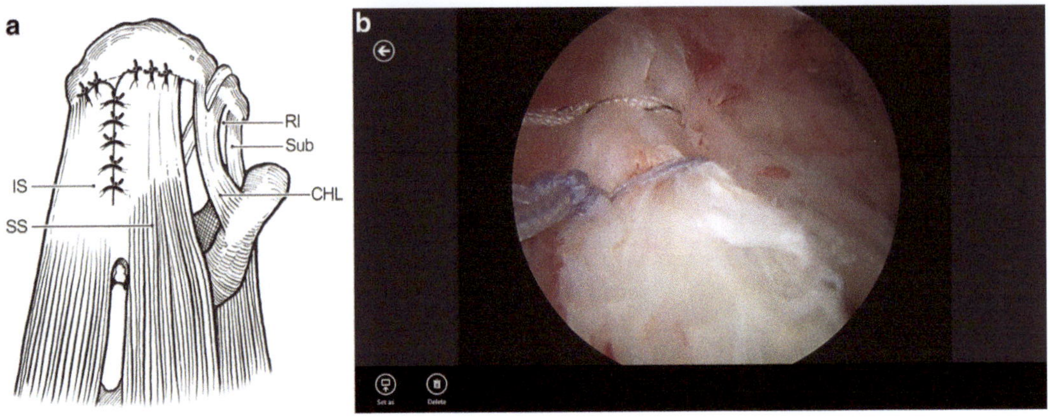

Fig. 20.1 A and B. Margin convergence. Side-to-side sutures are used to close down the defect and take tension off of the repair to the bone (Figure 20.1A reprinted from Burkart SS, Lo IKY. Arthroscopic Rotator Cuff Repair. Journal of the American Academy of Orthopaedic Surgeons. 2006; 14(6) with permission from Wolters Kluwer Health Inc.)

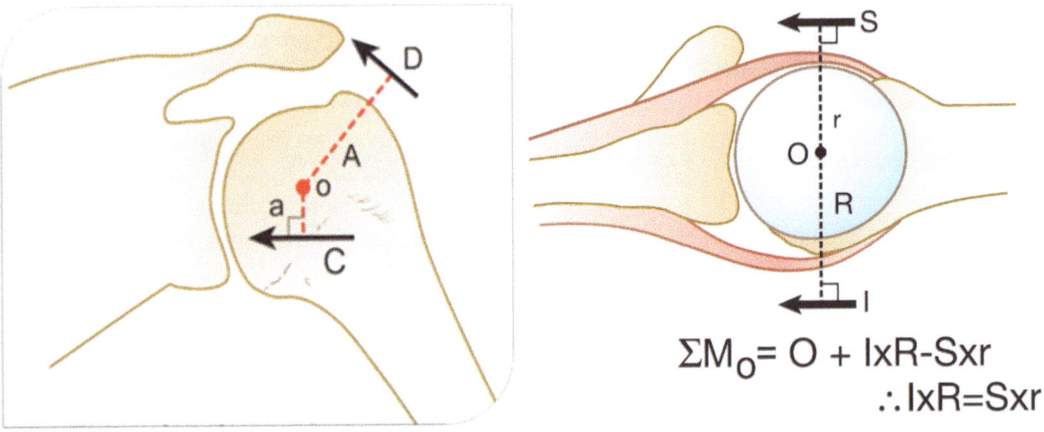

Fig. 20.2 Diagram demonstrating the concept of the force couple. All shoulder forces must remain in balance in order to maintain a stable fulcrum of motion (Reprinted from Burkart SS, Lo IKY. Arthroscopic Rotator Cuff Repair. Journal of the American Academy of Orthopaedic Surgeons. 2006; 14(6) with permission from Wolters Kluwer Health Inc.)

using surgical techniques that ignore the innate biomechanics of the shoulder, it is destined to fail. Function can be restored even in the presence of a persistent defect as long as the anterior and posterior forces are rebalanced.

Visualizing the Tear

The senior author prefers the lateral decubitus position, as it affords excellent visualization of the entire cuff, including the subscapularis.

A posterior portal is made in standard fashion with the portal established slightly lateral to the convexity of the humeral head. The camera is placed in the subacromial space through the posterior portal, and a thorough bursectomy is performed. A lateral working portal is then established under direct visualization. The portals should be place low enough such that the cannulas are parallel with the rotator cuff tendons. A second lateral portal can be established for large tears in order to obtain a "50-yard line view" of the tear.

Tear Pattern Recognition

In order to perform a successful repair of a massive tear one must first be able to recognize the tear pattern. Most massive rotator cuff tears can be broadly classified into various patterns: crescent-shaped tears, "L"-shaped tears, "reverse L"-shaped tears, and U-shaped tears. L-, reverse L-, and U-shaped tears comprise approximately 40 % of all tears and 85 % of the large and massive tears [31]. They comprise the majority of large and massive tears and extend further medial than crescent-shaped tears. The apex often extends medial to the glenoid rim. Again, it is important to realize that this medial extension of the tear does not represent retraction but rather represents the resting shape that a large tear assumes under physiologic load from its muscle-tendon components [10, 30]. Recognizing the tear pattern is critical because attempting to medially mobilize and repair the apex of the tear to a lateral bone bed will result in extreme tensile stresses in the middle of the repaired cuff margin, causing tensile overload and subsequent failure. Crescent-shaped tears, even large and massive tears, typically pull away from the bone but do not retract far. Therefore, they can be repaired directly to the bone with minimal tension.

Repairing the Crescent-Shaped Tear

Crescent-shaped tears usually can be easily repaired to the bone without tension. The senior author prepares a bleeding bone bed on the humerus just adjacent to the articular margin. A power shaver is used to achieve this. Care is taken not to decorticate the bone as this will weaken anchor fixation. A bleeding bone bed is all that is needed to promote tendon healing to the bone [21]. Suture anchors placed at 45° to the bone surface are the preferred means of fixation as studies have demonstrated that bone fixation by suture anchors is stronger than fixation by trans-osseous bone tunnels [33]. The goal is to avoid tension. Therefore, the suture anchors should be placed in a crescent shape just off the articular surface [10]. Viewing from a posterolateral portal allows excellent visualization while an anterograde suture shuttling device may be deployed from a direct lateral portal. Alternatively, a "50-yard line" view may be employed and sutures may be retrieved via a retrograde fashion using percutaneous instruments anteriorly and posteriorly, or the Neviaser portal may be utilized.

Principles of Repair: Large Tears

The senior author has amassed much experience in negotiating and overcoming failure paths and has compiled a list of helpful "pearls" which should serve the shoulder arthroscopist well.

1. Start with low distention.

   It is easy to "blow up" the shoulder joint and make visualization difficult. Therefore, it is important to start the intra-articular portion of the surgery with a low inflow pressure.
2. Release the inferior capsule.

   Since humeral head migration often ensues after long-standing cuff tears, the senior author has found inferior capsule release reduces tension on the repair and helps effect a proper tear reduction. The use of fine-tip electrocautery and hugging the glenoid works well in effecting a release of the entire IGHL.
3. Release the CHL.

   The senior author does not advocate large interval "slides" as this may further compromise tissue integrity. However, release of the CHL off the coracoid may afford significantly increased lateral excursion of the cuff. CHL release may be done intra-articularly, especially in the presence of a subscapularis tear, by skeletonizing the neck of the coracoid. Alternatively, in the subacromial space, while viewing laterally, an accessory anterolateral portal may be employed to liberate the posterior aspect of the coracoid and thereby release the CHL.
4. Place traction sutures.

   Traction sutures placed in anterior and posterior tear limbs not only help mobilization greatly but also help discern tear "reduction." For subscapularis tears, traction sutures in the "comma tissue" are invaluable (Fig. 20.3).

5. Excavate the cuff.

   As Burkhart has described, the cuff must be "excavated" from scar tissue and adhesions in the subacromial space. With a side-viewing portal, thermal devices can be applied to the acromion working posteriorly and medially so that the scapular spine is visualized. Bands of scar that do not insert directly on the humerus are termed "bursal leaders" by Burkhart and should be removed.

6. Repair the subscapularis.

   Subscapularis tears are under-recognized and hold the key to repair of many large cuff tears. Not only is the subscapularis a significant humeral head depressor, it also contains the anterior insertion of the condensation of tissue labeled by Burkhart as the "cable." The cable tissue is essential to maintaining a stable force couple. Only by repairing the subscapularis with its attendant cable tissue (CHL, SGHL) can abduction power be restored. This principle is elaborated further in the next section.

7. Preserve the comma.

   Again, only by recognizing and preserving the comma tissue can a force couple be restored. Furthermore, restoration of the comma tissue allows retracted posterior cuff tissue to be sewn to or "converged" to. The skilled arthroscopist must recognize the comma tissue and maintain its integrity in order to effect a successful massive cuff tear repair.

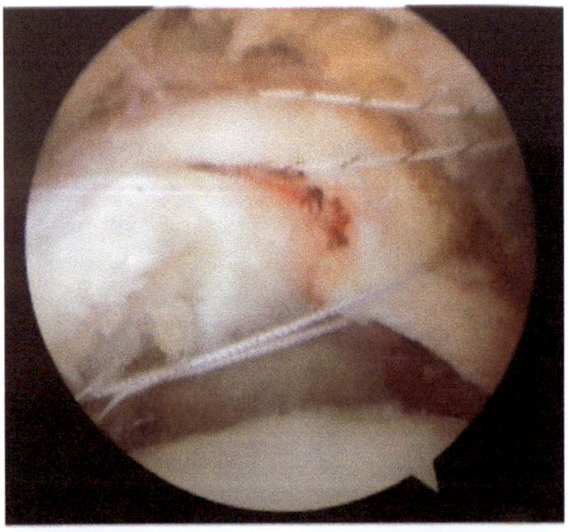

Fig. 20.3 Arthroscopic picture of traction stitch placed in order to facilitate lateral mobility of the supraspinatus and infraspinatus tendons

8. Reduce the tear.

   Proper tear reduction ensures at least a partial repair may be effected. The power of margin convergence cannot be overstated. This technique should not be abandoned in favor of adding more anchors or more suture.

9. Accept a partial repair.

   Contemporary authors describe results of partial repair as approaching complete repair [34]. If the cable tissue is restored, abduction is greatly enhanced.

10. Improve biology.

    While the results of PRP augmentation are controversial, the senior author believes in the "crimson duvet" principle proposed by Snyder [35]. Using an awl in the uncovered tuberosity may allow marrow progenitor cells to transform into cuff-like tissue and fortify the repair.

11. Use "ripstop" sutures.

    Poor tissue may need some help in holding suture. The use of some of the newer "tape" type of suture serves well as a "ripstop" to prevent anchor suture tearing through tissue. Ripstop sutures are placed first with anchor sutures subsequently placed medially (Fig. 20.4).

12. Obtain multiple fixation points.

    The more fixation points, the stronger the construct. The senior author prefers double- and even triple-loaded anchors for this reason. In the setting of massive cuff tears, there is seldom occasion to employ "double-row" fixation, since this would introduce undue tension. Burkhart's diamondback and rescue anchor repairs [36] utilize medial anchor suture limbs to obtain fixation points laterally (Fig. 20.5).

13. Use a "buddy anchor."

    In the presence of poor bone stock, Denard and Burkhart introduced the concept of a "buddy anchor" in order to secure fixation [36]. In the presence of weak pullout strength, stacking an anchor adjacent to the previously inserted one will greatly increase resistance to failure and add fixation points (Fig. 20.6).

Repairing the U-Shaped Tear

When initially assessing U-shaped tears, they may appear formidable. However, side-to-side sutures often allow dramatic convergence of the cuff to the margin, resulting in a simple repair to the bone. Again, traction sutures placed in both anterior and posterior cuff limbs help with mobilization. If the basic biomechanical principles of balanced force couples and margin convergence are adhered to when addressing the massive U-shaped tear, the patient can achieve a successful clinical and functional outcome.

Repairing the L-Shaped Tear

As noted earlier in the chapter, L-shaped and reverse L-shaped tears are similar to U-shaped tears. The difference is that L-shaped tears have one leaf that is more mobile than the other and therefore can be more easily mobilized to the bone bed. The apex of the L must be identified, and the longitudinal split then sutured in a side-to-side manner. It is critical to note that, when dealing with L and reverse L tears, the mobile limb is brought obliquely (approximately at a 45° angle) to the immobile limb. Tear reduction can be assessed by the absence of a "dog ear." A "dog ear" should not merely be eliminated with "another anchor" or more suture. They indicate poor reduction and should be revised. After side-to-side sutures are placed, causing margin convergence, the rotator cuff can be repaired to the bone.

Subscapularis and the "Comma Sign"

Multiple studies have reported on repair of combined or isolated subscapularis muscle tears [37–39]. Historically, the subscapularis muscle has been ignored when studying massive rotator cuff tears. However, the subscapularis plays an integral role in the function of the shoulder. The subscapularis seems to be unique among the rotator cuff tendons in that a significant part of its function

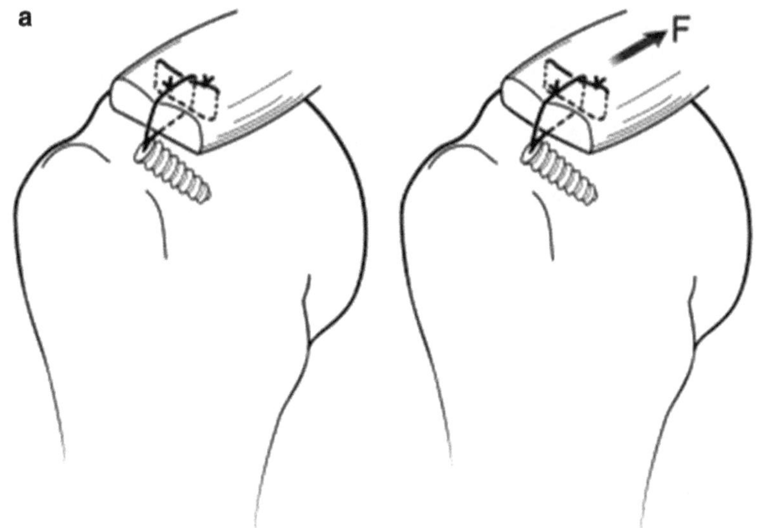

Fig. 20.4 (**a**) Ripstop stitch (Reprinted from Denard PJ, Burkhart SS. Techniques for Managing Poor Quality Tissue and Bone During Arthroscopic Rotator Cuff Repair. Arthroscopy: The Journal of Arthroscopic and Related Surgery. 2011; 27(10):1409–1421 with permission from Elsevier.). (**b**) Suture limbs from anchor passed medial to ripstop stitch (Reprinted from Denard PJ, Burkhart SS. Techniques for Managing Poor Quality Tissue and Bone During Arthroscopic Rotator Cuff Repair. Arthroscopy: The Journal of Arthroscopic and Related Surgery. 2011; 27(10):1409–1421 with permission from Elsevier.)

b

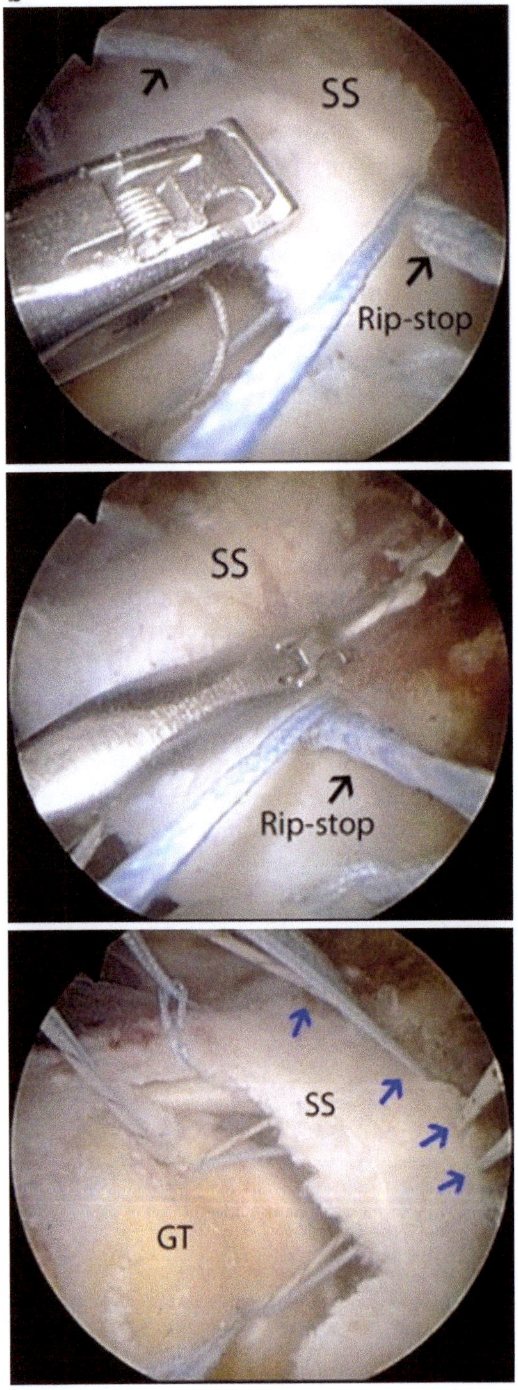

Fig. 20.4 (continued)

is a tenodesis function, and it is needed as an anterior restraint [40]. Even without contractile capabilities, it still can help provide a stable fulcrum of motion.

Surgeons may have ignored the subscapularis historically because identifying tears of the subscapularis has been difficult out of merely a lack of awareness. With a chronic isolated or combined complete tear, the tendon is often retracted medially and scarred to the deltoid fascia. Burkhart et al. described the "comma sign," which is a marker of the torn subscapularis stump and can be useful even when tackling chronic retracted subscapularis tears [41]. Locating the "comma sign" is integral in differentiating the subscapularis from the conjoined tendon and the coracoacromial ligament. The humeral insertion of the subscapularis, superior glenohumeral ligament, and the coracohumeral ligament is in close proximity and is interconnected, so the entire complex is torn together when the subscapularis tears from the lesser tuberosity. The comma tissue usually remains attached to the superolateral corner of the subscapularis tendon. This residual tissue appears as a comma shape at the superolateral border of the muscle and reliably directs the surgeon to the superolateral portion of the subscapularis (Fig. 20.7) [42, 43]. Subscapularis repair is critical as restoration of the comma tissue (coracohumeral and superior glenohumeral ligaments) will restore the anterior aspect of the "cable" tissue as well as afford tissue to sew to for the superior cuff repair. Retracted infraspinatus tears can be sewn to comma tissue once the subacromial space is entered.

Although the subscapularis tendon can be repaired using an open technique, the senior author favors arthroscopic treatment for its better visualization of the intra-articular subscapularis tendon, as well as for the increased mobilization it provides [43]. Occasionally, a 70° arthroscope is necessary to adequately visualize the entire subscapularis footprint. A diagnostic arthroscopy is performed, and careful inspection of the subscapularis tendon is carried out. Abduction and internal rotation of the arm can facilitate the visualization of the subscapularis footprint. The "posterior lever push" maneuver has been described by Burkhart to improve visualization. In this technique, the elbow is grasped while a posterior force is placed on the humerus. This movement allows the intact subscapularis fibers to pull away from the footprint, allowing the surgeon to better see the subscapularis insertion site. Burkhart and Brady report that this technique may increase the field of view by 5–10 mm [42].

The size and tear pattern are then assessed. In cases of retracted tears, the "comma sign" is identified which helps delineate the superolateral subscapularis margin. Once the subscapularis insertion site is evaluated, a thorough assessment of the medial sling and bicipital groove must also be performed. Medial dislocation of the biceps secondary to a tear of the insertion of the sling can often be seen with tears of the upper subscapularis. The biceps tendon can be assessed by inserting a probe through an anterior portal and tugging on the tendon. If appreciable medial subluxation is present, a biceps tenotomy or tenodesis is required in order to enhance visualization and protect the repair.

After a tear of the subscapularis has been identified, subsequent repair should be performed before other shoulder areas are addressed. Burkhart describes three portals to repair the

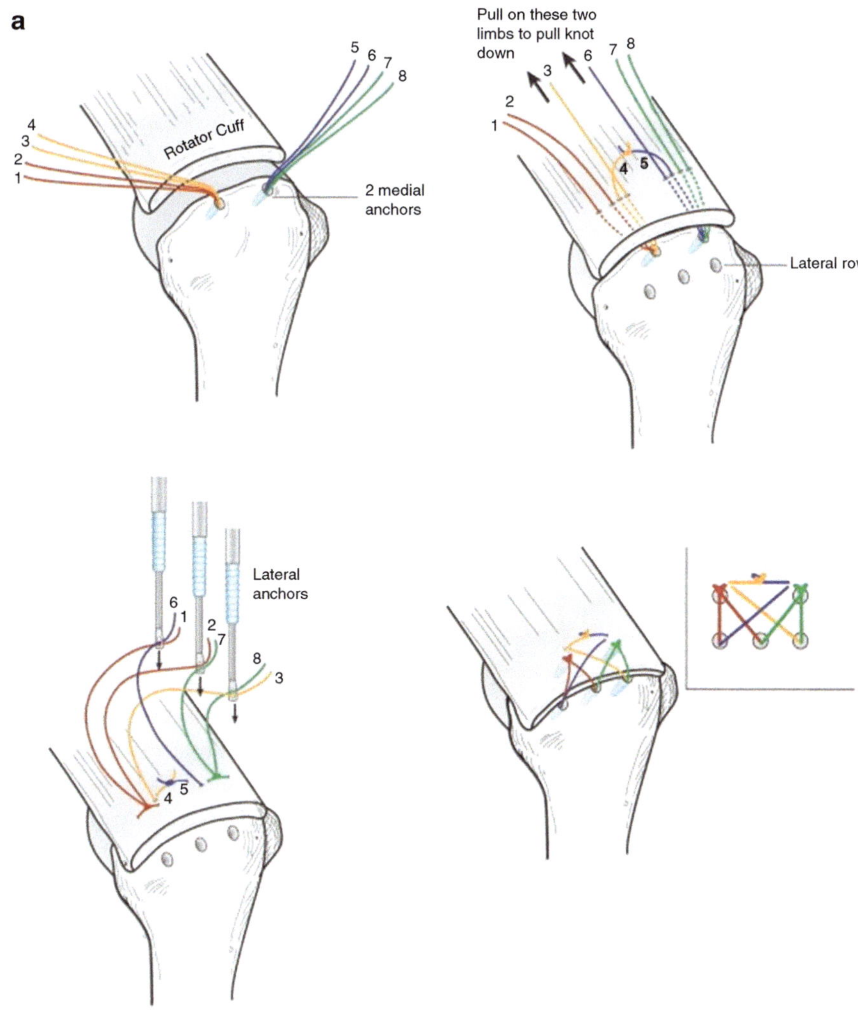

Fig. 20.5 (**a**) "Diamondback repair" (Reprinted from Burkhart SS, Denard PJ, Obopilwe E, Massocca AD. Optimizing Pressurized Contact Area in Rotator Cuff Repair: The Diamondback Repair. Arthroscopy: The Journal of Arthroscopic and Related Surgery. 2012; 28(2):188–195 with permission from Elsevier.). (**b**) Rescue anchor technique (Reprinted from Denard PJ, Burkhart SS. Techniques for Managing Poor Quality Tissue and Bone During Arthroscopic Rotator Cuff Repair. Arthroscopy: The Journal of Arthroscopic and Related Surgery. 2011; 27(10):1409–1421 with permission from Elsevier.)

b

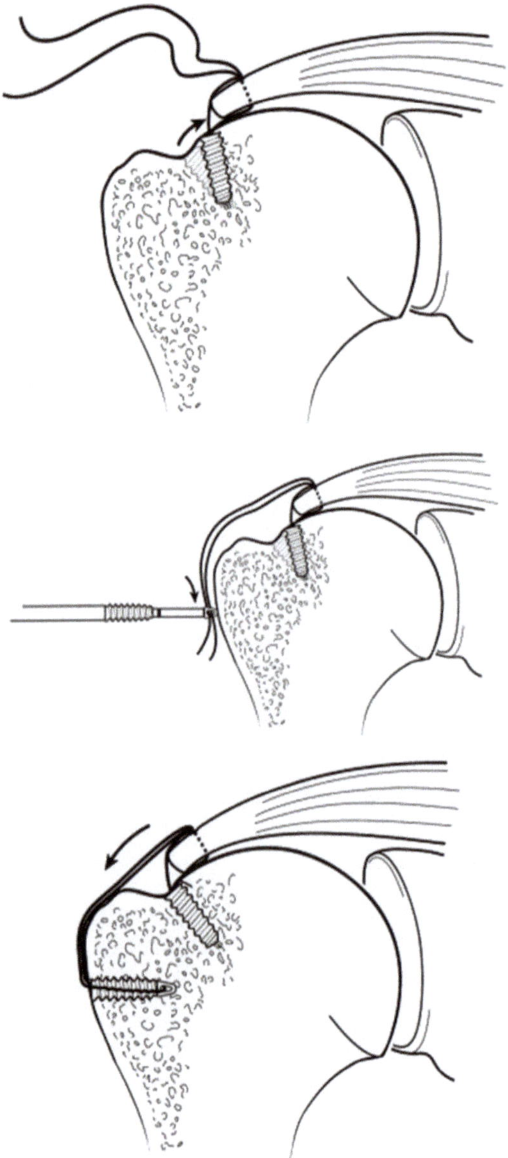

Fig. 20.5 (continued)

subscapularis [44]. The technique is described in more detail in another chapter. The posterior portal is the primary viewing portal. An anterosuperolateral portal is made just anterior to the biceps tendon and anterolateral edge of the acromion which is used to prepare the footprint and repair the tear. An anterior portal, just lateral to the coracoid, is used for anchor placement.

In the case of chronic retracted tears, mobilization techniques are required. To accomplish this, the coracoid tip and neck are skeletonized with elevators and cautery in order to free attachments of the retracted tendon. Lo and Burkhart describe the "interval slide in continuity" in which part of the rotator interval is resected while maintaining the integrity of the comma tissue in order to increase mobility of the subscapularis tendon [44, 45]. This technique involves peeling away the coracohumeral ligament from the lateral coracoid, which provides the subscapularis with greater excursion. Ide et al. recommend that a coracoplasty be performed in patients with a tight coracohumeral interval (<6 mm) to allow sufficient space for the subscapularis tendon and a large enough working area to perform the repair [46] (Fig. 20.8).

Preferred Surgical Technique

Preoperatively, a scalene block is placed to aid with postoperative pain. Examination under anesthesia is performed to assess shoulder range of motion and stability. The patient is placed in the lateral decubitus position. The extremity is placed in 10 pounds of traction with the shoulder held at 45° of abduction and 15° of forward flexion. A posterior portal is made in the standard fashion with the portal established slightly lateral to the convexity of the humeral head. Massive cuff tears are evident once the joint is entered. Gentle mobilization of the cuff off the labrum is commenced at this point. Subscapularis tears, complete with the attached "comma sign," are repaired at this time.

If superior migration of the humeral head is appreciable, an inferior capsular release is performed to minimize strain on the repair.

The camera is then placed in the subacromial space through the posterior portal, and a thorough bursectomy is performed via a lateral working portal. The portals should be placed low enough such that the cannulas are parallel with the rotator cuff tendons. A second lateral portal can be established for large tears in order to obtain a "50-yard line view" of the tear. Thermal

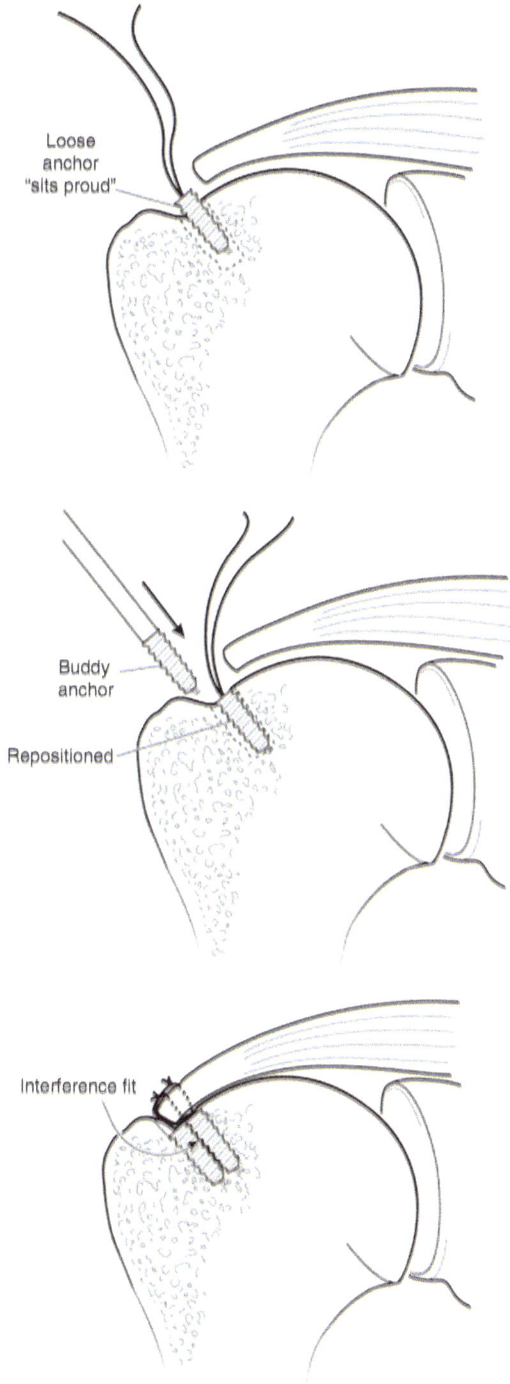

Fig. 20.6 "Buddy anchor" insertion technique from Denard and Burkhart (Reprinted from Denard PJ, Burkhart SS. Techniques for Managing Poor Quality Tissue and Bone During Arthroscopic Rotator Cuff Repair. Arthroscopy: The Journal of Arthroscopic and Related Surgery. 2011; 27(10):1409–1421 with permission from Elsevier.)

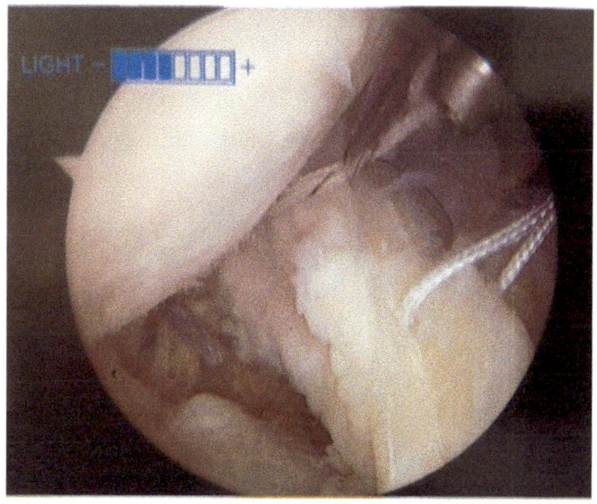

Fig. 20.7 Arthroscopic view of the comma tissue while repairing a subscapularis tear

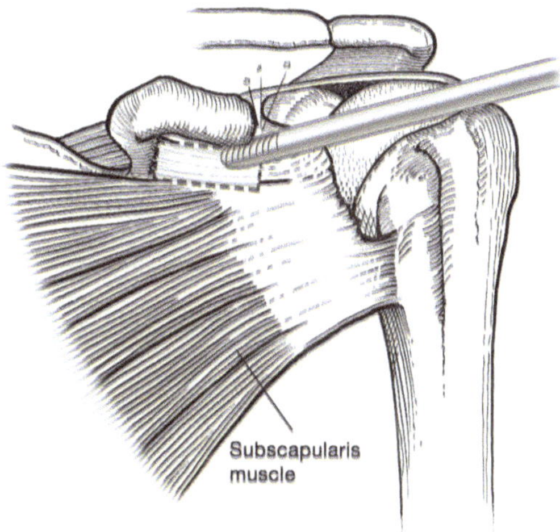

Fig. 20.8 Coracoplasty and "interval slide" in continuity allow sufficient mobilization for the subscapularis tendon while maintaining the all-important "comma tissue" (Reprinted from Lo IKY, Burkart SS. The interval slide in continuity: a method of mobilizing the anterosuperior rotator cuff without disrupting the tear margins. Arthroscopy: The Journal of Arthroscopic and Related Surgery. 2004; 20(4):435–441 with permission from Elsevier.)

ablation is used to excavate the rotator cuff to the scapular spine while viewing laterally. An acromioplasty is performed, making sure to remove the anterior-inferior hook while protecting the coracoacromial ligament. The senior author prefers to perform a Mumford procedure in most cases as the procedure is quick, and acromioclavicular joint arthritis is usually present.

The coracohumeral ligament is then released if the subscapularis tendon is not involved. This maneuver increases the lateral mobility of the supraspinatus and infraspinatus tendons (ISPs). Traction sutures are placed in opposing cuff edges in order to facilitate approximation. The biceps tendon is then visualized and addressed. The biceps tendon is usually frayed or subluxated medially if a tear of the subscapularis tendon is present. Generally, a tenodesis is performed in patients younger than 60. In patients over the age of 60, a biceps tenotomy is usually preferred.

The tear is visualized and a tear pattern is determined. After boney and biceps work, it is helpful to view from the posterior portal with a 70° scope. The mobile limb of the tear indicates the pattern of tear extension. U-shaped tears have anterior and posterior limbs that are equally mobile. The cuff tears are repaired using margin convergence. This technique involves placing side-to-side sutures in the tear which shifts the adjacent tissue into the cuff defect. This technique shortens the medial-lateral dimension as the free margin "converges" toward the tuberosity. This results in decreased strain in the rotator cuff margin.

Immobile Tears

In rare instances a large or massive tear may be contracted and truly nonmobile. Authors have reported on arthroscopic interval slides for the management of these patients. Tauro was the first to describe an interval slide for release of the rotator interval from the supraspinatus tendon [33]. The anterior interval slide involves the release of the supraspinatus tendon from the rotator interval from lateral to medial. The surgeon should start at the free margin of the tendon tear and progress to the base of the coracoid. The release also involves the incision of the coracohumeral ligament. This technique typically provides an additional 1–2 cm of lateral excursion [45]. The posterior interval slide releases the interval between the supraspinatus and infraspinatus. The technique of combining an anterior and posterior interval slide is coined the "double interval slide" and can be utilized when more mobility of the tendon is desired. The double interval slide is reserved to situations when more mobility is required than gained with an anterior interval slide alone.

Burkhart reported that an arthroscopic release of the coracohumeral ligament sometimes may result in an addition 1–2 cm of lateral excursion [10]. The extra mobility will allow a partial repair that may not have been possible otherwise. However, recent results of this technique have yielded variable clinical results [47]. As stated previously, the senior author does not recommend true interval slides, with tissue violation a suspected consequence. Rather, coracohumeral ligament release, traction sutures, and thorough "excavation" of the cuff tissue serve as the principal means of mobilization. The senior author has not been impressed by the excursion of tissue that peri-labral capsular release affords and thus does not routinely perform this.

Partial Repair

If the cuff cannot be fully mobilized to its footprint after margin convergence without over-tensioning the repair, then partial repair can be performed. The force couple still can be effective even though a hole is left in the superior portion of the cuff. Such partial cuff repairs have been shown to be effective if at least 1/2 of the infraspinatus can be repaired to the bone [48, 49]. "Ripstop" sutures are employed in cases of very weak tissue. The senior author favors "tape" type suture as reinforcement for massive cuff tears. We also prefer to use a single row of anchors to reattach the tendons to the footprint. Care is taken to minimize tension across the repair. Double-row configurations are not favored as they do not effect a proper "reduction" of the tear pattern. Secondly, undue tension disturbs biology and is to be avoided. If full coverage is not achieved, an awl is used to punch holes into the tuberosity in order to enhance biology at the repair site. More recently, the senior author has augmented deficient tissue with dermal allograft secured with "four corner" arthroscopic fixation with promising

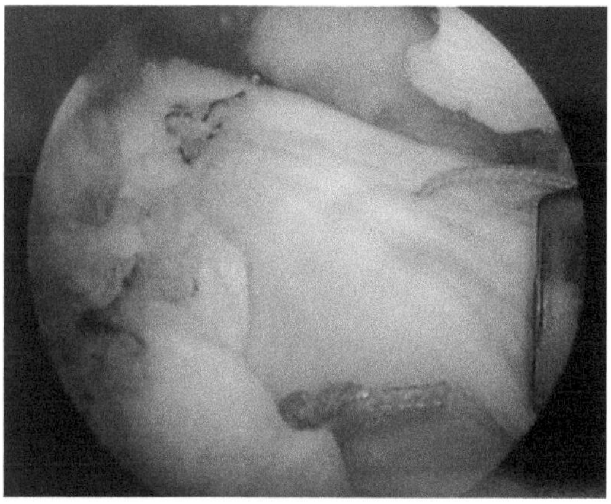

Fig. 20.9 Arthroscopic photo of dermal allograft

early results (Fig. 20.9). Mihata has shown promising results using fascia lata to reconstruct the superior capsule in large irreparable cuff tears. This clever means of resisting superior humeral head migration has biomechanical merit and may prove to be a worthy salvage procedure (Fig. 20.10) [50].

Results of Arthroscopic Repair

Favorable results have been reported with arthroscopic repair of massive rotator cuff tears. Studies have reported that pseudoparalysis can be reversed by arthroscopic means. Denard et al. reported that arthroscopic repair of MRCTs with advanced mobilization techniques can lead to reversal of preoperative pseudoparalysis in 90 % of patients who have not had previous surgery. These results were achieved with low complication rates [5]. Likewise, Oh et al. looked at 195 large-to-massive cuff tears and showed that recovery from pseudoparalysis after rotator cuff repair was evident in a large portion of the study group and postoperative function and cuff healing were not different according to the presence of pseudoparalysis [51].

Good to excellent outcomes have been reported even in patients who do not maintain cuff integrity after arthroscopic rotator cuff repair [3, 4]. One study reviewed a series of 108 patients who underwent arthroscopic repair of a massive cuff tear. They cited a 39.8 % anatomic failure rate but noted functional improvement in VAS, ASES, Constant, and SST scores in all patients. No preoperative factor was able to predict poor functional outcome. However, reduced postoperative AHD was the only relevant functional determinant in the patients' eventual functional outcome [3].

Burkhart et al. reported on 22 patients with grade 3 or 4 Goutallier degeneration of the infraspinatus [29]. They found improvements in the mean UCLA and Constant scores, as well as increases in forward elevation and external rotation after arthroscopic repair. The even reported functional improvement in two out of five patients with >75 % fatty degeneration. These results may demonstrate that arthroscopic repair may even be useful in patients with significant amounts of fatty degeneration that historically may have been treated with other more invasive surgical options.

In some instances, complete repair of massive rotator cuff tears may not be possible. In these situations, a partial repair may be indicated. Wellman et al. found that the mean Constant score significantly increased from 56 points before surgery to 71 points after surgery, the mean age- and sex-adjusted Constant score significantly improved from 63 to 90 % at a mean follow-up of 47 months after arthroscopic partial rotator cuff repair, and the subcategories pain and activity significantly improved. Furthermore, the active range of motion improved from 133° of flexion and 111° of abduction before surgery to 163° of forward flexion and 156° of abduction after surgery [34].

Mori et al. compared patch autograft repair (A) with that of partial repair (B). In their series, the clinical findings were significantly improved at the final follow-up in both groups ($p<0.001$). However, a significant difference was found between groups A and B in terms of postoperative Constant and American Shoulder and Elbow Surgeons scores ($p=0.001$ and $p=0.021$, respectively). There was a significant difference in the re-tear rate for the ISP between the two groups (8.3 % in group A vs. 41.7 % in group B, $p=0.015$). At the final follow-up, there was a significant difference in the affected side versus the unaffected side muscle strength

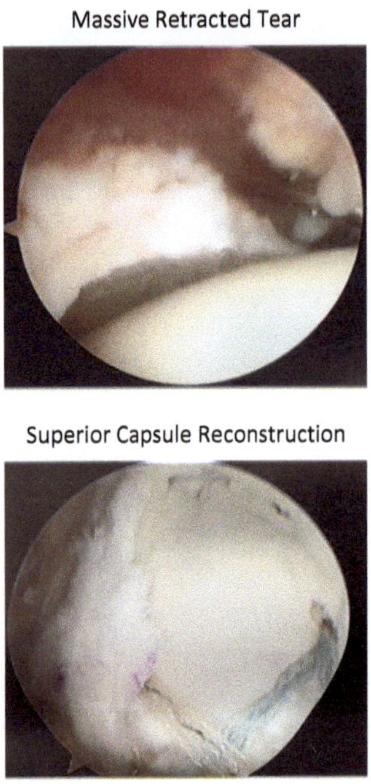

Fig. 20.10 Superior capsular reconstruction with allograft sutured to glenoid

ratios for abduction and external rotation between group A and group B ($p<0.001$ for both). Shoulders with re-tears of the infraspinatus showed significantly inferior clinical outcomes compared with those without re-tear ($p<0.001$) [52]. These findings support the role of patch autograft when addressing large difficult tears although patients undergoing partial repair did show clinical improvement.

Kim et al. reported on a series of 41 patients who either underwent complete repair with a posterior interval slide and side-to-side repair of the interval slide edge or partial repair with margin convergence. They demonstrated that no better clinical or structural outcomes compared with the partial repair group with margin convergence alone for large-to-massive contracted rotator cuff tears at 2-year follow-up. In addition, the complete repair with posterior interval slide group had a 91 % re-tear rate and a greater defect on follow-up MRA images [47].

Conclusions

Arthroscopic repair of massive rotator cuff tears is a minimally invasive procedure that can improve pain and functional outcomes in patients with fewer complications than more extreme interventions such as RTSA. The new enthusiasm for RTSA may be premature in that it puts patients at an increased risk of complications. The advantage of arthroscopic repair is that it does not preclude further options and may afford significant pain relief and increased function. It is our belief that arthroscopic cuff repair, whether partial or complete, should be a main tool in the shoulder surgeon's armamentarium for the treatment of massive rotator cuff tears. The understanding of basic principles and the advanced surgical techniques available to aid in the repair is critical in achieving a good clinical outcome.

References

1. Bokor DJ, Hawkins RJ, Huckell GH, Angelo RL, Schickendantz MS. Results of nonoperative management of full-thickness tears of the rotator cuff. Clin Orthop Relat Res. 1993;294:103–10.
2. Itoi E, Tabata S. Conservative treatment of rotator cuff tears. Clin Orthop Relat Res. 1992;275:165–73.
3. Chung SW, Kim JY, Kim MH, Kim SH, Oh JH. Arthroscopic repair of massive rotator cuff tears: outcome and analysis of factors associated with healing failure or poor postoperative function. Am J Sports Med. 2013;41(7):1674–83.
4. Paxton ES, Teefey SA, Dahiya N, Keener JD, Yamaguchi K, Galatz LM. Clinical and radiographic outcomes of failed repairs of large or massive rotator cuff tears: minimum ten-year follow-up. J Bone Joint Surg Am. 2013;95(7):627–32.
5. Denard PJ, Ladermann A, Jiwani AZ, Burkhart SS. Functional outcome after arthroscopic repair of massive rotator cuff tears in individuals with pseudoparalysis. Arthroscopy. 2012;28(9):1214–9.
6. Arrigoni P, Fossati C, Zottarelli L, Ragone V, Randelli P. Functional repair in massive immobile rotator cuff tears leads to satisfactory quality of living: results at 3-year follow-up. Musculoskelet Surg. 2013;97 Suppl 1:73–7.
7. Carbonel I, Martinez AA, Aldea E, Ripalda J, Herrera A. Outcome and structural integrity of rotator cuff after arthroscopic treatment of large and massive tears with double row technique: a 2-year followup. Adv Orthop. 2013;2013:914148.

8. Ellman H, Kay SP, Wirth M. Arthroscopic treatment of full-thickness rotator cuff tears: 2- to 7-year follow-up study. Arthroscopy. 1993;9(2):195–200.
9. DeOrio JK, Cofield RH. Results of a second attempt at surgical repair of a failed initial rotator-cuff repair. J Bone Joint Surg Am. 1984;66(4):563–7.
10. Burkhart SS. Arthroscopic treatment of massive rotator cuff tears. Clin Orthop Relat Res. 2001;390: 107–18.
11. Ellman H, Hanker G, Bayer M. Repair of the rotator cuff. End-result study of factors influencing reconstruction. J Bone Joint Surg Am. 1986;68(8):1136–44.
12. Wolfgang GL. Surgical repair of tears of the rotator cuff of the shoulder. Factors influencing the result. J Bone Joint Surg Am. 1974;56(1):14–26.
13. Shinoda T, Shibata Y, Izaki T, Shitama T, Naito M. A comparative study of surgical invasion in arthroscopic and open rotator cuff repair. J Shoulder Elbow Surg. 2009;18(4):596–9.
14. Burkhart SS. Arthroscopic debridement and decompression for selected rotator cuff tears. Clinical results, pathomechanics, and patient selection based on biomechanical parameters. Orthop Clin North Am. 1993;24(1):111–23.
15. Cofield RH. Rotator cuff disease of the shoulder. J Bone Joint Surg Am. 1985;67(6):974–9.
16. Ellman H. Arthroscopic subacromial decompression: analysis of one- to three-year results. Arthroscopy. 1987;3(3):173–81.
17. Melillo AS, Savoie III FH, Field LD. Massive rotator cuff tears: debridement versus repair. Orthop Clin North Am. 1997;28(1):117–24.
18. Zvijac JE, Levy HJ, Lemak LJ. Arthroscopic subacromial decompression in the treatment of full thickness rotator cuff tears: a 3- to 6-year follow-up. Arthroscopy. 1994;10(5):518–23.
19. Hyun YS, Huri G, Garbis NG, McFarland EG. Uncommon indications for reverse total shoulder arthroplasty. Clin Orthop Surg. 2013;5(4):243–55.
20. Gerber C, Pennington SD, Nyffeler RW. Reverse total shoulder arthroplasty. J Am Acad Orthop Surg. 2009;17(5):284–95.
21. Rittmeister M, Kerschbaumer F. Grammont reverse total shoulder arthroplasty in patients with rheumatoid arthritis and nonreconstructible rotator cuff lesions. J Shoulder Elbow Surg. 2001;10(1):17–22.
22. Wall B, Nove-Josserand L, O'Connor DP, Edwards TB, Walch G. Reverse total shoulder arthroplasty: a review of results according to etiology. J Bone Joint Surg Am. 2007;89(7):1476–85.
23. Wierks C, Skolasky RL, Ji JH, McFarland EG. Reverse total shoulder replacement: intraoperative and early postoperative complications. Clin Orthop Relat Res. 2009;467(1):225–34.
24. Cuff D, Pupello D, Virani N, Levy J, Frankle M. Reverse shoulder arthroplasty for the treatment of rotator cuff deficiency. J Bone Joint Surg Am. 2008;90(6):1244–51.
25. Cheung E, Willis M, Walker M, Clark R, Frankle MA. Complications in reverse total shoulder arthroplasty. J Am Acad Orthop Surg. 2011;19(7):439–49.
26. Omid R, Lee B. Tendon transfers for irreparable rotator cuff tears. J Am Acad Orthop Surg. 2013;21(8):492–501.
27. Gerber C, Rahm SA, Catanzaro S, Farshad M, Moor BK. Latissimus dorsi tendon transfer for treatment of irreparable posterosuperior rotator cuff tears: long-term results at a minimum follow-up of ten years. J Bone Joint Surg Am. 2013;95(21):1920–6.
28. Namdari S, Voleti P, Baldwin K, Glaser D, Huffman GR. Latissimus dorsi tendon transfer for irreparable rotator cuff tears: a systematic review. J Bone Joint Surg Am. 2012;94(10):891–8.
29. Burkhart SS, Barth JR, Richards DP, Zlatkin MB, Larsen M. Arthroscopic repair of massive rotator cuff tears with stage 3 and 4 fatty degeneration. Arthroscopy. 2007;23(4):347–54.
30. McLaughlin HL. Lesions of the musculotendinous cuff of the shoulder. The exposure and treatment of tears with retraction. 1944. Clin Orthop Relat Res. 1994;304:3–9.
31. Burkhart SS, Athanasiou KA, Wirth MA. Margin convergence: a method of reducing strain in massive rotator cuff tears. Arthroscopy. 1996;12(3):335–8.
32. Burkhart SS. Arthroscopic treatment of massive rotator cuff tears. Clinical results and biomechanical rationale. Clin Orthop Relat Res. 1991;267:45–56.
33. Tauro JC. Arthroscopic "interval slide" in the repair of large rotator cuff tears. Arthroscopy. 1999;15(5): 527–30.
34. Wellmann M, Lichtenberg S, da Silva G, Magosch P, Habermeyer P. Results of arthroscopic partial repair of large retracted rotator cuff tears. Arthroscopy. 2013;29(8):1275–82.
35. Snyder S, Burns J. Rotator cuff healing and bone marrow "crimson duvet" from clinical observations to science. Techniques in Shoulder and Elbow Surgery. 2009. 10(4):130–137.
36. Denard PJ, Burkhart SS. Techniques for managing poor quality tissue and bone during arthroscopic rotator cuff repair. Arthroscopy. 2011;27(10):1409–21.
37. Gerber C, Hersche O, Farron A. Isolated rupture of the subscapularis tendon. J Bone Joint Surg Am. 1996;78(7):1015–23.
38. Denard PJ, Burkhart SS. Arthroscopic recognition and repair of the torn subscapularis tendon. Arthrosc Tech. 2013;2(4):e373–9.
39. Deutsch A, Altchek DW, Veltri DM, Potter HG, Warren RF. Traumatic tears of the subscapularis tendon. Clinical diagnosis, magnetic resonance imaging findings, and operative treatment. Am J Sports Med. 1997;25(1):13–22.
40. Burkhart SS, Morgan CD, Kibler WB. The disabled throwing shoulder: spectrum of pathology Part I: pathoanatomy and biomechanics. Arthroscopy. 2003;19(4):404–20.

41. Lo IK, Burkhart SS. The comma sign: an arthroscopic guide to the torn subscapularis tendon. Arthroscopy. 2003;19(3):334–7.
42. Burkhart SS, Brady PC. Arthroscopic subscapularis repair: surgical tips and pearls A to Z. Arthroscopy. 2006;22(9):1014–27.
43. Denard PJ, Burkhart SS. A new method for knotless fixation of an upper subscapularis tear. Arthroscopy. 2011;27(6):861–6.
44. Lo IK, Burkhart SS. The interval slide in continuity: a method of mobilizing the anterosuperior rotator cuff without disrupting the tear margins. Arthroscopy. 2004;20(4):435–41.
45. Lo IK, Burkhart SS. Arthroscopic repair of massive, contracted, immobile rotator cuff tears using single and double interval slides: technique and preliminary results. Arthroscopy. 2004;20(1):22–33.
46. Ide J, Tokiyoshi A, Hirose J, Mizuta H. Arthroscopic repair of traumatic combined rotator cuff tears involving the subscapularis tendon. J Bone Joint Surg Am. 2007;89(11):2378–88.
47. Kim SJ, Kim SH, Lee SK, Seo JW, Chun YM. Arthroscopic repair of massive contracted rotator cuff tears: aggressive release with anterior and posterior interval slides do not improve cuff healing and integrity. J Bone Joint Surg Am. 2013;95(16):1482–8.
48. Burkhart SS. Partial repair of massive rotator cuff tears: the evolution of a concept. Orthop Clin North Am. 1997;28(1):125–32.
49. Oh JH, McGarry MH, Jun BJ, et al. Restoration of shoulder biomechanics according to degree of repair completion in a cadaveric model of massive rotator cuff tear: importance of margin convergence and posterior cuff fixation. Am J Sports Med. 2012;40(11):2448–53.
50. Mihata T, Lee TQ, Watanabe C, et al. Clinical results of arthroscopic superior capsule reconstruction for irreparable rotator cuff tears. Arthroscopy. 2013;29(3):459–70.
51. Oh JH, Kim SH, Shin SH, et al. Outcome of rotator cuff repair in large-to-massive tear with pseudoparalysis: a comparative study with propensity score matching. Am J Sports Med. 2011;39(7):1413–20.
52. Mori D, Funakoshi N, Yamashita F. Arthroscopic surgery of irreparable large or massive rotator cuff tears with low-grade Fatty degeneration of the infraspinatus: patch autograft procedure versus partial repair procedure. Arthroscopy. 2013;29(12):1911–21.

21 The Use of Graft Augmentation in the Treatment of Massive Rotator Cuff Tears

Barbara Steele, Joshua Asher Gordon, and Marc Labbé

Introduction

Rotator cuff repair can be a challenging task. Large tears and poor tissue quality can compromise healing resulting in structural failures. High re-tear rates of 30–74 % have been reported [1–4]. In a 2007 multicenter study on the results of 576 arthroscopic rotator cuff repairs, a 25 % re-tear rate was detected by postoperative MR or CT arthrogram [5]. Good and excellent results were achieved in 94 % of patients; however, greater functional improvement in activity level, motion, and strength was seen in those patients with complete healing. Pain did not correlate with tendon healing, and function was improved in patients with and without an intact repair. Healing was influenced by the chronicity of the tear, retraction, fatty infiltration, delamination, and the age of the patient. Numerous other studies have also found improved functional results in patients with a complete repair compared to a partial repair or re-tear [6–8]. The use of biologic grafts to aid in these repairs is an area of increasing interest and continued research.

Improvements in surgical technique and equipment allow surgeons to repair almost any tear. Regardless, we know that not all repairs will heal. The failure occurs chiefly at the biological level. The healing is either too slow or deficient, and the structural failure occurs during the rehabilitation process.

The poor healing capacity of the rotator cuff is due, in part, to the diminished biologic environment. There is decreased blood flow at the terminal ends of the torn and diseased rotator cuff tendons which leads to a decreased supply of growth factors to the repair site [9, 10]. Tissue loss and stiffness may also be a factor for large and chronic tears. Without the force of the rotator cuff insertion applied to the greater tuberosity, the bone quality diminishes with ensuing osteopenia and cysts. Osteoblasts from the greater tuberosity of patients with large, chronic rotator cuff tears have a lack of response to mechanical stimulation [11]. Indeed, increasing age negatively influences healing with higher recurrence rates seen in patients over age 65 [2, 7, 12, 13]. More chronic tears lend themselves to higher rates of fatty infiltration which is associated with decreased healing rates [14]. Active smokers have a significantly reduced

B. Steele, MD
Orthopaedic Surgery Sports Medicine, University of Pennsylvania Health System, Philadelphia, PA, USA

J.A. Gordon, MD (✉)
Department of Orthopaedic Surgery, Hospital of the University of Pennsylvania, Philadelphia, PA, USA
e-mail: Joshua.gordon@uphs.upenn.edu

M. Labbé, MD
Department of Orthopaedic Surgery, Baylor College of Medicine, Houston, TX, USA

University of Texas Medical Branch, Galveston, TX, USA

J.D. Kelly IV (ed.), *Elite Techniques in Shoulder Arthroscopy*,
DOI 10.1007/978-3-319-25103-5_21

capacity to heal the repaired rotator cuff tendon and should be encouraged to abstain [15–17]. NSAIDs and immune-modifying agents can also negatively influence healing and should be stopped if possible [18–21].

It is a wonder we can get any healing as we are asking the body to heal poor tissue to poor bone and often in older patients with a decreased intrinsic ability to heal.

Adding graft material is a treatment option that can aid in rotator cuff repair by adding strength and collagen at the repair site. Early results with freeze-dried allograft rotator cuff tissue were promising in Neviaser's 1978 study where 14 out of 16 patients had good or excellent results, classified as abduction greater than 90° [22]. However in 1988, Nasca showed functional improvement in only two of seven patients in which freeze-dried allograft tissue was used [23]. More recently, Moore showed a lack of healing in 15 out of 15 massive, irreparable rotator cuff repairs in which the repair was spanned with tendon allograft. The functional results from this study were equivalent to the results from debridement and subacromial decompression alone for massive rotator cuff tears [24].

Despite poor early outcomes, grafting is still area of ongoing research and can be helpful in dealing with difficult tears. Augmenting a large or massive repair with graft material has been met with mixed results and appears to be largely dependent on the graft type and patient characteristics [23–29]. Using the appropriately selected graft material may enhance rotator cuff repair healing in patients where a complete repair was otherwise unattainable. In certain cases of irreparable tears, spanning the defect with a graft may be of significant benefit. It is important to note that the FDA currently approves the use of grafts in tears that are reparable to within 1 cm of the greater tuberosity.

Grafts

Numerous grafts and graft types have become available within the past 15 years, including allograft human cadaveric skin or tendon, xenograft skin or pericardium, porcine small intestine submucosa, and synthetic grafts [30]. Currently available grafts and their properties are listed in Table 21.1. Graft performance is affected by the origin of the source tissue, preparation and sterilization techniques, thickness, pliability, elasticity, and suture retention strength. Tissue grafts undergo various processing techniques, such as decellularization, cross-linking, lamination, or lyophilization depending on the graft type [55].

The ideal graft is replaced slowly enough to provide structural support to the repair as the native rotator cuff tendon heals, typically occurring over months. A graft that is too resistant to degradation, however, may lead to encapsulation and scar formation [28, 61]. A graft that rapidly degrades may promote an immunologic response which can lead to soft tissue swelling and inflammation mimicking an infection.

There are currently no randomized controlled trials comparing graft materials used for augmentation of rotator cuff repair in humans. Thinner grafts tend to have lower suture pullout strength [43]. Grafts that are cross-linked tend to have less elongation to failure, but cross-linking does not necessarily correlate to mechanical strength [62]. More pliable grafts are useful for arthroscopic graft augmentation so that the graft may be folded, pushed, and pulled through the cannula while resisting tearing.

Dermal allografts, such as the GraftJacket® graft (Wright Medical Technology, Arlington, TN), currently have the highest quality data supporting their safety and effectiveness [27, 39–42, 59]. Burkhead et al. reported early success in 2007 with dermal allograft used for open augmentation of massive rotator cuff tears, with pain scores improving in 64 % and near normal function in 70 % at 1.2-year follow-up in 17 patients [63]. A 2012 randomized, prospective study with 2-year follow-up also showed success with dermal allograft used for arthroscopic augmentation of large or massive rotator cuff tears. This study showed rotator cuffs to be more frequently intact, based on postoperative MRI when augmented with dermal allograft as compared to those that were not, 85 % versus 40 %, respectively, with associated improved function in those that were augmented [27].

Table 21.1 Available graft material categorized by material type and reported with associated literature, strengths, and weaknesses

Graft type (product name)	Material type	Surgical use reported	Reported strengths	Reported weaknesses	Literature cited with level of evidence	Current status
Mersilene mesh	Synthetic	Primary open massive cuff repair [31]	Improved clinical scores, pain relief, and performance of activities of daily living (ADLs) [31]	No level I–II evidence—comparisons only made pre- and postoperatively	Audenaert et al. [31]—level IV	Clinical use, case series
Porcine dermal xenograft (Permacol)	Biologic xenograft	Massive open cuff repair [32]	Improved clinical scores, pain, strength, and ROM postoperatively [32]	No level I–II evidence—comparisons only made pre- and postoperatively	Badhee et al. [32]—level IV	Clinical use, case series
Porcine small intestine xenograft (restore)[b]	Biologic xenograft	Massive open cuff repair [33]		RCT demonstrates no clinical improvements, not recommended [33] Worse clinical measures postoperatively in multiple patients [26] Poor overall outcomes reported in additional studies [25] Animal studies demonstrate porcine DNA and cell presence associated with in vivo inflammatory response [34]	Iannotti et al. [33]—level II Sclamberg et al. [26]—level IV	Clinical use, RCT
Platelet-rich plasma (PRP) loaded fibrin matrix (PRPFM) (cascade autologous platelet system)[c]	Biologic	Severe arthroscopic cuff repair [35] Full-thickness arthroscopic cuff repair [36] Small to medium arthroscopic repairs [37]	Lower re-tear rates reported with mixed results from clinical scores [36]	Level III—cohort study found no difference between groups [35] Not useful for small to medium size tears [37]	Bergeson et al. [35]—level III Barber et al. [36]—level III Castricini et al.—level I [37]	Clinical use, RCT
Platelet-rich plasma (PRP)[d] gel applied to suture (PDS) or other non-matrix material	Biologic/synthetic	Arthroscopic rotator cuff repair [38]	No advantages documented	No differences observed, study allowed patients to choose treatment, possibly suboptimal application technique [38]	Jo et al.—level II–III	Clinical use, cohort study
Acellular human dermal matrix (GraftJacket)[e] (GraftJacket Maxforce and Maxforce Extreme options)	Biologic	Primary, 2-tendon, >3 cm arthroscopic cuff repairs [27] Massive arthroscopic cuff repairs [39] Massive mini-open cuff repair [40] Massive arthroscopic cuff repair [41]	Multicenter RCT with positive results found decreased re-tear rates and improved clinical scores [27] compared to controls Safety established for human dermal matrix [42] with a different production method than GraftJacket Biomechanically favorable suture grasp when compared to other products for GraftJacket Maxforce Extreme [43]	Very small number of participants in RCT [27]	Barber et al. [27]—level II Bond et al. [39]—level IV Gupta et al. [40]—level IV Wong et al. [41]—level IV Rotini et al. [42]	Clinical use, RCT

(continued)

Table 21.1 (continued)

Graft type (product name)	Material type	Surgical use reported	Reported strengths	Reported weaknesses	Literature cited with level of evidence	Current status
Free total or partial coracoacromial ligament graft	Biologic	Massive mini-open cuff repair [44]	Improved ROM and improved clinical scores postoperatively [44]	No level I–II evidence—comparisons only made pre- and postoperatively	Bektaser et al. [44]—level IV	Clinical use, case series
Autologous bone marrow mononuclear cells	Biologic	Consecutive rotator cuff injuries at a single institution—mini-open cuff repair [45]	Improved functional scores and no re-tears in a 14 patient series [45]	No level I–II evidence—comparisons only made pre- and postoperatively Lack of clearly defined patient population and small study size Iliac crest donor site morbidity [45]	Ellera Gomes et al. [45]—level IV	Clinical use, case series
Reticulated polycarbonate polyurethane patch[f]	Synthetic	Consecutive supraspinatus tears—open cuff repair [46]	Decreased pain, improved clinical scores, and low re-tear rate [46]	No level I–II evidence—comparisons only made pre- and postoperatively Small case series	EncaladaDiazetal.[46]—level IV	Clinical use, case series
Gore-Tex soft tissue patch[g]	Synthetic	Consecutive medium to large cuff tears—mini open [47]	Decreased pain, improved clinical scores, and better abduction strength with small Gore-Tex patch [47]	Lower abduction strength with larger patches [47]	Hiooka et al. [47]—level IV	Clinical use, case series
Fascia lata allografts (freeze dried)[h]	Biologic	Massive open rotator cuff repair [48]	Similar clinical results to McLaughlin procedure, with lower re-tear rates [48]	Case series compared to heterogeneous patient population [48]	Ito and Morioko—level IV [48]	Clinical use, case series
Tendon allograft (heterogeneous tendon sources) [24] (rotator cuff tendon) [22]	Biologic	Massive open rotator cuff repair [24]	Reliable alleviation of pain	No single tendon used as allograft: patellar, Achilles, and quadriceps tendons [24] No apparent improvement in outcomes [23] Study conducted in 1978 limited subjects in a case series [22]	Moore et al.—level IV [24] Nasca et al. [23]—level IV Neviaser et al. [22]—level IV	Clinical use, case series
Polyester fiber mesh ligament (Dacron)[i]	Synthetic	Massive arthroscopic cuff repair and Dacron ligament construction [49]	Improved clinical score and improved range of motion [49]	No level I–II evidence—comparisons only made pre- and postoperatively	Nada et al. [49]—level IV	Clinical use, case series
Deltoid muscle transfer/flap	Biologic	Supraspinatus confirmed—open repair	Improved ROM, clinical scores, and strength. Long-term follow-up [50]	No level I–II evidence—comparisons only made pre- and postoperatively[a] Not recommended for massive tears or those including subscapularis [50]	Gedouin et al. [50]—level IV	Clinical use, case series

Carbon fiber (Intagraft)	Synthetic	Massive open cuff repairs [51]	Predominantly good to excellent reported outcomes in available series [51]	No level I–II evidence—comparisons only made pre- and postoperatively Risk of humeral cyst associated with graft placement	Visuri et al. [51]—level IV	Clinical use, case series
Periosteal flap	Biologic	Degenerated tears—open cuff repair [52]	Improved clinical scores and moderately low re-tear rate (20 %) [52]	No level I–II evidence—comparisons only made pre- and postoperatively Risk of rotator cuff calcification, not correlated with inferior clinical outcomes [52]	Sceibel et al. [52]—level IV	Clinical use, case series
Tenotomized biceps tendon	Biologic	Massive arthroscopic repair [53]	Reported improvement in some aspects of ROM, strength, and image- based healing [53]	No level I–II evidence—comparisons only made pre- and postoperatively	Cho et al. —level IV [53]	Clinical use, case series
SportMesh[j]—knitted polyurethane urea fabric[33]	Synthetic	Biomechanical studies		Most displacement in biomechanical studies of augmentation products [43] Lower load at failure than commercially available comparators described by Barber et al. [43]	Barber et al.—Preclinical study [43]	Clinical use, no formal investigation
Allopatch HD[k] 2, acellular human collagen matrix from fascia lata [43]	Biologic	Biomechanical studies	Higher reported load to failure in biomechanical tests and compared to several commercially available alternatives [43]	No clinical data	Barber et al.—Preclinical study [43]	Clinical use, no formal investigation
OrthAdapt[l], cross-linked equine pericardium [43]	Biologic xenograft	Biomechanical studies		Lower load at failure than commercially available comparators described by Barber et al. [43]	Barber et al.—Preclinical study [43]	Clinical use, no formal clinical investigation
RC Allograft[m]—freeze-dried rotator cuff cleansed allograft [43] is provided to Arthrex by Allograft Tissue Systems	Biologic	Biomechanical studies	Lower reported elongation during cyclical biomechanical testing [43]	No clinical data	Barber et al.—Preclinical study [43]	Clinical use, no formal clinical investigation
CuffPatch[n]—porcine small intestine	Biologic xenograft	Biomechanical studies		Studies of restore, with a similar tissue origin raise concerns for inflammatory reactions associated with this product [34]	Zheng et al.—Preclinical study [34]	Clinical use, no formal clinical investigation

(continued)

Table 21.1 (continued)

Graft type (product name)	Material type	Surgical use reported	Reported strengths	Reported weaknesses	Literature cited with level of evidence	Current status
TissueMend[o]—highly processed fetal bovine skin graft, non-artificially cross-linked 99 % non-denatured bovine collagen [54]	Biologic xenograft	Biomechanical studies	High levels of remnant DNA in tested specimens [55]	No clinical data	Barber et al.—Preclinical study [43]	Clinical use, no formal clinical investigation
Leeds-Keio artificial ligament[p]	Synthetic	RCT of shoulder arthroplasty in patients with rheumatoid arthritis with and without rotator cuff reconstruction and augmentation	Good biomechanical profile RCT demonstrating superior pain and function scores in augmented reconstructions paired with shoulder arthroplasty [56] Findings mainly limited by the study population	Clinical studies for rotator cuff augmentation limited to arthroplasty cases requiring reconstruction, historically largely used for reconstruction of the anterior cruciate ligament of the knee, met with mixed but fairly positive results	Tanaka et al.—level II [56]	Clinical use, RCT
X-repair[q], poly-l-lactic acid (PLLA) mesh	Synthetic	Biomechanical studies [57]	Superior biomechanical performance of repairs in cadaveric studies [57]	Complications associated with PLLA implants may be of concern in proximity to the shoulder joint [58]	McCarron et al.—level IV [57]	Preclinical, few public studies

Information adapted from cited references and review articles [28, 43, 59, 60]
[a]Article not in English, results reported in abstract and cited literature (only abstract available in English)
Product sources as indicated in Table 21.1
[b]Restore Orthobiologic Implant; DePuy, Warsaw, Indiana
[c]Cascade Autologous Platelet System (Musculoskeletal Transplant Foundation, Edison, New Jersey)
[d]COBE spectra LRS Turbo, Caridian BCT, Lakewood, Colorado
[e]GraftJacket allograft (Wright Medical Technology, Arlington, TN)
[f]Biomerix, Fremont, CA
[g]Gore-Tex Expanded PTFE Patch: W.L. Gore & Associates, Flagstaff, AZ, USA
[h]Biodynamics, Germany
[i]Xirox plc, Leeds, United Kingdom
[j]Biomet Sports Medicine, Warsaw, IN
[k]Musculoskeletal Tissue Foundation, Edison, NJ
[l]Pegasus Biologics, Irvine CA
[m]Bonita Springs, FL
[n]Arthrotek, Warsaw, IN
[o]TEI Biosciences, Boston, MA; licensed to Stryker Howmedica Osteonics, Kalamazoo, MI
[p]Yufu Itonaga Co Ltd, Tokyo, Japan; Polyester Mesh Ligament
[q]Synthasome, San Diego, CA

Porcine xenografts have also been studied for rotator cuff augmentation. Porcine small intestine submucosa xenograft has been proposed as a graft material for rotator cuff augmentation; however, multiple studies have shown poor results with this material [25, 26, 33, 34]. A 2007 clinical study did not demonstrate a benefit for the use of porcine small intestine submucosa xenograft in rotator cuff augmentation. The xenograft group actually had decreased functional results and equal re-tear rates at 2-year follow-up compared with conventional rotator cuff repair. Also, 21 % of patients in the xenograft group developed a pseudoseptic inflammatory reaction requiring repeat surgery for irrigation and debridement [25]. Similar negative results were seen in a 2004 study with a 90 % re-tear rate seen on postoperative MRI [26]. However, porcine *dermal* xenograft may prove efficacious as a 2007 clinical study demonstrated improved functional results and 80 % intact grafts on postoperative imaging, with no adverse events reported [32].

Synthetic grafts have also been used and studied for augmentation of rotator cuff tears. Successful results were reported with the use of Gore-Tex (polytetrafluoroethylene) materials with improved functional results following rotator cuff augmentation. There was however greater abduction strength in the small patch group (≤2 cm) compared with the large patch group (>2 cm) and a 10 % re-tear rate between the rotator cuff and the graft, which required reoperation [47]. The Leeds-Keio artificial ligament is another synthetic graft, which is composed of polyester and has a mesh structure. This graft was studied in a 2006 prospective, randomized controlled study supporting its use in augmented subscapularis transposition for rheumatoid arthritis patients undergoing total shoulder arthroplasty [56].

Clinical Evaluation

Before considering graft augmentation, it is imperative to perform a detailed history and physical examination of the affected shoulder. Is the tear acute, chronic, or acute-on-chronic? An acute tear, even if it is large, is typically easier to reduce and has greater healing capacity than a chronic tear. Chronic tears typically have poor tissue quality due to degeneration and fatty infiltration. Large, chronic tears may develop atrophy that is visible on gross inspection of the supraspinatus and/or infraspinatus fossa. Acute-on-chronic tears may be caused by a new large tear in the setting of poor tissue quality from the chronic smaller tear, making the tear easier to reduce but still more difficult to heal because of the degenerative tissue.

Physical Examination

Evaluate both passive and active range of motion. Decreased active range of motion can be caused by pain, weakness, or secondary capsular contraction from lack of use. Capsular contraction causing limited passive motion needs to be addressed for a successful repair, either by preoperative physical therapy or intraoperative capsular release. The function of each specific cuff muscle should be tested individually.

Profound external rotation weakness coupled with a positive "hornblower's sign" indicates a large retracted posterior superior tear.

Imaging

Imaging tests are very helpful for evaluating the size of a suspected rotator cuff tear and determining whether or not a graft should be considered. Plain shoulder X-rays can show acromial morphology, acromioclavicular joint arthritis, and cystic changes in the greater tuberosity. In addition, there can be signs that a tear is large or massive with chronic elevation of the humeral head, acetabularization of the acromion, and arthrosis of the glenohumeral joint. Even though plain shoulder X-rays are important, MRI gives more detailed information about the soft tissues in the shoulder. MRI allows for better evaluation of the specific tendon involvement, degree of retraction, muscle atrophy, fatty infiltration, and degree of glenohumeral arthrosis. These factors help determine the possibility of successful repair and possible return of function. Erosion of the inferior acromion and significant glenohumeral arthritis portend a poor outcome for rotator cuff repair: in this case superior capsular reconstruction or reverse shoulder arthroplasty should be considered.

For patients who cannot undergo an MRI, ultrasound and CT arthrogram are other imaging options that can be helpful although the same degree of tissue detail cannot be achieved.

Treatment

The treatment plan for a patient with a rotator cuff tear should involve a shared decision making process between the orthopedic surgeon and the patient. The natural history of full-thickness rotator cuff tears is to increase in size over time; this can lead to worsening function, increased pain, and eventual pseudoparalysis. Therefore, continued follow-up is recommended for patients who wish to delay surgery. Some patients may be able to achieve a high level of function despite a large rotator cuff tear so long as there is good balance between the anterior and posterior joint force couples. Nonsurgical management includes activity modification, injection, and exercise. Avoiding overhead activities, especially with any resistance, can help limit the patient's exposure to painful stimuli and may lessen the chance of sudden tear progression. Steroid injections can provide temporary relief of pain and facilitate rehabilitative efforts. Strength exercises focusing on the anterior deltoid, remaining cuff tendons, and periscapular muscles can improve shoulder function. The decision for surgical repair of a rotator cuff tear should be based on the patient's goals and surgical risks. When indicated, the possible need for a graft during the repair should be discussed preoperatively with the patient who can then weigh the risks and benefits and share in the decision making process.

Graft Indications

The indications to use a graft include revision rotator cuff surgery and primary tears that are at an increased risk for failure. Risk factors for failure include size of the tear, degree of fatty infiltration, age (over 65 y.o.), and smoking [2, 5, 7, 12–17]. The goal of the graft is to provide additional strength and improve the biological environment by adding collagen, and possibly growth factors, at the site of repair. The FDA has approved the use of graft materials to augment rotator cuff repairs that can be repaired to within 1 cm of the tuberosity.

Though not currently FDA approved, new research supports the use of graft materials for reconstruction (filling in the defect) of an otherwise irreparable rotator cuff tear. Young, motivated patients with painful, irreparable tears are the best candidates to consider for this procedure. A recent case series demonstrated significant improvement in functional scores with a mini-open rotator cuff reconstruction using human dermal allograft. Follow-up ultrasounds at a mean of 3-years postoperative revealed a fully intact tendon in 76 % of patients [40]. Similar improvements in functional scores were seen when this bridging technique was performed arthroscopically with human dermal allograft [41].

Contraindications for the use of graft materials either as augmentation or replacement include rotator cuff arthropathy, unresolved infection, inflammatory arthropathy, or an immunocompromised state.

Surgical Treatment

Ideally, rotator cuff repair occurs relatively quickly; however, good preoperative management is critical to success. When appropriate, a preoperative medical evaluation needs to be performed to assess surgical risks. In addition, smoking needs to be specifically addressed. Patients need to understand that smoking is a direct cause for surgical failure and may need to seek medical assistance in quitting preoperatively. Shoulder stiffness should be addressed preoperatively through range of motion exercises or therapy as indicated to minimize the amount of surgical intervention necessary. The use of preoperative corticosteroid injections should be minimized to avoid tendon degradation. When the preoperative care has been maximized, repair should occur as soon as reasonable. Delaying surgery only increases the risk of tear propagation, further atrophy, and degeneration, thus increasing the risk of failure.

Surgical Technique

Arthroscopic augmentation begins with a standard quality cuff repair. Typically large and massive tears require a combination of margin convergence and anchor repair. Every attempt should be made to affect a partial repair of the remaining cuff to the tuberosities. Careful vigilance must be directed at the subscapularis as not only is it a significant humeral head depressor but its anatomic repair will advance the coracohumeral ligament and increase superior humeral head coverage. There are no special instruments required for augmentation. Two high tensile strength suture strands (no needles) and two anchors will be added after the partial repair for the augmentation. Suture passage can be performed with either antegrade or retrograde suture passers.

The first step is to create a framework of suture within the subacromial space using suture strands medially and anchors laterally. The sutures and anchors should be beyond the "edges" of the repair in all directions if possible to cover the repair completely. With the scope in the lateral portal, suture passage occurs through the anterior and posterior portals. Two mattress sutures are placed medial in the cuff muscle-tendon junction with one anterior and one posterior. There are multiple methods for passing these sutures using both antegrade and retrograde passers.

The author prefers a retrograde passer that goes in and out of the tendon with a suture loop coming through an opposing portal on a locking grasper. The loop is then grabbed and the suture pulled through the tendon in a retrograde direction. The suture grasper is then used to shuttle the suture out of the opposing portal (i.e., posterior medial mattress sutures come out the anterior portal) for later use. Two anchors are placed in the lateral tuberosity, one anteriorly and one posteriorly. These four corners (two medial sutures and two lateral anchors) now create the frame through which the graft will be placed (Fig. 21.1). The scope is moved to the posterior portal and a short 8.5 mm cannula is placed into the lateral portal. The sutures from each corner are retrieved through the lateral cannula. The next steps are key to achieving success in deploying the graft. Each pair of sutures must be kept separate from the others with meticulous suture management. Whichever suture pair is first retrieved is pulled out of the lateral cannula placed in its respective direction (anterior medial sutures pulled out and clipped to drapes anterior to cannula and toward the patient's feet if in lateral position). Tension is then placed on the sutures while the retriever goes back into the lateral cannula. Tensioning the sutures allows the retriever to pass through the cannula and avoiding crossing the sutures. The sutures should be on one side of the cannula, and the retriever should slide down the opposite side of the cannula and not pass through the sutures to retrieve the second pair. The process is repeated until the four pairs of sutures are out of the cannula and clipped to the drapes. The scope can be used to visualize the sutures which should be seen to enter the cannula separately (Fig. 21.2).

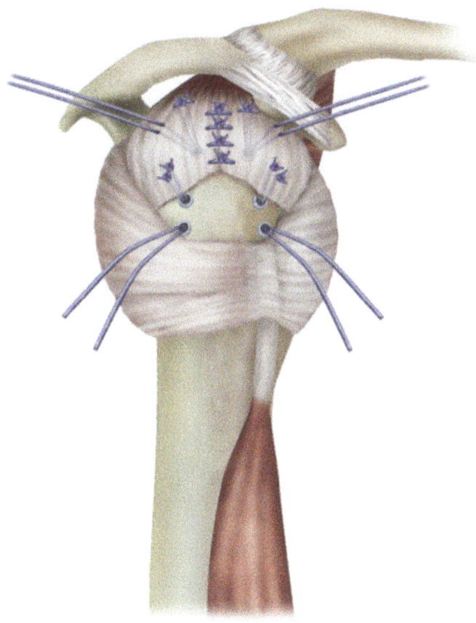

Fig. 21.1 Repaired rotator cuff with the four corners in place

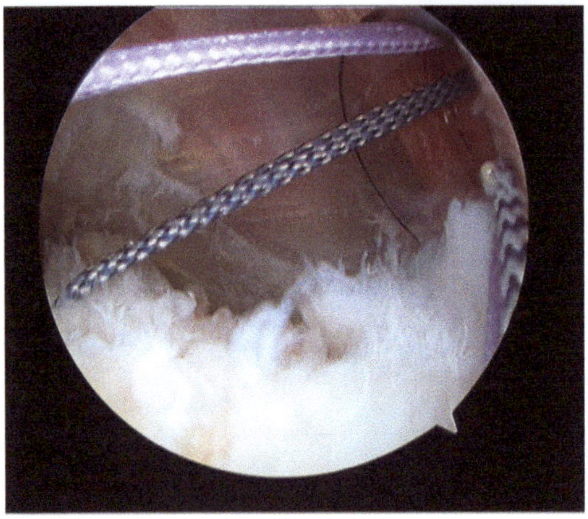

Fig. 21.2 View from the posterior portal as the sutures from the four corners can be seen entering the lateral cannula in an orderly fashion

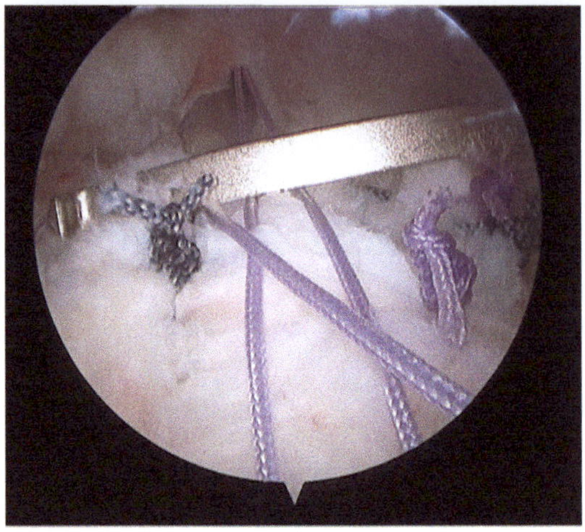

Fig. 21.3 View from the posterior portal while measuring the medial to lateral dimension of the repair

The size of the graft can now be determined. Using an arthroscopic ruler, the length and width of the graft framework is measured (Fig. 21.3). The shape of the graft can be variable and will range from square to rectangular or to trapezoidal depending on the shape of the tear repaired and the configuration of the corner sutures placed. The graft is then prepared according to the manufacturer's specifications and is cut to fit the measurement from the four corners. Most grafts have some degree of pliability and will be stretched. The stitches are now ready to be passed through the graft. Hemostats are placed in the corners of the graft and sutures are passed using free needles. For some dermal grafts, cutting needles are preferred as tapered needles have a difficult time passing and dull quickly. The sutures are passed from inferior to superior through the graft in mattress fashion matching their respective positions in the subacromial space (i.e., anterior medial sutures through anterior medial part of the graft). When passing the medial sutures, take a quick look arthroscopically to see if the tail is the most anterior or posterior of the two, and be sure the orientation stays the same as it passes through the graft.

When all eight suture tails are passed, preliminary knot tying can begin. Tie a sliding or sliding-locking knot and place a hemostat on the post-limb. Ensure the knot is sliding well using a knot pusher if needed. When all four knots are tied, grasp the medial edge of the graft in an arthroscopic grasper and hold the hemostats attached to the post-limbs. The hemostats should have been removed from the corners of the graft. Push the graft down the cannula and pull the post-limbs (Fig. 21.4). The graft can be observed entering the subacromial space arthroscopically. Once it is completely within the subacromial space, a knot pusher can be passed down each medial post-limb to "deploy" the graft and reduce the loop laxity within the knot. Through a separate cannula, the sutures can be retrieved and the arthroscopic knots completed (Fig. 21.5). The hemostats on the post-limbs help to identify the post-limb during this portion of the case. Once all knots are tied, the graft should be fixed to the cuff medially and the tuberosity laterally with some tension. If there is a portion of the graft not tensioned over the cuff, another suture can be passed using the same side-to-side technique when passing the medial mattress sutures. An antegrade or retrograde passer is passed throughout the cuff and graft, and either a suture leader is deployed or a suture looped is captured by the retriever. The limbs are then brought together in a knot tying cannula, and an arthroscopic knot is tied. The goal is to cover the cuff repair with the graft and have good contact between the graft and cuff in all areas (Fig. 21.6a, b).

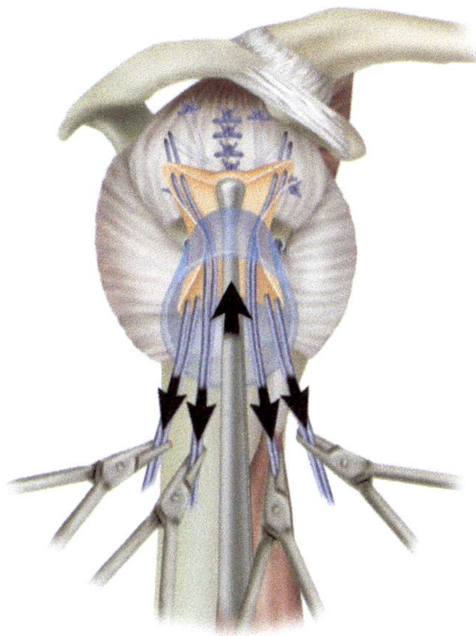

Fig. 21.4 Graft entering through the lateral cannula. In this illustration, the knots are not pre-tied but they can be. Tension on the post-limbs will then reduce the knot onto the graft holding the graft in place

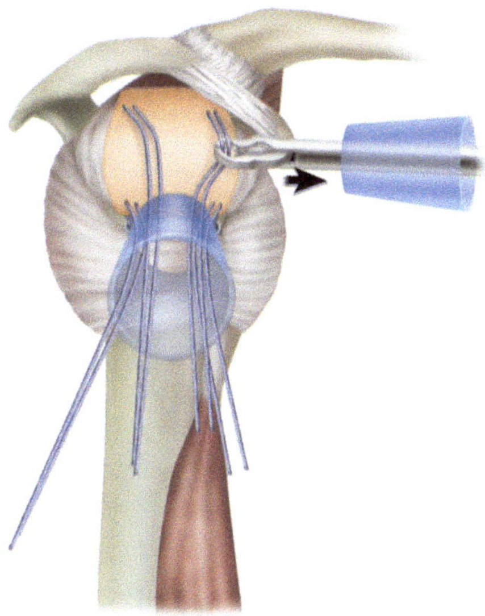

Fig. 21.5 Suture retrieval through separate cannula for knot tying

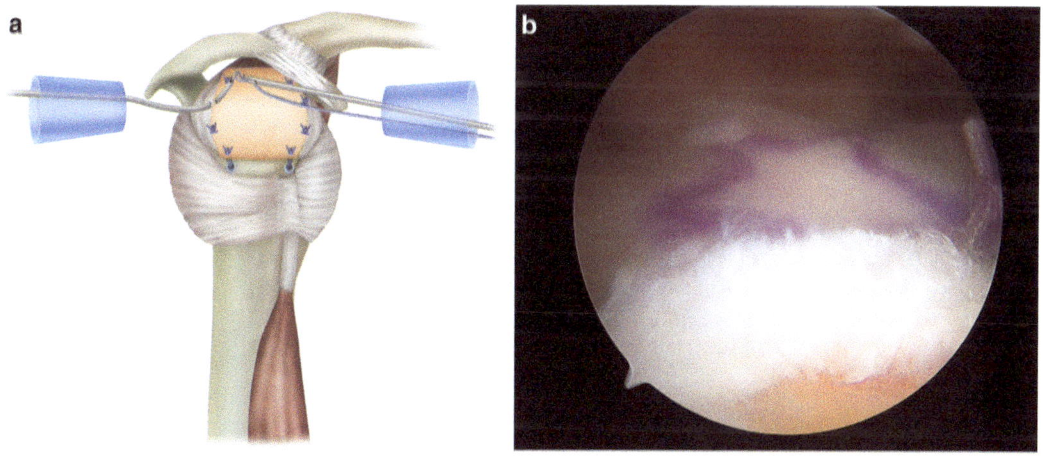

Fig. 21.6 (**a**) Extra sutures can be applied to the edges of the graft for further fixation or to reduce small wrinkle so that the graft has good circumferential contact. (**b**) View of the final construct from the lateral portal. Markings on the graft help to preserve orientation

Postoperative Management

Following the repair, patients are placed into a sling with an abduction pillow for approximately 4 weeks. Pendulum exercises may begin during this initial 4 weeks depending on the repair strength and tissue quality. Active elbow motion and scapular retraction exercises are performed 2–3 times a day. After 4–6 weeks formal physical therapy commences focusing on increasing range of motion. Motion is passive until 6 weeks. Active-assisted and active motion with formal periscapular strengthening starts at week 6. At 12 weeks postoperatively, rotator cuff strengthening may begin with larger muscle group strengthening. Pectoralis and deltoid strengthening can begin at 4–5 months postoperatively.

Complications

An inflammatory reaction, which presents similarly to an infection, has been associated with graft augmentation. This inflammatory reaction is most commonly seen with small intestine submucosa grafts, causing some to recommend against the use of this type of graft [25].

Disease transmission is also a potential risk when using allograft or xenograft. Due to the screening process performed prior to obtaining graft material, in addition to the acellular nature of the grafts and/or the sterilization processes used, no disease transmission has been reported from the use of these grafts in rotator cuff surgery. Likewise, the infection rate following rotator cuff repair with and without graft augmentation is comparable.

Postoperative shoulder stiffness is a complication associated with rotator cuff repair surgery with or without graft use. The overall incidence of shoulder stiffness following graft augmentation has not been reported. It is important to evaluate shoulder range of motion preoperatively and treat patients with limited motion with physical therapy before surgery. With large and massive rotator cuff tears, there may be a perception of loss of motion postoperatively as the humeral head can no longer subluxate through the torn cuff. Capsular releases should be performed as indicated at the time of grafting and repair surgery.

Technical Challenges

The first challenge when performing a rotator cuff repair with graft augmentation arthroscopically is dealing with the rotator cuff repair itself. The surgeon must be adept at multiple techniques that may be necessary when dealing with large and massive tears including tissue mobilization, suture management, and knot tying. Suture management is the biggest technical challenge for successful arthroscopic graft placement. The arthroscopic technique involves multiple sutures passing through a single cannula into the subacromial space. The use of sutures of different colors as well as proceeding in a preconceived order helps identify each suture and avoid entanglement. The suture should be tensioned and pulled to one side once it is brought through the cannula. The retriever should then go down the opposite side of the cannula to grab the next suture and not entangle the prior suture.

This chapter describes one technique of arthroscopic rotator cuff graft augmentation focusing on suture management. There are other methods that will also achieve the same goal, and each surgeon should use the method with which he/she is most comfortable. The key to performing this technique is practice. First, observing the procedure will not only help the surgeon familiarize himself/herself with the steps but also give insight as to how assistants in the case can facilitate the procedure. Next, the surgeon should practice the procedure either with a plastic model or cadaver specimen focusing on suture management. Once this is accomplished, the procedure can be performed with ease and predictability.

The Future

The use of these graft materials for rotator cuff repair surgery will continue to evolve as more procedures are developed and more research is performed on this subject. Currently, there is one prospective, multicenter, single-blinded study on the use of GraftJacket® (Wright Medical, Memphis, Tenn.) in rotator cuff surgery. The data from this study may help guide its use within the orthopedic community. The data available on the various types of grafts has not led to a consensus on a "best graft"; however, some types of grafts have shown inferior results with respect to rotator cuff repair surgery. Currently, acellular dermal grafts have shown the best clinical success. As these materials continue to be used, improvements can be expected in both surgical technique and instrumentation.

Theoretically, these grafts add mechanical strength and collagen at the rotator cuff repair site. The future use of the graft as a vehicle for platelet-rich plasma, stem cells, and/or growth factors at the repair site may also aid in the healing process [64–66]. Growth factors, such as transforming growth factor, fibroblast growth factor, cartilage-derived morphogenic protein, and bone morphogenic protein, stem cells, or platelet-rich plasma, may be injected at the repair site, or the graft may be pre-seeded prior to implantation. These adjuncts are discussed further in another chapter.

The future is very bright for the use of grafts aiding in rotator cuff repair surgery as more research into this new and powerful technology emerges.

References

1. Bishop J, et al. Cuff integrity after arthroscopic versus open rotator cuff repair: a prospective study. J Shoulder Elbow Surg. 2006;15:290–9.
2. Boileau P, et al. Arthroscopic repair of full-thickness tears of the supraspinatus: does the tendon really heal? J Bone Joint Surg Am. 2005;87:1229–40.
3. Cho NS, Yi JW, Lee BG, Rhee YG. Retear patterns after arthroscopic rotator cuff repair: single-row versus suture bridge technique. Am J Sports Med. 2010;38:664–71.
4. Koh KH, Kang KC, Lim TK, Shon MS, Yoo JC. Prospective randomized clinical trial of single- versus double-row suture anchor repair in 2- to 4-cm rotator cuff tears: clinical and magnetic resonance imaging results. Arthroscopy. 2011;27:453–62.
5. Flurin P-H, et al. Cuff Integrity after arthroscopic rotator cuff repair: correlation with clinical results in 576 cases. Arthroscopy. 2007;23:340–6.
6. Harryman 2nd DT, et al. Repairs of the rotator cuff. Correlation of functional results with integrity of the cuff. J Bone Joint Surg Am. 1991;73:982–9.
7. Björnsson HC, Norlin R, Johansson K, Adolfsson LE. The influence of age, delay of repair, and tendon involvement in acute rotator cuff tears: structural and clinical outcomes after repair of 42 shoulders. Acta Orthop. 2011;82:187–92.
8. Iannotti JP. Full-thickness rotator cuff tears: factors affecting surgical outcome. J Am Acad Orthop Surg. 1994;2:87–95.
9. Longo UG, et al. Histopathology of the supraspinatus tendon in rotator cuff tears. Am J Sports Med. 2008;36:533–8.
10. Longo UG, Berton A, Khan WS, Maffulli N, Denaro V. Histopathology of rotator cuff tears. Sports Med Arthrosc Rev. 2011;19:227–36.
11. Simon DWN, et al. Identifying the cellular basis for reimplantation failure in repair of the rotator cuff. J Bone Joint Surg (Br). 2008;90:680–4.
12. Mall NA, Tanaka MJ, Choi LS, Paletta Jr GA. Factors affecting rotator cuff healing. J Bone Joint Surg Am. 2014;96:778–88.
13. Castagna A, et al. Arthroscopic repair of rotator cuff tear with a modified Mason-Allen stitch: mid-term clinical and ultrasound outcomes. Knee Surg Sports Traumatol Arthrosc. 2008;16:497–503.
14. Goutallier D, Postel J-M, Gleyze P, Leguilloux P, Van Driessche S. Influence of cuff muscle fatty degeneration on anatomic and functional outcomes after simple suture of full-thickness tears. J Shoulder Elbow Surg. 2003;12:550–4.
15. Carbone S, et al. The impact of preoperative smoking habit on rotator cuff tear: cigarette smoking influences rotator cuff tear sizes. J Shoulder Elbow Surg. 2012;21:56–60.
16. McRae S, Leiter J, Walmsley C, Rehsia S, Macdonald P. Relationship between self-reported shoulder function/quality of life, body mass index, and other contributing factors in patients awaiting rotator cuff repair surgery. J Shoulder Elbow Surg. 2011;20:57–61.
17. Mallon WJ, Misamore G, Snead DS, Denton P. The impact of preoperative smoking habits on the results of rotator cuff repair. J Shoulder Elbow Surg. 2004;13:129–32.
18. Chechik O, et al. Timing matters: NSAIDs interfere with the late proliferation stage of a repaired rotator cuff tendon healing in rats. Arch Orthop Trauma Surg. 2014;134:515–20.
19. Caro AC, et al. Efficacy of various analgesics on shoulder function and rotator cuff tendon-to-bone healing in a rat (*Rattus norvegicus*) model. J Am Assoc Lab Anim Sci. 2014;53:185–92.
20. Connizzo BK, et al. The detrimental effects of systemic ibuprofen delivery on tendon healing are time-dependent. Clin. Orthop. 2013. doi:10.1007/s11999-013-3258-2.
21. Cohen DB, Kawamura S, Ehteshami JR, Rodeo SA. Indomethacin and celecoxib impair rotator cuff tendon-to-bone healing. Am J Sports Med. 2006;34:362–9.
22. Neviaser JS, Neviaser RJ, Neviaser TJ. The repair of chronic massive ruptures of the rotator cuff of the shoulder by use of a freeze-dried rotator cuff. J Bone Joint Surg Am. 1978;60:681–4.
23. Nasca RJ. The use of freeze-dried allografts in the management of global rotator cuff tears. Clin Orthop. 1988;228:218–26.
24. Moore DR, Cain EL, Schwartz ML, Clancy Jr WG. Allograft reconstruction for massive, irreparable rotator cuff tears. Am J Sports Med. 2006;34:392–6.
25. Walton JR, Bowman NK, Khatib Y, Linklater J, Murrell GAC. Restore orthobiologic implant: not recommended for augmentation of rotator cuff repairs. J Bone Joint Surg Am. 2007;89:786–91.
26. Sclamberg SG, Tibone JE, Itamura JM, Kasraeian S. Six-month magnetic resonance imaging follow-up of

large and massive rotator cuff repairs reinforced with porcine small intestinal submucosa. J Shoulder Elbow Surg. 2004;13:538–41.
27. Barber FA, Burns JP, Deutsch A, Labbé MR, Litchfield RB. A prospective, randomized evaluation of acellular human dermal matrix augmentation for arthroscopic rotator cuff repair. Arthroscopy. 2012; 28:8–15.
28. Ricchetti ET, Aurora A, Iannotti JP, Derwin KA. Scaffold devices for rotator cuff repair. J Shoulder Elbow Surg. 2012;21:251–65.
29. Aurora A, et al. The biomechanical role of scaffolds in augmented rotator cuff tendon repairs. J Shoulder Elbow Surg. 2012;21:1064–71.
30. Chen J, Xu J, Wang A, Zheng M. Scaffolds for tendon and ligament repair: review of the efficacy of commercial products. Expert Rev Med Devices. 2009;6:61–73.
31. Audenaert E, Van Nuffel J, Schepens A, Verhelst M, Verdonk R. Reconstruction of massive rotator cuff lesions with a synthetic interposition graft: a prospective study of 41 patients. Knee Surg Sports Traumatol Arthrosc. 2006;14:360–4.
32. Badhe SP, Lawrence TM, Smith FD, Lunn PG. An assessment of porcine dermal xenograft as an augmentation graft in the treatment of extensive rotator cuff tears. J Shoulder Elbow Surg. 2008;17:S35–9.
33. Iannotti JP, et al. Porcine small intestine submucosa augmentation of surgical repair of chronic two-tendon rotator cuff tears. A randomized, controlled trial. J Bone Joint Surg Am. 2006;88:1238–44.
34. Zheng MH, et al. Porcine small intestine submucosa (SIS) is not an acellular collagenous matrix and contains porcine DNA: possible implications in human implantation. J Biomed Mater Res B Appl Biomater. 2005;73:61–7.
35. Bergeson AG, et al. Effects of platelet-rich fibrin matrix on repair integrity of at-risk rotator cuff tears. Am J Sports Med. 2012;40:286–93.
36. Barber FA, Hrnack SA, Snyder SJ, Hapa O. Rotator cuff repair healing influenced by platelet-rich plasma construct augmentation. Arthroscopy. 2011;27:1029–35.
37. Castricini R, et al. Platelet-rich plasma augmentation for arthroscopic rotator cuff repair: a randomized controlled trial. Am J Sports Med. 2011;39:258–65.
38. Jo CH, et al. Does platelet-rich plasma accelerate recovery after rotator cuff repair? A prospective cohort study. Am J Sports Med. 2011;39:2082–90.
39. Bond JL, Dopirak RM, Higgins J, Burns J, Snyder SJ. Arthroscopic replacement of massive, irreparable rotator cuff tears using a GraftJacket allograft: technique and preliminary results. Arthroscopy. 2008;24:403–409.e1.
40. Gupta AK, et al. Dermal tissue allograft for the repair of massive irreparable rotator cuff tears. Am J Sports Med. 2012;40:141–7.
41. Wong I, Burns J, Snyder S. Arthroscopic GraftJacket repair of rotator cuff tears. J Shoulder Elbow Surg. 2010;19:104–9.
42. Rotini R, et al. Human dermal matrix scaffold augmentation for large and massive rotator cuff repairs: preliminary clinical and MRI results at 1-year follow-up. Musculoskelet Surg. 2011;95 Suppl 1:S13–23.
43. Barber FA, Aziz-Jacobo J. Biomechanical testing of commercially available soft-tissue augmentation materials. Arthroscopy. 2009;25:1233–9.
44. Bektaşer B, et al. Free coracoacromial ligament graft for augmentation of massive rotator cuff tears treated with mini-open repair. Acta Orthop Traumatol Turc. 2010;44:426–30.
45. Ellera Gomes JL, da Silva RC, Silla LMR, Abreu MR, Pellanda R. Conventional rotator cuff repair complemented by the aid of mononuclear autologous stem cells. Knee Surg Sports Traumatol Arthrosc. 2012;20: 373–7.
46. Encalada-Diaz I, et al. Rotator cuff repair augmentation using a novel polycarbonate polyurethane patch: preliminary results at 12 months' follow-up. J Shoulder Elbow Surg. 2011;20:788–94.
47. Hirooka A, et al. Augmentation with a Gore-Tex patch for repair of large rotator cuff tears that cannot be sutured. J Orthop Sci. 2002;7:451–6.
48. Ito J, Morioka T. Surgical treatment for large and massive tears of the rotator cuff. Int Orthop. 2003;27:228–31.
49. Nada AN, Debnath UK, Robinson DA, Jordan C. Treatment of massive rotator-cuff tears with a polyester ligament (Dacron) augmentation: clinical outcome. J Bone Joint Surg (Br). 2010;92:1397–402.
50. Gédouin JE, et al. Deltoid muscle flap for massive rotator cuff tears: 41 cases with a mean 7-year (minimum 5 year) follow-up. Rev Chir Orthop Réparatrice Appar Mot. 2002;88:365–72.
51. Visuri T, Kiviluoto O, Eskelin M. Carbon fiber for repair of the rotator cuff. A 4-year follow-up of 14 cases. Acta Orthop Scand. 1991;62:356–9.
52. Scheibel M, Brown A, Woertler K, Imhoff AB. Preliminary results after rotator cuff reconstruction augmented with an autologous periosteal flap. Knee Surg Sports Traumatol Arthrosc. 2007;15: 305–14.
53. Cho NS, Yi JW, Rhee YG. Arthroscopic biceps augmentation for avoiding undue tension in repair of massive rotator cuff tears. Arthroscopy. 2009;25: 183–91.
54. Barber FA, Herbert MA, Coons DA. Tendon augmentation grafts: biomechanical failure loads and failure patterns. Arthroscopy. 2006;22:534–8.
55. Derwin KA, Baker AR, Spragg RK, Leigh DR, Iannotti JP. Commercial extracellular matrix scaffolds for rotator cuff tendon repair: biomechanical, biochemical, and cellular properties. J Bone Joint Surg. 2006;88:2665–72.
56. Tanaka N, Sakahashi H, Hirose K, Ishima T, Ishii S. Augmented subscapularis muscle transposition for rotator cuff repair during shoulder arthroplasty in patients with rheumatoid arthritis. J Shoulder Elbow Surg. 2006;15:2–6.

57. McCarron JA, Milks RA, Chen X, Iannotti JP, Derwin KA. Improved time-zero biomechanical properties using poly-L-lactic acid graft augmentation in a cadaveric rotator cuff repair model. J Shoulder Elbow Surg. 2010;19:688–96.
58. McCarty 3rd LP, Buss DD, Datta MW, Freehill MQ, Giveans MR. Complications observed following labral or rotator cuff repair with use of poly-L-lactic acid implants. J Bone Joint Surg Am. 2013;95:507–11.
59. Papalia R, et al. Augmentation techniques for rotator cuff repair. Br Med Bull. 2013;105:107–38.
60. Edwards SL, Lynch TS, Saltzman MD, Terry MA, Nuber GW. Biologic and pharmacologic augmentation of rotator cuff repairs. J Am Acad Orthop Surg. 2011;19:583–9.
61. Badylak SF, Gilbert TW. Immune response to biologic scaffold materials. Semin Immunol. 2008;20:109–16.
62. Johnson W, Inamasu J, Yantzer B, Papangelou C, Guiot B. Comparative in vitro biomechanical evaluation of two soft tissue defect products. J Biomed Mater Res B Appl Biomater. 2007. doi:10.1002/jbm.b.30816.
63. Burkhead WZ, Schiffern SC, Krishnan SG. Use of graft jacket as an augmentation for massive rotator cuff tears. Semin Arthroplasty. 2007;18:11–8.
64. Angeline ME, Rodeo SA. Biologics in the management of rotator cuff surgery. Clin Sports Med. 2012;31:645–63.
65. Gulotta LV, Rodeo SA. Growth factors for rotator cuff repair. Clin Sports Med. 2009;28:13–23.
66. Seeherman HJ, et al. rhBMP-12 accelerates healing of rotator cuff repairs in a sheep model. J Bone Joint Surg Am. 2008;90:2206–19.

Suprascapular Nerve Release: General Principles

22

Arash A. Dini, Michael J. O'Brien, and Felix H. Savoie III

Introduction

Suprascapular nerve neuropathy is a cause of shoulder pain and dysfunction that is often overlooked in the diagnosis of long-standing shoulder pain. Previously regarded as a diagnosis of exclusion, increased attention to the condition has resulted in specific diagnostic techniques and treatment plans tailored to this previously elusive diagnosis. The condition can be caused both by traction or manipulative injury to the nerve, as well as from compression from normal anatomic structures and pathologic masses. Conservative treatments as well as surgical treatments, both open and arthroscopic, have been well described and shown to be effective treatments. Suprascapular nerve neuropathy should be part of the differential diagnosis for shoulder pain refractory to treatment in certain populations.

Anatomy

The suprascapular nerve receives its major contribution from the C5 nerve root, with minor contributions from C4 to C6. The nerve exits the upper trunk of the brachial plexus near the supraclavicular fossa and enters the suprascapular notch beneath the transverse scapular ligament (Fig. 22.1), dividing into two branches which innervate the supraspinatus and infraspinatus, respectively [2]. The potential for compression and traction injury in the suprascapular notch has been well studied [29]. The two branches are comprised of a nerve to the supraspinatus muscle which exits medially (Fig. 22.2); the second branch continues across the floor of the supraspinatus fossa of the scapula toward the junction of the scapular spine and the posterior–superior neck of the glenoid. The nerve continues around the bone junction under the spinoglenoid ligament (when present) and travels medially across the superior aspect of the infraspinatus fossa of the scapula, innervating and terminating in the infraspinatus (Fig. 22.3) [8]. Some investigators describe a third sensory branch that arises near the suprascapular notch and courses laterally to supply the glenohumeral joint.

Recent attention has been given to anatomic variants of the course of the suprascapular nerve and its associated artery and vein, with particular attention toward how these variants may be associated with compression and injury. Polguj et al. performed anatomic studies of 106 cadaveric specimens showing the constant path of the suprascapular nerve beneath the transverse scapula ligament in all specimens [19]. However, the course of the artery and vein was found to

A.A. Dini, MD • M.J. O'Brien, MD
F.H. Savoie III, MD (✉)
Department of Orthopaedics, Tulane University School of Medicine, New Orleans, LA, USA
e-mail: fsavoie@tulane.edu

J.D. Kelly IV (ed.), *Elite Techniques in Shoulder Arthroscopy*, DOI 10.1007/978-3-319-25103-5_22

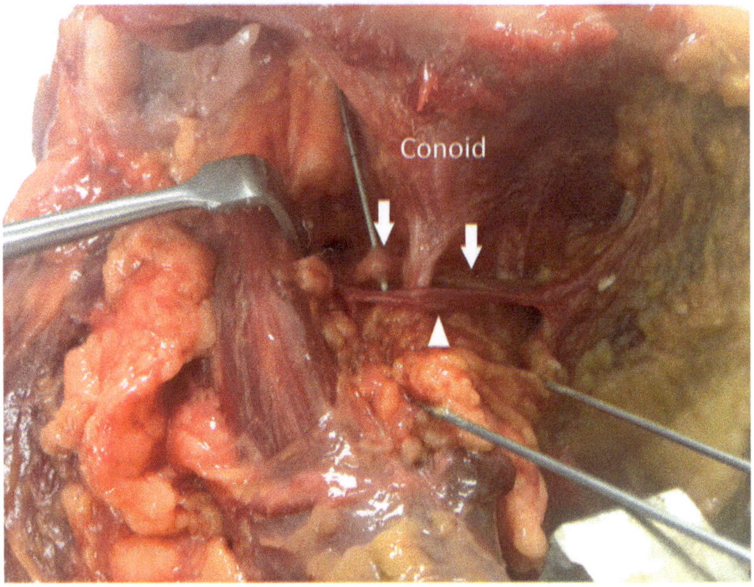

Fig. 22.1 The anatomic course of the suprascapular nerve. The suprascapular nerve (*white arrows*) leaves the brachial plexus and travels posteriorly under the transverse scapular ligament with the vein, while the artery (*white arrowhead*) travels over the ligament. The transverse scapular ligament can be identified at the base of the coracoid, just medial and posterior to the coracoclavicular ligaments. The retractor is retracting the supraspinatus muscle posteriorly. (Published with the permission of ©Felix H. Savoie, III 2015)

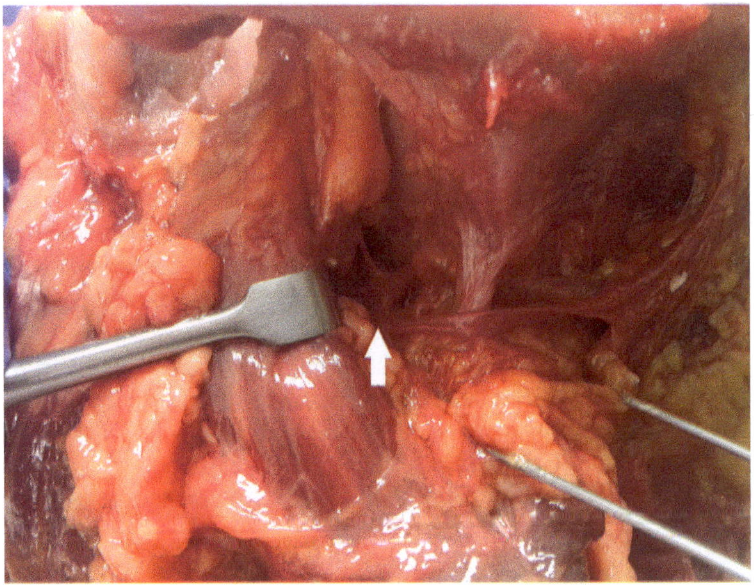

Fig. 22.2 Cadaveric dissection demonstrates the nerve branching at the *white arrow*, with a medial branch innervating the supraspinatus muscle, a branch diving deep along the floor of the supraspinatus fossa that continues to the spinoglenoid notch, and a small lateral sensory branch to the glenohumeral joint. (Published with the permission of ©Felix H. Savoie, III 2015)

be highly variable, and a proposed classification system was offered. The majority of specimens (61 %) were found to have the suprascapular artery pass above the transverse scapular ligament and the vein below the transverse scapular ligament in type I of this classification (Fig. 22.1). Type II specimens showed both the artery and vein passing above the transverse scapular ligament; this configuration was present in about 17 % of specimens. Type III specimens showed both the artery and vein passing below the ligament (12 %). A type IV classification was reserved for other variants including double veins and vessels that passed below the anterior coracoscapular ligament (a ligament found in over half of the specimens dissected).

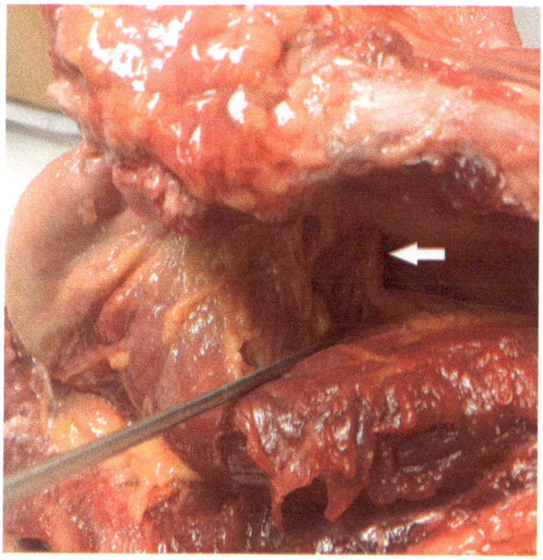

Fig. 22.3 The suprascapular nerve continues around the spinoglenoid notch at the base of the scapular spine (*white arrow*) and courses medially to innervate the infraspinatus muscle. In this photograph, the nerve can be seen branching out on the superior surface of the infraspinatus. (Published with the permission of ©Felix H. Savoie, III 2015)

Pathogenesis

Extrinsic compression and traction of the suprascapular nerve has been shown to cause neuropathy. The suprascapular notch and the spinoglenoid notch are the two implicated locations of compression. Aiello et al. were able to distinguish between entrapment of the nerve at the spinoglenoid notch and the suprascapular notch, usually as a result of a ganglion cyst in the spinoglenoid notch [1]. Repetitive microtrauma as a result of overhead activities and sports may lead to direct or indirect traction-type injury to the nerve and nearby vasculature, resulting in ischemic injury to the nerve [22]. Iatrogenic injury to the suprascapular nerve has been reported during distal clavicle resection, positioning during spine surgery, and other surgeries on or near the shoulder. Acute trauma in the case of glenohumeral dislocations, proximal humerus fractures, and scapula fractures have also been implicated [4, 5, 25]. All of these above mentioned mechanisms of injury are likely to cause compression at the suprascapular notch due to the limited translational freedom of the nerve around the narrow confines of the notch, predisposing it to injury in extreme positions of scapular depression, retraction, or abduction [26]. Compression-related neuropathy as a result of the ganglion cyst or tumor is more often a result of compression at the spinoglenoid notch [10]. The ganglion cyst may be a result of labral or capsular violations with associated extravasation of synovial fluid. This association has been challenged, yet most experienced clinicians relate that a labral tear is usually found in the presence of paralabral cysts [9, 27].

The treatment of isolated spinoglenoid compression will be elaborated further in a subsequent chapter.

Presentation

Often mimicking rotator cuff pathology, suprascapular neuropathy presents as diffuse pain over the lateral and posterior aspects of the shoulder with associated weakness. Referred symptoms can be as far as the lateral aspect of the arm, ipsilateral neck, and anterior chest well. A careful history is necessary to reveal any episodes of trauma, such as a fall on outstretched extremity, or other direct force. Trauma may include a hyper-external rotational movement, such as seen in volleyball, tennis, and water polo. The athlete may complain of resultant "soreness and weakness" that may mimic an infraspinatus tendonitis.

Physical Exam

Inspection of the shoulder may reveal atrophy in the supraspinatus and infraspinatus fossae. In the very early stages, the upper infraspinatus, just below the scapular spine, is often the first place to note subtle atrophy. Looking downward at the scapular spine on a seated patient helps discern subtle spinati atrophy. Long-standing proximal compression may show wasting of both the supraspinatus and infraspinatus, with the deltoid maintaining its bulk. Compression at the spinoglenoid notch will often show isolated wasting of the infraspinatus. Symptoms, in this case, are often vague and diffuse without an obvious associated weakness in strength attributed to the posterior deltoid and teres minor compensation [7]. Strength comparison with the contralateral arm will often demonstrate a strength difference between the two sides. Provocative maneuvers can be utilized to further assess the severity of the symptoms, including the Whipple test (Fig. 22.4), whereby the patient positions the arm in 90° of forward flexion and maximal adduction and resists downward pressure. The infraspinatus strength may be assessed by resisted external rotation with the arm adducted or with positioning the arm in 90° of abduction and full external rotation. These tests are often positive early in the disease course. Impingement tests including the Neer sign and Hawkins test are often positive, secondary to weakness in the supraspinatus and infraspinatus muscles.

The suprascapular nerve stretch test (Fig. 22.5) has been described in order to reproduce the posterior shoulder pain associated with compression of the nerve at the suprascapular notch [12]. This test is performed by the examiner rotating the head of the patient laterally and away from the affected shoulder while retracting the shoulder with gentle traction, applying stretch to the nerve. A positive test elicits posterior shoulder pain.

Imaging

Patients will often receive a full set of shoulder radiographs as part of their workup to exclude other causes of shoulder pain. In the absence of concomitant pathology, radiographs are usually normal. Occasionally one might see slight superior migration of the humeral head on the glenoid due to loss of the humeral head depression effect of the posterior cuff. Radiographs of the cervical spine may be warranted to exclude radicular causes of the patient's symptoms. In the post-traumatic setting, radiographs of the scapula and clavicle may demonstrate callus formation from healing fractures resulting in compression of the nerve. Post and Mayer described a radiograph taken from anterior to posterior of the scapula with the beam directed caudally 15–30° for a view of the suprascapular notch [21]. Depending on the severity of any bony deformity, a computed tomography (CT) scan may be indicated.

Magnetic resonance imaging (MRI) is generally indicated as the next step in imaging workup subsequent to radiographs. MRI allows for definition of the course of the nerve, associated muscle atrophy, space-occupying lesions, and view of concomitant pathology such as rotator cuff tears and labral pathology. Edema followed by atrophy of the supraspinatus and infraspinatus is the first sign of compression distinguishable on an MRI (Fig. 22.6a, b) [14]. Long-standing compression

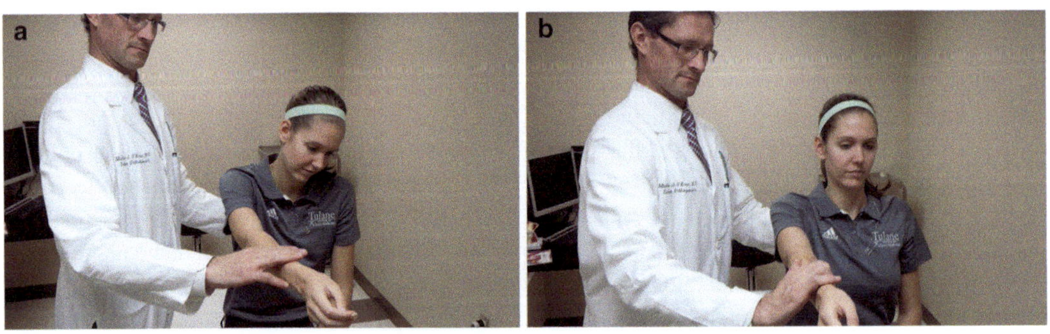

Fig. 22.4 The Whipple test is performed with the affected arm in 90° of forward flexion and full adduction, resisting a downward pressure. Pain and weakness indicate supraspinatus pathology. If the patient has poor posture and a protracted shoulder (**a**), the test is repeated holding the shoulder in a retracted position (**b**). Improved strength in this position is indicative of scapular dyskinesia. (Published with the permission of ©Felix H. Savoie, III 2015)

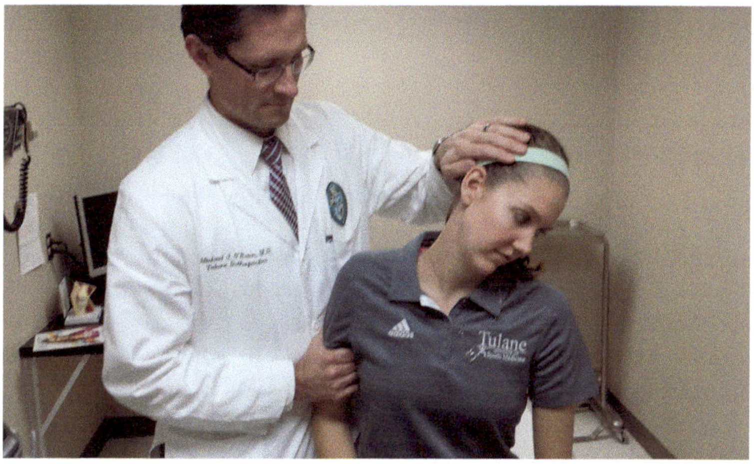

Fig. 22.5 The suprascapular nerve stretch test is performed by rotating the head of the patient laterally and away from the affected shoulder while retracting the shoulder with gentle traction, applying stretch to the nerve. (Published with the permission of ©Felix H. Savoie, III 2015)

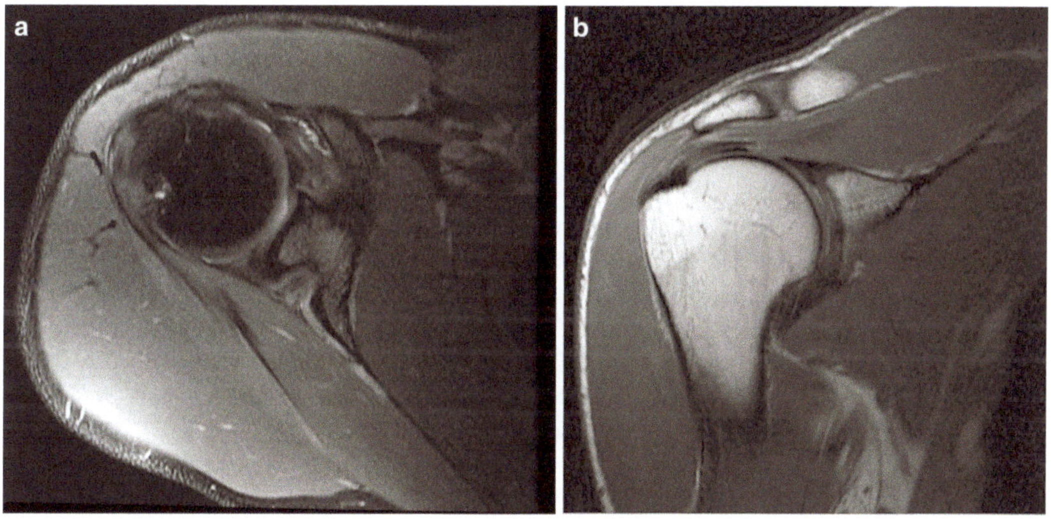

Fig. 22.6 MRI showing atrophy of the supraspinatus and infraspinatus muscles from long-standing compression of the suprascapular nerve in a young baseball pitcher. (**a**) Axial (**b**) Coronal (Published with the permission of ©Felix H. Savoie, III 2015)

will show marked atrophy of the associated rotator cuff musculature.

Electromyographic nerve conduction studies may help specifically define the site of compression if questions still remain after the previous imaging studies are inconclusive. Severe atrophy in the musculature is associated with increased false-negative electrodiagnostic studies as the superficial electrical signal may be picked up by the more bulky deltoid muscle. In addition, the expertise of the electromyographer is paramount in the utility of electrodiagnostic studies, as a high degree of experience is required in order to properly execute the study [24].

Suprascapular diagnostic nerve blocks with local anesthetic have been described in certain cases to aid in diagnosis, with a positive test being defined as elimination of associated shoulder pain after local injection of the anesthetic [1]. The use of this test may be more practical with the use of ultrasound guidance, which has been well described for the suprascapular nerve as a diagnostic tool despite its limited appearance in the literature [17].

Nonoperative Treatment

The success of nonoperative treatment for suprascapular nerve-related symptoms is most closely related to the etiology of the problem. Injury to the nerve unrelated to direct compression has the best likelihood of recovery without surgery [20]. Symptoms that can be attributed to a defined site of compression are less likely to experience any improvement without surgical intervention. In the setting of non-compressive causes of nerve injury, a structured therapy program can be used with specific emphasis on scapula retraction, maintaining proper posture, and glenohumeral range of motion [23]. The appropriateness of duration of nonoperative treatment remains controversial. The correct diagnosis of a suprascapular nerve entrapment is often delayed, and it is common that several modalities of conservative treatment may have been administered to the patient over an extended period of time. This has led some authors to suggest operative treatment as soon as the correct diagnosis is made [20]. Others have suggested to administer a full 1-year course of conservative treatment in the absence of an obvious compressive lesion [16]. In cases where a clear spinoglenoid cyst is identifiable, aspiration of the cyst can result in sufficient decompression to permit nerve healing with sufficient rehabilitation. However, recurrence rates have been reported to be high [9, 27]. In more advanced cases, surgical decompression of either the suprascapular notch or spinoglenoid notch should be performed.

Operative Treatment

Indications for operative treatment include symptoms refractory to appropriate conservative treatment, and/or an identifiable compressive lesion to the suprascapular nerve [6]. Surgical decompression of the entrapped nerve has been shown to be successful in many series. Several open approaches have been described and have accompanying good outcomes. Vastamaki has described the open approach in which an incision is made directly over the supraspinatus fossa. The trapezius is split, allowing access to the supraspinatus muscle and fossa. The supraspinatus muscle can be retracted posteriorly to allow access to the suprascapular notch and the area of compression directly released. In most cases, the supraspinatus can also be retracted anteriorly, allowing access to decompress the spinoglenoid notch as well [28].

Lafosse et al. described the arthroscopic technique for decompression at the suprascapular notch with excellent short-term results [13]. The technique specifically described an all arthroscopic approach for resection of the transverse scapular ligament in a small cohort of patients (10), all of whom had resolution of symptoms postoperatively. Plancher et al. have described the arthroscopic decompression at the spinoglenoid notch in a cadaveric model [18]. Mall et al. have described an open approach to the spinoglenoid notch via deltoid splitting approach at the level of the scapular spine [15]. The senior author prefers arthroscopic decompression, which will be described in detail.

Technique

Suprascapular Notch Decompression

The suprascapular notch decompression is approached arthroscopically with the arthroscope in the lateral subacromial portal. An anterolateral working portal is established as well. The base of the coracoid is identified and forms the floor of the area of surgery (Fig. 22.7A, B).

A Neviaser portal is established and a switching stick is placed via this portal to retract the suprascapular nerve and artery, while a careful removal of the soft tissues between the coracoclavicular (CC) ligaments and the supraspinatus muscle is accomplished (Fig. 22.8A, B).

The lateral view then allows one to enter a "room with walls" where the floor is formed by

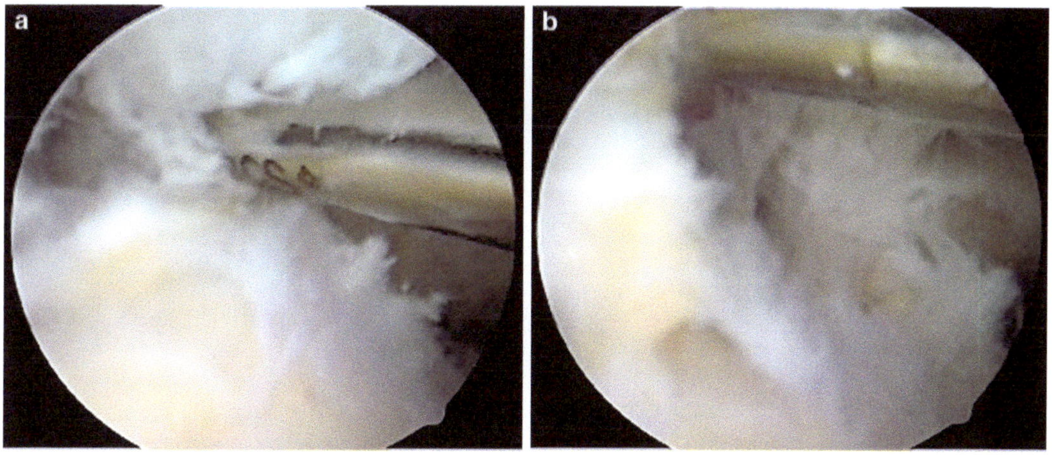

Fig. 22.7 Exposure of coracoid base (Published with the permission of ©Felix H. Savoie, III 2015)

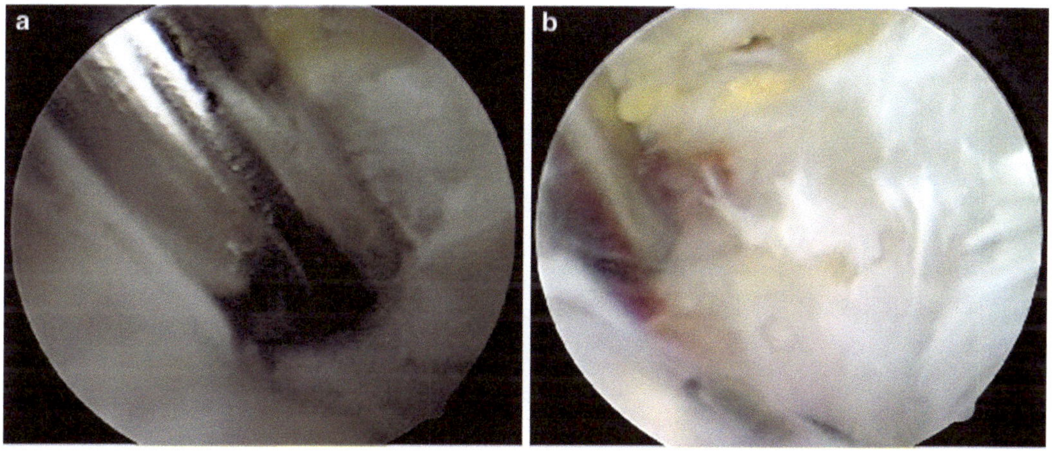

Fig. 22.8 Placement of switching stick and retractor through Neviaser portal (Published with the permission of ©Felix H. Savoie, III 2015)

the coracoid base and supraspinatus fossa; the posterior wall is the supraspinatus muscle and the anterior wall is the coracoclavicular ligaments.

A second Neviaser portal is created 2 cm medial to the first, and a second switching stick placed into this area (Fig. 22.9).

The switching stick can be placed directly into the suprascapular notch to protect the artery and nerve. The lateral Neviaser portal can then be used for instrumentation to release and remove the ligament, freeing the nerve (Fig. 22.10A, B, C). One should always check anteriorly and posteriorly for additional adhesions, especially in revision cases.

Spinoglenoid Notch Decompression

The notch is approached by visualization via a standard lateral subacromial portal. A standard posterior portal is used for instrumentation, and a second more medial and inferior portal used for protection of the nerve (accessory posterior–inferior portal) (Fig. 22.11). The scapular spine is located and followed inferiorly. As the spinoglenoid ligament is inconsistent, one should keep a switching stick at the spinoglenoid notch area to prevent inadvertent resection of the nerve. As one gets closer to the base of the spine, the dissection is mostly with blunt probe via the more medial

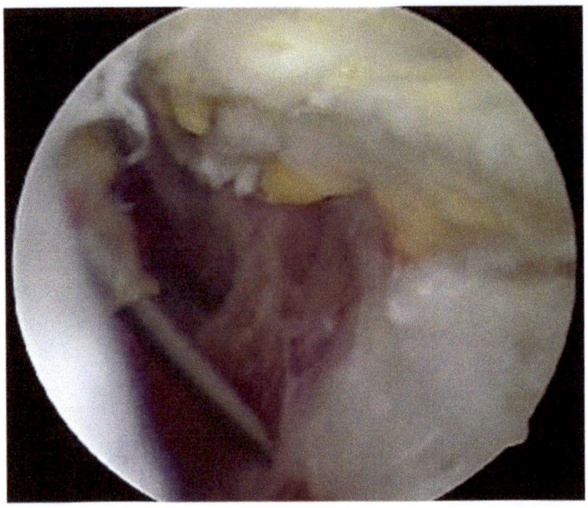

Fig. 22.9 Spinal needle showing position of second (medial) Neviaser portal (Published with the permission of ©Felix H. Savoie, III 2015)

portal until the nerve is identified (Fig. 22.12). There is usually two or more adhesions medial to the notch that will need to be released in addition to the spinoglenoid ligament.

Postoperative Care

Patients receive brief period of rest in a postoperative sling and begin early therapy and range of motion, provided no other pathology was addressed intraoperatively. A home nerve stimulator may be used and rehabilitation should stress the importance of posture and scapular position. Most patients will have an immediate decrease in their pain and improvement in their strength, yet

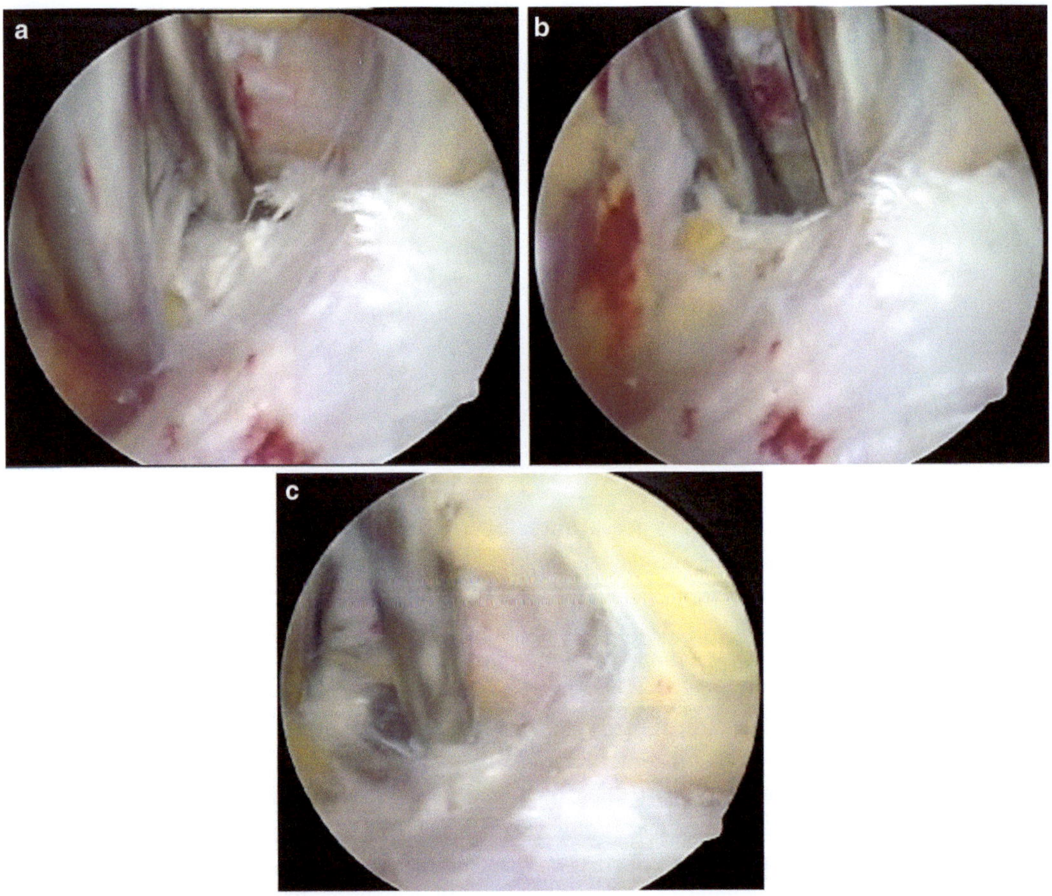

Fig. 22.10 Retractor protecting the suprascapular nerve and shaver preparing to resect the transverse scapular ligament. (C) shows the resected ligament. (Published with the permission of ©Felix H. Savoie, III 2015)

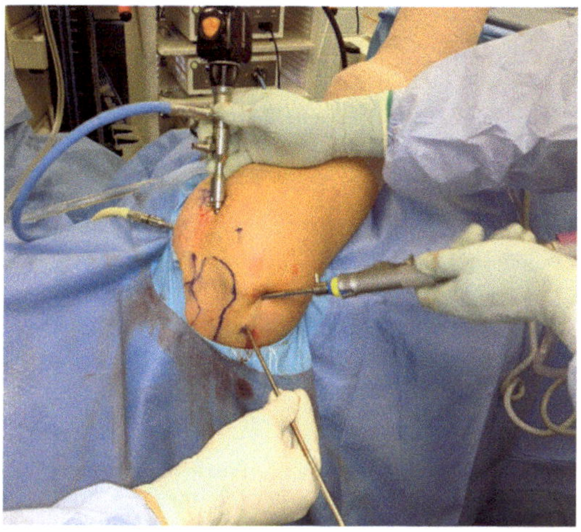

Fig. 22.11 Arthroscope in the lateral portal (camera). Posterior portal is used for instrumentation (shaver handle). Accessory posterior–inferior portal is used for retracting of the nerve (switching stick). (Published with the permission of ©Felix H. Savoie, III 2015)

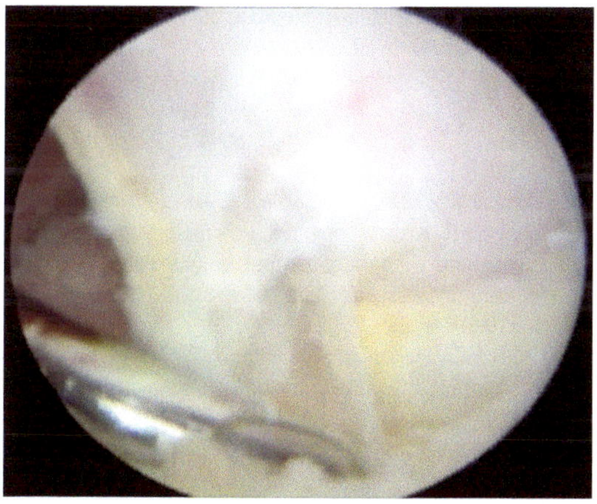

Fig. 22.12 Identification of the suprascapular nerve in the spinoglenoid notch (Published with the permission of ©Felix H. Savoie, III 2015)

a full 6–12 months of observation is required to assess their true strength recovery.

Results

Lafosse et al. have reported excellent results with arthroscopic decompression of the suprascapular notch [13]. In his series, 10 patients with defined symptoms of suprascapular nerve compression and positive electrodiagnostic studies were treated with arthroscopic release of the transverse scapular ligament. Postoperative course included brief immobilization (48–72 h) and early range of motion and rehabilitation. All patients had decreased postoperative pain scores and improved muscle strength. Eight of 10 patients received postoperative EMG testing as well, with 7 of them showing normalization of their conduction velocities, distal latency, and amplitude. These results are comparable to previous studies showing the improvement in patients' symptoms that can be expected from an open decompression. In the largest reported series (31 patients), Kim et al. were able to show significant improvement in strength and reduced pain in all subjects [11].

Mall et al. have also reported satisfactory results with open spinoglenoid decompression. In a series of 29 patients who underwent an open approach to the spinoglenoid notch with subsequent decompression, a mean increase in ER strength of 1.3 grades was seen, as well as a mean increase in manual muscle strength of at least 1 grade. Patients where a ganglion cyst was found, experienced quicker return to strength compared with patients who had no specific cysts found at the time of surgery [15].

Plancher et al. have similar results with a novel arthroscopic technique. Details of his unique approach are discussed in another chapter [18].

Discussion

The main challenge with suprascapular nerve (SSN) neuropathy is recognition and formation of a timely diagnosis. Rather than suprascapular nerve neuropathy (a diagnosis of exclusion), a thorough history and physical exam may lead to diagnosis of compression of this unique nerve. Subtle elements to the history and activity status of the patient, in addition to direct visualization of the patient's spinati muscle bulk, should aid in diagnosis. MRI and EMG protocols have become specific enough to also provide earlier and accurate diagnosis. The differential diagnosis should include Parsonage–Turner syndrome, as well as concurrent ganglion cysts. Neuropathy due to a compressive lesion or stenotic pathway will reliably respond quite well to decompression.

Associated pathology with concomitant compression of the suprascapular nerve can also be encountered, which deserves mention. Nerve entrapment in the setting of massive rotator cuff tears can result in pain, weakness, and atrophy just as it would in cases of direct compression with a mass. Both cases can complicate the diagnosis and treatment. Nerve compression is a result of tendon retraction which conceivably tethers the nerve at the transverse scapular ligament or spinoglenoid notch. A high index of suspicion and attention is required to discern the diagnosis of nerve compression in these cases. Lafosse, in a series of 75 patients with massive rotator cuff tears (still in review), demonstrated 39 % of patients had positive EMG change consistent with SSN neuropathy [12]. Some authors agree in the identification of the SSN compression with the massive rotator cuff tear but do not necessarily decompress the nerve at the time of surgery. Costouros et al. performed rotator cuff repairs for patients with massive tears, and in all cases patients (6) had improvement in their postoperative EMG studies without the nerve being decompressed at the time of surgery [3]. While the controversy continues as to whether reduction of the tear truly decompresses nerve tethering, at our institution we perform decompression of the SSN in the setting of massive tears and revision cases if we suspect a clinically significant compression.

References

1. Aiello I, Serra G, Traina GC, Tugnoli V. Entrapment of the suprascapular nerve at the spinoglenoid notch. Ann Neurol. 1982;12:314–6.
2. Avery BW, Pilon FM, Barclay JK. Anterior coracoscapular ligament and suprascapular nerve entrapment. Clin Anat. 2002;15:383–6. doi:10.1002/ca.10058.
3. Costouros JG, Porramatikul M, Lie DT, Warner JJ. Reversal of suprascapular neuropathy following arthroscopic repair of massive supraspinatus and infraspinatus rotator cuff tears. Arthroscopy. 2007;23:1152–61. doi:10.1016/j.arthro.2007.06.014.
4. De Laat EAT, Visser CPJ, Coene LNJEM, Pahlplatz PVM, Tavy DLJ. Nerve lesions in primary shoulder dislocations and humeral neck fractures: A prospective clinical and EMG study. J Bone Joint Surg Br. 1994;76:381–3.
5. Edeland HG, Zachrisson BE. Fracture of the scapular notch associated with lesion of the suprascapular nerve. Acta Orthop Scand. 1975;46:758–63.
6. Fehrman DA, Orwin JF, Jennings RM. Suprascapular nerve entrapment by ganglion cysts: A report of six cases with arthroscopic findings and review of the literature. Arthroscopy. 1995;11:727–34.
7. Ferretti A, Cerullo G, Russo G. Suprascapular neuropathy in volleyball players. J Bone Joint Surg Am. 1987;69(2):260–3.
8. Gossline KL, Krivickas LS. Proximal neuropathies of the upper extremity. Neurol Clin. 1999;17:525–47.
9. Hawkins RJ, Piatt BE, Fritz RC, Wolf E, Schickendantz M. Clinical evaluation and treatment of spinoglenoid notch ganglion cysts [abstract]. J Shoulder Elbow Surg. 1999;8:551.
10. Inokuchi W, Ogawa K, Horiuchi Y. Magnetic resonance imaging of suprascapular nerve palsy. J Shoulder Elbow Surg. 1998;7:223–7.
11. Kim DH, Murovic JA, Tiel RL, Kline DG. Management and outcomes of 42 surgical suprascapular nerve injuries and entrapments. Neurosurgery. 2005;57:120–7. doi:10.1227/01.NEU.0000163406.14384.4F.
12. Lafosse L, Piper K, Lanz U. Arthroscopic suprascapular nerve release: indications and technique. J Shoulder Elbow Surg. 2011;20(2):S9–13. doi:10.1016/j.jse.2010.12.003.
13. Lafosse L, Tomasi A, Corbett S, Baier G, Willems K, Gobezie R. Arthroscopic release of suprascapular nerve entrapment at the suprascapular notch: technique and preliminary results. Arthroscopy. 2007;23(1):34–42. doi:10.1016/j.eats.2012.07.004.
14. Linda DD, Harish S, Stewart BG, Finlay K, Parasu N, Rebello RP. Multimodality imaging of peripheral neuropathies of the upper limb and brachial plexus. Radiographics. 2010;30(5):1373–400. doi:10.1148/rg.305095169.
15. Mall NA, Hammond JE, Lenart BA, Enriquez DJ, Twigg SL, Nicholson GP. Suprascapular nerve entrapment isolated to the spinoglenoid notch: surgical technique and results of open decompression. J Shoulder Elbow Surg. 2013;22(11):e1–8. doi:10.1016/j.jse.2013.03.009.
16. Martin SD, Warren RF, Martin TL, Kennedy K, OÕBrien SJ, Wickiewicz TL. Suprascapular neuropathy: results of non-operative treatment. J Bone Joint Surg Am. 1997;79:1159–65.
17. Martinoli C, Bianchi S, Pugliese F, Bacigalupo L, Gauglio C, Valle M, Derchi LE. Sonography of entrapment neuropathies in the upper limb (wrist excluded). J Clin Ultrasound. 2004;32(9):438–50. doi:10.1002/jcu.20067.
18. Plancher KD, Luke TA, Peterson RK, Yacoubian SV. Posterior shoulder pain: a dynamic study of the

spinoglenoid ligament and treatment with arthroscopic release of the scapular tunnel. Arthroscopy. 2007;23(9):991–8. doi:10.1016/j.arthro.2007.03.098.
19. Polguj M, Rożniecki J, Sibiński M, Grzegorzewski A, Majos A, Topol M. The variable morphology of suprascapular nerve and vessels at suprascapular notch: a proposal for classification and its potential clinical implications. Knee Surg Sports Traumatol Arthrosc. 2014. doi:10.1007/s00167-014-2937-1.
20. Post M, Grinblat E. Suprascapular nerve entrapment: Diagnosis and results of treatment. J Shoulder Elbow Surg. 1993;2:190–7.
21. Post M, Mayer J. Suprascapular nerve entrapment: Diagnosis and treatment. Clin Orthop. 1987;223:126–36.
22. Ringel SP, Treihaft M, Carry M, Fisher R, Jacobs P. Suprascapular neuropathy in pitchers. Am J Sports Med. 1990;18:80–6.
23. Romeo AA, Rotenberg DD, Bach Jr BR. Suprascapular neuropathy. J Am Acad Orthop Surg. 1999;7(6): 358–67.
24. Savoie FH, Field LD. Arthroscopic release of nerve entrapment. In: Wiesel SW, editor. Operative techniques in orthopaedic surgery, vol. 1. Philadelphia: Wolters Kluwer; 2011. ISBN-13: 978-0781763707.
25. Shaffer BS, Conway J, Jobe FW, Kvitne RS, Tibone JE. Infraspinatus muscle splitting incision in posterior shoulder surgery: an anatomic and electromyographic study. Am J Sports Med. 1994;22:113–20.
26. Ticker JB, Djurasovic M, Strauch RJ, et al. The incidence of ganglion cysts and other variations in anatomy along the course of the suprascapular nerve. J Shoulder Elbow Surg. 1998;7:472–8.
27. Tirman PFJ, Feller JF, Janzen DL, Peterfy CG, Bergman AG. Association of glenoid labral cysts with labral tears and glenohumeral instability: Radiologic findings and clinical significance. Radiology. 1994; 190:653–8.
28. Vastamäki M. Suprascapular nerve entrapment. Duodecim. 1986;102(6):369–75.
29. Zehetgruber H, Noske H, Lang T, Wurnig C. Suprascapular nerve entrapment: a meta-analysis. Int Orthop. 2002;26:339–43. doi:10.1007/s00264-002-0392-y.

Distal Suprascapular Nerve Compression: Spinoglenoid Ligament Release

23

Kevin D. Plancher and Stephanie C. Petterson

Suprascapular nerve entrapment is a diagnosis to consider when presented with a patient with posterior shoulder pain [1]. While posterior shoulder pain is often mistaken as rotator cuff or cervical disc disease, one must consider compression of the suprascapular nerve as a possible underlying pathologic condition. Suprascapular nerve compression not only contributes to pain in the posterior shoulder girdle, but also weakness and possible subtle or significant muscle wasting in the supraspinatus and infraspinatus fossa. A prolonged course of symptoms, whether ignored by the patient or the result of a misdiagnosis, can contribute to a protracted disease course, significant symptomatology, and loss of function in young individuals. Two common sites of compression of the suprascapular nerve include the transverse scapular ligament and spinoglenoid ligament [2–5] (Fig. 23.1). An improved understanding of the pathophysiology of this entity, as well as utilization of advanced arthroscopic techniques, will hopefully translate to improved outcomes and patient satisfaction. This chapter's primary focus will be on compression of the suprascapular nerve at the spinoglenoid notch.

K.D. Plancher, MD, MS (✉)
Clinical Professor, Department of Orthopaedic Surgery, Albert Einstein College of Medicine, New York, NY, USA
e-mail: kplancher@plancherortho.com

S.C. Petterson, MPT, PhD
Orthopaedic Foundation, Stamford, CT, USA

Anatomy Suprascapular Nerve

The suprascapular nerve has been classically thought to arise from the upper trunk of the brachial plexus (C5–C6) at Erb's point; however, in 25 % of individuals, the C4 nerve root also contributes to this nerve [6, 7] (Fig. 23.2). As the nerve approaches the suprascapular notch, the accompanying suprascapular artery diverges [8]. At this point, the suprascapular nerve travels *under* the transverse scapular ligament as it enters the suprascapular notch. The suprascapular artery traverses *over* the transverse scapular ligament; however, in rare instances, the artery travels with the nerve [9]. As the nerve then courses laterally along the supraspinatus fossa, it approaches the posterior glenoid rim, travels around the scapular spine, and descends into the infraspinatus fossa after it passes under the spinoglenoid ligament (inferior transverse scapular ligament) [10] (Fig. 23.3). The suprascapular nerve then gives rise to 2–4 branches to the infraspinatus muscle belly.

Some authors have described two types of spinoglenoid ligaments: Type I, a thin indistinct band of tissue, and Type II, a well-formed ligament. We performed a cadaveric study and found that the spinoglenoid ligament was present in 100 % of specimens. We also found that it has attachments to the glenohumeral joint capsule which can contribute to compression of the suprascapular nerve at the spinoglenoid ligament upon

J.D. Kelly IV (ed.), *Elite Techniques in Shoulder Arthroscopy*,
DOI 10.1007/978-3-319-25103-5_23

internal rotation of the shoulder. The nerve itself is approximately 2.5 cm away from the glenoid rim (posterior superior) and is located approximately 4 cm from the posterolateral corner of the spine of the scapula [4]. The spinoglenoid ligament is quadrangular in shape and originates from the posterior glenoid neck and glenohumeral capsule to insert as a bilaminar "ligament" into the scapular spine (Fig. 23.4). Recent clinical studies together

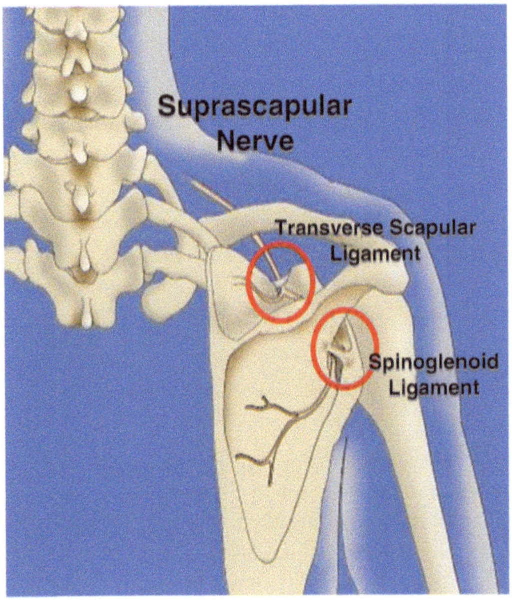

Fig. 23.1 Right shoulder posterior view artwork demonstrating the two compression sites for the suprascapular nerve (Copyright Kevin D. Plancher MD 2015)

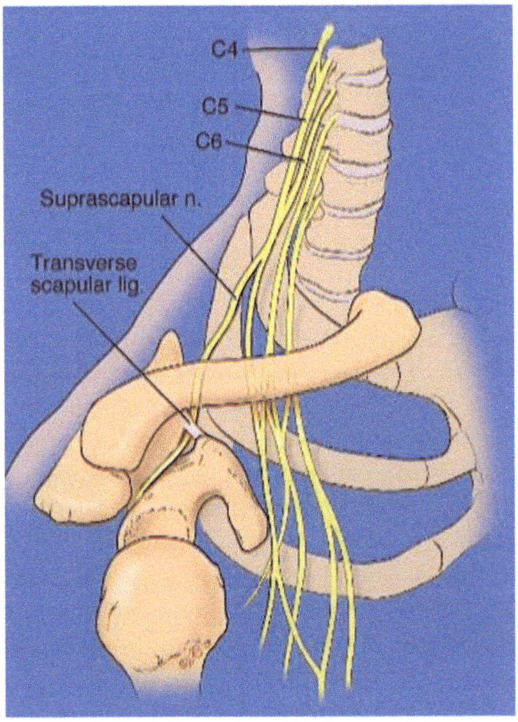

Fig. 23.2 Right shoulder anterior view artwork of the suprascapular nerve arising from the upper trunk of the brachial plexus (Copyright Kevin D. Plancher MD 2015)

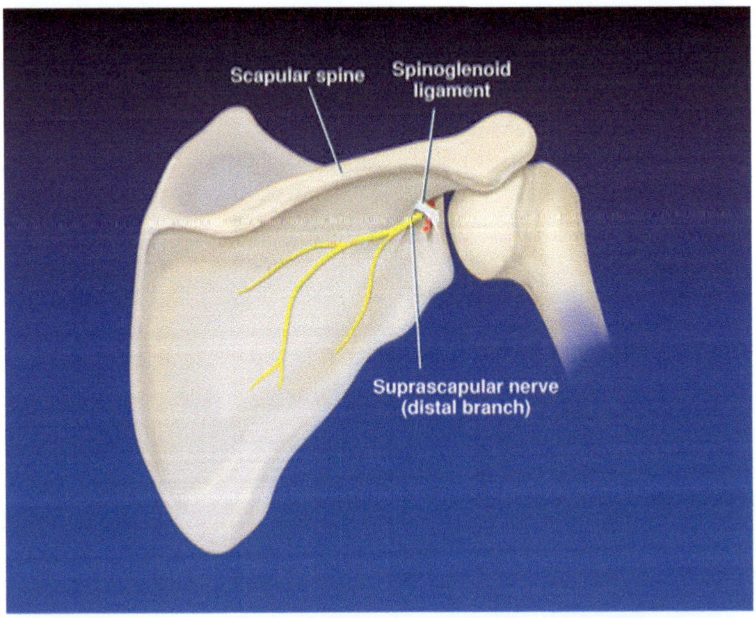

Fig. 23.3 The suprascapular nerve descending into the infraspinatus fossa passing under the spinoglenoid ligament (Copyright Kevin D. Plancher MD 2015)

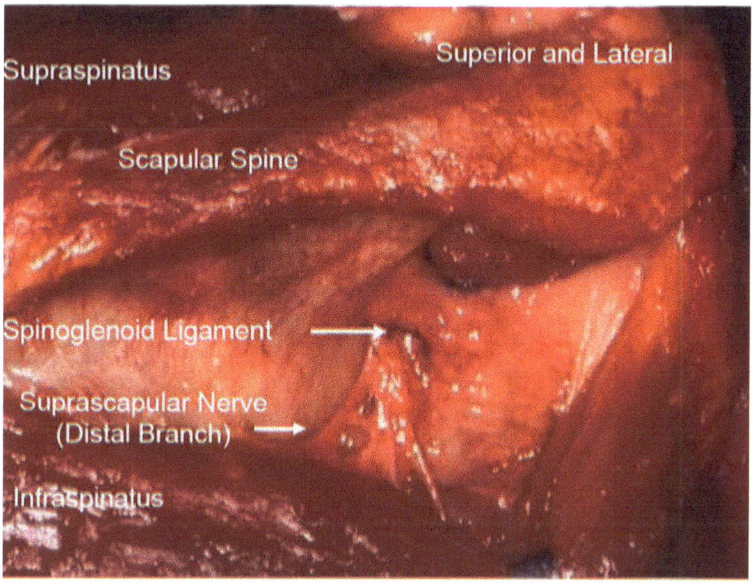

Fig. 23.4 The spinoglenoid ligament, *quadrangular* in shape, demonstrated in the posterior view of a right shoulder dissection. Note the distal branch of the suprascapular nerve compressed (Copyright Kevin D. Plancher MD 2015)

with previous anatomic dissections suggest that the suprascapular nerve contributes an appreciable sensory innervation to the shoulder AC joint. These sensory contributions may explain pain upon traction or compression of the nerve as well as upon repair of a massive rotator cuff tear with advancement [11].

Pathophysiology

Isolated compression or injury to the suprascapular nerve may occur at the spinoglenoid ligament (Fig. 23.5). While the more common site of suprascapular entrapment neuropathy is at the transverse scapular ligament in the suprascapular foramen or notch, clinical presentation and diagnosis of compression at the most distal site have been well recorded (Fig. 23.6). Several mechanisms have been proposed and previously discussed above. While most commonly thought of in the overhead athletes, injury to this nerve may occur from repetitive traction and microtrauma [3, 4, 12–14]. The spinoglenoid ligament has also been demonstrated to tighten when the shoulder is in a position for overhead throwing, resulting in increased pressure on the suprascapular nerve [15] (Fig. 23.7). Early investigators speculated that injury to this nerve occurred by intimal damage from

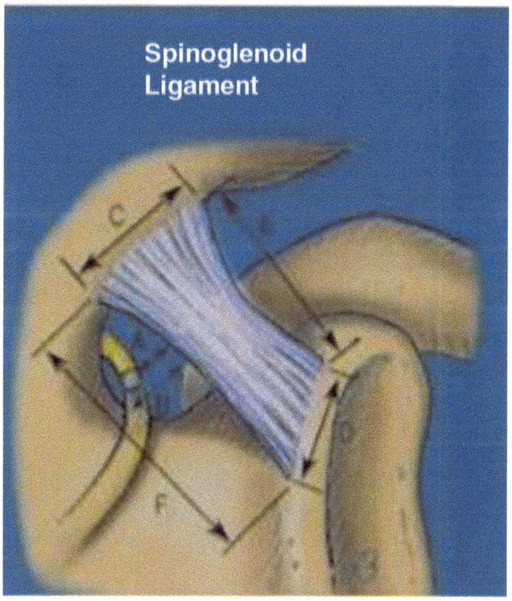

Fig. 23.5 Artwork demonstrating the relationship of the spinoglenoid ligament in a previous published study with investigation of space available between the suprascapular nerve and the spinoglenoid ligament. Note the attachment to the spine of the scapula (Copyright Kevin D. Plancher MD 2015)

microemboli in the vasa nervorum [16]. While intriguing, there is no firm science to support this contention. A stenotic suprascapular notch, an ossified spinoglenoid ligament, or even superiorly

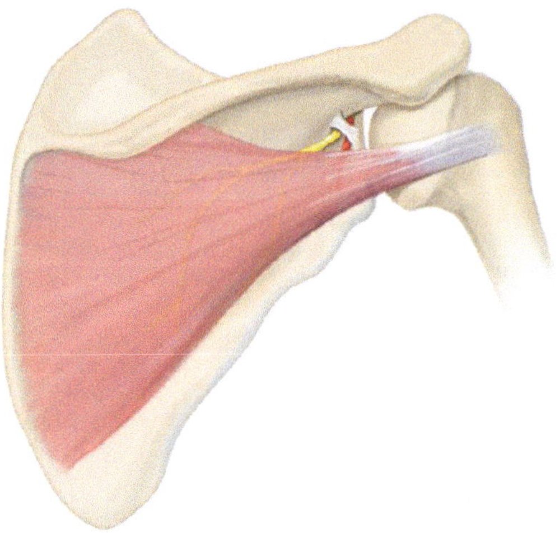

Fig. 23.6 Artwork demonstrating suprascapular nerve entrapment at the spinoglenoid ligament. Note the medial course of the nerve as it wraps around the spinoglenoid notch (Copyright Kevin D. Plancher MD 2015)

oriented fibers of the subscapularis muscle may cause a suprascapular nerve compression [8, 17]. Compression of the nerve at the spinoglenoid ligament has been noted by many authors to be caused by a soft tissue mass or ganglion cyst as a result of some form of a labral or capsule injury. While previously treatment of a cyst-associated compression was labral repair [18, 19], the senior author recommends decompressing the ganglion from the posterior aspect of the shoulder without labral repair to yield excellent results (Fig. 23.8a–f). Compression by a ganglion cyst or soft tissue mass has been known to occur because of the relatively fixed position of the suprascapular nerve combined with the close proximity of the infraspinatus muscle to the glenohumeral joint. A ganglion cyst may form when the labral-glenoid junction tears and synovial fluid is transported into the soft

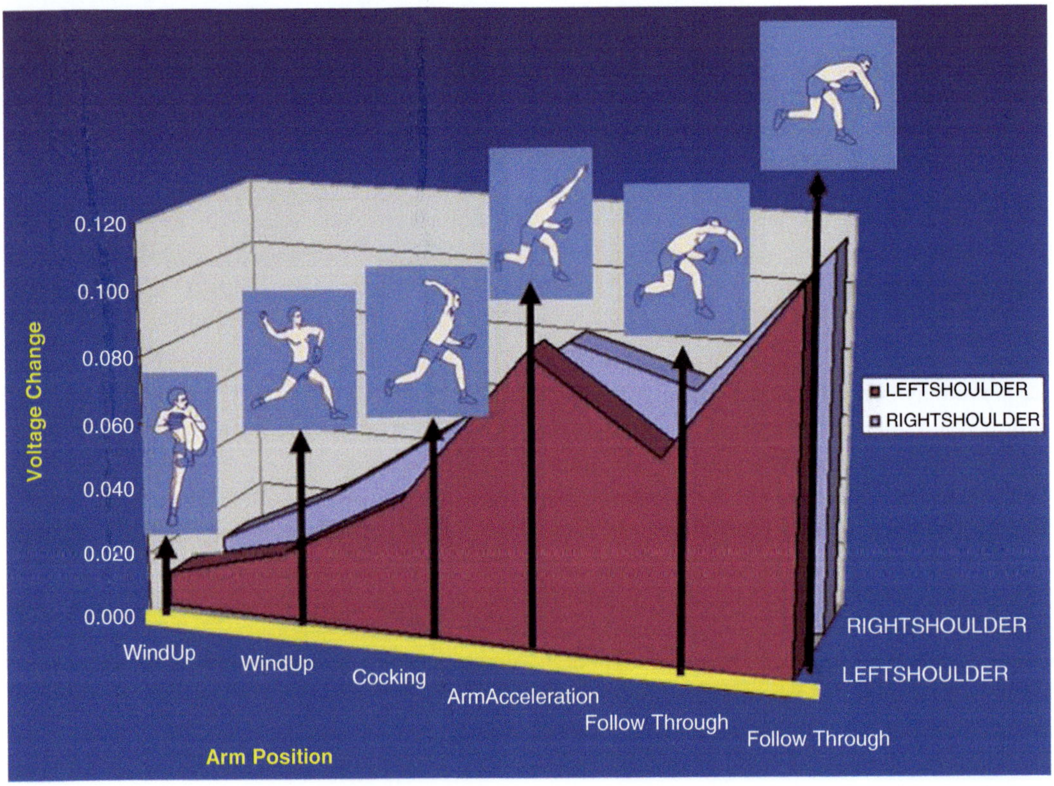

Fig. 23.7 The voltage change with throwing motion with intact spinoglenoid ligament. Note the follow-through or crossed-arm adduction position yields the highest pressure change at the spinoglenoid ligament [(Copyright Kevin D. Plancher MD 2015) Previously published in Plancher et al. Posterior shoulder pain: A dynamic study of the spinoglenoid ligament and treatment with an arthroscopic release of the scapular tunnel. Arthroscopy 23(9): 2007 991–998; Fig. 4]

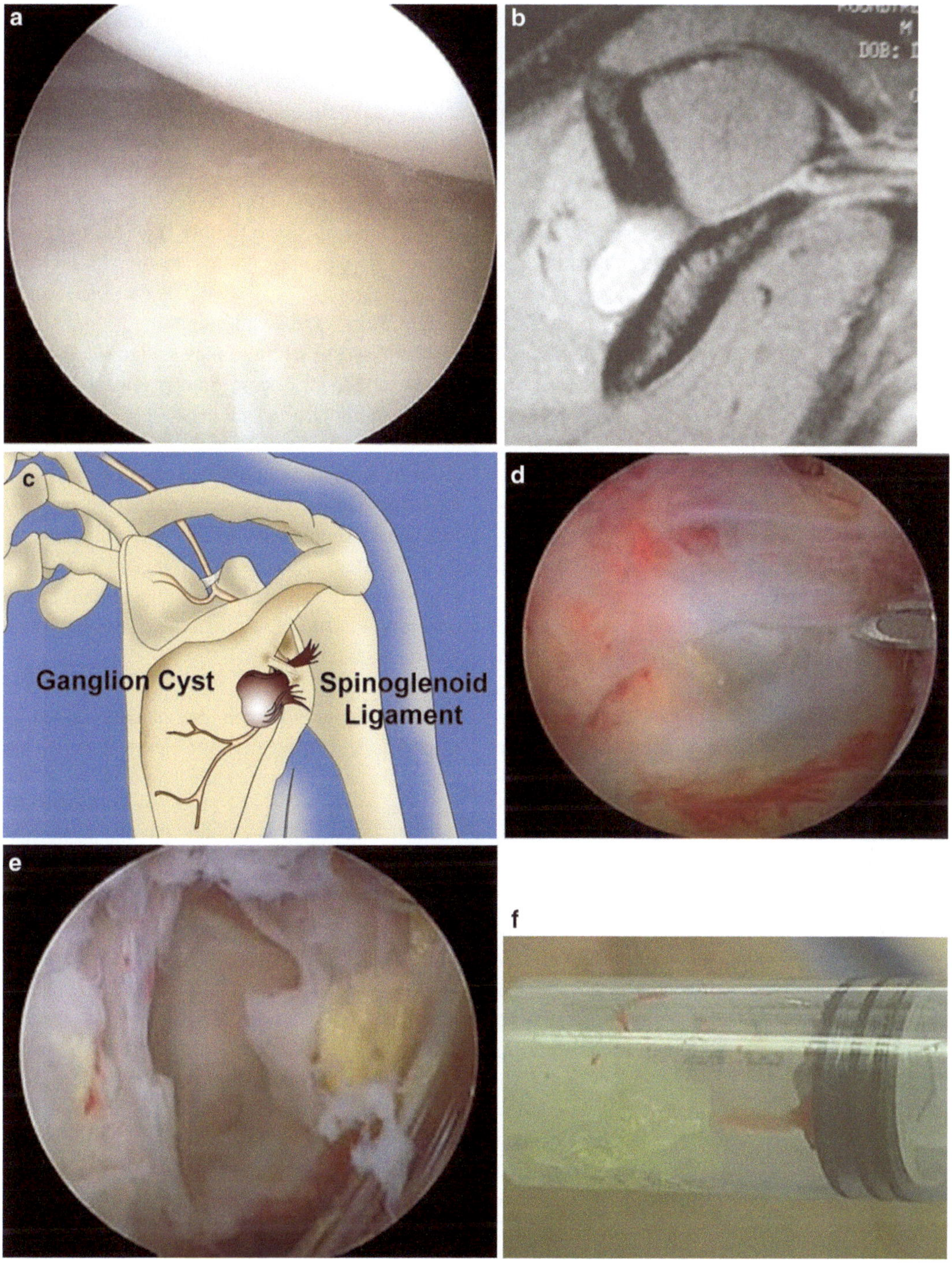

Fig. 23.8 (**a**) Arthroscopic view of a ganglion cyst decompressed from the outside emitting its contents intra-articularly through a posterior inferior perforation in the labrum. (**b**) Sagittal oblique MRI demonstrating a ganglion cyst compressing the suprascapular nerve at the spinoglenoid notch. (**c**) Artwork of posterior view of right shoulder demonstrating a classic ganglion compressing the spinoglenoid ligament at its notch. (**d**) Posterior view of bulging ganglion cyst located at the spinoglenoid notch. (**e**) Decompressed ganglion cyst at the spinoglenoid notch prior to complete excision of its root. (**f**) Syringe containing the contents of the ganglion cyst commonly seen on MRI compressing the suprascapular nerve at the spinoglenoid ligament (Copyright Kevin D. Plancher MD 2015) (Reprinted with permission from Jonathan Ticker, MD)

tissues via a one-way valve effect. This mechanism is very similar to the formation of meniscal cysts in the knee [20].

While rare, a patient may sustain a neuropathy from a parsonage Turner syndrome, although it is more common for this viral neuritis to attack other nerves. Whatever the mechanism, compression or injury to the suprascapular nerve at the spinoglenoid ligament will result in infraspinatus weakness. If sustained long term, atrophy of the infraspinatus muscle will ensue with little if any probability of return to normal muscle strength expected.

Patient Profile

History

Patients with compression of the suprascapular nerve at the spinoglenoid notch comprise a unique group of individuals, more commonly overhead athletes and laborers that perform a preponderance of their activities above the shoulder. These individuals are usually young, well developed, and complain of a diffuse ache around the posterior shoulder region. Their pain is more localized to approximately 4 cm medial to the posterolateral corner of the acromion as well as near the posterior aspect of the glenohumeral joint.

A patient may complain of weakness on attempts of external rotation and abduction which may confuse the examiner since no different than compression at the transverse scapular ligament, the patient with rotator cuff disease or even cervical disc disease may present in a similar fashion. However, patients with compression of the suprascapular nerve at the spinoglenoid ligament usually have more profound weakness on external rotation and a longer, protracted, chronic history, often the result of a missed diagnosis.

There are other unique possibilities that can result in suprascapular nerve compression. Forced, sudden humeral internal rotation, as seen in many racquet sports, can produce a stretch on the suprascapular nerve at the bony notch compression point, irrespective of the ligament dimensions. In such a scenario, activities across the body are often difficult, and the motion of a follow-through, whether throwing a baseball or spiking a volleyball, can be quite painful leading the athlete to avoid those movements. The position of follow-through or adduction in an extended position has been shown by our group to increase the tension and pressure within the spinoglenoid notch [3]. Common sports encompassing this motion include golf, volleyball, basketball, tennis, weight lifting, and swimming.

While sports activities may lead to suprascapular neuropathy, the heavy laborer may be plagued with this affliction as well because of all the repetitive overhead work duties they may perform, no different than those laborers with compression of the suprascapular nerve at the transverse scapular ligament. Compression at the spinoglenoid ligament is often insidious in onset, and a delay in diagnosis is the single biggest impediment to full restoration of muscle strength, alleviation of pain, and reversal of atrophy.

As stated previously, the suprascapular nerve at the spinoglenoid notch may be compressed by a ganglion cyst because the nerve is relatively immobile as it traverses the lateral edge of the scapular spine and is in close proximity of the posterior glenohumeral joint. Diagnosis by history can be difficult because the findings overlap considerably with rotator cuff and labral pathology. Certain findings though will help the clinician discern the diagnosis. One example is weakness on external rotation. The patient may complain that their infraspinatus fossa appears different in comparison to the opposite side. Often the chronic posterior ache or pain will increase and may even become constant and interrupt sleeping. Spinoglenoid compression, rather than compression at the transverse scapular ligament, is more commonly associated with complaints of catching, locking, or clicking because of the frequent association of a labral tear. As a final consideration, increased sports participation by females has caused the incidence of compression of the suprascapular nerve at the spinoglenoid ligament to have no appreciable gender bias.

Physical Examination

Clinical examination often has nonspecific findings in the early stages of this disease process. Symptoms are often less severe with suprascapular neuropathy at the spinoglenoid notch as opposed to more proximal compression. Some athletes present with isolated painless wasting of the infraspinatus. Surprisingly, palpation at the spinoglenoid notch can be very painful. Some patients may describe micro-instability as a part of their complaints although confirmatory physical findings will not be found.

Completion of a cervical spine examination and a standard exam of both shoulders with a full neurological assessment must be completed. The patient, when placed in a shoulder gown with the complete scapula in full view, may demonstrate subtle or severe atrophy to the infraspinatus fossa (Fig. 23.9). Atrophy though in a well-developed individual who participates in a weight-training program may at times be difficult to discern due to the overlying trapezius and large bulk of the deltoid muscle.

Range of motion and strength must be assessed. There may be only a subtle loss of external rotation as well as abduction strength in young, overhead athletes. Strength of external rotation should be tested with the arm at the side, and weakness will often be present without any significant pain. The painless strength deficit is due to the fact that the sensory portion of the suprascapular nerve may be unaffected at the spinoglenoid notch. We have found that in long-standing disease, the teres minor and serratus anterior muscle may hypertrophy as compensation for the loss of the infraspinatus, hiding any strength deficit.

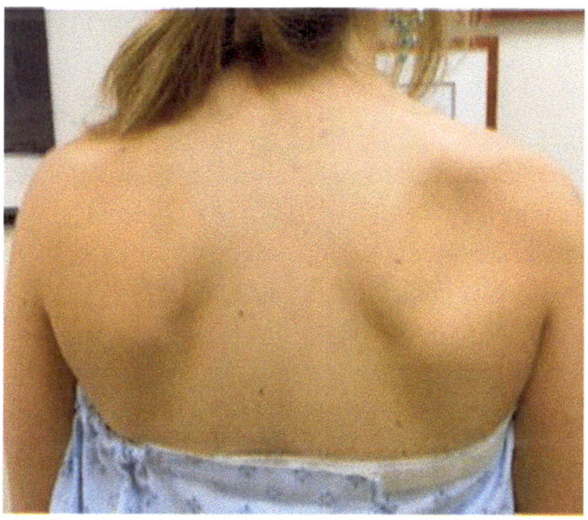

Fig. 23.9 Clinical photo and posterior view of the right shoulder demonstrating severe atrophy in a 21-year-old female tennis player with chronic wasting of the infraspinatus since age 9 with no apparent diagnosis (Copyright Kevin D. Plancher MD 2015)

Provocative tests for labral pathology must be performed as labral tears with associated paralabral cysts may be found in conjunction with a suprascapular neuropathy at the spinoglenoid ligament.

A cross-arm adduction test, as described above, must be performed and recorded and correlated with a Zanca view X-ray in order to rule out acromioclavicular (AC) joint arthritis (Fig. 23.10a, b). If cross-body adduction reproduces the patient's symptoms with the arm extended or internally rotated and the pain is primarily felt in the posterior aspect of the shoulder but the X-ray is negative, then the diagnosis of AC joint arthritis can be ruled out with an injection of lidocaine. A diagnosis of suprascapular nerve entrapment can now be claimed [21].

The differential diagnosis for suprascapular neuropathy at the spinoglenoid notch includes the same conditions considered for compression of the nerve at the transverse scapular ligament, i.e., cervical disc disease, a brachial neuritis, Parsonage–Turner syndrome, rotator cuff tendinopathy, labral pathology with or without a ganglion cyst, mild adhesive capsulitis, osteoarthritis of the glenohumeral joint, subacromial bursitis with or without impingement syndrome, AC degeneration disease, posterior glenohumeral instability, quadrilateral space syndrome, triangular space and interval disease or thoracic outlet syndrome, and the rare Pancoast tumor. The astute clinician recognizes that the lack of reproducible signs on physical exam for other common diagnoses and the overlapping symptoms with other shoulder problems often leads to a correct diagnosis.

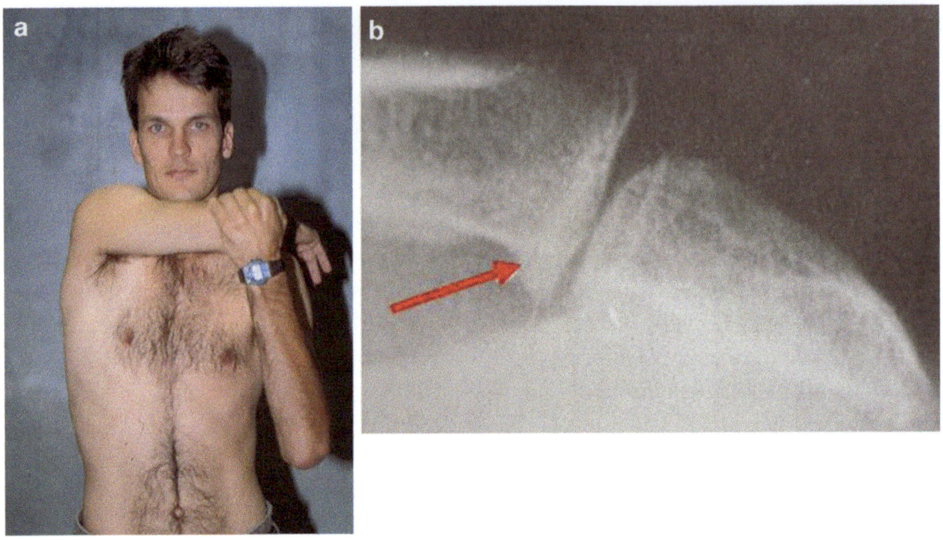

Fig. 23.10 (**a**) Clinical photo of the cross-arm adduction test. (**b**) Zanca view of a left shoulder showing classical osteoarthritis of the acromioclavicular joint with an osteophyte which would preclude a diagnosis of suprascapular nerve entrapment (Copyright Kevin D. Plancher MD 2015)

Radiographic Examination

Plain radiographs including an anteroposterior (AP), axillary lateral, and the Y or supraspinatus outlet view should always be obtained (Fig. 23.11a–c). Special views such as a Stryker notch view can be ordered when necessary [5]. This plain series will identify any fracture or significant trauma to the scapula, clavicle, coracoid, or glenoid neck.

Magnetic resonance imaging (MRI) and identification of soft tissue masses such as a ganglion cyst are critically important when evaluating compression of the suprascapular nerve at the spinoglenoid ligament (Fig. 23.12). The MRI can identify a true ganglion with a homogenous signal, low T1 intensity, with high T2 intensity and rim enhancement if contrast is utilized [22]. The MRI will also detect labral tears arising from the posterosuperior quadrant of the glenoid with the ganglion cyst attached (Fig. 23.13). Controversy exists as to whether the cyst truly arises from associated labral tears. Those that believe that this is the case insist on treatment to the labrum to minimize recurrence, while others advocate leaving the labrum alone after the cyst has been excised or decompressed.

The presence of a soft tissue mass or ganglion cyst on MRI does not necessarily indicate suprascapular neuropathy. However, abnormal signal intensity within the infraspinatus muscle will indicate significant suprascapular nerve compression at the spinoglenoid notch. Some patients will demonstrate increased signal intensity on T2 fast spin echo with fat saturation with a normal muscle mass implying subacute denervation of the muscle leading to neurogenic edema. Chronic denervation, seen best on T1 spin echo with increased signal intensity within the muscle mass, will demonstrate muscle atrophy with fatty infiltration (Fig. 23.14).

Newer modalities such as ultrasound may be helpful as well to identify ganglion cysts. This operator-dependent test can be very helpful not only in making a diagnosis but in assisting surgeons to complete an ultrasound-guided aspiration of the ganglion cyst. Compression sites can be readily visualized and aid in making a definitive diagnosis.

Selective Injections

A 1 % lidocaine anesthetic injection may be placed into the spinoglenoid notch to confirm the diagnosis of suprascapular nerve entrapment

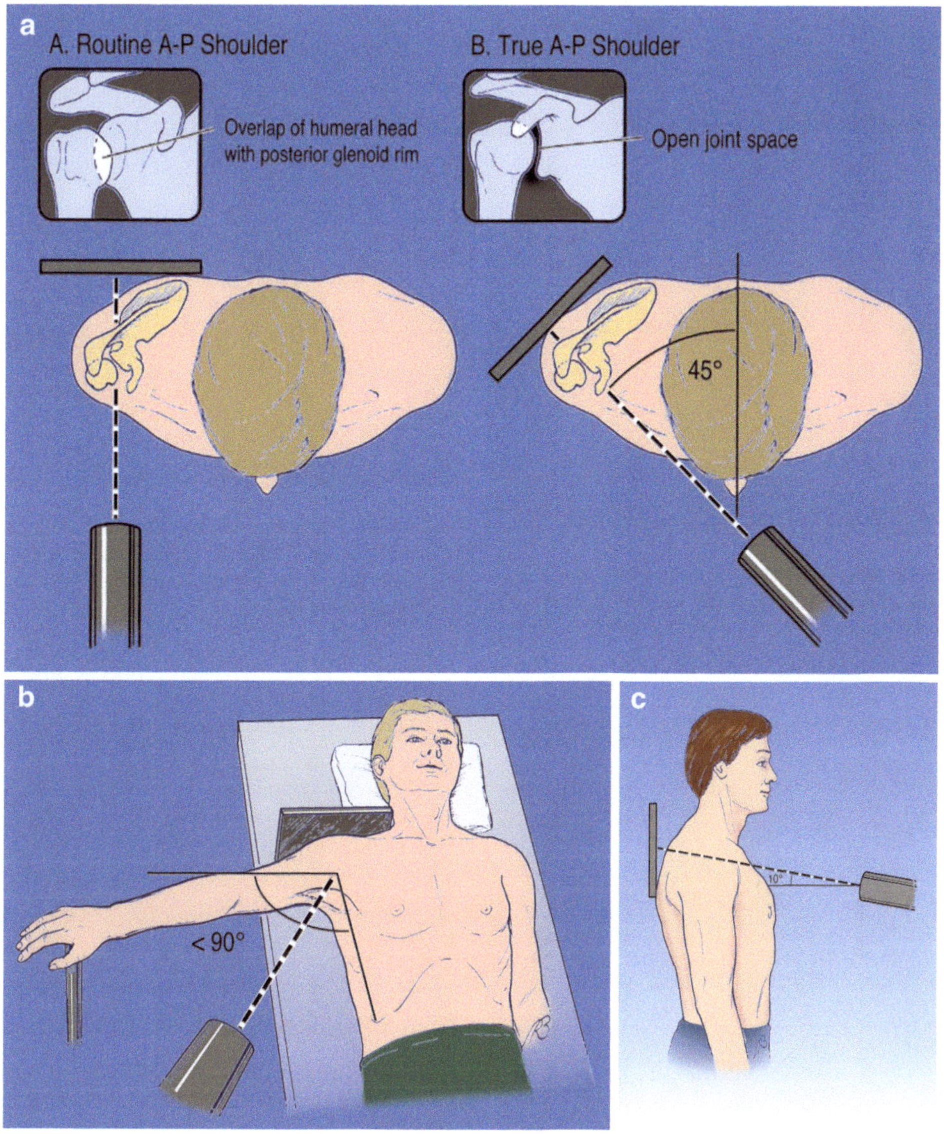

Fig. 23.11 (**a**) Artwork demonstrating the difference and correct way to obtain a true versus routine anteroposterior (AP) view of the shoulder. (**b**) Supine axillary view artwork demonstrated. (**c**) Artwork demonstrating the direction of the X-ray beam to obtain an X-ray of the acromioclavicular joint with a Zanca view (Copyright Kevin D. Plancher MD 2015)

(Fig. 23.15). The needle is placed 4 cm medial to the posterolateral corner of the acromion. The patient is then asked if there is any change in the chronic ache that may have been present prior to injection. A cross-arm adduction test is then performed, and, if preinjection symptoms dissipate, the test is considered positive.

We have found pain relief to be dramatic and almost immediate with properly placed injections. Ultrasound may be used as an adjunct to guide the needle to ensure accuracy. This injection technique is simple; one feels the spine of the scapula and drops inferior to it by 1–2 cm and then, while aspirating, easily falls into the spinoglenoid

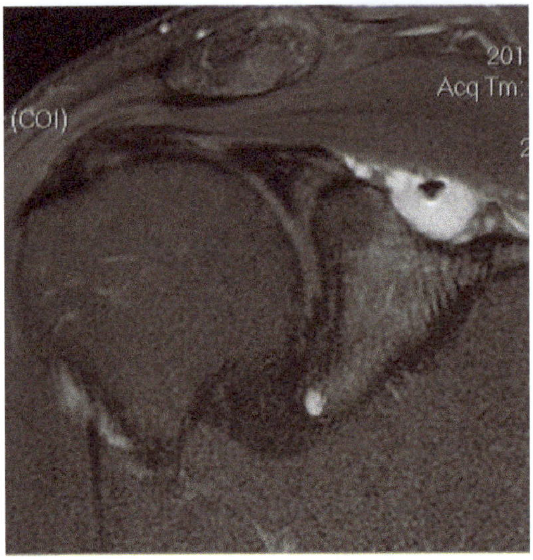

Fig. 23.12 MRI coronal view demonstrating ganglion cyst displacing the suprascapular nerve at the spinoglenoid notch (Copyright Kevin D. Plancher MD 2015)

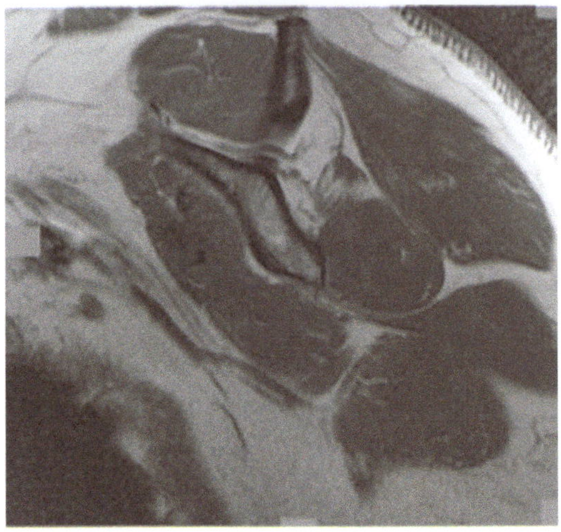

Fig. 23.14 Oblique MRI demonstrating isolated infraspinatus atrophy in this volleyball player. Note the course of the nerve in this T2-weighted image (Copyright Kevin D. Plancher MD 2015)

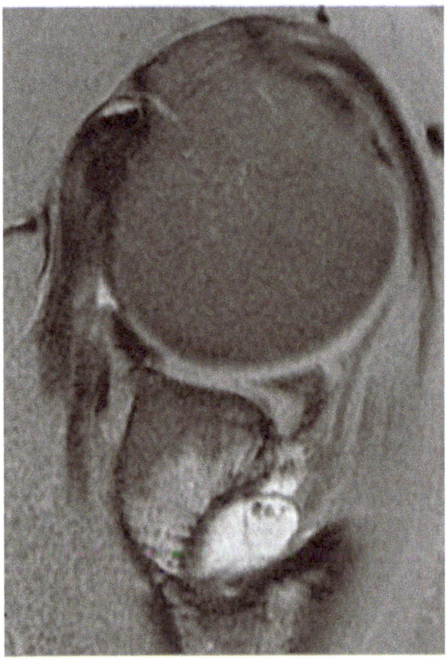

Fig. 23.13 MRI axial view demonstrating labral tear as well as ganglion cyst compressing the suprascapular nerve at the spinoglenoid notch (Copyright Kevin D. Plancher MD 2015)

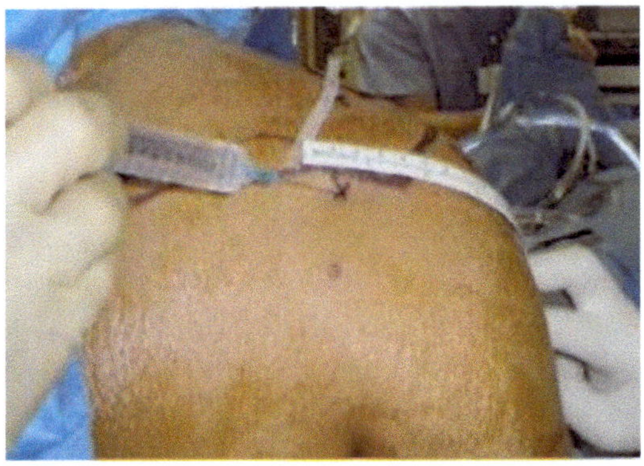

Fig. 23.15 Clinical photo of a lidocaine injection to be placed at the spinoglenoid ligament, 4 cm medial to the posterolateral corner of the acromion (Copyright Kevin D. Plancher MD 2015)

notch. A negative injection test in conjunction with the absence of atrophy, a negative EMG, no evidence of a labral tear or ganglion cyst, yet weakness and pain, mandates at least a 6-month course of nonoperative treatment before considering any type of operative intervention.

Electrodiagnostic Testing

Electrodiagnostic testing replete with electromyography (EMG) and nerve conduction studies can help to confirm compression of the suprascapular nerve at the spinoglenoid notch. When the suprascapular nerve is compressed by a ganglion cyst or soft tissue mass at the spinoglenoid notch, the nerve will show decreased innervation of the infraspinatus muscle with normal innervation of the supraspinatus muscle. The stimulation point is typically performed at Erb's point. Motor distal latency and motor response amplitude at the supraspinatus and infraspinatus muscles are measured. An increased latency beyond 3.3 ms (range 2.4–4.2 ms) is considered definitive for compression to the infraspinatus [23].

A classic positive electrodiagnostic study that detects compression at the spinoglenoid notch will demonstrate a dramatic motor loss to the infraspinatus if atrophy is present without changes in the supraspinatus muscle. Patients without visible atrophy present may still have compression of the nerve to the infraspinatus and hopefully on EMG will demonstrate a delayed terminal latency to the inferior branch of the suprascapular nerve. Side-to-side electrodiagnostic measurement differences are important [24]. Evaluation of the sensory velocities is less useful as the sensory innervation of this nerve is not as well defined.

Some investigators report that the only early finding may be increased nerve conduction time of the suprascapular nerve. This positive finding will allow the physician to discern that the neural compression is not in the cervical spine but rather located distally. This finding will enable the clinician to identify the compression point with selective injections and hopefully avoid irreversible damage to the suprascapular nerve. Decreases in the amplitude and spontaneous or marked polyphasicity of the evoked potentials are significant findings in confirming the presence of suprascapular entrapment at either the transverse scapular ligament or spinoglenoid ligament [5].

It has been shown that EMG and nerve conduction velocity may only be accurate 91% of the time in detecting nerve injury associated with muscle weakness [25, 26]. We believe that suprascapular nerve dysfunction can exist in the presence of a normal nerve conduction study and electromyography. EMG testing of the infraspinatus may be even more confusing as only one division of the muscle can be affected, while the rest of the muscle may be unaffected, leading the physician to think that suprascapular nerve entrapment is not present.

Compression of the suprascapular nerve has been shown to be a dynamic disease. The EMG is often negative, no different than in the cubital tunnel to detect disease in the elbow. A negative EMG of the suprascapular nerve does not dissuade us from surgical intervention upon confirmation of the disease by selective injections. Therefore, we also encourage the examiner to test multiple locations. Needle recording better detects compression than surface recordings because stimulation of other periscapular muscles, common with surface EMG electrodes, leads to volume interference. The suprascapular nerve, as mentioned previously, is a mixed motor and sensory nerve which makes detection of a partial compression even more difficult since sensation may be spared, even in the face of significant neuronal injury. We encourage all clinicians to communicate with the neurologist prior to allowing the patient to undergo an EMG and nerve conduction velocity testing so that the most accurate outcome of this type of testing is obtained.

Physical Therapy and Nonoperative Treatment

It is reasonable to initiate nonoperative measures as first-line treatment for an isolated suprascapular nerve compression, especially when no space-occupying lesion is present. These conservative measures include rest, activity modification, anti-inflammatory medications, physical therapy in order to maintain range of motion, and strengthening of the shoulder girdle. The therapist should target scapular stability, promote proper static and dynamic posture, and initiate a resistive strengthening program to the trapezius, rhomboids, and the serratus musculature prior to any consideration of operative intervention. Return to sport is permitted after proprioceptive and plyometric exercises are mastered. In the absence of a direct compressive lesion, most neuropathies will improve, but the symptoms of pain and weakness may take more than a year to reach full resolution.

The natural history of suprascapular nerve entrapment at the spinoglenoid notch is poorly known; therefore, it is uncertain how long to recommend a nonoperative course. If there is a space-occupying lesion, we would forego any nonoperative treatment. The majority of these space-occupying lesions are ganglion cysts and may be associated with labral tears. Several studies have supported our general approach to avoid a prolonged nonoperative regime. Hawkins et al. reported that only 2 out of 19 patients with a spinoglenoid cyst resolved their symptoms with nonsurgical (aspiration) treatment [27]. Hawkins further found patient satisfaction was much higher with surgical intervention. Specifically, they reported a meager 18 % success rate for aspiration of the cyst with 48 % of aspirated cysts demonstrating recurrence.

Ultrasound-guided aspiration of the ganglion cysts has in fact been reported with inconsistent results by others. Some authors have reported recurrence rates up to 75 %, and while generally a safe technique, we do not recommended this to our patients [27, 28].

We believe that all patients that present with visible atrophy to the infraspinatus should have minimal nonoperative treatment, as we have found that good results most predictably come with early intervention. Prompt release of the suprascapular nerve may halt progression of atrophy. The reversibility of atrophy after release is inconsistent and depends on severity and duration of nerve compression [29].

While many authors believe that a program of physical therapy that concentrates on scapular stabilization, shoulder motion, and strengthening is disease altering, we maintain that this theory is incorrect. These measures may sustain a young athlete because increased recruitment of serratus anterior or teres group of muscles will support shoulder abduction and mitigate symptoms in the short term. Unfortunately, these same patients often return 10 years later (as witnessed in our practice) with marked atrophy and irreversible muscle damage to the supraspinatus or infraspinatus. We hold that surgical intervention is essential in most cases and should be performed arthroscopically. We maintain that our approach when a mass is present or absent will arrest the disease process and allow the athlete or laborer to return to their sport of job in a very short period of "down" time [5, 30]. We do not encourage therapy for more than 6–8 weeks.

In advanced and long-standing cases with profound spinati atrophy that almost assuredly will never recover completely without intervention, we recognize that shoulder pain can improve with cessation of activity. However, with resumption of activity, the pain predictably returns. Prior to the evolution of the arthroscopic approach, because of the limited experience of many surgeons and an attitude of hesitancy because of unfamiliarity with anatomy, many surgeons were not very familiar with the diagnosis of suprascapular neuropathy. In other words, concerning this diagnosis, "it may have seen you, but you have not seen it." It is our hope that this chapter will help patients be afforded the opportunity to be diagnosed in a timely fashion and treated promptly so that long-term sequelae of this potentially disabling condition may be averted.

Endoscopic Release of the Spinoglenoid Ligament

Understanding Ganglion Cysts and Our Treatment Regime

The arthroscopic technique described below will enable surgeons to treat and excise paralabral ganglion cysts as well as decompress the spinoglenoid ligament in an atraumatic fashion. Avoiding traditional infraspinatus musculature detachment offers a huge benefit to the patient [27, 31]. Much debate exists whether cyst decompression alone is sufficient or if it is more appropriate to perform cyst decompression *and* labral debridement or repair [32]. Recently, some investigators have recommended mere repair of the labrum without cyst decompression with the expectation that cystic contents will slowly regress [33]. However, there exists no high-level evidence to support superiority of one technique over another.

This section will discuss the literature as well as stating our recommendations for effectively treating a patient with atrophy in the infraspinatus fossa, pain, weakness, and an MRI with evidence of a ganglion cyst in the spinoglenoid notch and a concomitant labral tear. In addition, patients who present with persistent compression of the suprascapular nerve at the spinoglenoid notch without any demonstrable space-occupying lesion may also benefit from this technique.

Advocates for treating intra-articular lesions alone (labral tear) believe that if you correct the one-way valve mechanism, the cyst will spontaneously dissipate [34]. Thus, these authors, as noted above, singularly treat the SLAP tear and simply ignore the cyst as they expect spontaneous cystic regression will logically follow. Other authors recommend investigation of the type of labral tear present and advocate arthroscopic decompression of the cyst and debridement of a frayed labrum or repair of a type 2 SLAP lesion [35]. Therefore, if the labrum is intact, these investigators advocate incision of the capsule adjacent to the labrum just posterior to the biceps in order to effect ganglion cyst decompression. Other authors advocate a subacromial method of cyst decompression by finding the raphe between the supraspinatus and infraspinatus which is lateral to the spinoglenoid notch. They advocate incision of the capsule in this location and then proceed with a decompression of the ganglion cyst with an accessory posterolateral portal [31]. Some authors hold that addressing any coexisting pathology, the glenoid labrum in most patients with a spinoglenoid ganglion cyst offers the best outcome and may confer the lowest recurrence rate [19, 21, 36].

We believe that direct decompression of the spinoglenoid notch with a posterior approach is much more efficacious. We have performed this method for several years and have had only one patient where the pain did not resolve. This one failure occurred in a multiply operated worker's compensation case. In addition, we have not noted a single recurrence of any cyst after several years of follow-up. We acknowledge that every patient in our series group undergoes a thorough arthroscopic exam in search of any intra-articular pathology. We advocate that the presence of an intact labrum obviates the need for a capsulotomy posterior and superior to the glenoid rim to decompress the stalk of the ganglion cyst. Those authors who support this type of decompression understand that no dissection should proceed beyond 1 cm medial to the superior capsule attachment to the glenoid to avoid the nerve as it course through the spinoglenoid notch. Again, we caution surgeons who attempt to decompress a ganglion cyst at the spinoglenoid notch to be wary of the capsulotomy technique in order to avoid neural injury and consider a more direct approach. Injury to the suprascapular nerve indeed may occur with dissection medial to the glenoid as the average distance to the suprascapular nerve from the posterior glenoid rim is 1.8 cm with the motor branches found to be approximately 2.0 cm medial from the glenoid margin. We have encountered patients with injured nerves subsequent to surgery who present with profound external rotation weakness. Sadly, we can only offer them a latissimus dorsi transfer as a means to salvage function.

The last matter worthy of further discussion concerns the patient treated with labral repair and no cyst decompression. As stated earlier, some authors hold that spinoglenoid cyst excision is unnecessary and avoids undue risk of injury to the suprascapular nerve during surgery. Although good results were reported with resolution of pain, we do not concur with this approach since many patients demonstrated a persistent cyst on repeat MRI. The presence of a cyst may conceivably continue to affect nerve conduction and ultimately cause irreversible muscular atrophy in the infraspinatus fossa with permanent external rotation weakness.

Recurrence of ganglion cysts with other approaches other than a direct posterior approach to the spinoglenoid notch has been reported. As stated, Hawkins has shown nonoperative techniques with aspiration lead to an unacceptable recurrence rate with continued compression of the suprascapular nerve [27]. Recurrence of the cyst due to failure of the SLAP repair to heal or inadequate initial resection of the cyst has convinced us that a more direct approach is needed [19]. A far medial approach with cyst resection off the glenoid neck may be inadequate. Injury to the suprascapular nerve is difficult to avoid as visualization is difficult. Understanding the appropriate depth of resection when working with such an oblique angle of approach and tight space may pose a challenge even for the most skilled surgeon. While the cyst is traditionally located adjacent to the posterior and superior quadrant of the glenoid at the 10:30–11:00 position on a right shoulder and at 2:00–2:30 position on the left shoulder, identification of the exact location of the cyst using the medial approach presents challenges. Finally, the failure of the labral repair to heal is not an issue with our direct posterior approach as described below. Our direct approach is not reliant on the labrum developing a firm seal to the glenoid in order to facilitate cyst resorption.

Rehabilitation is also more challenging with the intra-articular technique as opposed to our posterior approach with no labrum repair. If a concomitant SLAP repair is performed, then the patient must remain in a sling for 3–4 weeks. If no SLAP repair is performed, then a mere 7 days of a sling is utilized with the patient commencing progressive range of motion exercises and strengthening with return to full overhead activities by 6 weeks. We acknowledge that sometimes labral repair is necessary in the higher-performance overhead athlete, but we maintain that a direct isolated cyst decompression will resolve symptoms for most patients with suprascapular nerve compression. Future studies and meticulous follow-up will be needed to truly confirm our opinions.

Technique

Arthroscopic release of the suprascapular nerve at the spinoglenoid notch should be performed using a posterior only approach. We utilize both a posteromedial and posterolateral portal in the infraspinatus fossa (Fig. 23.16a, b). As stated above, others have advocated a subacromial approach [37]. However, we submit that the ability to visualize anatomy and return to sport or activity of daily living is much faster and simpler than proceeding with the open or subacromial technique. We maintain that the morbidity and postoperative recovery are much simpler and more pleasant for the patient as well.

We place the patient in the beach chair position with arm laid at the side. It is essential to prep and drape from the mid-sternum to the mid-posterior spine with the complete scapula included. We encourage the anesthesiologist to maintain a systolic blood pressure slightly below 100 mmHg. Our pump pressure is kept low at 45 mmHg to avoid unnecessary swelling.

The portals selected include two portals: (1) the viewing portal which is placed 8 cm medial to the posterolateral corner of the acromion just inferior to the scapula spine and (2) the working portal which is placed 4 cm medial to the posterolateral corner of the acromion just inferior to the scapula spine (Fig. 23.16a, b).

Release of the spinoglenoid ligament precedes any work done within the glenohumeral joint. We recommend that ultimately this part of the procedure should take no more than 10 min to ensure a limited amount of swelling to occur in the limb.

The blunt trocar is introduced into the viewing (medial) portal and heads straight toward the infraspinatus fossa (Fig. 23.17). The tissue under the spine of the scapula is swept away, and the

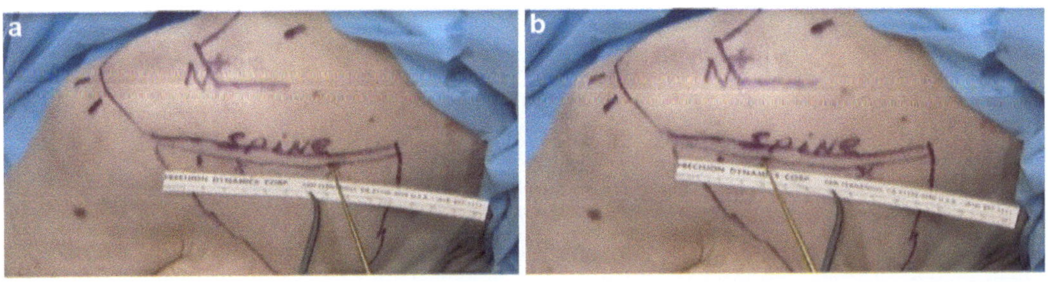

Fig. 23.16 (a) Clinical photo of a left shoulder posterior view. The gold probe is pointing 8 cm medial to the posterolateral corner of the acromion. This portal is the viewing portal for release of the spinoglenoid ligament compressing suprascapular nerve at the spinoglenoid notch. (b) Clinical photo of a left shoulder posterior view. The gold probe is pointing 4 cm medial to the posterolateral corner of the acromion. This portal is the working portal for release of the spinoglenoid ligament compressing suprascapular nerve at the spinoglenoid notch (Copyright Kevin D. Plancher MD 2015)

trocar heads to the working portal passing above the suprascapular nerve heading and falling into the spinoglenoid notch. The key to this step, which allows for visualization, is to ensure that the trocar sweeps under the roof of the infraspinatus spine while feeling its curvature.

The arthroscope replaces the trocar, and our first view of the spinoglenoid ligament is appreciated (Fig. 23.18a, b). Identification of the various landmarks is completed. Success with this procedure will occur with visualization of the spine of the scapula to be maintained throughout the release of the ligament and decompression of the nerve.

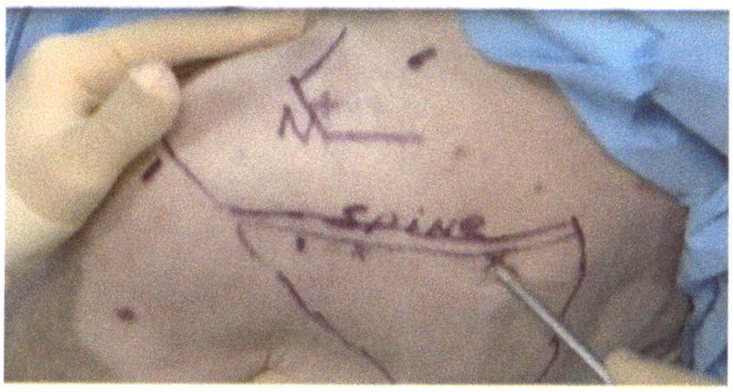

Fig. 23.17 Clinical photo of a left shoulder posterior view. The trocar is introduced in the following fashion. The tip of the blunt trocar palpates the spine of the scapula. The trocar is then moved inferiorly and gently swept to clear a space with the infraspinatus posterior and the tip of the trocar on the infraspinatus fossa. The tip of the trocar is then moved laterally toward the working portal 4 cm medial to the posterolateral corner of the acromion. The trocar as it is moved laterally sweeps the infraspinatus under the arch of its fossa to create a path for the arthroscope to allow visualization of the spinoglenoid ligament (Copyright Kevin D. Plancher MD 2015)

A spinal needle is used followed by a trocar into the working (more lateral) portal, and the soft tissue is teased away laterally as the course of the nerve can always be located in the medial side of the spinoglenoid notch (Fig. 23.19a, b). A radio-frequency wand or small radius nonaggressive shaver with the suction turned off can be utilized at this point to clear the tissue and more specifically identify the spinoglenoid ligament (Fig. 23.20a, b). The ligament can be resected by staying on the spine of the scapula to avoid any bleeding. The ligament can be followed to the glenohumeral joint at its insertion to understand and appreciate a complete resection.

The blunt tip trocar is utilized now to assess the mobility and adequate release of the suprascapular nerve (Fig. 23.21a–d). We then head into the spinoglenoid notch to note any aberrations in anatomy such as a ganglion cyst or the existence of a bifid nerve (Fig. 23.22a, b). Decompression of the ganglion and excision of the stalk can now be easily completed. It is important to understand that the ganglion root may be heading toward the posterior inferior quadrant of the glenohumeral joint. Observation

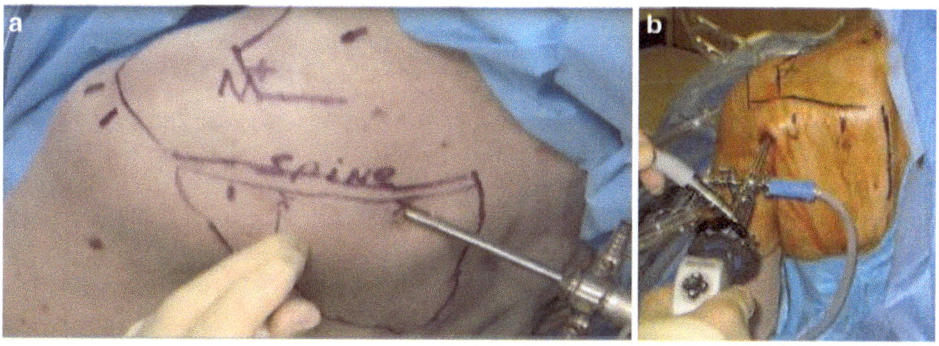

Fig. 23.18 (**a**) Clinical photo of a left shoulder posterior view. The 30° arthroscope is introduced into the viewing portal located 8 cm medial to the posterolateral corner of the acromion. Note the anesthesiologist is instructed to maintain a systolic blood pressure no higher than 100 mg Hg mindful of the patient's health if this is not possible. We have always released the spinoglenoid ligament prior to proceeding with any intra-articular work or if needed any release of the transverse scapular ligament to avoid any undue swelling that will make this procedure more difficult. (**b**) Clinical photo of a left shoulder, posterior view, with the spinoglenoid portals marked out (SG). The arthroscope is in the standard posterior portal for intra-articular glenohumeral joint inspection. Note the relationship of the normal posterior portal to the spinoglenoid ligament portals. "X" represents Nevaiser's portal (Copyright Kevin D. Plancher MD 2015)

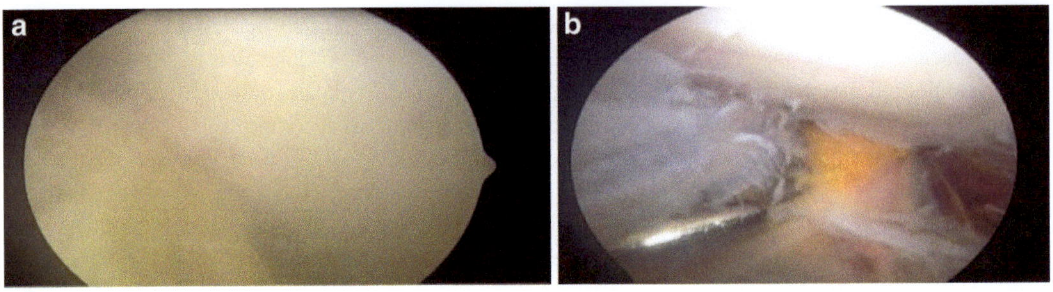

Fig. 23.19 (**a**) Arthroscopic picture of the same left shoulder after initial sweeping of the soft tissue away to expose the adipose around the spinoglenoid ligament. Clarity of the pictures occurs once the water is turned on. (**b**) Intraoperative photo of the same left shoulder showing perineural fat with trocar teasing the spinoglenoid ligament off the suprascapular nerve. The *white* above represents the spine of the scapula. The glenohumeral joint would be off to the left (Copyright Kevin D. Plancher MD 2015)

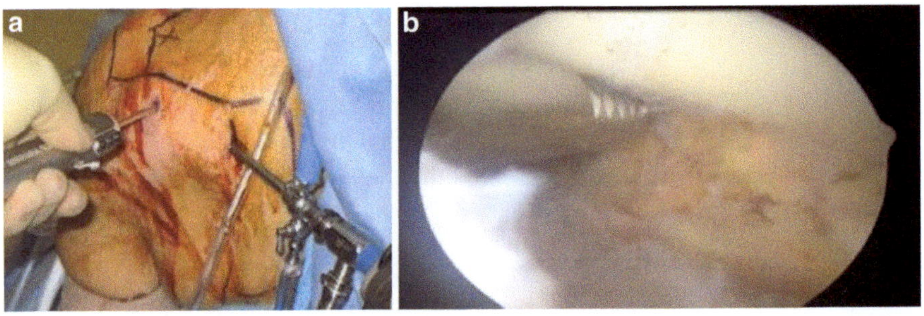

Fig. 23.20 (**a**) The arthroscope and shaver are now moved into the appropriate spinoglenoid portals for decompression of the suprascapular nerve at the spinoglenoid notch. (**b**) Intraoperative photo of the same left shoulder, posterior view. The spine of the scapula is above. The shaver is taking the spinoglenoid ligament directly off the spine of the scapula. All work is being completed lateral to the suprascapular nerve. No different than resecting the ligamentum mucosa/infrapatellar plica in a knee, all work is done on the bone or the notch (the knee), thereby safely avoiding injury to the nerve anterior and medially (Copyright Kevin D. Plancher MD 2015)

of the released suprascapular nerve with the artery can now be seen hugging tightly as it wraps around the notch and heads medially giving its 2–4 muscular branches to the infraspinatus (Fig. 23.23) Upon completion and full inspection, and after joint arthroscopic visualization, the equipment is removed from the body, and the portals are closed in routine fashion. The patient should wear a sling for 7 days for comfort. Thereafter, all activities can be resumed depending on any other work that may have been performed to this same shoulder.

Our experience with this technique has been exceptionally favorable when a patient has failed conservative treatment and has EMG-proven compression and visual atrophy in the infraspinatus fossa. The patient's pain profile (dull ache posteriorly) the next day after release is often described as "completely gone", and while we have not witnessed full restoration of the infraspinatus muscle belly, we have seen, in those whose disease has not been present for more than 2 years, significant and measurable strength gains in external rotation. This technique, we believe, is safe and effective as it approaches the anatomy directly without violation of any nonessential or essential muscular planes. We have also used this approach successfully in the 20 patients who did not exhibit any infraspinatus wasting but had a chronic ache and exhibited a positive crossed arm adduction test and external rotation weakness on physical exam with a negative Zanca view on plain radiographs and proactive selective injections. These patients enjoyed essentially immediate relief and return to overhead sport and activities of daily living.

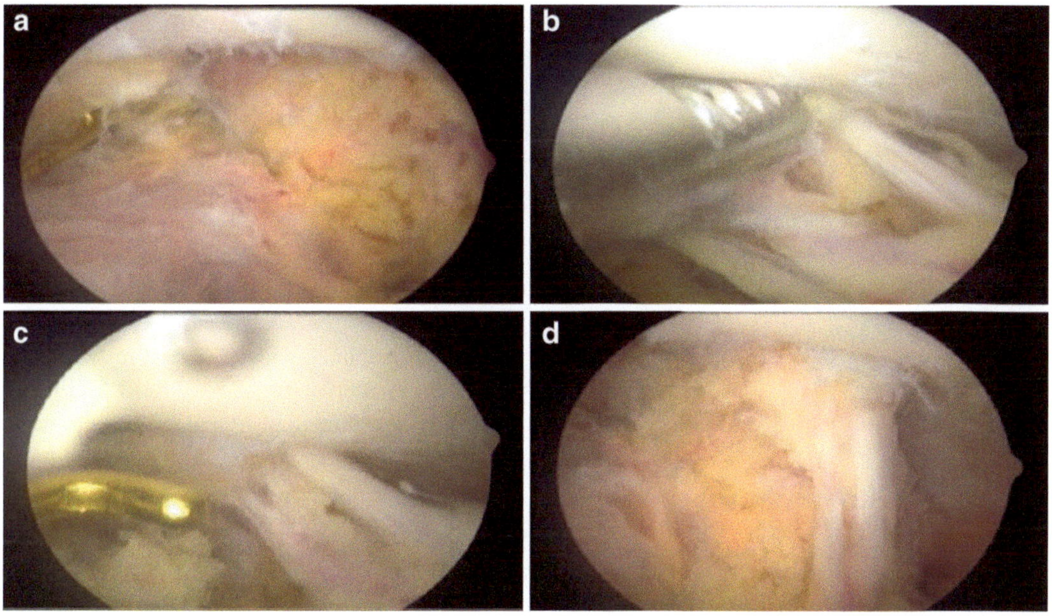

Fig. 23.21 Intraoperative photo of the same left shoulder, posterior view. The spine of the scapula is above (*white*). (**a**) The probe is teasing the spinoglenoid ligament off of the glenohumeral attachment laterally. The suprascapular nerve will reveal itself in the perineural fat with blunt dissection. (**b**) The dull trocar has been used to tease the tissue and expose the suprascapular nerve seen at the tip of the shaver moving obliquely to the right. (**c**) In this arthroscopic view, the suprascapular nerve is clearly seen off to the right, and the slightly anterior to the nerve is the suprascapular artery. The gold probe on the left is being used to tease any remaining remnants of the spinoglenoid ligament or the tissues compressing the suprascapular nerve. (**d**) The suprascapular nerve is now freed and fully mobile as it exits the spinoglenoid notch to move medially now that it has been decompressed (Copyright Kevin D. Plancher MD 2015)

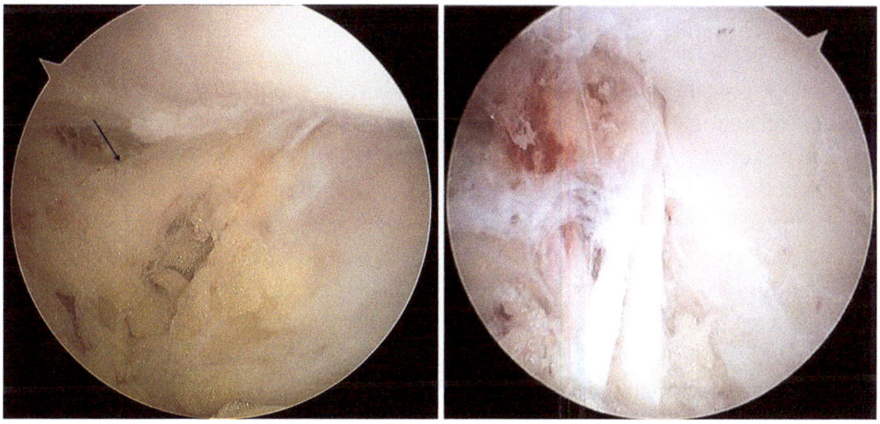

Fig. 23.22 (**a**) Arthroscopic view of the left shoulder, posterior view, with the *arrow* pointing to the suprascapular nerve heading medially. Note the bulging tissue to the *left*, representing a ganglion cyst not yet decompressed. The spine of the scapular (*white*) is above. (**b**) Arthroscopic view of a left shoulder, posterior view. Note the relationship of the suprascapular nerve as it always hugs tightly the suprascapular notch. This suprascapular nerve represents an anomaly which is yet to be described because of its bifid nature. The nerve branches will head medially toward the *right*. Arthroscopic decompression of the spinoglenoid ligament can be safely performed by staying lateral to the nerve which is fixed in position in the spinoglenoid notch (Copyright Kevin D. Plancher MD 2015)

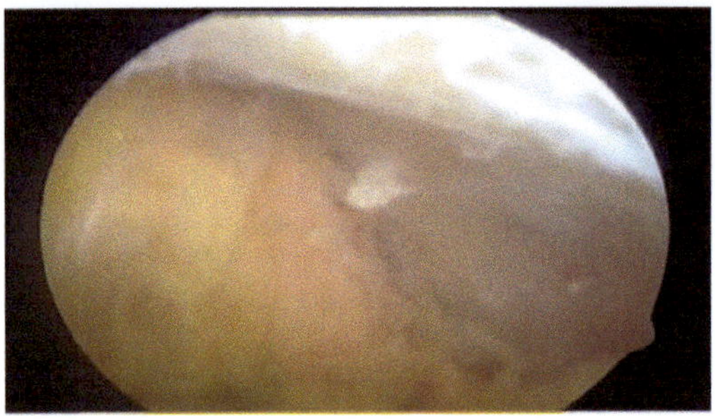

Fig. 23.23 Intraoperative photo of the same left shoulder demonstrating the most medial aspect of the spinoglenoid notch. This is the danger zone as the suprascapular nerve will always hug the most medial aspect of the notch as it heads midline giving off 2–4 muscular branches to the infraspinatus. Note the spine of the scapular up above (*white*). Note the curvature of the infraspinatus fossa seen to the right of the perineural fat surrounding the suprascapular nerve (Copyright Kevin D. Plancher MD 2015)

Outcomes

Literature on this topic is sparse. There are very few series with long-term follow-up including our own data. We are awaiting at least a 3-year average follow-up before reporting to ensure confidence that the ganglion cyst has not returned and that the athlete or laborer has in fact returned to all activities without pain. Satisfactory treatment of persistent chronic atrophy has proved elusive. We remain hopeful a solution to stubborn, persistent atrophy looms in the near future.

Historically, Warren et al. reviewed their results with nonoperative treatment. They recommended that if no ganglion cyst or soft tissue mass was present and no compression of the suprascapular nerve was detected, then nonoperative measures were indicated. This series did not focus solely on the spinoglenoid notch [38]. Post et al. reported on open surgical decompression without evaluation of the labrum and felt one could expect excellent or good results in 88 % of the patients [26]. Fehrman reported in a small series of patients who failed nonoperative treatment. He described surgical success with complete pain relief by addressing the intra-articular lesion in addition to an open resection of the ganglion [21]. Chen and Lichtenberg independently both reported on a small series of patients who underwent concomitant arthroscopic repair of a SLAP lesion and excision of the ganglia [39, 40]. All patients in both studies had complete pain relief and improvement in strength and excellent function at their reported follow-up.

Schroder et al. reported on a series of labral repair alone without decompression of the cyst and noted excellent results. Again, as stated previously, resolution of the cyst was not confirmed in all cases [33]. Curiously, there is a case report of debridement of a labral tear and cyst aspiration with radiographic evidence of cyst resolution as well as reinnervation shown by EMG [36]. However, we remain skeptical of the long-term prognosis of this approach.

Reports from our group are forthcoming with direct posterior decompression as well as others who advocate other means of arthroscopic nerve decompression. However, the early data presented in many meetings across the globe are very promising.

Summary

Compression of the suprascapular nerve at the spinoglenoid ligament is an affliction of a young overhead laborer or avid athlete. This chapter will help the reader to recognize its existence as this disease entity "has seen us but we have not seen it" because of its infrequent occurrence. The patient's complaints can often be confused with rotator cuff disease, but by following the guidelines written above, it is our hope that physicians will identify this condition and perhaps consider, after much practice in a lab setting, endoscopic release of the spinoglenoid ligament, cyst excision, and decompression of the suprascapular nerve in order to facilitate rapid resolution of symptoms.

References

1. Thompson WA, Kopell HP. Peripheral entrapment neuropathies of the upper extremity. N Engl J Med. 1959;260:1261–5.
2. Cummins CA, Messer TM, Nuber GW. Suprascapular nerve entrapment. J Bone Joint Surg Am. 2000;82: 415–24.

3. Plancher KD, Luke TA, Peterson RK, Yacoubian SV. Posterior shoulder pain: a dynamic study of the spinoglenoid ligament and treatment with arthroscopic release of the scapular tunnel. Arthroscopy. 2007;23:991–8.
4. Plancher KD, Peterson RK, Johnston JC, Luke TA. The spinoglenoid ligament. Anatomy, morphology, and histological findings. J Bone Joint Surg Am. 2005;87:361–5.
5. Post M, Mayer J. Suprascapular nerve entrapment. Diagnosis and treatment. Clin Orthop Relat Res. 1987;223:126–36.
6. Rengachary SS, Burr D, Lucas S, Hassanein KM, Mohn MP, Matzke H. Suprascapular entrapment neuropathy: a clinical, anatomical, and comparative study. Part 2: anatomical study. Neurosurgery. 1979;5:447–51.
7. Yan J, Horiguchi M. The communicating branch of the 4th cervical nerve to the brachial plexus: the double constitution, anterior and posterior, of its fibers. Surg Radiol Anat. 2000;22:175–9.
8. Bigliani LU, Dalsey RM, Mccann PD, APRIL EW. An anatomical study of the suprascapular nerve. Arthroscopy. 1990;6:301–5.
9. Tubbs RS, Smyth MD, Salter G, Oakes WJ. Anomalous traversement of the suprascapular artery through the suprascapular notch: a possible mechanism for undiagnosed shoulder pain? Med Sci Monit. 2003;9:BR116–9.
10. Warner JP, Krushell RJ, Masquelet A, Gerber C. Anatomy and relationships of the suprascapular nerve: anatomical constraints to mobilization of the supraspinatus and infraspinatus muscles in the management of massive rotator-cuff tears. J Bone Joint Surg Am. 1992;74:36–45.
11. Matsumoto D, Suenaga N, Oizumi N, Hisada Y, Minami A. A new nerve block procedure for the suprascapular nerve based on a cadaveric study. J Shoulder Elbow Surg. 2009;18:607–11.
12. Ferretti A, De Carli A, Fontana M. Injury of the suprascapular nerve at the spinoglenoid notch. The natural history of infraspinatus atrophy in volleyball players. Am J Sports Med. 1998;26:759–63.
13. Lajtai G, Pfirrmann CW, Aitzetmuller G, Pirkl C, Gerber C, Jost B. The shoulders of professional beach volleyball players: high prevalence of infraspinatus muscle atrophy. Am J Sports Med. 2009;37:1375–83.
14. Lajtai G, Wieser K, Ofner M, Raimann G, Aitzetmuller G, Jost B. Electromyography and nerve conduction velocity for the evaluation of the infraspinatus muscle and the suprascapular nerve in professional beach volleyball players. Am J Sports Med. 2012;40:2303–8.
15. Plancher KD, Johnston JC, Peterson RK, Hawkins RJ. The dimensions of the rotator interval. J Shoulder Elbow Surg. 2005;14:620–5.
16. Ringel SP, Treihaft M, Carry M, Fisher R, Jacobs P. Suprascapular neuropathy in pitchers. Am J Sports Med. 1990;18:80–6.
17. Bayramoglu A, Demiryurek D, Tuccar E, Erbil M, Aldur MM, Tetik O, Doral MN. Variations in anatomy at the suprascapular notch possibly causing suprascapular nerve entrapment: an anatomical study. Knee Surg Sports Traumatol Arthrosc. 2003;11:393–8.
18. Abboud JA, Silverberg D, Glaser DL, Ramsey ML, Williams GR. Arthroscopy effectively treats ganglion cysts of the shoulder. Clin Orthop Relat Res. 2006;444:129–33.
19. Westerheide KJ, Dopirak RM, Karzel RP, Snyder SJ. Suprascapular nerve palsy secondary to spinoglenoid cysts: results of arthroscopic treatment. Arthroscopy. 2006;22:721–7.
20. Moore TP, Fritts HM, Quick DC, Buss DD. Suprascapular nerve entrapment caused by supraglenoid cyst compression. J Shoulder Elbow Surg. 1997;6:455–62.
21. Fehrman DA, Orwin JF, Jennings RM. Suprascapular nerve entrapment by ganglion cysts: a report of six cases with arthroscopic findings and review of the literature. Arthroscopy. 1995;11:727–34.
22. Fritz RC, Helms CA, Steinbach LS, Genant HK. Suprascapular nerve entrapment: evaluation with MR imaging. Radiology. 1992;182:437–44.
23. Khalili AA. Neuromuscular electrodiagnostic studies in entrapment neuropathy of the suprascapular nerve. Orthop Rev. 1974;3:27–8.
24. Ogino T, Minami A, Kato H, Hara R, Suzuki K. Entrapment neuropathy of the suprascapular nerve by a ganglion. A report of three cases. J Bone Joint Surg Am. 1991;73:141–7.
25. Nardin RA, Rutkove SB, Raynor EM. Diagnostic accuracy of electrodiagnostic testing in the evaluation of weakness. Muscle Nerve. 2002;26:201–5.
26. Post M, Grinblat E. Suprascapular nerve entrapment: diagnosis and results of treatment. J Shoulder Elbow Surg. 1993;2:190–7.
27. Piatt BE, Hawkins RJ, Fritz RC, Ho CP, Wolf E, Schickendantz M. Clinical evaluation and treatment of spinoglenoid notch ganglion cysts. J Shoulder Elbow Surg. 2002;11:600–4.
28. Hashimoto BE, Hayes AS, Ager JD. Sonographic diagnosis and treatment of ganglion cysts causing suprascapular nerve entrapment. J Ultrasound Med. 1994;13:671–4.
29. Post M. Diagnosis and treatment of suprascapular nerve entrapment. Clin Orthop Relat Res. 1999;368:92–100.
30. Callahan JD, Scully TB, Shapiro SA, Worth RM. Suprascapular nerve entrapment. A series of 27 cases. J Neurosurg. 1991;74:893–6.
31. Iannotti JP, Ramsey ML. Arthroscopic decompression of a ganglion cyst causing suprascapular nerve compression. Arthroscopy. 1996;12:739–45.
32. Youm T, Matthews PV, EL Attrache NS. Treatment of patients with spinoglenoid cysts associated with superior labral tears without cyst aspiration, debridement, or excision. Arthroscopy. 2006;22:548–52.
33. Schroder CP, Skare O, Stiris M, Gjengedal E, Uppheim G, Brox JI. Treatment of labral tears with associated spinoglenoid cysts without cyst decompression. J Bone Joint Surg Am. 2008;90:523–30.

34. Pillai G, Baynes JR, Gladstone J, Flatow EL. Greater strength increase with cyst decompression and SLAP repair than SLAP repair alone. Clin Orthop Relat Res. 2011;469:1056–60.
35. Black KP, Lombardo JA. Suprascapular nerve injuries with isolated paralysis of the infraspinatus. Am J Sports Med. 1990;18:225–8.
36. Chochole MH, Senker W, Meznik C, Breitenseher MJ. Glenoid-labral cyst entrapping the suprascapular nerve: dissolution after arthroscopic debridement of an extended SLAP lesion. Arthroscopy. 1997;13:753–5.
37. Ghodadra N, Nho SJ, Verma NN, Reiff S, Piasecki DP, Provencher MT, Romeo AA. Arthroscopic decompression of the suprascapular nerve at the spinoglenoid notch and suprascapular notch through the subacromial space. Arthroscopy. 2009;25:439–45.
38. Martin SD, Warren RF, Martin TL, Kennedy K, O'brien SJ, Wickiewicz TL. Suprascapular neuropathy. Results of non-operative treatment. J Bone Joint Surg Am. 1997;79:1159–65.
39. Chen MJ, Lew HL, Hsu TC, Tsai WC, Lin WC, Tang SF, Lee YC, Hsu RC, Chen CP. Ultrasound-guided shoulder injections in the treatment of subacromial bursitis. Am J Phys Med Rehabil. 2006;85:31–5.
40. Lichtenberg S, Magosch P, Habermeyer P. Compression of the suprascapular nerve by a ganglion cyst of the spinoglenoid notch: the arthroscopic solution. Knee Surg Sports Traumatol Arthrosc. 2004;12:72–9.

Part V

Post Op Care

Maximizing Return to Activity Post Cuff and Instability Surgery

24

Marisa Pontillo and Brian Leggin

Introduction

Designing a rehabilitation program after a patient has had surgical intervention should take several factors into account: the degree and type of mechanical disruption, the type and strength of the surgical procedure, the chronicity of the problem, the strength and endurance of the rotator cuff and scapular musculature, the flexibility of the soft tissues around the shoulder, and the patient's anticipated level and type of activity post-rehabilitation. Postoperative guidelines which respect tissue healing timelines should be followed; at the same time, the patient should be progressed through the phases of rehabilitation only when the criteria of each phase are met.

The examination of the postoperative patient is determined by the time period from surgery. Tissue fixation and healing principles must be followed when assessing ROM and strength. Strength assessment requiring significant resistance should be avoided until the relevant tissue can maintain its integrity. Typically, 4–6 weeks are sufficient for capsular tissues to achieve adequate physiologic healing (depending on tissue quality and degree of tension), with a considerably longer times necessary for tendon repair. Additionally, for patients who have undergone a procedure for instability, the contralateral upper extremity should be examined for the degree of gross connective tissue hyperelasticity (e.g., using the Beighton scale). Typically, the patient with multidirectional instability (MDI) will demonstrate hypermobility of other joints. The degree of hypermobility that a patient exhibits should guide the therapist as to how aggressive postoperative range of motion (ROM) should be attained.

Regardless of underlying pathology, the goal of rehabilitation is functional recovery and returning the patient to their previous level of activity. With the shoulder complex, it is important to work from less to more provocative positions. For example, external rotation performed with the arm by the side will potentially be less provocative than if performed at 90° of abduction for instability repairs. However, in the case of overhead athletes, the patient will need to progress to therapeutic activities more rapidly in this position. Return to sport activities should be incorporated in final phases of rehabilitation. Once a patient demonstrates sufficient strength and neuromuscular control to be cleared for plyometric exercises, these exercises will improve power and encourage maximal firing of

M. Pontillo, PT, DPT, SCS (✉)
GSPP Penn Therapy and Fitness,
Penn Sports Medicine Center, Philadelphia, PA, USA
e-mail: marisa.pontillo@uphs.upenn.edu

B. Leggin, PT, DPT, OCS
Penn Therapy and Fitness at Valley Forge,
Berwyn, PA, USA

J.D. Kelly IV (ed.), *Elite Techniques in Shoulder Arthroscopy*,
DOI 10.1007/978-3-319-25103-5_24

the rotator cuff and scapular muscles to provide a necessary transition to high-speed activities. Additionally, interval sports programs (ISPs) will train the musculature to the specific demands of individual sports. Rehabilitation should focus on the elimination of pain and the restoration of functional movement through dynamic stability of the rotator cuff and scapular musculature.

Rehabilitation following Arthroscopic Rotator Cuff Repair

Rehabilitation following rotator cuff repair may vary based on surgical technique, cuff tear size, tissue quality, amount of tension at the repair site, patient age, patient goals, functional demands of the patient, and systemic disease processes. The prognosis following repair has been correlated to the rotator cuff tear size, preoperative atrophy, and ROM restrictions. The amount of postoperative interaction the patient has with the surgeon and therapist is dictated by individual patient need. Ideally, the therapist sees the patient at the time of postoperative visits with the surgeon. Visits with the surgeon usually occur at 7–10 days, 6 weeks, 3 months, and 6 months postoperatively for all patients. Some patients are able to begin passive ROM at that first postoperative visit, whereas the initiation of these exercises may be delayed in other patients.

Recent work by Soslowsky demonstrating that immobilization resulted in superior structural, compositional, and viscoelastic properties, as well as improved tendon to bone healing has lead us to a delayed approach to rehabilitation following rotator cuff repair. An assessment of whether to begin ROM in the first 6 weeks after surgery is made by the surgeon at the first postoperative visit. Patients are expected to achieve 100° of passive forward elevation and 30° of passive external rotation at that initial encounter. Patients who meet that motion threshold with medium to massive rotator cuff repairs will be held immobilized for the next 4–6 weeks postoperatively. The goal in these patients is to allow sufficient healing of the rotator cuff prior to mobilization of the extremity. Any stiffness accumulated during this time period has been shown to be transient. Patients who do not meet those criteria or who have repair of a partial or small rotator cuff tear will most likely be sent to therapy immediately. Patients who are seen in therapy are expected to reduce any muscle guarding, gain 10° of passive forward elevation, and demonstrate the exercises independently. Patients meeting those criteria will be allowed to exercise with a home program until the next postoperative visit with the surgeon at 6 weeks. Patients who do not meet those criteria will be seen in therapy on at least a weekly basis until the ROM improves sufficiently.

The rehabilitation program we are presenting consists of a basic set of stretching and strengthening exercises. The timing of when these exercises are introduced to the patient depends on the type of procedure performed and size of the rotator cuff tear. We will discuss the rehabilitation process after rotator cuff repair through four phases.

Phase I

When beginning rehabilitation after rotator cuff repair, a therapist must know the size of the tear and tendon involvement, quality of the tissue and ease of tendon mobilization, surgical technique, presurgery treatment, and the patient's goals. Patients who have had repair of a small cuff tear will most likely be immobilized in a sling to be used for comfort and when they are in public places. As long as the patient is comfortable, they are able to go without the sling as early as the first postoperative day. Patients who have had repair of a large or massive rotator cuff tear are usually immobilized in a sling in slight abduction for the first 3–6 weeks postoperatively.

Patients with small tears begin with pendulum exercises, elbow AROM, and hand squeezes within the first week after surgery. At the first postoperative visit, patients are instructed in phase I stretching exercises which are supine passive forward elevation with the opposite hand and external rotation with a cane or stick (Fig. 24.1). Emphasis is placed on the patient achieving a tolerable, submaximal stretch several times per day

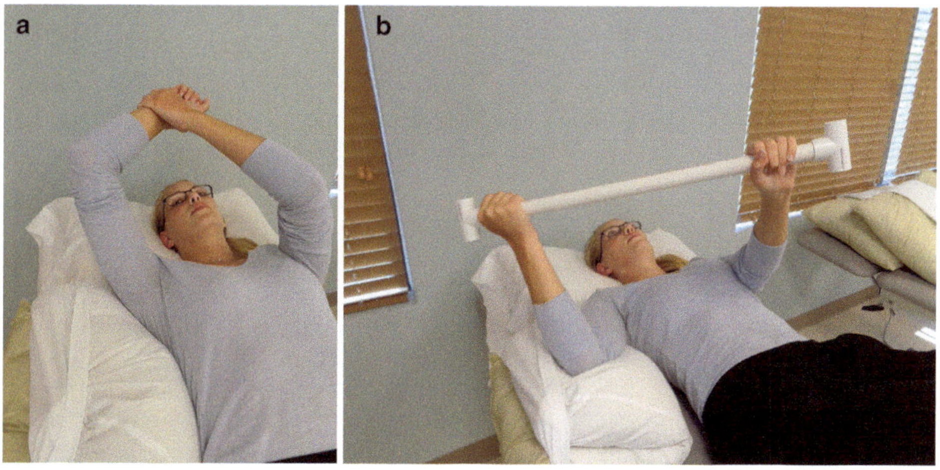

Fig. 24.1 (**a**) Phase I ROM: forward elevation. (**b**) Phase I ROM: ER

rather than aggressive short bouts of stretching. The patient is asked to perform 10–20 repetitions with at least a 10-second (s) hold, 4–6 times per day at home. The therapist also must assess whether the patient requires more supervised physical therapy during these initial 6 weeks after surgery. We have found that patients who achieve greater than 100° of passive forward elevation or a 10° improvement in forward elevation during the first visit do well continuing with the home program on their own. In addition, patients must be able to demonstrate independence with the performance of these exercises. Patients who do not fit these criteria will be recommended for more supervised therapy. Muscle guarding and pain must be managed at this time. Patients may have difficulty and pain attempting to perform supine passive forward elevation due to a heavy arm or a weak opposite extremity. We have found "unweighting" the arm with a chair stretch to be useful in these patients. The patient stands behind a chair with both hands on the backrest, and they walk backwards until they experience a slight stretch. This position is held for 10 s and repeated 10 times. Some patients have also benefited from using transcutaneous electrical nerve stimulation (TENS) prior to exercising for pain modulation.

As stated earlier, the surgeon may delay beginning these ROM exercises until 4–6 weeks post-op for some patients with medium, large, or massive cuff tears. In these patients, the program remains the same, but the time frame for the implementation of the exercises is changed to correspond with the start date of the exercises.

Phase II

This stage typically begins 6–8 weeks after surgery for partial and small repairs and 8–12 weeks for medium, large, or massive tears. Patients are asked to continue performing the phase I ROM exercises. The supine forward elevation exercise may now be performed with a cane or stick to achieve end-range forward elevation PROM. Patients are instructed in phase II ROM exercises (Fig. 24.2) and Phase I strengthening exercises at this time (Fig. 24.3). Caution must be employed with patients who have had large or massive rotator cuff tears. Restrictions in internal rotation ROM are to be expected due to the nature of the repair. Therefore, this exercise must be performed submaximally. Pain or weakness with the strengthening exercises may necessitate shorter arcs of motion. In some cases of a complex repair or where the integrity of the repair may be in question, rotator cuff strengthening may not be initiated until 10–12 weeks post-surgery.

Patients who are not progressing as expected may be referred to supervised therapy.

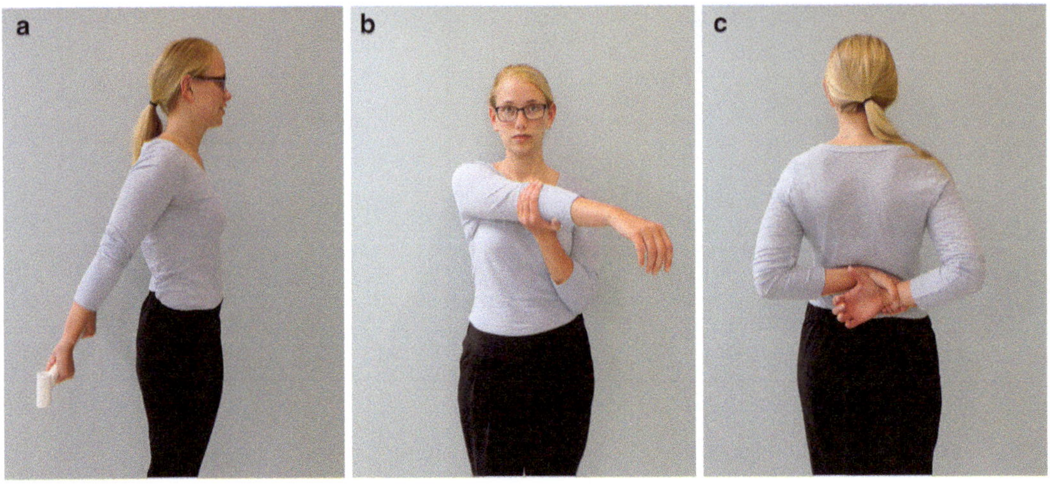

Fig. 24.2 (**a**) Phase II ROM: extension. (**b**) Phase II ROM: cross body adduction. (**c**) Phase II ROM: internal rotation

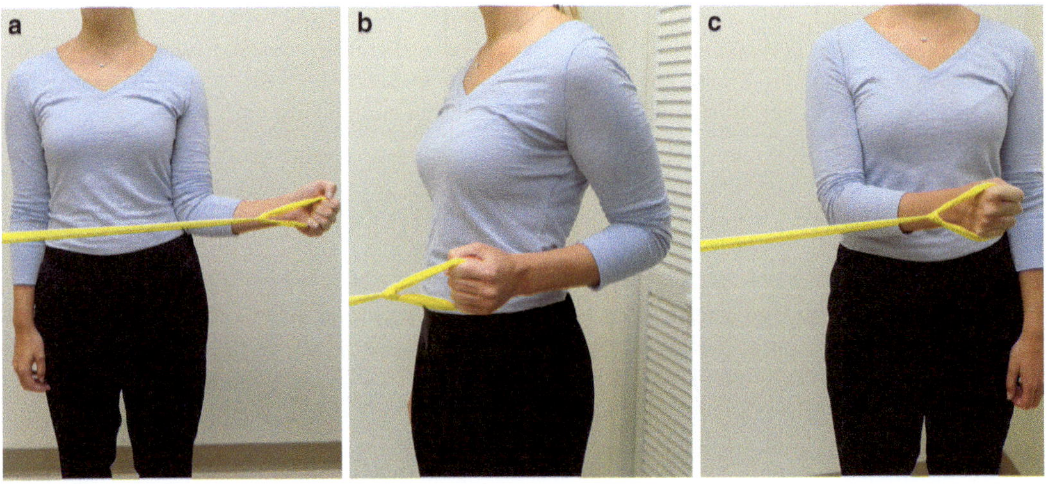

Fig. 24.3 (**a**) Phase I strengthening: external rotation. (**b**) Phase I strengthening: extension. (**c**) Phase I strengthening: internal rotation

Strengthening exercises may be delayed if the patient continues to have pain and stiffness. To help advance PROM, glenohumeral mobilizations and gentle, relatively pain-free manual stretching can be performed. To augment strengthening, manual resistance can be applied with alternating isometrics beginning with the arm supported at 45° in the plane of the scapula (POS) and neutral rotation. Scapular strengthening exercises can also begin at this time period. Exercises should be performed with the arms below shoulder height to avoid increasing pain.

Phase III

This phase begins 12–16 weeks after surgery for small/medium tears and 16–24 weeks for large/massive tears. The patient should have full PROM for FE and ER. It should be expected that internal rotation ROM will be only slightly better than at

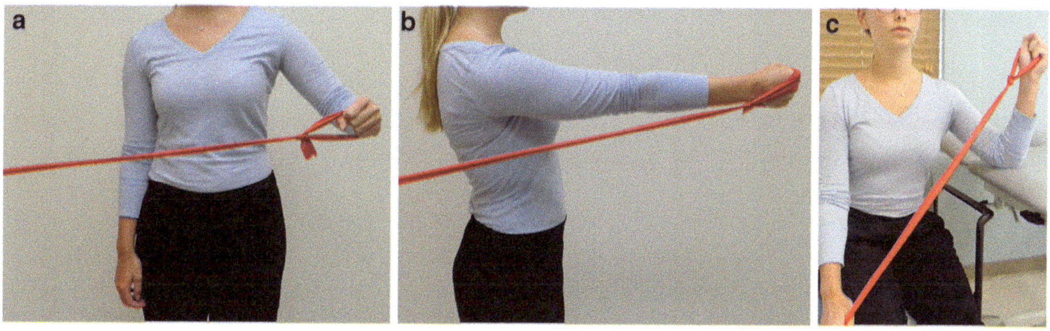

Fig. 24.4 (**a**) Phase II strengthening: abduction to 45. (**b**) Phase II strengthening: forward elevation. (**c**) Phase II strengthening: external rotation supported at 45

the beginning of phase II. It is important to assess active ROM at this point.

Patients who are able to raise their arm against gravity and are able to perform the phase I strengthening exercises with green resistance band will be instructed in phase II strengthening exercises (Fig. 24.4). These exercises are designed to begin training the rotator cuff and deltoid for functional demands. However, as always, pain is respected and the intensity of the exercises must be monitored.

Phase IV

This phase typically begins 16–24 weeks postoperative and continues for up to 9 months postoperatively. Patients will be progressed to Phase II scapular strengthening which includes a backhand and forehand motion with elastic resistance as well as horizontal abduction with ER. Patients are encouraged to approach overhead activities with caution, and whenever possible reposition their upper extremity so that the elbow can remain below shoulder level. They are again instructed in the biomechanics of lifting in efforts to reduce the risk of rotator cuff overload.

For the athlete, sport-specific training can begin utilizing plyometrics to enhance neuromuscular control, strength, and proprioception. Recommendations and instruction for proper use of gym equipment should also be done at this time.

Rehabilitation following Arthroscopic Stabilization

Success during rehabilitation following any orthopedic surgical procedure is dependent upon the appropriate application of stress to the repaired structures. Initially minimal stress is required for beginning healing, followed by a progressive gradual increase in stress over several months to the surgical repair to protect it while the repair matures. Four principles are of critical importance for the rehabilitation professional to understand and successfully apply to be able manipulate stress and facilitate healing in capsulolabral repairs of the shoulder and promote a safe return to function: (1) a basic understanding of the surgical procedure; (2) an understanding of the anatomic structures which must be protected, how they are stressed, and the rate at which they heal; (3) the identification and skilled application of the methods used during rehabilitation to manipulate stress to the surgical repair; and (4) identifying the appropriate length of immobilization and rate of return to full ROM.

Phase I

The goals of this early phase include protecting the structures that were repaired and improving ROM in a slow controlled manner. Rapid and excessive progression of ROM may lead to a poor outcome. The evaluation is limited to passive forward elevation and passive external rotation with the arm at approximately 20° of abduction in the POS. It is also important to administer a self-report outcome tool such as the Penn Shoulder Score or ASES Shoulder Score Index at 2- to 4-week intervals in order to track progress. Patient education is important in the early phases following surgery. Patients are instructed to use their arm for waist level activities when tolerated. They are cautioned about using the arm away from the body, sleeping on the operated side, leaning on that side, and making sudden movements. When sitting, the patient is encouraged to position the arm in neutral rotation and the POS supported by a pillow.

Patients may begin their rehabilitation program at any time during the first six postoperative weeks. Surgeons may wish to hold off on beginning ROM exercises depending on the patient's connective tissue elasticity in order to allow healing and protect the repair. We begin with pendulum exercises, hand squeezes, and elbow active ROM. Phase I passive ROM exercises are also begun at this time. These include supine forward elevation in the POS utilizing the opposite hand and external rotation supported at 45° in the POS utilizing a cane or stick. The goal for PROM FE is 135° and 45° for external rotation with the arm below 45° of abduction. Patients who rapidly regain ROM in this phase may be told to hold off performing these exercises during this time period. In addition, scapular retraction and scapular retraction with downward rotation exercises without resistance can be added at this time.

Phase II

Phase II of the rehabilitation process begins at approximately postoperative week 6 and extends to approximately week 12. The criteria for progression to phase II include appropriate healing of the surgical repair by adhering to the precautions and immobilization guidelines, and the staged ROM goals are met *but not significantly exceeded.* During this stage, phase II ROM exercises are added, which include extension behind the back with a stick, cross body adduction, and internal rotation up the back with the opposite hand or a towel. Rotator cuff strengthening exercises with elastic resistance are also introduced for smaller tears with solid structural repair. These are called phase I strengthening exercises, and include external rotation, internal rotation, and extension, all with the arm by the side (Fig. 24.3). Patients are asked to begin by performing one set of 10 repetitions. When they have no difficulty or discomfort with that first set, they can add a set with the goal of achieving three sets of 10 repetitions without difficulty. When they are able to achieve three sets of 10 without difficulty, they can move to the next level of elastic resistance. Manual resistance to external and internal rotation with the patient in supine and the arm supported at 45° in the POS can be initiated using alternating isometrics and short arc rotation.

Scapular muscle integration and appropriate scapulohumeral rhythm is encouraged in all strengthening exercises. Scapular retraction with elastic resistance at waist level and from overhead may be added for the middle and lower trapezius muscles. When the patient is able to achieve the third level of elastic resistance, phase II strengthening exercises can be added to the program. These include abduction with the elbow bent to 90° in the POS and staying below 60°, forward elevation to 60°, and external rotation supported at 45° in the POS (Fig. 24.4).

Phase III

Phase III of the rehabilitation program begins approximately at week 12 and extends to approximately week 24. The criteria to begin phase III include full active ROM for forward elevation, the ability to perform strengthening exercises without difficulty, and the ability to demonstrate good scapular control during the exercises and functional activities. Manual resistance can be

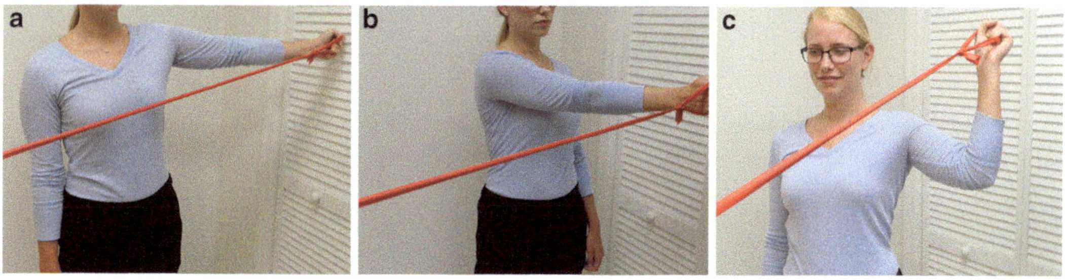

Fig. 24.5 (**a**) Scapular retraction: backhand. (**b**) Scapular protraction: forehand. (**c**) Horizontal abduction with retraction and external rotation: cocking position

progressed to unsupported positions, combinations of movement, and functional positions. Diagonal patterns (D1 and D2) can be incorporated into the manual resistance program. The isotonic strengthening exercises now progress to combination movements and functional patterns. Elastic resistance for "backhand" and "forehand" type motions to strengthen the scapular protractors and retractors can be added (Fig. 24.5). A useful exercise to help the throwing athlete prepare for return to throwing is the combination of horizontal abduction, scapular retraction, and external rotation against elastic resistance (Fig. 24.5). Functional internal rotation with elastic resistance mimicking the throwing motion is helpful to prepare for return to throwing (Fig. 24.6). We will also introduce one-arm rows for the latissimus dorsi and the lat pulldown machine to the front of the body.

A useful device for rehabilitating overhead athletes is the Bodyblade (Hymanson Inc., Playa Del Ray, CA) (Fig. 24.7). The Bodyblade is a flexible fiberglass rod ranging from two-and-a-half feet to 5 feet with a handgrip in the middle. With a gentle oscillating force, the ends will flex back and forth challenging the muscles to co-contract to resist the movement of the blade. Oscillating the blade requires short excursion, high-speed co-contraction muscle activity of the rotator cuff, deltoid, biceps, and scapular muscles. The patient can perform this exercise in multiple positions and therefore achieving dynamic stability throughout the throwing motion especially at the position of 90° of abduction and 90° of external rotation.

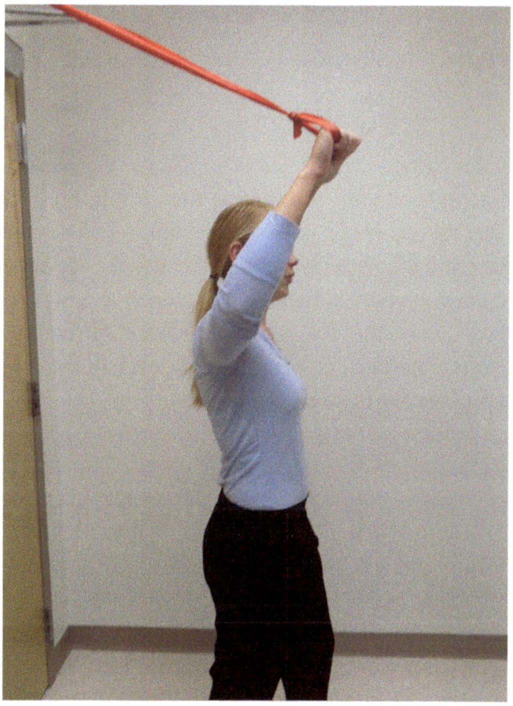

Fig. 24.6 Functional internal rotation

Plyometric training using weighted balls can be used to enhance neuromuscular control, strength, dynamic stability, and proprioception by reproducing the physiologic stretch-shortening cycle of muscle in multiple shoulder positions. Plyometric exercise employs three phases, all intended to use the elastic and reactive properties of the muscle to generate maximum force production. The first phase is the eccentric phase,

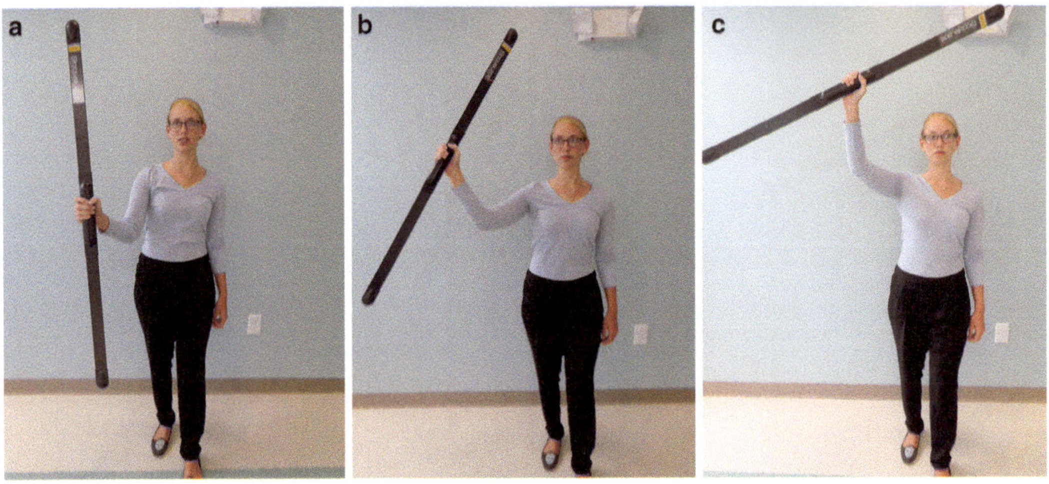

Fig. 24.7 (**a**) Bodyblade position 1. (**b**) Bodyblade position 2. (**c**) Bodyblade position 3

where a rapid prestretch is applied to the musculotendinous unit, stimulating the muscle spindle. The second phase is the amortization phase, representing the time between the eccentric and concentric phases. This time should be as short as possible so that the beneficial effects of the prestretch are not lost. The final phase is the resultant concentric contraction.

Wilk et al. established a plyometric exercise program for the overhead thrower. The initial plyometric program consists of two-handed exercise drills such as a chest pass, overhead soccer throw, and side throws. The goal of the plyometric drills is the transfer of energy from the legs and trunk to the upper extremity. Once the two-handed exercises are mastered, the athlete is progressed to one-handed drills in a functional throwing position. To improve strength and coordination during the deceleration phase of throwing, the athlete can catch a weighted ball from a vertical drop while in sidelying or standing. This can be progressed to catching the ball thrown over the throwing shoulder to mimic the deceleration and follow-through phases. A 6-week plyometric training program resulted in enhanced joint position sense, enhanced kinesthesia, and decreased time to peak torque generation during isokinetic testing.

Return to Sport

Interval Sports Programs

Once an athlete meets the advanced phase of rehabilitation, an interveal sports program (ISP) may be considered. Prior to initiation of an ISP, the patient must exhibit full, pain-free ROM and strength of at least 80 % symmetry versus the contralateral side. Ideally, both the rotator cuff and scapulothoracic musculature should be assessed.

ISPs are developed to increase the amount of an athletic skill in a systematic manner. For example, an interval throwing program will increase the number of pitches, the distance pitched, and the velocity of the pitches over several weeks. Similar programs have been described in the literature for golf, tennis, softball, volleyball, and swimming [1–3].

An example of a typical step one for a pitcher is as follows:

45′ phase
Warm-up throws
Twenty five throws (at 45′)
Rest for 15 min
Warm-up throwing
Twenty five throws (at 45′)

Proper warm-up, stretching, and soreness rules should be included with the patient education when administering an ISP. Of note, ISPs are usually performed concurrently with formal physical therapy/home exercise program and strength and conditioning workouts.

Upper Extremity Functional Testing

Upper extremity functional testing is important to provide objective information about how the athlete uses her upper extremity during a task by testing several constructs simultaneously (strength, speed, and stabilization) and aids in determining return-to-play readiness. These include, but are not limited to, the upper quarter Y-balance test, the single arm shot put, and closed kinetic chain upper extremity stability test. For unilateral tests, limb symmetry should be calculated.

The upper quarter Y-balance test is the upper extremity counterpart of Y-balance test. The patient is to maintain push-up position with feet 12 in. apart and, with one hand stabilized, performs maximal effort reaches with opposite hand in three directions (medial, superolateral, and inferolateral). The test score (reach distance) is normalized to upper limb length. This test has a good test-retest reliability with an $ICC_{(2,2)}>0.90$ and demonstrates a moderate association with side plank and closed kinetic chain upper extremity stability test (CKCUEST) [4, 5].

For the CKCUEST (Fig. 24.8), patients' scores should be compared to normative values. The CKCUEST has high test-retest reliability, with an $ICC_{(2,2)}$ of 0.92 [6]. This test correlates with rotator cuff strength by handheld dynamometer for both elevation ($r=0.68$) and internal rotation ($r=0.75$) [7]. Additionally, normative values have been reported for collegiate athletes; female collegiate athletes ($n=206$) scored an average of 21.8 touches (SD=3.9), and male collegiate athletes ($n=270$) scored an average of 26.0 touches (SD=4.1). Individual scores are listed by sport (Tables 24.1 and 24.2). For the CKCUEST test, two lines of tape are placed 36 in. apart on the floor. Patients start the test in a standard push-up position, with one hand on each line of tape (Fig. 24.8a). Using

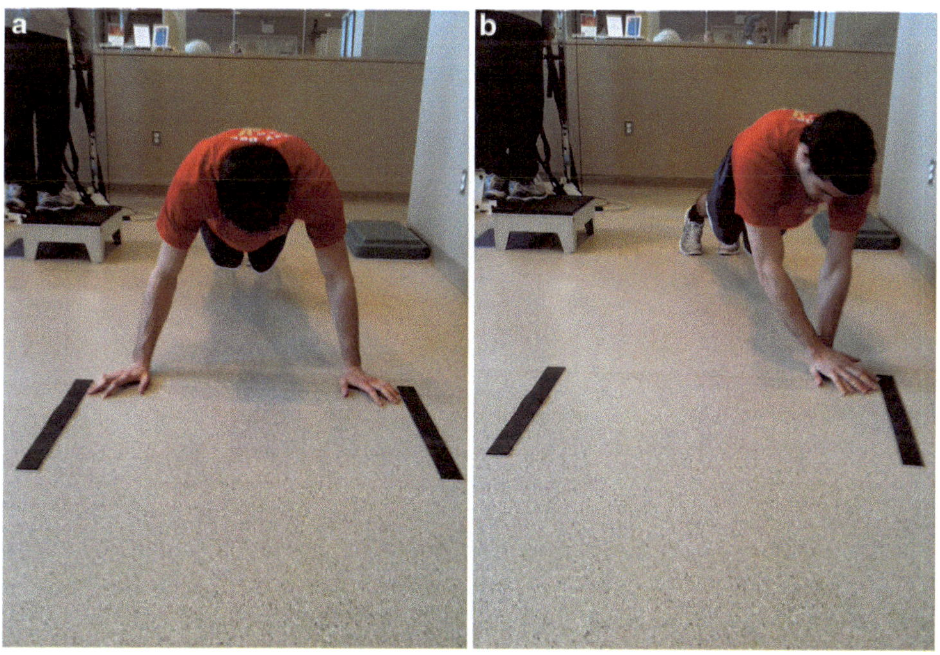

Fig. 24.8 (**a**) Closed kinetic chain upper extremity stability test (CKCUEST) start position. (**b**) CKCUEST in progress

Table 24.1 Normative values by sport, men

Sport	CKCUEST average
Squash	23.7
Track	25.7
Lacrosse	25.9
Tennis	26.3
Crew	26.3
Basketball	27.3
Fencing	27.9
Swimming	27.9
Wrestling	28.1
Baseball	28.8
Football	29.0
Diving	29.8

Table 24.2 Normative values by sport, women

Sport	CKCUEST average
Diving	17.5
Squash	18.0
Field hockey	20.8
Cheerleading	21.3
Crew	21.5
Swimming	21.6
Fencing	22.4
Track/XC	22.4
Golf	23.2
Lacrosse	23.3
Tennis	23.7
Basketball	23.9
Soccer	23.9
Softball	24.1
Gymnastics	26.8

their right hand, the patients are instructed to touch the tape under their left hand (Fig. 24.8b), then return their right hand to the start position, and complete alternating touches. The score is the number of touches achieved in 15 s.

The single arm shot put (Fig. 24.9) is used to assess isolated upper extremity power. It is performed seated, with the patient in a chair and his or her legs propped on second chair. The patient is secured with two straps to eliminate motion at the torso (Fig. 24.9a). The patient is asked to "put" a 2.72 kg medicine ball (Fig. 24.9b). This test has excellent test–retest reliability, with $ICC_{(3,1)}=0.98$ [8]. Reference values for healthy, active individuals are 234.95 cm for the dominant upper extremity and 212.37 cm for the nondominant upper extremity [9].

Other Considerations/Red Flags

Strength and Conditioning

Especially at the collegiate and professional levels, the athletic population is likely to participate in strength and conditioning programs. The injured athlete and strength and conditioning staff must be aware of any restrictions that they have. Additionally, it is the role of the physical therapist to have frequent communication with the strength and conditioning team and/or athletic training to discuss potential limitations and alternatives. With upper extremity injuries, it is essential that lower body lifting is performed without the use of the upper extremity in the acute and subacute phases. For example, a back squat may not be safe for a patient with anterior glenohumeral instability, and leg press or safety squat may provide safe alternatives, to avoid the "high five" position [10]. Upper body strength training should be carefully monitored. Overhead activities are often unsafe until the later phases of rehabilitation. Certain exercises, such as the bench press, may be limited to a certain ROM to avoid undue stress on healing structures (i.e., avoidance of full horizontal abduction for anterior instability and avoidance of locking out the arms at the top of the motion for posterior glenohumeral instability or elbow instability). Integration of the athlete into a strength and conditioning program to improve performance and maintain total arm strength is encouraged; however, respect for healing tissues and prevention of reinjury should be a focus.

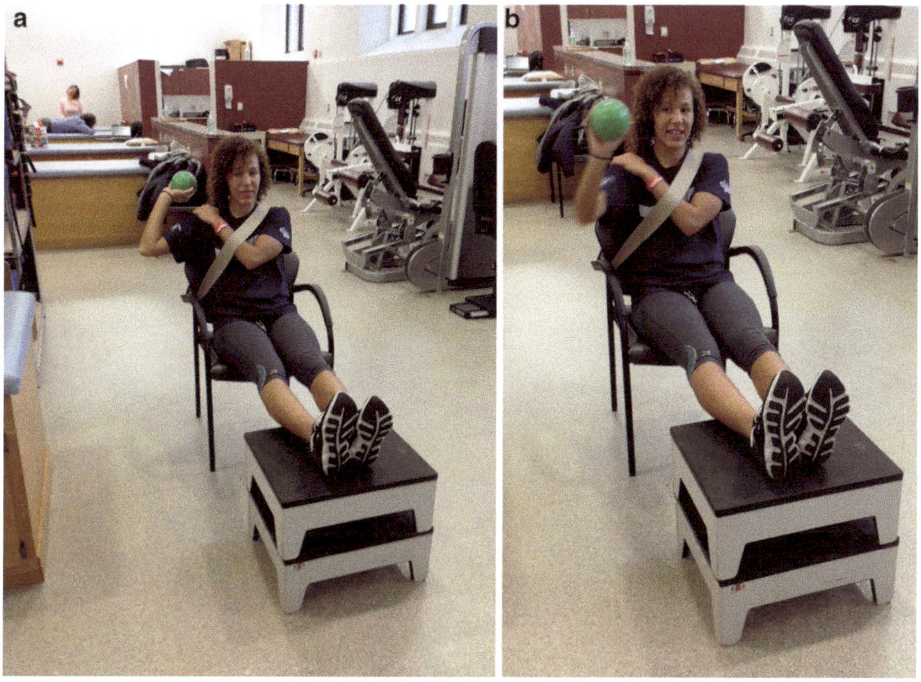

Fig. 24.9 (A and B) Single arm shot put

References

1. Hurd W, Hunter-Giordano A, Axe M, Snyder-Mackler L. Data-based interval hitting program for female college volleyball players. Sports Health. 2009;1(6):522–30.
2. Reinold MM, Wilk KE, Reed J, Crenshaw K, Andrews JR. Interval sport programs: guidelines for baseball, tennis and golf. J Orthop Sports Phys Ther. 2002;32(6):293–8.
3. Axe M, Windley T, Snyder-Mackler L. Data-based interval throwing programs for collegiate softball players. J Athl Train. 2002;37(2):194–203.
4. Gorman PP, Butler RJ, Plisky PJ, Kiesel KB. Upper quarter Y balance test: reliability and performance comparison between genders in active adults. J Strength Cond Res. 2012;26(11):3043–8.
5. Westrick RB, Miller JM, Carow SD, Gerber JP. Exploration of the Y-balance test for assessment of upper quarter closed kinetic chain performance. J Sports Phys Ther. 2002;7(2):139–47.
6. Ellenbecker TS, Manske R, Davies GJ. Closed kinetic chain testing techniques of the upper extremities. Orthop Phys Ther Clin North Amer. 2000;9:219–29.
7. Pontillo M, Sennet BJ, Horneff JG. Profile of upper extremity rotator cuff strength and function in division 1 collegiate athletes. J Orthop Sports Phys Ther. 2011;41(1):A45.
8. Pontillo M, Horneff JG, Huffman GR, Sennett BJ. Relationship between upper extremity strength, functional testing, and self-reported disability in collegiate athletes. J Orthop Sports Phys Ther. 2010;40(1):A108.
9. Negrete RJ, Hanney WJ, Kober MJ, Davies GJ, Riemann B. Can upper extremity functional tests predict the softball throw for distance: a predictive validity investigation. J Sports Phys Ther. 2011;6(2):104–11.
10. Wilk KE, Meister K, Andrews JA. Current concepts in the rehabilitation of the overhead throwing athlete. Am J Sports Med. 2002;30(1):136–51.

When Is the Patient Truly "Ready to Return," a.k.a. Kinetic Chain Homeostasis

25

Aaron Sciascia and Michele Monaco

Introduction

There are different rehabilitation approaches for treating patients following shoulder surgery including targeting only the site of symptoms (such as only performing therapeutic measures at or around the shoulder) or targeting all potential regions or segments which could be contributing to or creating the symptoms. The latter is known as the kinetic chain framework approach for rehabilitation and has been previously described in detail [1, 2]. It is advocated as an ideal tactic for treating patients with musculoskeletal injury because of its comprehensive treatment design. The kinetic chain framework describes five logically arranged key areas of focus to be addressed during the treatment process (proper motion, core stability and strength, stability of energy transfer links, closed-chain exercise implementation, and use of multiple planes). Similar to the kinetic chain description of functional performance, the kinetic chain rehabilitation philosophy specifically utilizes global muscles to facilitate local muscle activation and function throughout the course of treatment. An understanding of kinetic chain function is critical and serves as the foundation for this treatment approach.

The kinetic chain is a coordinated sequencing of activation, mobilization, and stabilization of body segments to produce a dynamic activity [3]. The kinetic chain has several functions [4]: (1) using integrated programs of muscle activation to temporarily link multiple body segments into one functional segment (i.e., the back leg in cocking stance and push-off during throwing; lower extremity weight shifting in arm forward tasks) in order to decrease the degrees of freedom in the entire motion; (2) providing a stable proximal base for distal arm mobility; (3) maximizing force development in the large muscles of the core and transferring it to the hand; (4) producing interactive moments at distal joints that develop more force and energy than the joint alone could develop while decreasing the magnitude of the applied loads at the distal joint; and (5) producing torques that decrease deceleration forces.

Each body part has one or more specific roles in the entire motion of any dynamic task [5]. The feet are contact points with the ground and allow maximum ground reaction force for proximal stability and force generation. The legs and core are the mass for the stable base and the engine for the largest amount of force generation. The shoulder is the funnel for force regulation and transmission and the fulcrum for stability during

A. Sciascia, MS, ATC, PES (✉)
Lexington Clinic, Shoulder Center of Kentucky, Lexington, KY, USA
e-mail: ascia@lexclin.com

M. Monaco, DSC, ATC
Department of Human Movement Science, Immaculata University, Immaculata, PA, USA

J.D. Kelly IV (ed.), *Elite Techniques in Shoulder Arthroscopy*,
DOI 10.1007/978-3-319-25103-5_25

the rapid motion of the arm. The arm and hand is the rapidly moving delivery mechanism of the force to the projectile or instrument.

A deficit within one or more of the individual anatomical segments can negatively affect performance and potentially lead to reinjury, even after surgical repair has been performed [3]. In fact, dysfunction of one proximal link in the kinetic chain leads to "catch up" or increased demands distally. Therefore, a clinician has good reason to implement injury rehabilitation and prevention programs which will initially eliminate physical deficits in critical anatomical segments. This strategy is followed by a focus on increasing a patient's functional longevity while simultaneously decreasing the risk of injury [2]. After restoration of any existing impairment or deficit, the clinician must assist the patient in reestablishing functional patterns and task-specific skills. This can be done with a logical progressive rehabilitation approach which begins and ends with integrated muscle activation and movement.

Kinetic Chain Function

Three components required to obtain optimal kinetic chain function have been previously described [3]. The first component is to have optimal integrity of native anatomy and physiology in critical structures. Following the restoration of disrupted tissue through surgical intervention, functional restoration is initiated in the rehabilitation setting. In order to assure safe return to activity, clinicians routinely implement postsurgical programs designed to restore physical function through the gradual improvement of anatomic and physiological elements. For example, after labral repair, all surgeons oversee rehabilitation aimed at return of shoulder motion and rotator cuff strength. While different approaches for addressing this first component of kinetic chain restoration exist, the specific details of accomplishing this task will be discussed in subsequent sections of this chapter.

Once the anatomy and physiology have been restored to adequate levels of performance, clinicians should address the second component necessary for optimizing kinetic chain function by attempting to recreate the expected preprogrammed muscle activations which are necessary to produce anticipatory postural adjustments (APAs). APAs position the body to withstand the perturbations to balance created by the forces of throwing or arm forward task execution [6–8]. The APAs create the proximal stability for distal mobility. The muscle activations create interactive moments that develop and control forces and loads at joints. Interactive moments are moments at joints that are created by motion and position of adjacent segments [9]. They are developed in the central body segments (known as the core) and are keys to developing proper force at distal joints and for creating relative bony positions that minimize internal loads at the joint. When this proximal-to-distal pattern of activation is operating off of optimized anatomy, it allows the segmented system to operate in an efficient manner where not only maximal speed is produced but forces to joints are reduced and thus risk of injury is lessened. This is considered a biomechanical protection mechanism.

Biomechanically, tasks performed in overhead sports (baseball, tennis, softball, etc) and in the workforce (assembly line or overhead work such as automobile mechanics) occur as a result of the summation of speed principle which states that in order to maximize the speed at the distal end of a linked system, the movement should start with the proximal segments (the hips and core) and progress to the distal segments (shoulder, elbow, wrist) [9]. One action resulting from the summation of speed principle is upper extremity long axis rotation. Upper extremity long axis rotation consists of coupled shoulder internal rotation and elbow pronation around the long axis of the arm extending from the glenohumeral joint to the hand and is accentuated by maximum elbow extension before maximum arm rotation. Marshall and Elliot have shown that long axis rotation is a key biomechanical event just prior to ball release/ball impact [10]. This coupled motion generates internal rotation around the almost straight long axis of the brachium, incorporating the shoulder to the hand. Furthermore, freely mobile long axis rotation minimizes the valgus loads that may be generated at the elbow. Thus, truly effective rehabilitation programs aim to restore all the links responsible for generation of optimal long axis rotation.

Since each segment in this linked system can influence motions of its adjacent segments, rehabilitation should encourage maneuvers and exercises which incorporate the concept of the body working as a unit. For example, during a baseball pitch, stability of the back and stride legs allow rotation of the trunk which in turn allows for maximal throwing arm external rotation. The stable lower extremity serves as a platform for trunk and upper extremity motion, whereas the amount of trunk rotation is proportionate to the amount of arm motion generated. Variations in motor control and physical fitness components such as strength, flexibility, or muscle endurance can affect the efficiency and effectiveness of the linked system [11, 12]. Thus, a treatment approach which encourages functional positions of standing in order to utilize the lower extremity muscles to both stabilize and propel the arm in a designated direction would more closely parallel kinetic chain function.

The final component in the kinetic chain framework is the neuromuscular system via Bernstein's theory of motor control. Nikolai Bernstein noted that there are many degrees of freedom or possible segment positions and motions from the foot to the hand during specified tasks [13]. This so-called redundancy is built into the human system intentionally in order to adjust to both internal and external stimuli such as fatigue, soreness, and/or environmental changes which can occur during task execution. This has been demonstrated in studies examining the effects of fatigue where altered muscle activations, joint kinematics, or task error increased following the onset of fatigue [14, 15].

Bernstein defined motor control as the process of mastering redundant degrees of freedom [12]. Proper kinetic chain sequencing can reduce the possible degrees of freedom in the entire motion, maximizing the efficiency of force production (less energy use) and interactive moment production (optimal joint motion and minimal joint load) and minimizing muscle activation. Efficient kinetic chains have been shown to demonstrate certain key segment positions and motions that can be correlated with decreased joint loads, maximum velocity, and maximal force production [13, 16, 17]. It has been postulated that pitchers who seem to throw "effortlessly" enjoy more career longevity than those who seem to "muscle" the ball.

To effectively enhance kinetic chain function and reduce the risk of reinjury to the arm following shoulder surgery, it must be understood that focusing solely on one of the three specific components would be an incomplete method of management. Just as improvements in scapular function alone do not directly reduce the incidence of injury to the shoulder, improvements in a single component or anatomical segment do not necessarily reduce the incidence of injury.

It has been suggested that deficits within the kinetic chain such as a lack of strength, flexibility, and/or proprioception at specific segments (hips, core, scapula, etc.) place the upper extremity at risk for injury because the stability and force generation capabilities of the different segments create increased ("catch up") loads on the tissues of the arm [3]. Recent investigations have found that the presence of core instability, as determined through decreased single-leg balance performance, negatively affects arm function [18]. The deficits in both core function and motor control are more prevalent in individuals with shoulder pain [19, 20]. These findings support the idea that shoulder function is dependent upon the function of the segments which precede it in regard to overhead tasks.

Ascribing to the kinetic chain model of function, the logical assumption would be that improvement of common deficiencies within the links of the chain (immobility of the pelvis, hip, trunk, and/or scapula, muscular weakness of the same areas, and alterations in muscle recruitment and timing) would decrease the risk of injury to the upper extremity. This rationale has been applied successfully in nonoperative, rehabilitation scenarios [1, 2] and can be implemented following shoulder surgery.

In addition to the individual patient needs, the complexity of the shoulder, both in anatomical composition and dynamic function, can create challenges for clinicians in developing postoperative shoulder rehabilitation programs. To overcome these potential difficulties, a rehabilitation method which utilizes the components of optimal kinetic chain function would be recommended.

Rehabilitation

There are five key areas of focus to be addressed during the treatment process—proper motion, core stability and strength, stability of energy transfer links, closed-chain exercise implementation, and use of multiple planes. Proper motion must be obtained as the first step in the comprehensive kinetic chain approach. It is not uncommon to have flexibility deficits in both global and local musculature in both upper and lower extremities. Flexibility can be increased via standard static, dynamic, and/or ballistic stretching. Based on previous findings regarding flexibility deficits in the overhead athlete, the hamstring, hip flexor, hip adductors, hip rotator, and gastrocsoleus muscle groups should be targeted for the lower extremity, while the pectoralis minor, biceps short head, scalenes, latissimus dorsi, and posterior shoulder muscles should be the point of focus for the upper extremity [21–24]. Improving lower extremity muscle flexibility has been linked to improving lower body movement patterns and improving overall athletic performance [25–27].

The kinetic chain approach utilizes the abovementioned proximal-to-distal sequencing model where the larger proximally positioned central muscles of the body (legs and trunk) generate and transfer energy to the smaller distally positioned muscles of the upper extremity (scapula and shoulder). The centralized muscles are often collectively termed the "core." Two terms which are at times interchanged but actually have different meanings are "core strength" and "core stability." Core strength is the physiological capability of the centralized muscles to generate force. Conversely, core stability is the ability to control the position and motion of the trunk over the pelvis and leg in order to allow optimum production, transfer, and control of force and motion to the terminal segment in integrated kinetic chain activities [11]. In order to create a stable base, the rehabilitation protocols start with the primary stabilizing musculature such as the transverse abdominus and multifidi. These groups are responsible for segmental spinal stability and provide the foundation for adequate trunk stability due to their direct attachment to the spine and pelvis; they are responsible for the most central portion of the core stability. The internal/external obliques, erector spinae, rectus abdominis, and the quadratus lumborum should then be incorporated for trunk stability. These local and global stabilizers together provide ultimate core stability. The larger global muscles including the abdominal muscles, erector spinae, and hip abductors are vital to power generation and stability for upper extremity function. The incorporation of core strengthening into rehabilitation regimens has been shown to increase hip extensor muscle strength balance [28]. This stage of rehabilitation is not only to restore core function by itself but also is the first stage of extremity rehabilitation as the core, being the most proximal component of the kinetic chain (in relation to the arm), is the critical link between the development and transfer of energy.

The next key goal is to gain stability in the energy transfer links, typically, the pelvis and the scapula. The pelvis is usually naturally addressed in rehabilitation since it is an integral part of the core. However, it is the responsibility of the clinician to implement exercises which both strengthen the pelvic muscles but also allow for progressively integrated movements where synchronous stability and energy transfer involving the pelvis can occur. Movement patterns of the scapula are considered essential in the kinetic chain process because scapular function facilitates shoulder function. Peri-scapular muscles such as the serratus anterior and lower trapezius should be a point of focus in early training and rehabilitation. Early training should incorporate the trunk and hip in order to facilitate the kinetic chain proximal-to-distal sequence of muscle activation. Little stress is placed on the shoulder

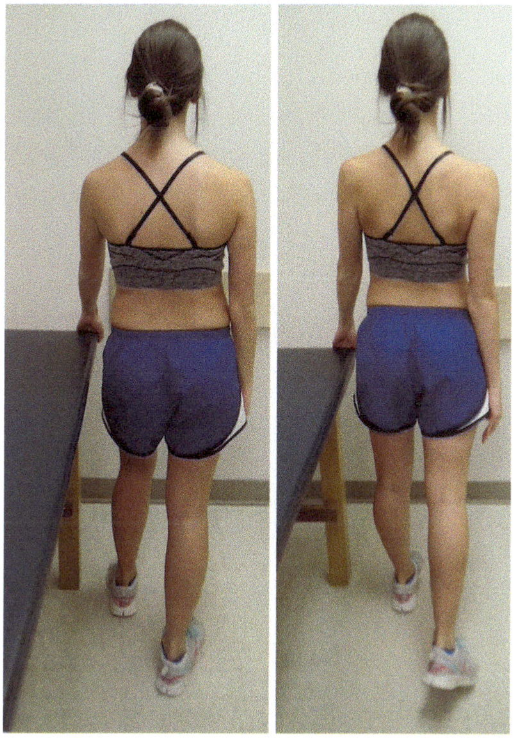

Fig. 25.1 Low row exercise for serratus anterior and lower trapezius strengthening

during the movements of hip and trunk extension combined with scapular retraction. All exercises are started with the feet on the ground and involve hip extension and pelvic control. The patterns of activation are both ipsilateral and contralateral. Diagonal motions involving trunk rotation around a stable leg simulate the normal pattern of throwing. As the shoulder heals and is ready for motion and loading in the intermediate or recovery stage of rehabilitation, the patterns can include arm motion as the final part of the exercise. Specific exercises known as the scapular stability series (Figs. 25.1, 25.2, 25.3 and 25.4)—low row, inferior glide, "lawnmower," and "robbery"—have been shown to activate the serratus and lower trapezius at safe levels of muscle activation and arm position and may be used in the early phases of rehabilitation [29].

The utilization of closed kinetic chain maneuvers can be implemented as a means of providing feedback and less loading through the affected extremity. Typically, when tissue is compromised, inflamed, or irritated, closed-chain exercises are implemented early in the rehabilitation process due to the decreased amount of shear force and stress they confer to the involved joints. These types of exercises are best suited for reestablishing the proximal stability and control in the links of the kinetic chain such as the scapula and pelvis. Open-chain exercises, which generate greater joint loads in comparison to closed-chain activities, should be utilized later in rehabilitation programs due to the increased joint reactive forces resulting from the longer arm levers inherent in these exercises.

Another rationale behind the initial closed-chain emphasis is that the shoulder functions as a true closed chain to transfer forces [30, 31], and in such training it is the optimal method to restore activation in inhibited and weak muscles. Specific training of inhibited muscles is accomplished by placing the extremity in a closed-chain position, emphasizing normal activation patterns, and focusing on the muscle of interest by deemphasizing compensatory muscle activation. For example, if a patient presents with shrugging during arm elevation, it can be assumed that the lower trapezius and/or serratus anterior are not working effectively dynamically. A closed-chain exercise such as the low row should be utilized because this "short lever" positioning would selectively emphasize those muscles which would decrease the upper trapezius' ability to activate. Once the normal activation pattern of the inhibited muscles has been restored, more challenging exercises which promote larger ranges of motion and multiple planes can be employed.

The preceding areas of the kinetic chain approach focused on alleviating underlying impairments/deficits, creating a sound foundation of muscle activation, and introducing strength through safe lower load maneuvers. The final key aspect of the kinetic chain approach for rehabilitation is the incorporation of multi-planar exercises which will utilize the gains made in the preceding areas in order to prepare patients to perform more complex tasks. The lower extremity and core should be challenged to perform in its natural capacity as a base of support and generator of power during recreational and labor-intensive

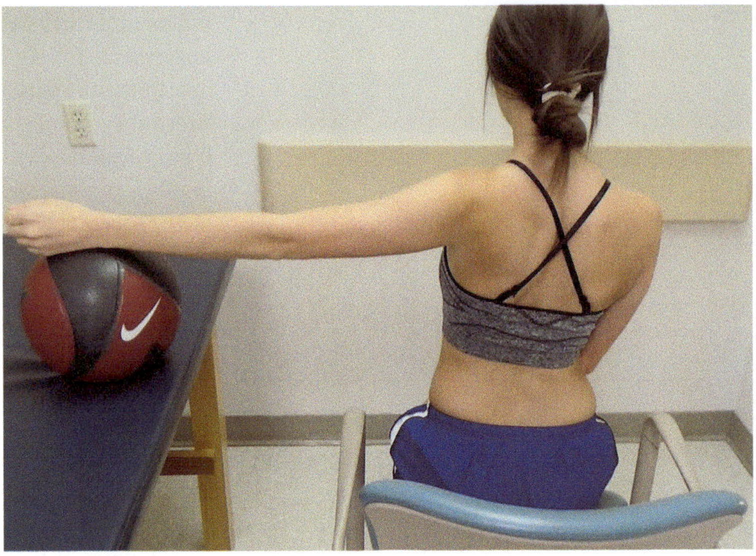

Fig. 25.2 Inferior glide exercise utilizing co-contraction of shoulder stabilizers

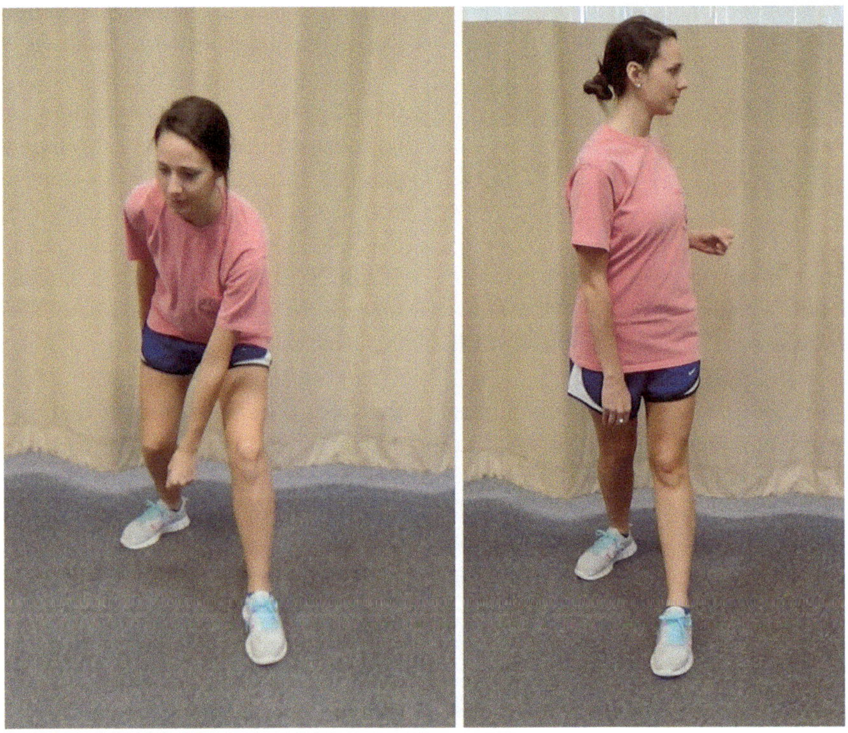

Fig. 25.3 Lawnmower maneuver utilizes multiple kinetic chain segments to improve scapular stability

tasks, while the focus for the upper extremity should be to serve as a funnel for the energy generated from the preceding anatomical segments. Since upper extremity tasks utilize rotary motion from the core and shoulders throughout the entire sequence of throwing and swinging, this strategy is logically employed as it is more functional. For example, to properly mimic and thereby enhance the throwing motion, a two-phase exercise known as the power position step back (Fig. 25.5), which

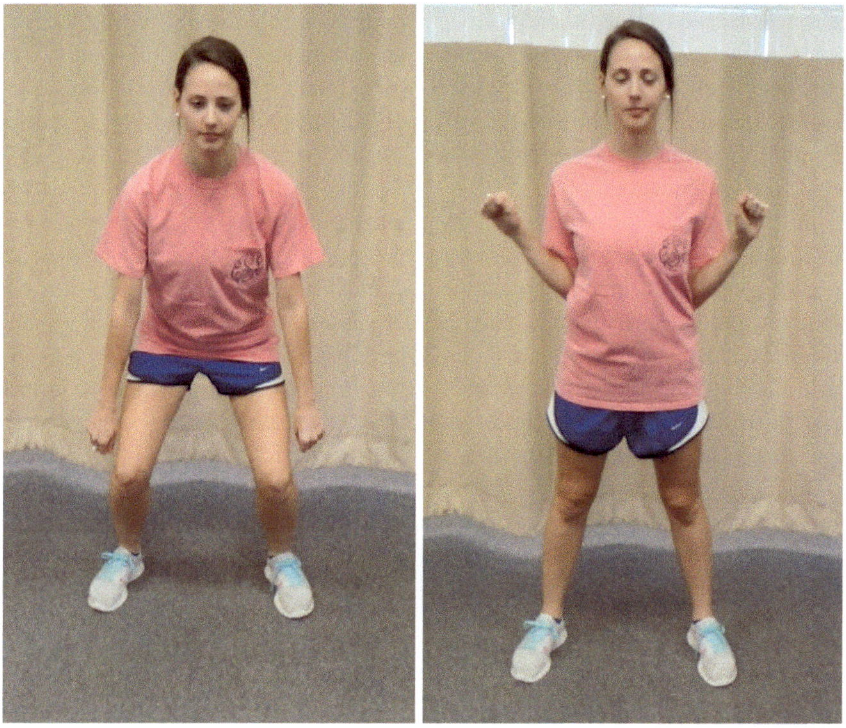

Fig. 25.4 The robbery maneuver helps regain adequate scapular retraction and depression by instructing the patient to "place the elbows in the back pockets"

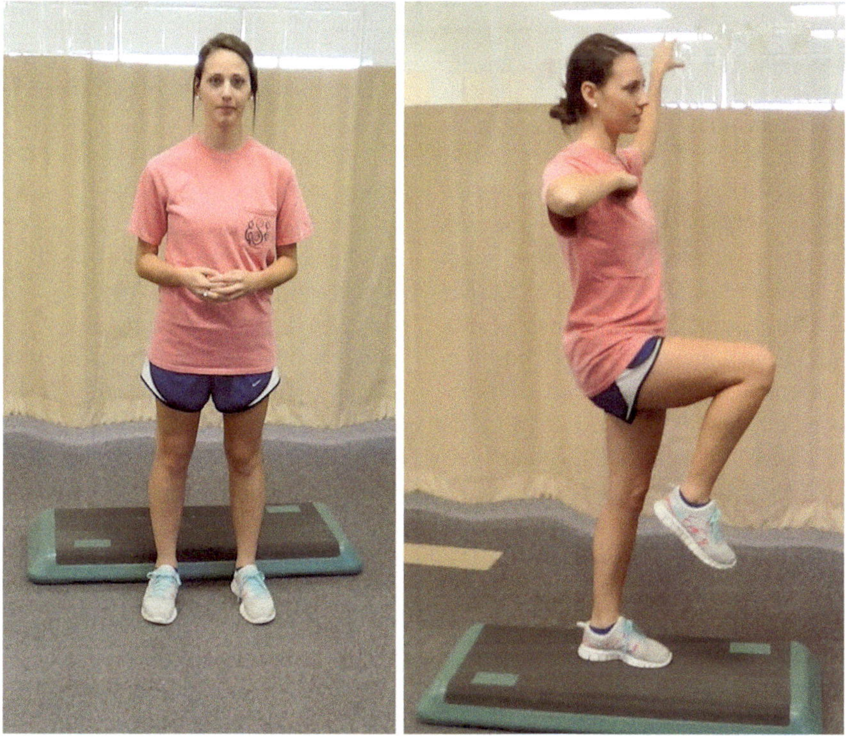

Fig. 25.5 Power position step back. This exercise helps retrain the motor system to simultaneously perform stability and complex, challenging motion at multiple kinetic chain segments

encourages single-leg and trunk stability along with scapular retraction and arm placement, can be prescribed. Each phase of the maneuver should be introduced individually then progressed to more functional stages where the actions are performed sequentially.

Proper safe progression is the primary concern in rehabilitation. In the kinetic chain rehabilitation process, multiple segments are active. Each exercise movement must be of quality in nature and integrate safe and appropriate movement patterns. The movement patterns prescribed progress from proximal-to-distal segments of the kinetic chain. As loading occurs in the distal segments, the exercise choices also progress from a static exercise to a dynamic choice of movements. In order to attain successful movement patterns, the patients must be provided feedback both verbal and tactile to avoid compensatory movements that hinder the kinetic chain. The feedback enables the person to identify the errors and correct the movements and commit the patterns to muscle memory. Slow removal of feedback can occur as the patient progresses to a more independent awareness of segmental function. Additional progression includes various resistance tools, change in movement patterns, and variable surfaces. As a precaution, the clinician overseeing the rehabilitation protocol must monitor the patient closely in order to prevent harmful overload. In preventing kinetic chain rehabilitation pitfalls, the clinician must also monitor some of the most common areas of weakness which transfer to compensatory movements. For example, scapulothoracic rhythm monitoring is essential as it is a primary indicator of compensation. Fatigue is a common concern that hinders the kinetic chain rehabilitation process. Thus, the goal of each exercise is performed without compensatory movement patterns.

Functional Readiness

The final consideration in postoperative shoulder rehabilitation is to determine the patient's ability to return to desired activities. Using dynamic performance measurements beyond traditional impairment testing may help reduce or eliminate premature return to activity (i.e., return prior to the optimization of functional capability necessary to perform sport-specific or work-specific tasks) [32]. This is especially challenging for clinicians because no universal method of functional assessment for the shoulder has been accepted or adopted for clinical practice. This is likely due to the numerous assessment maneuvers and test batteries that have been developed in order to assess shoulder function, most of which have been shown to have acceptable levels of inter-tester and/or intra-tester reliability [33–36]. Thus, the selection of the most appropriate method of testing is indeed difficult. Further complicating the matter, existing testing methods have been designed to assess only one component of physical function (strength, flexibility, power, etc.) or have been designed for specific populations only [32].

With the absence of a universal performance measures, some experts have suggested that interval programs, specific to individual sports or vocations, may be useful for assessing skills and for qualitatively assessing performance under controlled conditions [37–39]. Interval programs can be described as sports-specific return to play progressions designed to mimic the basic maneuvers and demands of a specific sport [37]. The programs are often implemented in the controlled, rehabilitation setting so the patient can be carefully monitored yet challenged without influence or pressure from external parties (coaches, teammates, etc.). Periodic testing throughout the rehabilitation process may give all involved parties insight as to whether patient expectations are being achieved, biomechanical improvements are being made, and if set goals are possibly being reached. The shortcomings of interval programs are their inherent subjectivity and that they serve as progressive supplements to rehabilitation, rather than as testing regimens. The lack of a grading scale or scoring metric within the interval program construct does not assist clinicians in making return to activity determinations. In order to overcome the individual limitations of dynamic performance testing and interval programs, a comprehensive approach is recommended which integrates multiple components including the use of patient self-reported function, impairment measures (strength, range of motion, etc.), dynamic performance testing, and interval programs as well as biomechanical assessments [32]. This ideal comprehensive approach utilizes information from various sources and allows kinetic chain-based factors to be considered and accounted for, aiding clinicians in identifying adequacies and/or deficiencies within the system [32, 40].

To optimize determination of function, clinicians should first select a dynamic performance measure that is both closely related to the activity the patient is attempting to return to and assists in measuring patient-specific goals established prior to the beginning of rehabilitation. Next, a biomechanical assessment should be conducted to determine if the patient can adequately perform the task in question and to assess the quality of the motion. Mechanical nodes have been described where recommended motions have been advocated for optimal performance and injury reduction during athletic tasks [4, 41]. "Nodes" are specific segment positions and motions that are determined to be fundamental for efficient linkage and sequencing of multiple segments in a kinetic chain [5]. An example of a sequential series of nodes would be the achievement of adequate knee flexion when initiating the cocking motion of the serve in tennis which is then followed by hip and trunk counterrotation and scapular retraction and concludes with propulsion of the body up and through the ball and long axis rotation of the arm following ball contact [5, 41]. The posttreatment mechanical examination is important in identifying anatomical and/or mechanical abnormalities as well as a lack of node achievement because the motor system has not been regularly exposed to the specific tasks required to perform the sport or job due to the constraints of the rehabilitation process. Additionally, improvements in strength and/or flexibility may lead to altered performance initially because the athlete is not familiar with how to best utilize the new gains. Clinicians should allot an adequate time to retrain the motor system in order to perform under the additional or constrained degrees of freedom. Finally, in order to routinely utilize the proper mechanics and to restore muscular endurance, clinicians should utilize the interval task program specific to individual patient needs. The programs should not be standardized but be developed and advanced based on individual patient improvement and physiological adaptation.

Summary

The rehabilitation process of the shoulder has many variables that must be considered, especially the kinetic chain complex. The shoulder is one of many interdependent links in the kinetic chain. In contrast to traditional rehabilitation protocols which include single planar range of motion and muscle strengthening exercises, the kinetic chain approach integrates various body sections into the rehabilitation process and allows the neuromuscular system to activate the biomechanical sequencing of the upper extremity. The kinetic chain approach reliably provides a successful rehabilitation program for return to function activity. This approach further allows for the retraining and reeducation of the body as a unit which in turn creates more opportunities for the patient to experience a successful rehabilitation outcome.

References

1. McMullen J, Uhl TL. A kinetic chain approach for shoulder rehabilitation. J Athl Train. 2000;35(3): 329–37.
2. Sciascia A, Cromwell R. Kinetic chain rehabilitation: a theoretical framework. Rehabil Res Pract. 2012; 2012:1–9.
3. Sciascia AD, Thigpen CA, Namdari S, Baldwin K. Kinetic chain abnormalities in the athletic shoulder. Sports Med Arthrosc Rev. 2012;20(1):16–21.
4. Kibler WB, Wilkes T, Sciascia A. Mechanics and pathomechanics in the overhead athlete. Clin Sports Med. 2013;32(4):637–51.
5. Lintner D, Noonan TJ, Kibler WB. Injury patterns and biomechanics of the athlete's shoulder. Clin Sports Med. 2008;27(4):527–52.
6. Cordo PJ, Nashner LM. Properties of postural adjustments associated with rapid arm movements. J Neurophysiol. 1982;47(2):287–308.

7. Bouisset S, Zattara M. A sequence of postural movements precedes voluntary movement. Neurosci Lett. 1981;22:263–70.
8. Zattara M, Bouisset S. Posturo-kinetic organisation during the early phase of voluntary upper limb movement. 1 Normal subjects. J Neurol Neurosurg Psychiatry. 1988;51:956–65.
9. Putnam CA. Sequential motions of body segments in striking and throwing skills: description and explanations. J Biomech. 1993;26:125–35.
10. Marshall R, Elliott BC. Long axis rotation: the missing link in proximal to distal segment sequencing. J Sports Sci. 2000;18(4):247–54.
11. Kibler WB, Press J, Sciascia AD. The role of core stability in athletic function. Sports Med. 2006;36(3): 189–98.
12. Sporns O, Edelman GM. Solving Bernstein's problem: a proposal for the development of coordinated movement by selection. Child Dev. 1993;64:960–81.
13. Davids K, Glazier PS, Araujo D, Bartlett R. Movement systems as dynamical systems: the functional role of variability and its implications for sports medicine. Sports Med. 2003;33(4):245–60.
14. Ebaugh DD, McClure PW, Karduna AR. Effects of shoulder muscle fatigue caused by repetitive overhead activities on scapulothoracic and glenohumeral kinematics. J Electromyogr Kinesiol. 2006;16:224–35.
15. Tripp B, Uhl TL, Mattacola CG, Srinivasan C, Shapiro R. Functional multijoint position reproduction acuity in overhead athletes. J Athl Train. 2006;41(2):146–53.
16. Hirashima M, Kadota H, Sakurai S, Kudo K, Ohtsuki T. Sequential muscle activity and its functional role in the upper extremity and trunk during overarm throwing. J Sports Sci. 2002;20:301–10.
17. Girard O, Micallef JP, Millet GP. Lower-limb activity during the power serve in tennis: effects of performance level. Med Sci Sports Exerc. 2005;37(6):1021–9.
18. Radwan A, Francis J, Green A, Kahl E, Maciurzynski D, Quartulli A, et al. Is there a relation between shoulder dysfunction and core instability? Int J Sports Phys Ther. 2014;9(1):8–13.
19. Reeser JC, Joy EA, Porucznik CA, Berg RL, Colliver EB, Willick SE. Risk factors for volleyball-related shoulder pain and dysfunction. Phys Med Rehabil. 2010;2(1).27–35.
20. Baierle T, Kromer T, Petermann C, Magosch P, Luomajoki H. Balance ability and postural stability among patients with painful shoulder disorders and healthy controls. BMC Musculoskelet Disord. 2013; 14:282.
21. Tyler TF, Nicholas SJ, Roy T, Gleim GW. Quantification of posterior capsule tightness and motion loss in patients with shoulder impingement. Am J Sports Med. 2000;28:668–73.
22. Tyler TF, Nicholas SJ, Lee SJ, Mullaney M, McHugh MP. Correction of posterior shoulder tightness is associated with symptom resolution in patients with internal impingement. Am J Sports Med. 2010;38(1):114–9.
23. Lephart SM, Smoliga JM, Myers JB, Sell TC, Tsai YS. An eight-week golf-specific exercise program improves physical characteristics, swing mechanics, and golf performance in recreational golfers. J Strength Cond Res. 2007;21(3):860–9.
24. Tsai YS, Sell TC, Smoliga JM, Myers JB, Learman KE, Lephart SM. A comparison of physical characteristics and swing mechanics between golfers with and without a history of low back pain. J Orthop Sports Phys Ther. 2010;40(7):430–8.
25. Worrell TW, Smith TL, Winegardner J. Effect of hamstring stretching on hamstring muscle performance. J Orthop Sports Phys Ther. 1994;20:154–9.
26. Bandy WD, Irion JM, Briggler M. The effect of time and frequency of static stretching on flexibility of the hamstring muscles. Phys Ther. 1997;77(10):1090–6.
27. Bandy WD, Irion JM, Briggler M. The effect of static stretch and dynamic range of motion training on the flexibility of the hamstring muscles. J Orthop Sports Phys Ther. 1998;27:295–300.
28. Nadler SF, Malanga GA, Bartoli LA, Feinberg JH, Prybicien M, DePrince M. Hip muscle imbalance and low back pain in athletes: influence of core strengthening. Med Sci Sports Exerc. 2002;34(1):9–16.
29. Kibler WB, Sciascia AD, Uhl TL, Tambay N, Cunningham T. Electromyographic analysis of specific exercises for scapular control in early phases of shoulder rehabilitation. Am J Sports Med. 2008;36(9): 1789–98.
30. Veeger HEJ, van der Helm FCT. Shoulder function: the perfect compromise between mobility and stability. J Biomech. 2007;40:2119–29. doi:10.1016/j.jbiomech.2006.10.016.
31. Worsley P, Warner M, Mottram S, Gadola S, Veeger HEJ, Hermens H, et al. Motor control retraining exercises for shoulder impingement: effects on function, muscle activation, and biomechanics in young adults. J Shoulder Elbow Surg. 2012. doi:10.1016/j.jse.2012.06.010.
32. Reiman MP, Manske RC. The assessment of function: how is it measured? A clinical perspective. J Man Manip Ther. 2011;19(2):91–9.
33. MacDermid JC, Ghobrial M, Quirion KB, St-Amour M, Tsui T, Humphreys D, et al. Validation of a new test that assesses functional performance of the upper extremity and neck (FIT-HaNSA) in patients with shoulder pathology. BMC Musculoskelet Disord. 2007;8(42):1–11.
34. Goldbeck TG, Davies G. Test-retest reliability of the closed chain upper extremity stability test: a clinical field test. J Sport Rehabil. 2000;9:35–45.
35. Negrete RJ, Hanney WJ, Kolber MJ, Davies G, Ansley MK, McBride AB, et al. Reliability, minimal detectable change, and normative values for tests of upper extremity function and power. J Strength Cond Res. 2010;24(12):3318–25.

36. Negrete RJ, Hanney WJ, Kolber MJ, Davies GJ, Riemann B. Can upper extremity functional tests predict the softball throw for distance: a predictive validity investigation. Int J Sports Phys Ther. 2011;6(2):104–11.
37. Reinold MM, Wilk KE, Reed J, Crenshaw K, Andrews JR. Interval sports programs: guidelines for baseball, tennis, and golf. J Orthop Sports Phys Ther. 2002; 32(6):293–8.
38. Axe MJ, Hurd WJ, Snyder-Mackler L. Data-based interval throwing programs for baseball players. Sports Health. 2009;1(2):145–53.
39. Shaw L, Domanski S, Freeman A, Hoffele C. An investigation of a workplace-based return-to-work program for shoulder injuries. Work. 2008;30:267–76.
40. Sciascia AD. A basic construct for improving outcomes in rehabilitation. Int J Athl Ther Train. 2013;18(3):14–9.
41. Kovacs M, Ellenbecker T. An 8-stage model for evaluating the tennis serve: implications for performance enhancement and injury prevention. Sports Health. 2011;3:504–13.

Index

J.D. Kelly IV (ed.), *Elite Techniques in Shoulder Arthroscopy*,
DOI 10.1007/978-3-319-25103-5

T

MIX
Papier aus verantwortungsvollen Quellen
Paper from responsible sources
FSC® C105338

If you have any concerns about our products,
you can contact us on
ProductSafety@springernature.com

In case Publisher is established outside the EU,
the EU authorized representative is:
Springer Nature Customer Service Center GmbH
Europaplatz 3, 69115 Heidelberg, Germany

Printed by Libri Plureos GmbH
in Hamburg, Germany